THE PEDIATRIC DIAGNOSTIC EXAMINATION

Editors

Donald E. Greydanus, MD

Professor, Pediatrics & Human Development
Michigan State University College of Human Medicine
Pediatrics Program Director
Michigan State University/Kalamazoo Center for Medical Studies
Kalamazoo, Michigan

Arthur N. Feinberg, MD

Professor, Pediatrics & Human Development
Michigan State University College of Human Medicine
Pediatric Clinic Director
Michigan State University/Kalamazoo Center for Medical Studies
Kalamazoo, Michigan

Dilip R. Patel, MD

Professor, Pediatrics & Human Development
Michigan State University College of Human Medicine
Michigan State University/Kalamazoo Center for Medical Studies
Kalamazoo, Michigan

Douglas N. Homnick, MD, MPH

Professor, Pediatrics & Human Development
Michigan State University College of Human Medicine
Director, Division of Pediatric Pulmonology
Cystic Fibrosis Center Director
Pediatrics Program
Michigan State University/Kalamazoo Center for Medical Studies
Kalamazoo, Michigan

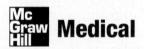

*New York Chicago San Francisco Lisbon London Madrid Mexico City
Milan New Delhi San Juan Seoul Singapore Sydney Toronto*

The **McGraw·Hill** Companies

The Pediatric Diagnostic Examination

Copyright © 2008 by The McGraw-Hill Companies, Inc. All rights reserved. Printed in China. Except as permitted under the United States Copyright Act of 1976, no part of this publication may be reproduced or distributed in any form or by any means, or stored in a data base or retrieval system, without the prior written permission of the publisher.

1 2 3 4 5 6 7 8 9 0   CTP/CTP   0 9 8 7

ISBN 978-0-07-147176-3
MHID 0-07-147176-6

This book was set in Palatino by International Typesetting and Composition.
The editors were Anne M. Sydor and Robert Pancotti.
The production supervisor was Catherine Saggese.
Project management was provided by International Typesetting and Composition.
The cover designer was Mary McKeon.
Cover Photos: top right: A female doctor examines the throat of a young patient. Credit: Phanie / Photo Researchers, Inc.Bottom left: Ear examination. Credit: Adam Gault / Photo Researchers, Inc.
China Printing & Translation Services was printer and binder.

This book is printed on acid-free paper.

Library of Congress Cataloging-in-Publication Data

  The pediatric diagnostic examination / [edited by] Donald E. Greydanus ... [et al.].
      p. ; cm.
    ISBN 978-0-07-147176-3;
    1. Children—Diseases—Diagnosis.   2. Children—Medical examinations.
    I. Greydanus, Donald E.
    [DNLM: 1. Diagnosis, Differential.   2. Adolescent.   3. Child.
  4. Infant.   5. Physical Examination—methods. WS 141 P3677   2008]
  RJ50.P43   2008
  618.92'0075—dc22   2007016002

International Edition ISBN 978-0-07-128727-2
International Edition MHID 0-07-128727-2

Copyright © 2008. Exclusive rights by The McGraw-Hill Companies, Inc., for manufacture and export. This book cannot be reexported from the country to which it is consigned by McGraw-Hill. The International Edition is not available in North America.

Dedication

Donald E. Greydanus dedicates this book in loving memory of his parents, **John** and **Margaret Greydanus**, and to his loving wife, **Katherine**, and his wonderful children, **Marissa, Elizabeth, Suzanne,** and **Megan.** I am eternally grateful for your love and support. Amor vincit omnia!

Arthur N. Feinberg dedicates this book in memory of his parents, **Milton** and **Rena Feinberg,** as the product of their futile attempts to teach him grammar and syntax, and to his wife, **Marilyn,** and children, **Lisa** and **Daniel,** in appreciation of their mutual and unconditional love.

Dilip R. Patel dedicates this book to **Ranjan** and **Neil** for their enduring love and support.

Douglas N. Homnick dedicates this book to his wife, **Tamara** (pediatric nurse), son, **Benjamin,** daughters, **Emily** and **Hannah,** and his parents, **Virginia** and **Myron** (pediatrician), whose love and support have always been there. Family (and especially children) has played the most important role in our lives both in and out of the office.

Contents

Contributors/Authors ix

Foreword xv

Preface xvii

1. **TAKING A HISTORY IN INFANTS, CHILDREN, AND ADOLESCENTS** 1
Arthur N. Feinberg, Melissa A. Davidson, and Artemis K. Tsitsika

2. **PERFORMING A PHYSICAL EXAMINATION IN INFANTS, CHILDREN, AND ADOLESCENTS** 25
Arthur N. Feinberg and Thomas Melgar

3. **VITAL SIGNS** 45
Vinay N. Reddy

4. **DEVELOPMENT OF A DIFFERENTIAL DIAGNOSIS FROM THE HISTORY AND PHYSICAL EXAMINATION** 59
Arthur N. Feinberg and Vinay N. Reddy

5. **THE TERM NEWBORN** 69
Arthur N. Feinberg

6. **THE PEDIATRIC DYSMORPHOLOGY DIAGNOSTIC EXAMINATION** 111
Bryan D. Hall and Helga V. Toriello

7. **THE EYES, EARS, NOSE, THROAT, NECK, AND ORAL EXAMINATION** 137
Elyssa R. Peters, Monte Del Monte, Jonathan Gold, Ashir Kumar, and Joseph A. D'Ambrosio

8. **THE RESPIRATORY SYSTEM** 189
Douglas N. Homnick

9. **THE CARDIOVASCULAR SYSTEM** 227
Eugene F. Luckstead

10. **THE GASTROINTESTINAL TRACT, LIVER, GALL BLADDER, AND PANCREAS** 267
Arthur N. Feinberg and Lisa A. Feinberg

11. THE MUSCULOSKELETAL SYSTEM   301
Dilip R. Patel

12. THE NEUROLOGY SYSTEM   349
Arthur N. Feinberg

13. THE ENDOCRINE SYSTEM   403
Martin B. Draznin and Manmohan K. Kamboj

14. THE RENAL SYSTEM   443
Alfonso D. Torres and Donald E. Greydanus

15. THE HEMATOLOGY-ONCOLOGY SYSTEM   489
Elna N. Saah, Renuka Gera, Ajovi B. Scott-Emuakpor,
and Roshni Kulkarni

**16. THE INTEGUMENT SYSTEM—SKIN,
HAIR, NAILS**   541
Arthur N. Feinberg

17. THE PSYCHODIAGNOSTIC EXAMINATION   599
Joseph L. Calles Jr.

**18. PRINCIPLES OF DEVELOPMENTAL
DIAGNOSIS**   629
Dilip R. Patel

19. THE MALE GENITOURINARY SYSTEM   645
Julian H. Wan

**20. THE GYNECOLOGY SYSTEM AND
THE CHILD**   685
Jennifer Johnson

**21. THE GYNECOLOGY SYSTEM AND
THE ADOLESCENT**   701
Donald E. Greydanus, Artemis K. Tsitsika,
and Michelé J. Gains

22. LABORATORY TESTING OVERVIEW   751
Vinay N. Reddy

Appendix   759
Index   773

Contributors

Medical Student Reviewer

Daniel Olson, BS
Fourth Year Medical Student
Michigan State University/Kalamazoo Center for Medical Studies
Kalamazoo, Michigan

Pediatrics Resident Reviewer

Elena J. Lewis, MD
Pediatric Residency Program
Michigan State University/Kalamazoo Center for Medical Studies
Kalamazoo, Michigan

Medical Illustrator

Megan M. Greydanus, BFA
Portage, Michigan

Authors

Jay E. Berkelhamer, MD
2006 President, American Academy of Pediatrics
Senior Vice President for Medical Affairs
Children's Healthcare of Atlanta
Clinical Professor of Pediatrics
Emory School of Medicine
Atlanta, Georgia

Joseph L. Calles, Jr., MD
Clinical Associate Professor of Psychiatry
Michigan State University College of Human Medicine
Director, Child and Adolescent Psychiatry
Psychiatry Residency Training Program
Michigan State University/Kalamazoo Center for Medical Studies
Kalamazoo, Michigan

Joseph D'Ambrosio, DMD, MD
Assistant Professor, Internal Medicine and Pediatrics & Human
    Development
Michigan State University College of Human Medicine
Transitional Internship Program Director
Michigan State University/Kalamazoo Center for Medical Studies
Kalamazoo, Michigan

Melissa A. Davidson, MD
Assistant Professor, Internal Medicine and Pediatrics & Human
    Development
Michigan State University College of Human Medicine
Combined Medicine-Pediatrics Program
Michigan State University/Kalamazoo Center for Medical Studies
Kalamazoo, Michigan

Monte A. Del Monte, MD
Skillman Professor of Pediatric Ophthalmology
Department of Ophthalmology and Visual Science and Pediatrics
Professor of Pediatrics
Department of Pediatrics and Communicable Diseases
Director of Pediatric Ophthalmology and Adult Strabismus
W. K. Kellogg Eye Center
University of Michigan
Ann Arbor, Michigan

Martin B. Draznin, MD
Professor, Pediatrics & Human Development
Michigan State University College of Human Medicine
Director, Pediatric Endocrine Division
Pediatrics Program
Michigan State University/Kalamazoo Center for Medical Studies
Kalamazoo, Michigan

Arthur N. Feinberg, MD
Professor, Pediatrics & Human Development
Michigan State University College of Human Medicine
Pediatric Clinic Director
Michigan State University/Kalamazoo Center for Medical Studies
Kalamazoo, Michigan

Lisa A. Feinberg, MD
Clinical Associate, Department of Pediatric Gastroenterology
Cleveland Clinic Foundation
Cleveland, Ohio

Michelé J. Gains, MD
Associate Professor Clinical-UCLA, Pediatrics
Chief, Adolescent Medicine Services
Martin Luther King/Charles R. Drew Medical Center
Los Angeles, California

Renuka Gera, MD
Professor and Associate Chair, Department of Pediatrics/Human
  Development
Division of Pediatric and Adolescent Hematology/Oncology
Michigan State University College of Human Medicine
East Lansing, Michigan

Jonathan Gold, MD
Assistant Professor, Department of Pediatrics & Human Development
Michigan State University College of Human Medicine
East Lansing, Michigan

Donald E. Greydanus, MD
Professor, Pediatrics & Human Development
Michigan State University College of Human Medicine
Pediatrics Program Director
Michigan State University/Kalamazoo Center for Medical Studies
Kalamazoo, Michigan

Bryan D. Hall, MD
Emeritus Professor of Pediatrics
Past Chief, Division of Genetics and Dysmorphology
Department of Pediatrics, Kentucky Clinic
University of Kentucky
Lexington, Kentucky

Douglas N. Homnick, MD, MPH
Professor, Pediatrics & Human Development
Michigan State University College of Human Medicine
Director, Division of Pediatric Pulmonology
Cystic Fibrosis Center Director
Pediatrics Program
Michigan State University/Kalamazoo Center for Medical Studies
Kalamazoo, Michigan

Jennifer Johnson, MD
Senate emerita
Department of Pediatrics
University of California, Irvine
Irvine, California

Manmohan K. Kamboj, MD
Assistant Professor, Pediatrics & Human Development
Michigan State University College of Human Medicine
Division of Pediatric Endocrinology, Pediatrics Program
Michigan State University/Kalamazoo Center for Medical Studies
Kalamazoo, Michigan

Roshni Kulkarni, MD
Professor and Division Chief,
Pediatric & Adolescent Hematology/Oncology
Director (Pediatric), MSU Center for Bleeding & Clotting Disorders
Pediatrics & Human Development
Michigan State University College of Human Medicine
East Lansing, Michigan;
Director, Division of Hereditary Blood Disorders
National Center on Birth Defects and Developmental Disabilities
Centers for Disease Control & Prevention
Atlanta, Georgia

Ashir Kumar, MD
Professor, Pediatrics & Human Development
Michigan State University College of Human Medicine
Pediatric Infectious Diseases Division
East Lansing, Michigan

Eugene F. Luckstead, MD
Professor, Pediatrics and Cardiology
Department of Pediatrics
Texas Tech Medical School–Amarillo
Amarillo, Texas

Thomas Melgar, MD
Associate Professor, Internal Medicine and Pediatrics & Human
  Development
Michigan State University College of Human Medicine
Program Director, Combined Medicine-Pediatrics Program
Michigan State University/Kalamazoo Center for Medical Studies
Kalamazoo, Michigan

Dilip R. Patel, MD
Professor, Pediatrics & Human Development
Michigan State University College of Human Medicine
Pediatrics Program
Michigan State University/Kalamazoo Center for Medical Studies
Kalamazoo, Michigan

Elyssa R. Peters, MD
Instructor, Department of Ophthalmology and Visual Science
W. K. Kellogg Eye Center
University of Michigan
Ann Arbor, Michigan

Vinay N. Reddy, MD, MS, MSE
Assistant Professor, Pediatrics and Human Development
Michigan State University College of Human Medicine
Director, Inpatient Pediatrics
Pediatrics Program
Michigan State University/Kalamazoo Center for Medical Studies
Kalamazoo, Michigan

Elna N. Saah, MD
Division of Pediatric & Adolescent Hematology/Oncology
Pediatrics & Human Development
Michigan State University College of Human Medicine
East Lansing, Michigan

Ajovi F. Scott-Emuakpor, MD, PhD
Professor, Department of Pediatrics/Human Development
Director, Pediatric & Adolescent Sickle Cell Program
Division of Pediatric and Adolescent Hematology/Oncology
Michigan State University College of Human Medicine
East Lansing, Michigan

Helga V. Toriello, PhD
Professor, Pediatrics and Human Development
Michigan State University College of Human Medicine
Genetics Services, Spectrum Health
Grand Rapids, Michigan

Alfonso D. Torres, MD
Director, Pediatric Nephrology
Pediatrics Program
Michigan State University/Kalamazoo Center for Medical Studies
Kalamazoo, Michigan

Artemis K. Tsitsika, MD, PhD
Pediatrics-Adolescent Medicine
Scientific Supervisor/Adolescent Health Unit (AHU)
Second Department of Pediatrics
University of Athens
"P & A Kyriakou" Children's Hospital
Mesogion 24,11527
Athens, Greece

Julian H. Wan, MD
Associate Professor, Pediatric Urology
University of Michigan Medical Center
Ann Arbor, Michigan

Foreword

Those who are faced with diagnosing disease states in newborns, children, and adolescents will find this text a complete and accurate compendium of critical information that will complement other sources that focus more on various treatments available. The emphasis on the physical signs and symptoms is important in a time when so many advances have occurred in the laboratory and in imaging. We are truly blessed by the advances in science that have made it possible to measure and peer deeply into the bodies of our patients. However, the art and science of the physical examination are an inseparable part of a careful and detailed history and diagnostic testing leading to a differential diagnosis and the ultimate correct diagnosis.

Often there is an urge to move from the history to diagnostic testing without adequately pausing to assess the key signs and symptoms to ensure an appropriate differential diagnosis, risking delays, unnecessary discomfort, and increased cost of care. The physical examination can be done carefully and quickly, adding to the overall efficiency and quality of the care of the patient. This is particularly true in the case of the newborn, child, and adolescent.

The Pediatric Diagnostic Examination provides the reader with compact and digestible material that serves as both a reference for the more experienced diagnostician and a readable text for students and residents. The tables and diagrams provide concise information that can be used to prepare for presentations to colleagues and instructors.

At the beginning of this text, there are important topics of an overarching nature that define the unique features of pediatrics as a specialty and set this text apart from other textbooks on the diagnostic examination. The editors and authors are experienced pediatricians who are widely regarded as among the best in their respective subspecialty areas.

As a physician who has spent the past 40 years honing my skills as a diagnostician, I see this book as a welcome addition to my personal library and recommend it enthusiastically to all those who desire to improve their personal effectiveness in getting children the right care at the right time.

Jay E. Berkelhamer, MD, FAAP
President, American Academy of Pediatrics
Senior Vice President for Medical Affairs
Children's HealthCare of Atlanta
Atlanta, Georgia

Preface

Medicine should begin with the patient, continue with the patient, and end with the patient.

—William Osler, MD

With the advent of modern technology and specialization, there have been major advances in medicine that have greatly improved the accuracy and timeliness of diagnosis. However, with these good things come caveats:

1. A significant improvement does not mean perfection.
2. Technology is expensive, and physicians must use it with discretion.
3. We still must employ the art of clinical diagnosis with a thorough and skillful history and physical examination to help choose among our many technical options.
4. Primary care pediatricians taking care of children must learn when it is appropriate to refer to a specialist and how to present the specialist with relevant and useful information.

There are many excellent standard textbooks of pediatrics and of adult physical diagnosis, including De Gowin's, a timeless systematic approach to diagnosis. However, there remains a need for a more general yet concise systematic overview of *pediatric* diagnosis geared toward the student and resident but useful to anyone caring for children. The goal of this book is to present a diagnostic framework on which a learner can build his or her "databank" of diagnostic facts. The format of each systems-based chapter consists of an "Introduction," "Physiology and Mechanics," "Functional Anatomy," "History," "Physical Examination," "Synthesizing a Diagnosis," "Laboratory and Imaging," and "When to Refer." We have attempted in the "Synthesizing a Diagnosis" sections to present the material in tabular form whenever possible so that the learner has more concise and digestible information. There is some variability among the chapters because different systems lend themselves to different approaches. For example, dermatology is more of a "visual art" with less emphasis on history. Probably the most "divergent" chapter is Chapter 17, "The Psychodiagnostic Examination." The author felt that the reader should learn to "think like a psychiatrist."

For conciseness, we are limited in selecting the most common diagnoses, which we feel all practitioners, beginners and advanced, should "have in their heads." However, this should never discourage anyone from consulting books and online resources for any clinical encounter.

Keeping the preceding in mind, we *dedicate* this book to all our past, present, and future residents and students at the Michigan State University College of Human Medicine (MSUCHM)/Kalamazoo Center for Medical Studies (KCMS)—you are constantly a true inspiration to us. With this book we hope you will maintain and improve your "morning reportsmanship" skills and continue to keep us even further on edge!

This book would not have been possible without the help of very significant people. We are most appreciative of the efforts of Daniel Olson, BS, fourth-year student at MSUCHM rotating through our campus, and Elena J. Lewis, MD, one of our pediatric residents, who both reviewed the chapters and gave many constructive suggestions from their perspective as learners of pediatric medicine. We are indebted to our medical illustrator, Megan M. Greydanus, BFA, for her excellent artistry. We recognize Dr. Tor Shwayder, pediatric dermatologist at Henry Ford Hospital in Detroit, Michigan, for providing the dermatology photos and reviewing chapter 16. We also recognize Dr. Gerald Fenichel, pediatric neurologist at Vanderbilt University, Nashville, Tennessee, for editing Chapter 12 and whose framework in his textbook *Clinical Pediatric Neurology* served as a foundation for that chapter. We thank our many distinguished authors for taking time from their busy lives to contribute to this book. Finally, we are indebted to Anne M. Sydor, PhD, senior editor at McGraw-Hill Medical Publishers, for her steadfast encouragement and professional guidance in this exciting work.

In conclusion, old-fashioned clinical diagnosis should never become a lost art!

Finis Coronat Opus

Donald E. Greydanus, MD
Arthur N. Feinberg, MD
Dilip R. Patel, MD
Douglas N. Homnick, MD, MPH

1 Taking a History in Infants, Children, and Adolescents

Arthur N. Feinberg, Melissa Davidson, and Artemis Tsitsika

A full and accurate history is paramount to making a reliable diagnosis. It is critical to obtain as much information as possible at the initial interview regarding the patient's medical and psychosocial past. Verify and update this information at subsequent visits. We will present first the format for the initial history for all new patients. In the next section we build a focused history of the present illness from infancy, ages 1 month to 2 years, to childhood, ages 2 to 12 years, to adolescence, ages 12 to 21 years, with the assumption that this patient was seen at birth and remained a patient throughout. The pediatrician should obtain all past history for new patients appearing at any age, either through old records or through an interview. At times it may be necessary to obtain information from other sources, such as hospitals, schools, psychologists, and social agencies. In the focused history section, we lay out a format for gathering data and will devote subsequent chapters to synthesizing this information into diagnoses. Focused histories elicit pertinent facts with little superfluous information, which becomes necessary as the clinician faces the reality of time constraints with every patient visit and must operate as efficiently as possible.

We consider infants, children, and adolescents as separate entities and devote the final section of this chapter to eliciting information from them and their caretakers. Because much of pediatric history is based on caretaker perceptions, we prefer the term *problem* to *symptom* and will use it throughout the book.

Initial Interview

Data Gathering

Since time is precious, a patient or caretaker may complete a standard intake history form prior to the office visit. Some may need help from the office staff if they are unable to complete it accurately. Obtain demographic information first, including languages spoken and cultural, religious, and spiritual needs. Gestational, obstetrical, and birth information have a significant effect on children's outcomes. Obtain a maternal health history, both medical and psychosocial. Does the mother smoke or consume alcohol? Assess the mother's family support systems. When did she start prenatal care? If prenatal care was delayed, why? Was there a lack of access to physicians because the pregnancy was unplanned or because of substance abuse or homelessness? Include the standard screens, such as VDRL, rubella, hepatitis B, human immunodeficiency virus (HIV), and group B streptococcus. Did the mother sustain any injuries or illness during the pregnancy, e.g., hyperemesis, infections, or bleeding? How long was the gestation? Were there any problems during the labor specifically related to fetal distress? How long was the labor? Was the delivery vaginal or cesarean section? Did the membranes rupture prematurely? Record the birth weight, and determine its appropriateness for gestational age. What were the initial Apgar scores? How was the newborn's hospital stay? Did jaundice, infection, or any other problems prolong it? Ask specifically if the baby had any diagnoses at the hospital other than normal-term newborn.

In the first 2 years of life, most visits are hopefully well-child care, anticipatory guidance, and immunizations. It is beyond the scope of this chapter to cover all aspects of growth and development, but the physician must obtain a growth chart and enter gross motor, fine motor, adaptive, language, and personal-social skills into the intake history for all new patients not followed from birth. Growth charts and a capsule summary of developmental landmarks appear in TABLES 1–1 through 1–3 and the Appendix.

Past Medical History

Obtain the past medical history. Were there any hospitalizations or surgeries? All past medical diagnoses should be cataloged and readily available on the patient chart. What medications has the patient taken or is still taking? Are there any allergies or intolerances to food or medication? Assess exposures such as smoke, pets, use of fluoride, and lead risk. Does the home meet standard safety requirements, specifically the presence of smoke and carbon monoxide detectors? Are immunizations current? List all immunizations in the chart in a readily accessible area. With the advent of computerized tracking systems and electronic medical records, this is becoming much easier. Review all completed caretakers' forms.

Review of Systems

All new patients must have a review of systems, including both symptoms and diagnoses. Update this on subsequent patient visits. Organize the review of systems as illustrated in TABLES 1–4 and 1–5 for infants, children, and adolescents.

Family History

Family history is of critical importance. Do this in the format of the review of systems. Include all family members. Note any diagnoses that may have any bearing on the patient in the chart, thus making them easily accessible to the reader.

TABLE 1-1 *Developmental Timeline, Ages 2 to 9 Months*

	2 Months	4 Months	6 Months	9 Months
Gross motor	Lifts head (prone)	Head control while sitting; lifts to chest (prone); rolls over front to back	Rolls over both ways; sits with support; no head lag	Sits without support; pulls to stand; cruises
Fine motor	Losing grasp reflex	Holds hands in midline	Reaches, transfers	Bangs two objects; primitive pincer grasp
Adaptive	Follows past midline	Follows 180 degrees	Turns to sound	Feeds self with fingers; imitative games (bye-bye)
Language	Coos; reciprocal vocalizations	Squeals	Babbles; imitates speech	Mama-dada not specific; understands name
Personal-social	Regards object; smiles	Laughs out loud; initiates social contact	Stranger anxiety and night waking	Recognizes key people and objects; more stranger anxiety and night waking

TABLE 1–2 *Developmental Timeline Ages 12 to 24 Months*

	12 Months	15 Months	18 Months	24 Months
Gross motor	Two to three steps with help	Walks, stoops, and recovers	Runs (totter)	Stairs (holding); kicks ball; jumps up
Fine motor	Neat pincer	Horizontal line; scribbles; cube in a cup	Casts ball; two-cube stack; puts shapes in holes	Four- to six-cube stack; vertical line
Adaptive	Drink from cup (held)	Point and grunt; drinks from cup (holds own)	Uses spoon; conveys dirty diaper	Wash and dry hands; remove clothes; put on hat; uses fork
Language	3 words	6–10 words	10–15 words; simple body parts	50 words; few double words
Personal-social	Simple games (peek-a boo); stranger anxiety; plays give and take	Single commands; more stranger anxiety	Imitates housework; more and more stranger anxiety and tantrums	Expresses needs; points to picture; maximal stranger anxiety and tantrums

TABLE 1-3 *Developmental Timeline Ages 3 to 6 Years*

	3 Years	4 Years	5 Years	6 Years
Gross motor	Pedals tricycle; broad jump; stands on one foot for 3 seconds	Walks up and down stairs; hops; stands on one foot for 3 seconds	Skips; tandem walks; hops well	Rides bicycle
Fine motor	Tower of eight cubes; vertical stroke with pencil	Copies circle and cross; draws person (4-year-old)	Draws person (5-year-old); copies square; grasps pencil maturely; prints letters	Ties shoelaces; writes name; copies two-part figure
Adaptive	Puts on tee shirt	Dresses without help; brushes teeth	Prepares bowl of cereal	Knows left from right
Language	50–75% intelligent; five- to eight-word sentences; simple adjectives; stuttering	Four colors; relates events; asks questions "what," "when," and "why"	Counts five objects	Counts 10 objects
Social	Imaginary friends; gullible	Pretend play; sassy mouthy; antisocial	Plays simple board games	Able to relate impact of events

Source: Pediatrics in Review 1999–2003 Self-Assessment Curriculum.

TABLE 1-4 *Review of Systems for Infants, Ages 1 Month to 2 Years*

Skin	Rashes, jaundice, dryness, scaling, eczema, impetigo, bruising, birthmarks, pigment change, hemangiomas, warts
Lymphatics	Lymphadenopathy
Orthopedic	Fractures, dislocations, injuries, weakness, muscle wasting or hypertrophy, congenital deformities
Hemopoietic	Anemia, history of white blood cell or platelet problems, bleeding tendency
Endocrine	Newborn screening abnormalities (TSH, CAH), ↑ or ↓ blood glucose
Allergy and immunology	Eczema, urticaria, food allergy (GI sx, cough), wheezing, reaction to insect bites, conjunctivitis, itching, recurrent infections, growth pattern
Head and neck	Micro/macrocephaly, malformations (suture, fontanelle closure), injuries, neck masses (branchial cleft problems, hygroma, torticollis
Eyes	Visual acuity, cataracts, abnormal light reflex, trauma, tumors, strabismus, retinopathy of prematurity
Ears, nose, and throat (ENT)	Ear infections, colds, coryza, cough, sore throats, sinus infections, hearing assessment, malformations
Respiratory	Bronchiolitis, asthma, pneumonia, congenital chest or lung malformations, bronchopulmonary dysplasia
Cardiovascular	Exercise tolerance, cough, dyspnea, cyanosis, heart murmurs, known congenital malformations, pulmonary edema, hepatomegaly, arrhythmias
Gastrointestinal	Feeding, weight gain, colic, vomiting, diarrhea, constipation, distension, jaundice, bleeding, hepatosplenomegaly, congenital anomalies, pyloric stenosis, intussusceptions, volvulus, fissures, anal malformations
Genitourinary	Infection, known congenital malformation, urinary stream and output
Breasts	Gynecomastia, agenesis
Neurologic	Gait, use of all four extremities, weakness, malformations of brain and cord, seizures, developmental milestones, metabolic disease (NB screen)

Abbreviations: TSH = thyroid-stimulating hormone, CAH = congenital adrenal hyperplasia. GI sx = gastrointestinal symptoms, NB screen = newborn screen.

The family personal and social history provides much useful information. Is the child's father actively involved? If not, is he providing financial support? Is there extended family support or other day-care arrangements? What is the employment and health insurance status of the family? Has there been any involvement with social workers or child

TABLE 1–5 *Review of Systems for Children, Ages 2 to 12 Years*

Skin	Same as in infants plus moles, warts, scarlet fever, purpura
Lymphatics	Lymphadenopathy, lymphoma
Orthopedic	Same as infants plus pain, stiffness, heat, swelling, arthritis, atrophy, joint mobility (hyper or hypomobile)
Hemopoieitic	Anemia, leukopenia, thrombocytopenia, bleeding diathesis
Endocrine	Growth, puberty stage, signs of hyper/hypothyroidism (dry skin, cold intolerance, sluggishness, thick hair/exophthalmos, sweating, heat intolerance, thin hair), hypo/hyperadrenalism (skin pigmentation, hypotension, vomiting/Cushing signs), hypo/hyperparathyroidism (tetany/abdominal pain, polydipsia, polyuria), and diabetes mellitus or insipidus (polyuria, polydipsia, weight loss)
Allergy and immunology	Same as infants plus seasonal allergies (hay fever, vernal conjunctivitis), allergy to x-ray contrast material, food, or environmental allergies documented by skin or RAST testing
Head and neck	Same as infants plus headache, migraine, masses, infections, stiffness
Eyes	Same as infants plus myopia, hyperopia, astigmatism, diplopia, color blindness
Ear, nose, and throat (ENT)	Same as infants plus tinnitus, vertigo, perforations, history of PE tube placement, tonsillectomy/adenoidectomy
Respiratory	Same as infants plus tuberculosis status
Cardiovascular	Same as infants plus known cardiac disease, rheumatic fever, palpitation, chest pain, edema, hepatomegaly
Gastrointestinal	Same as infants plus appendicitis, known GBD, pancreatitis, past need for TPN, acholic stools, hemorrhoids
Genitourinary	Same as infants
Breasts	Gynecomastia in boys, breast development in girls
Neurologic	Same as infants plus headache, migraine, vertigo, hemiparesis, paresthesias, pain radiating down extremities

Abbreviations: PE = polyethylene; GBD = gallbladder disease; TPN = total parenteral nutrition; RAST = radioallergosorbent test.

protective services in the past? Although it may not apply to children, adolescents may well partake in the decision-making process involving advance directives. Note this on the chart. FIGURE 1–1 represents the standard intake form we use in our pediatric outpatient clinic.

Today's Date:

PATIENT INFORMATION

Last Name:	First:		MI:	Date of Birth:	Sex:
Patient SS#:		Parent SS#:			
If married, name of spouse:					
Address of patient:			Apt. #		
City:	State:		Zip:		
Home phone #:					
Address of parent or guardian if different:					
Address:			Apt. #		
City:	State:		Zip:		
Home phone #:	Work phone #:		Cell phone/pager #:		
Emergency contact #:		Emergency contact name:			

What is the primary language of the household?	
Patient's school:	Do you or the patient have any cultural, religious or spiritual practices which affect your healthcare decisions? Yes ☐ No ☐ If yes, please explain:

FAMILY INFORMATION

Mother:	Father:	Other Guardian if applicable:
Sibling #1 Name: Age:	Sibling #2 Name: Age:	Sibling #3 Name: Age:
Sibling #4 Name: Age:	Sibling #5 Name: Age:	Sibling #6 Name: Age:

PAST MEDICAL HISTORY

Full-term birth: yes no	If premature, how many weeks:

Mother's complications during pregnancy? (please specify):

Mother's medications during pregnancy:
Any problems during delivery?

Mother's previous pregnancies #	# of live births

Any known developmental delays?   Slow to walk? Roll over? Crawl? Failure to thrive?
Other (please specify):

Name:

Please circle any conditions that apply to the patient or family member (**P for patient, F for family**):

Anemia	P	F	Asthma	P	F	Behavior problems	P	F
Bowel problems	P	F	Celiac disease	P	F	Cancer	P	F
Cerebral Palsy	P	F	Chicken pox	P	F	Cystic Fibrosis	P	F
Dental problems	P	F	Diabetes	P	F	Drug use	P	F
Chronic Fatigue	P	F	HIV	P	F	Headaches	P	F
Syndrome			Hearing difficulties	P	F	Heart condition	P	F
Hepatitis	P	F	High blood pressure	P	F	Kidney condition	P	F
Liver condition	P	F	Lupus	P	F	Mental illness	P	F
Meningitis	P	F	Recurrent Ear	P	F	Scarlet fever	P	F
Seizures	P	F	Infections			Vision problems	P	F
Tuberculosis	P	F	Speech problems	P	F	Thyroid condition	P	F
Ulcers	P	F	Urinary Tract	P	F	Other(please specify):		

Do you have documentation of your child's immunizations?	Yes ☐	No ☐
If yes, did you bring a copy with you today?	Yes ☐	No ☐
If no, did you request the records to be sent to us?	Yes ☐	No ☐

Is the patient experiencing any pain?	Yes ☐	No ☐

If yes, please give location(s) and describe:

Have there been any recent changes in the patient's mobility, use and function of arms or legs?	Yes ☐	No ☐
Any difficulty performing daily activities or problems speaking or swallowing?	Yes ☐	No ☐

If yes, please explain:

Have there been any changes in the patient's eating habits?	Yes ☐	No ☐

If yes, please explain:

How would you describe the patient's appetite:	Good ☐	Fair ☐

Picky ☐

MEDICATIONS

Please list all medications being taken by the patient. Include vitamins, prescriptions, herbal preparations and over-the-counter medications:

FIGURE 1–1 Example of Intake History Form.

Name:

ALLERGIES AND REACTIONS TO DRUG, FOOD OR ENVIRONMENT

Drug or food:	Reaction:
Drug or food:	Reaction:
Drug or food:	Reaction:

It is recommended that children do not receive aspirin. Do you give your child Aspirin?	Yes ☐	No ☐
It is recommended that children less than 12 months not receive honey. Did you know this?	Yes ☐	No ☐
Do you have a working smoke detector?	Yes ☐	No ☐
Do you have a carbon monoxide detector?	Yes ☐	No ☐
Does your child use fluoride?	Yes ☐	No ☐
Is your child around pets? If yes, what type?	Yes ☐	No ☐
Has your child's home been tested for lead?	Yes ☐	No ☐
Does your child live in an apartment, house, or mobile home? Please circle one.		
Does your child drink city, well, or bottled water? Please circle one.		

PSYCHOSOCIAL

If the patient has fears state them:
What comforts the patient?
How does the patient indicate pain?
Has the family has recent changes which may cause stress?
Has there ever been any domestic violence or incidents of physical, verbal, or sexual abuse in your household?
Are any community agencies assisting the patient? Please state contact person:
Do you need any additional information about the patient's health or illness? ☐ Yes ☐ No

Name:

List any operations, hospitalizations, or serious injuries and the approximate dates:	

Name of person completing this form (print):	
Signature:	Relationship to patient:

Physician signature: ———————————————————— Date:

Physician's comments:

FIGURE 1-1 *(Continued)*

History of Present Illness

General Comments

Taking a history from a child or parent goes well beyond asking clinically appropriate questions. Most sick visits to a pediatric clinic are frightening experiences for both patients and their caretakers. Most infants develop normal stranger anxiety around 6 months of age, and this often carries over through age 3. Often a screaming infant is an unnerving experience for both parent and physician. Children and adolescents also may be fearful, uncomfortable, or even angry and may not be forthcoming. It is important to set the tone for a calm and relaxed visit. The pediatrician should enter the exam room and sit down immediately. Studies demonstrate that parents perceive the duration of an office visit as longer when the provider sits as opposed to standing. The child should remain in the parent's lap and receive attention at all times. Close the door in order to maintain an aura of confidentiality.

Before asking your questions, it is important to review the intake history. Cultural and spiritual needs will play an important role in assessing the patient's outlook on the present situation. Questions should be open-ended and nonjudgmental. Allow patients to answer them without interruption. Occasionally, if a patient becomes verbose and repetitive, it may be necessary to redirect the conversation in a tactful fashion. Listening to and observing the patient are invaluable. As the physician gets to know a patient, he or she should recognize when the patient is feeling at ease and comfortable because this will promote more openness. Unease may manifest itself in many ways, ranging from overt hostility to silence. Try to make eye contact with the patient throughout. Some interviewers are able to do this while writing or typing; some are not. It is important to realize that patients are not familiar with medical language, so do not use any jargon. Furthermore, the average reading level for a patient is at about seventh grade, so tailor all communications to that. In certain situations, the reading level may be lower. If there is a language barrier, it is critical to obtain good translation. Studies demonstrate that family members should not be translators because they may omit or change questions based on their knowledge of the patient's vulnerabilities, perhaps to avoid repercussions after the visit. Professional translators can be most helpful.

Taking a Focused History

The history ascertains information to synthesize later into a full narrative with enough clues in it to make a diagnosis. In this chapter we will develop a format to analyze an individual problem. In subsequent chapters we will apply this format to each system, and through this approach the reader will learn appropriate questions to clarify individual problems. The reader also will learn to seek additional information about appropriate related problems that will lead to a correct diagnosis.

TABLE 1–6 The PQRST System for Clarification

P	Provocative or palliative measures
Q	Quality of the problem
R	Region involved
S	Severity of the problem
T	Temporal pattern of the problem

Always enter the chief complaint into the chart in the patient's or caretaker's own words. This is most important because it gives the best possible view of the patient's perception of his or her problem. The *PQRST mnemonic* is most helpful in analyzing a problem (TABLE 1–6).

Always let the patient supply the answers to these questions. Just listen and record. *Do not ask any other questions at this time.* Using this schema for a given problem, such as pain, we may ascertain the following:

- What makes the pain worse or better? The patient may tell you anything: eating, sleeping, walking, or belching.
- Describe the pain. The patient may say or imply sharp, dull, gnawing, deep, superficial, or intermittent.
- Location of the pain: arm, leg, abdomen, chest, etc. The patient may tell you if it migrates anywhere, but at this stage, do not ask any questions.
- How severe is the pain? This is a subjective question. The diagnosis and alleviation of pain have taken on a very high priority in recent times. Various scales quantify pain. We include one for children and adolescents in FIGURE 1–2. It should be posted in every exam room.
- Is there any particular time of the day that the pain changes? Does it affect work or sleep? If it comes and goes, how long do the episodes last? How much time is free of pain? Let the patient answer the question.
- What are the patient's (parents') goals for and means of pain relief?
- Are there any personal or cultural barriers to the ability to report pain?

After the patient has answered all the questions, now it is time for the physician to help elicit further information about the symptoms through the following methods:

- Clarification. Examples: The patient's information up to this point may be vague. If the patient states that he or she is "dizzy," it is necessary to ask if the patient feels that he or she is spinning or that the room is spinning. Subsequent chapters will present pertinent questions to ask to clarify specific problems that do not seem understandable.
- *Quantification.* Examples: How much blood has the patient been spitting up? How many drinks per day does the patient consume? Use pain scales to quantify pain. When you urinate frequently, are you producing more or less urine than normally at a given time?

PAIN ASSESSMENT SCALE

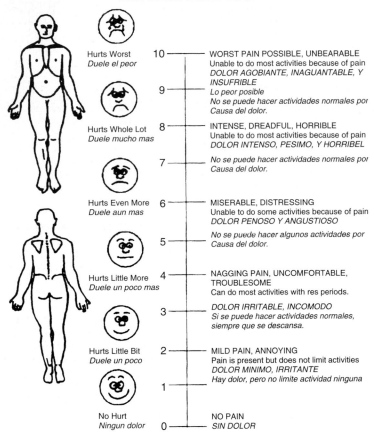

Hurts Worst	10	WORST PAIN POSSIBLE, UNBEARABLE
Duele el peor		Unable to do most activities because of pain
		DOLOR AGOBIANTE, INAGUANTABLE, Y
		INSUFRIBLE
	9	*Lo peor posible*
		No se puede hacer actividades normales por
		Causa del dolor.
Hurts Whole Lot	8	INTENSE, DREADFUL, HORRIBLE
Duele mucho mas		Unable to do most activities because of pain
		DOLOR INTENSO, PESIMO, Y HORRIBEL
	7	*No se puede hacer actividades normales por*
		Causa del dolor.
Hurts Even More	6	MISERABLE, DISTRESSING
Duele aun mas		Unable to do some activities because of pain
		DOLOR PENOSO Y ANGUSTIOSO
	5	*No se puede hacer algunos actividades por*
		Causa del dolor.
Hurts Little More	4	NAGGING PAIN, UNCOMFORTABLE,
Duele un poco mas		TROUBLESOME
		Can do most activities with res periods.
	3	*DOLOR IRRITABLE, INCOMODO*
		Si se puede hacer actividades normales,
		siempre que se descansa.
Hurts Little Bit	2	MILD PAIN, ANNOYING
Duele un poco		Pain is present but does not limit activities
		DOLOR MINIMO, IRRITANTE
	1	*Hay dolor, pero no limite actividad ninguna*
No Hurt		NO PAIN
Ningun dolor	0	*SIN DOLOR*

FIGURE 1-2   Example of Pain Assessment Scale.

- *Timing.* Examples: Patient logs are often very helpful in elucidating timing as well as quantification for headaches, food intake, and assessment of asthma (asthma action plans).

After clarifying, quantifying, and timing individual problems, it is now time to inquire about additional problems. This will serve two purposes:

- It may serve as a reminder to the patient of problems he or she or the caretaker forgot to mention. However, depending on the patient's suggestibility, some of these questions may become "leading questions," and the physician should take this into consideration.
- If the patient denies the problem mentioned, this serves as an important "pertinent negative."

As an example, suppose that a patient presents with a problem of abdominal pain and describes it clearly, quantitatively, and temporally.

It is now important to ask whether the patient has other problems, e.g., vomiting, diarrhea, jaundice, pruritus, or change in stool or urine color. At the earliest stages of training, it is conceivable that physicians may not know what questions to ask. Subsequent chapters of this book will help to build on this capability. Furthermore, a given problem may not be limited to one system. For example, vomiting may be due to infection or irritation of the gastrointestinal tract or due to increased intracranial pressure. In the ensuing chapters we will discuss problems that may originate from systems other than the one addressed in that chapter.

Special Considerations

Infants, Ages 0 to 2 Years

Since most infants are either nonverbal or their speech and language are rudimentary, we must view them in the context of their environment (caretakers). Caretakers, usually parents, will furnish most, if not all, medical histories. Although a newborn may be considered a *tabula rasa*, their parents are not; they bring with them all their past life experience—cognitive, affective, ethnic, cultural, and religious. It is critical that an open and trusting relationship exist between the physician and the entire family. In many instances, parents will interview pediatricians prior to the birth of a child in order to choose one with whom they feel most comfortable. Assessment begins at this point. The interviewer should present many potentially sensitive questions calmly and in a nonthreatening manner. What are the parents' expectations of their child? Was this a planned pregnancy? Are they feeling positively or negatively about having a baby? Are they anxious or worried? Are they feeling some or all of these emotions? How are these parents equipped to raise a child—cognitively, financially, and temperamentally? How will this child fit into the parents' priorities? Do both parents work outside the home? How much do their jobs keep them away from home? Do they have any other priorities that may conflict with parenting? How are the parents' support systems? Are there grandparents?

Once the baby is born, it is important to assess the mother's psychological state. Giving birth is an overwhelming experience, and approximately 70 percent of new mothers will report feeling "overwhelmed," "scared," "tearful," or "depressed" in the first few weeks after delivery. These are considered typical "baby blues" and should dissipate by 1 month postpartum. However, they may not, and therefore, the mother may be experiencing a postpartum depression. It is well known that maternal depression has a significantly negative impact on child well-being. It is wise for pediatricians to consider this in early office visits with new babies, and recent studies have shown that merely asking, "How are you feeling?" or observing a mother is not sufficient to identify postpartum depression. A standardized questionnaire such as the Edinburgh Postpartum Depression Scale is far more effective.

As the child grows and develops, it is critical to assess the entire family structure. How does the father participate in care? Is he actively involved? How do mother and father act together in the context of the child? What impact has the baby had on the marriage? How do they share responsibilities and decision making? If the father is not present, does he provide financial support? Are there siblings? How are they doing with the baby? How do they manifest their jealousy?

How are the parents equipped to handle a toddler's search for independence (i.e., walking, tantrums)? How do they stand on discipline? Both parents invariably have grown up with different approaches to these issues. Are they able to reconcile these differences?

Since parents are the primary historians in an infant's office visit, their backgrounds, as discussed earlier, bring much to bear on their interpretations of the baby's symptoms. They may reveal many hidden agendas. Do they comprehend the severity or not of the illness? If not, is it due to ignorance, guilt, anxiety, or parental strife? Is there any secondary gain for a parent when a child is ill? It is important to discern whether parents are displaying normal concern or mild overconcern as opposed to a misperception that a child is weaker than he or she is (vulnerable child) or suffering from Munchausen's syndrome by proxy. Are the parents able to trust the physician? Do they need an authoritarian approach, or do they prefer to be actively involved in decision making regarding the child? Does this mesh with the physician's outlook?

Thus one must address many "intangibles" when obtaining a medical history for an infant.

Children, Ages 2 to 12 Years

Gathering a medical history on children should take into account all the intangibles discussed earlier. Infants function mainly on basic trust. In contrast, children are at a point where they are attempting to strike out on their own and develop thinking patterns consistent with their age. After age 2, they start to develop cognition, language, and memory, and they like to apply these new skills. Thus they can provide a history that can be useful to the clinician, but only in the context of their thought processes. Struggles between parents and children over autonomy are inevitable. In the best of circumstances it is not easy for a parent to trust a 2-year-old going off by himself or herself. The constant reminders of "good boy/girl–bad boy/girl" coincide with the development of shame, guilt, and doubt at age 3. After this rudimentary development of right versus wrong, older children, starting as early as age 3, develop the earliest stages of cause-and-effect reasoning. Early on, it is egocentric, and they feel that they are the cause of every outcome. As they get older, around ages 3 to 6, they begin to see causes and effects based on outside events and observations, and then they draw conclusions from that. But because of their limited experience, the conclusions may be flawed. For example, a 3- or 4-year-old may see a ball of clay rolled into a snake-shaped object. He may conclude that the snake weighs more than the ball because it is longer. A 7-year-old with more experience may come to the conclusion that the clay weighs the same in both instances because the snake may be longer, but it is also thinner. An older child may reason that the weight is the same because reshaping the ball of clay neither adds nor takes away anything.

Children about age 5 develop the ability to assess how an event or an outcome affects them. As they get older, around age 10, they may develop empathy, i.e., how the same event affects others. Also, school-age children now begin to develop much richer language, and they develop the ability to pun or to tease early on, followed by subtlety and innuendo, when they develop more empathy or an understanding of the "golden rule." It is important for the physician taking a history from a child to determine his or her level of cognition and language in order to understand better the information.

Adolescents, Ages 12 to 21 Years

Adolescents want to be treated as adults, although neurodevelopmentally they are trapped between childhood and adulthood. This divides into early, middle, and late adolescence, followed by young adulthood, not based so much on age alone but rather on sexual maturity rating and cognitive psychosocial development. Self-esteem relates closely to the timing of a teen's pubertal advancement compared to that of his or her peers. Through these stages also is a transition from concrete to formal operations.

The nature of the interaction with the adolescent (i.e., questions asked, issues discussed, and information and guidance offered) always must match their psychosocial developmental stage (e.g., address alcohol abuse or protection from sexually transmitted diseases differently at different ages). Since chronological age is not always compatible with developmental status, the clinician must find ways to explore the developmental level before further proceeding. Chatting about topics of interest such as sports, music, books, hobbies, movies, etc. may provide information about psychosocial development, and this should match the adolescent's developmental level. Adolescents have certain characteristics and needs at every defined stage of development, as summarized in TABLE 1–7.

Family, school, and peer group all remain important for optimal psychosocial development, but the major developmental task of adolescence is initiating independence from the family. Therefore, teens expect to take an active role in their health care discussions and decisions, including advanced directives. They also have an increased wish for privacy.

Obtaining a medical history from an adolescent differs somewhat from eliciting either a pediatric or an adult history, and special skill is necessary to establish rapport with a teenager. The primary physician-patient relationship now lies with the adolescent, not with the parent or caregiver. The parents remain critical for accurate and complete health data collection; part of the art of the adolescent history taking is to gracefully both include and exclude the parents.

The birth history and early childhood milestones take on a lesser role during adolescence, but they are important if they are relevant to the complaint at hand. Information on hospitalizations, serious early childhood illnesses, and the family medical history also may be necessary. The social history is paramount in understanding the potential health risks of the adolescent, but this section of the history should wait until the parent leaves the room.

An adolescent will only share information with a provider if he or she feels respected and safe. Adolescents will be wary of new care providers,

TABLE 1-7 Development of Adolescent Thought Processes

Development	Early (11–14 Years)
Cognitive	Concrete thinking Inability to think hypothetically Attached to present tense, cannot appreciate the future and realize consequences
Psychological	Self-centered, preoccupied with physical changes, view of self and environment
Social	Same-sex relationships, still influenced by parents, starting exploratory behavior
Middle (15–17 Years)	
Cognitive	Starting abstract thinking, starting to see future consequences
Psychological	Testing limits, seeking identity and independence, peer interaction, opposition to parents
Social	Dating, opposite- or same-sex sexual experimentation, personal myth ("Won't happen to me"), peer pressure, high-risk behaviors
Late (>17 Years)	
Cognitive	Abstract thinkers, ability to see into the future
Psychological	Independent individuals, friends with parents
Social	Mature romantic and friend relationships, risk-taking reduced

and you will have to earn their trust. Make the exam environment as private and welcoming to teens as feasible. Allow them to remain clothed during the interview and afterwards before discussing the plan. Maintain a professional demeanor. Providers who are too stiff will inhibit patients from responding freely. Providers who are too casual will fail to instill confidence in their patients. Knock before entering the room, and introduce yourself to the teen first. Inquire as to how they would like you to address them, and document a preferred nickname on the chart for future reference. Ask the teen to introduce his or her parents or others who have accompanied him or her. Seat yourself at eye level with the adolescent as quickly as possible, and always address the questions first to him or her.

Early in the visit, thank the parent or parents for accompanying their teen, and ask them to share their concerns with the patient in the room. Explain that this is the policy of the clinic to listen to their concerns and gather the data, but then excuse them from the room. Inform them that you will call them back before the end of the visit so that they can hear your opinions and care plan recommendations. Do not inquire into sensitive information such as "Do you smoke or drink?" or "Are you sexually active?" before asking the parents to leave the room. This puts the adolescent in the uncomfortable position of either having to admit to things they may not have discussed with their parents or, worse, of lying to both his or her parents and the medical provider. This could be potentially dangerous, e.g., if a teen were going to surgery or needed medications that would be dangerous to a fetus but had denied being sexually active. Rarely, a parent will refuse to leave the room. In this situation, explore with the parent his or her concerns and emphasize your desire to provide the best care possible. Explain that trust is necessary in the parent-teen relationship, just as it is in the physician-patient relationship, and that your relationship needs to be primarily with the teen.

Health history forms may be useful aids in adolescent histories. If you develop your own forms (TABLE 1–8), be sure to use lay terms and write them at a level that an adolescent would understand. Also be sure to indicate who completed the form. Teens and their parents may have different agendas for the visit, or they may view the home situation or risk factors differently. The American Medical Association has standardized health history forms intended for separate completion by teens and their parents. These General Adolescent Preventative Services (GAPS) are available on the AMA website.

Typically, a parent or legal guardian must accompany an adolescent or give formal consent to treat until the adolescent is 18 years of age. There may be rare circumstance in which an adolescent is legally emancipated, meaning that he or she can act as his or her own guardian. Such circumstances may include legal marriage with consent of the parents, imprisonment, or enlistment in the military. There are, additionally, several medical conditions in which an adolescent younger than 18 years of age is considered temporarily emancipated and can seek care for that diagnosis without the knowledge or consent of the parent or guardian. These conditions are determined by individual state governments and therefore vary. Exceptions occur in cases of suicidal youth, sexual abuse, or intention of the adolescent to harm others. In these situations, it is mandatory to inform authorities, special services, and parents. It is important not to let personal beliefs and values compromise patient confidentiality in these situations. It is complicated at times to navigate insurance systems and ensure patient safety without eventually involving the families. These facilitated conversations can happen only with the consent of the patient.

The interview should begin with eliciting the chief complaint. Always be aware of hidden as well as obviously stated concerns. When interviewing, maintain as much eye contact as possible, and minimize writing or typing in front of the patient because it makes patients self-conscious. The history should be orderly but not rigid. Some of the most meaningful history from a teen may be whispered under the breath or appear on the surface to be off-subject. It is important to be flexible and follow up those pieces of information with additional questions. Keep questions open-ended at first: "What is bothering you today?" "How have you been feeling since your last visit?" or "Is there more you wanted to talk about today?" It may seem like the history has to be dragged from some teens, but overly directive questions typically will beget only monosyllabic "yes" or "no" answers. If time constraints intervene or getting the teen to interact is an issue, directive questions should be of the "when," "why," and "how" variety. At other times an adolescent might

TABLE 1–8 *Adolescent Health Questionnaire*

This questionnaire will help us to know you better. Sometimes it is easier to raise questions you have on your mind this way. Check "YES" or "NO" to the questions on this page; check the appropriate column for the problems listed on page 2. Hand this paper directly to your physician. You may have it back if you wish.

By what name do you like to be called? _____

Why are you coming to the doctor today? _____

	YES	NO
1. Do you have any other things needing medical attention?		
2. In general, do you think you are a healthy person?		
3. Have you ever had a serious illness, an operation, or stayed in the hospital?		
4. Do you worry that you might have heart trouble?		
5. Do you worry that you might have cancer?		
6. Have you ever had low blood or anemia?		
7. Are there any foods you can't eat or medicines you can't take because of allergies?		
8. Do you have any questions about pregnancy or birth control?		
9. Do you have any questions about drinking or using drugs?		
10. Do you have any questions about cigarette smoking?		
11. Do you have any questions about AIDS or other sexually transmitted diseases?		
12. Do you have any worries about how your body is developing?		
13. Are you happy with your weight?		
14. Are you happy with your height?		
15. Are you absent from school (or job) a lot?		
16. Are you having any trouble passing your courses at school?		
17. Does anything bother you about school (or job)?		
18. Do you get along with your parents?		

(*Continued*)

TABLE 1-8 Adolescent Health Questionnaire *(Continued)*

	YES	NO
19. Can you talk to your parents about important things or worries?		
20. Do you get along with your brothers and sisters?		
21. Are there any big problems at home?		
22. Do you have any problem making friends?		
23. Do you date?		
24. Do you go steady?		
25. Do you have any worries about your sex feelings or dating partner preferences?		

This is a list of conditions and problems that sometimes give young people trouble. Check each one as to whether you are troubled by it a lot, once in a while, or never.

	NEVER	A LOT	ONCE IN A WHILE
Skin problems: rashes, pimples			
Headaches			
Dizzy spells, fainting, blackouts			
Eye or vision problems			
Wear eye glasses or contact lenses			
Ear or hearing problems			
Stuffy, runny, or bleeding nose			
Colds or sore throats			
Trouble with teeth or gums			
Coughing or wheezing..........................			
Get out of breath more than friends			
Pain or aches in stomach......................			
Vomiting (throwing up)......................			
Diarrhea (loose bowels)........................			
Constipation..			
Frequency, pain, burning, blood with urination (passing water)			

(Continued)

TABLE 1–8 Adolescent Health Questionnaire (Continued)

	NEVER	A LOT	ONCE IN A WHILE
Pain or discharge or any other problems with your sex organs			
Girls: problems with your period (menstruation)			
Pain or aches in back, arms, leg, muscles, or joints			
Hay fever, hives, or asthma			
Feel upset or nervous			
Feel angry			
Feel lonely, sad, or depressed			
Feel tired all day; no energy			
Have problems sleeping			
Eat too much or too little			
Don't eat right foods			

Is there anything else your doctor should
know about you? .... Yes _____   No _____
Do you have any other health questions?...... Yes _____   No _____

Thank you

Source: From Hofmann A: Providing care to adolescents. In: Hofmann A, Greydanus DE
(eds.). *Adolescent Medicine.* Stamford, CT: Appleton and Lange, 1997, Chap. 3, p. 30–31.

tell a verbose tale, but it still may be far from the complete story. Feel
comfortable guiding or redirecting the history, e.g., "That's quite a story,
but can you tell me specifically how you came to hurt your leg?" At all
times avoid asking leading questions; they limit the patient's response
to what he or she thinks you want to know, e.g., "You haven't had sex
before, have you? This puts a value judgment on premarital intercourse,
and the obvious desired response would be "No, never."

Adolescents are even more sensitive to nonverbal communication
than are adults. They will be monitoring your facial expressions, posture, gestures, and touch. Similarly, you must listen with more than your
ears. Place your chair about 3 or 4 feet from the adolescent, a distance
that respects personal space boundaries but simultaneously shows that
you are interested in what they have to say. Avoid acting shocked, gri-
macing, or laughing at a response even though it may seem at times the
patient is trying to shock you. Do not patronize the adolescent, but do
make sure to ask questions in a way the teen understands. Avoid technical jargon. If a patient uses a term to describe an event or a symptom,
try to incorporate that term into your clarifying questions. It is great to
know some of the slang that teens use, but do not try to act as if you
are their friend—it will seem insincere and unprofessional to them.

After eliciting the chief complaint, proceed with the history of the
present illness in the PQRST format described in TABLE 1–6. Try to determine the functional impact of their concern. Assess whether the symptoms

have secondary gain for the patient (e.g., keeping them out of school or earning them special attention from home) or for the parent (e.g., granting them benefits of disability to care for an ill child so as not to motivate the child to get well).

A major point in the art of interviewing adolescents is the psychosocial history. Teenagers are a particularly vulnerable to environmental factors, and age group and teen morbidity relates closely to psychosocial factors (e.g., sexually transmitted diseases, unhealthy dieting, unwanted pregnancies, depression, violence, substance abuse, etc.). A useful tool for assessing the psychosocial history is the acronym *HEEADSSS* (first developed as HEADSS in 1972 and recently expanded in 2004). HEEADSSS is the acronym for the words *home, education, eating, activities, drugs, sexuality,* and *suicide,* as well as depression and safety, which are main domains of the adolescent life to explore carefully. Important points concerning HEEADSSS are

- Approach sensitive matters (i.e., sexuality, drug abuse, self-esteem, peer acceptance, etc.) in a discrete and respectful manner. The clinician initially may explore attitudes of peers and friends toward important issues (e.g., smoking or dating) and then ask the adolescent about his or her view and if he or she may have experienced something similar.
- Eating disorders (including overweight/obesity) are a very common in modern youth. Asking the relevant questions and revealing issues at an early stage can lead to better chances of a successful intervention. Weight changes in adolescence may be strongly associated with psychological or environmental dysfunction. However, exclude organic reasons; e.g., severe weight loss within a short time period may be precipitated by malignancy, inflammatory bowel disease, thyroid gland dysfunction, diabetes mellitus type 1, parasitosis, major depression, eating disorders, drug abuse, or traumatic social experience. Questions about accompanying symptoms such as vomiting, loose or bloody stools, polyuria, polydipsia, excessive appetite, exophthalmos, hand shaking, emotional bursts, etc. can reveal valuable information and direct further investigating.
- Questions about sexual abuse are very important. Without asking, it is most possible that the adolescent will volunteer nothing. Useful questions are the following: "Have you had any negative sexual experiences?" or "Has anyone ever touched you in parts of your body that made you feel uncomfortable without your permission?"
- School performance is an important issue to investigate. Consistently low school grades in a seemingly bright teenager may be the result of a neglected learning disorder. Sudden, impressive worsening of school performance may be the result of psychological distress, drug abuse, or environmental instability. Questions must be precise and persistent. For example, asking "How is school going?" will not work. The answer will not provide any information in most cases (most adolescents would answer "OK"). More useful questions are: "What are your grades this year?" "Are they better or worse than last year?" "Which is your favorite course?" and "Do you often miss school?" Some adolescents may

be employed, and it is equally important to assess how they function in the workplace.

- Direct investigation of suicidal thoughts is critical for every adolescent. Regardless of what might be the common perception, questions about suicidal intentions do not lead to attempts. On the contrary, revealing such a situation may result in a much better chance of successful intervention.

- Assuming that adolescents are heterosexual is incorrect. Most adolescents are exploring their sexual orientation; some are bisexual or homosexual. Questions such as "Do you have a boyfriend or a girlfriend?" or "Are you sexually attracted to someone?" are preferable.

- Always take cultural framework into consideration with respect. Strive to learn about diverse cultural norms.

- Adolescents are the age group on which prevention programs should mainly focus because the health knowledge obtained and the habits established during this time period will determine adult quality of life. It is a basic rule of adolescent medicine that every visit, no matter the chief complaint, is always a prevention visit as well.

Anticipate some blank stares, downcast eyes, and periods of silence. Keep questions short and simple. Give the adolescent time to gather his or her thoughts, and rephrase questions if you sense that the patient does not understand them. Avoid long periods of silence with adolescent patients; unlike adults, who may benefit from time for self-reflection, a teenager is more likely to become distracted or lose trust in you as an examiner and conclude that you do not know what you are doing. Since peer groups have significant influence, sometimes invoking them makes questions less threatening. For example, instead of answering directly, "Do you use drugs or alcohol?" you might instead state, "Many people your age are experimenting with drugs or drinking alcohol. Have you tried this or been pressured to try this?"

As the history progresses, frequently confirm with the patient that you have heard him or her correctly. Try to understand how the patient perceives a problem, and acknowledge how he or she might feel about this. End the adolescent history by asking if the patient has had the chance to voice all his or her concerns. Summarize what you have gleaned as the patient's most important concerns and what he or she can expect from the physical exam and decision-making process.

Adolescents often have appointments for a "sports physical." In addition to the general history, a sports-participation-specific history should be integrated into the visit. The key elements to be included in such a history are shown in TABLE 1–9.

TABLE 1–9 Key Elements of Sport Preparticipation History in Adolescents

Past History
- Known medical conditions, their status and treatment (such as asthma, epilepsy, sickle cell disease, hemophilia, cystic fibrosis, other chronic diseases)
- Surgeries (eye, chest, abdomen, spine, other)
- Febrile illness in recent past
- Details of previous musculoskeletal injuries
- Details of previous head and neck injuries

Allergies
- Medications, food, bees, other

Medications History
- Current therapeutic medications, dietary supplements, other drug use

Dietary History
- Current diet, perception of weight, attempts to gain or lose weight and how

Cardiovascular History
Past History
- Congenital heart disease, its treatment, follow-up, any activity restrictions
- History of rheumatic fever, Kawasaki disease

Family History
- Premature cardiac death before age 50 years in first-degree relatives
- Heart disease in surviving relatives age younger than 50 years
- Marfan syndrome, cardiomyopathy, hypertension, lipid disorders, diabetes mellitus

Personal History
- Exertion-related syncope or presyndcope
- Exertion-related undue fatigue, shortness of breath, chest pain
- Episodes of dizziness, palpitations
- Known history of heart murmur, high cholesterol, high blood pressure
- Recent febrile illness
- Use of medications, illicit drugs, performance-enhancing supplements or drugs

Pulmonary History
- Exercise-related cough or wheezing
- Smoking or smoke exposure

Neurologic History
- Details of head and neck injury including current symptoms
- Exercise-related headaches

Other
- Eye symptoms and visual acuity
- Any history of hearing impairment
- Recent musculoskeletal injuries and current symptoms
- Menstrual history in girls
- Immunizations

2 Performing a Physical Examination in Infants, Children, and Adolescents

Arthur N. Feinberg and Thomas Melgar

The goal of this chapter is to develop a framework with which to build a thorough and accurate physical examination. We will compare the physical examinations of infants, children, and adolescents in terms of developing diagnostic priorities but leave the details and techniques of examination to the individual chapters covering each system.

General Considerations

The four cornerstones to building data in a physical examination are observation, palpation, percussion, and auscultation. However, we must realize that we cannot perform these tasks without our basic senses: vision, hearing, olfaction, taste, and touch. Thus inspection depends on vision, olfaction, and taste; palpation, on touch; percussion, on touch; and auscultation, on hearing.

Inspection

General Visual Inspection (Gestalt)

Most experienced physicians begin the process of developing their differential diagnosis from the moment they walk into the examination room. Does anything strike you on immediate first impression? Are there any obvious malformations? Does the patient appear well or is he or she uncomfortable, appear to be in pain, or appear to have respiratory distress or seem listless or apathetic? Is there anything outstanding about the patient's behavior? Experience and knowledge are most helpful in tempering a clinician's interpretation of a patient's appearance. As a simple example, a less experienced clinician might be concerned that a patient's respiratory rate is 50 breaths per minute, whereas his more experienced colleague may state, "This is a newborn. A respiratory rate of 50 breaths per minute is normal." Thus the more experience we have, the more we develop a wider sense of "normal limits," therefore giving us more leeway in arriving at a conclusion without resorting to incorrect hypotheses and unnecessary tests.

Close Visual Inspection

It is important to maximize our ability to see patients by placing them in a room with adequate lighting. This is helpful in interpreting size, shape, and color nuances. It is generally accepted that certain tools to enhance vision may be used. A magnifying glass may be necessary to examine small skin lesions. Ophthalmoscopes and otoscopes are part of the primary physician's armamentarium. Other tools, such as laryngoscopes, may be used for visualization by personnel trained in advanced life support. Emergency medicine physicians and primary care physicians may be able to use a slit lamp to examine the anterior chamber of the eye. Gastroscopes, colonoscopes, thoracoscopes, and laparoscopes, for example, are best left to the specialty consultant.

Visualization may go beyond the patient. One may evaluate body fluids. Is the urine dark colored or cloudy? Is the cerebrospinal fluid bloody or cloudy? Are the stools red, black, or white? In the old days, when physicians made house calls, often observation of the patient's home environment was helpful in gathering useful information.

Olfaction

The sense of smell is an integral part of the clinical evaluation. For example, odors on the breath such as acetone may help to identify diabetic ketoacidosis. Foul odors may indicate bacterial infections such as strep throat or sinusitis, lung abscess, dental caries, or a nasal foreign body. Metabolic disorders may give representative odors to the skin, cerumen, or urine, such as maple syrup urine disease (branched-chain ketoaciduria) or the mousy or musty odor of phenylketonuria. Other bodily fluids such as vomitus, diarrhea, urine, and pus also may reveal useful information.

Palpation

The sense of touch has many aspects, e.g., tactile, temperature, and kinesthetic senses such as position and vibration. Unfortunately, it is doubtful that we reach anywhere near our maximal potential for this sense. This is illustrated by the well-known fact that individuals who are blind develop far keener senses of touch than the average person. Also, we must learn how to maximize our use of this sense. Specifically, the finger tip is the best part of the hand to use for tactile sense, whereas the dorsum of the hands or fingers best elicits temperature sense. The base of the fifth metacarpophalangeal area is the most sensitive part of the hand for vibration detection.

The examiner should ask many questions about what he or she is feeling. What is the texture? Is it coarse, thick, rough, or smooth? Is there crepitus? Is it wet or dry? Is the temperature warm or cold to the touch? Where are pulsations and vibrations located? How strong or weak are they? Does palpation elicit pain? How much force and in what direction caused this?

Percussion

Percussion is the art of striking the surface of the body in order to elicit tones with varying frequencies and is helpful in evaluating the density of the underlying tissue. FIGURE 8–7 demonstrates the method of indirect bimanual percussion. One places the palmar surface of the distal left middle finger on the surface (pleximeter). The tip of the right middle finger (plexor) strikes the pleximeter finger with a sharp blow to the distal interphalangeal joint by rapid and equal flexions of the right wrist. The examiner will then shift both hands up and down the area being percussed (e.g., abdomen or thorax) and listen carefully for changes in the tone and quality of the sound. Specifically, denser tissue under the fingers will yield a "flat" tone and quality (e.g., skeletal muscle). Less dense tissue (e.g., cardiac muscle) may yield a "dull" timbre. The normal thorax will produce "resonance" owing to air-filled lung tissue. In an emphysematous lung with more air than tissue, the sound is "hyperresonant." In the case of a hollow viscus such as a dilated air-filled stomach, the tone becomes "tympanitic." Since each individual examiner perceives stimuli in his or her own way, multiple examinations are necessary to develop a feel for these varying tones and timbres.

Movement of the pleximeter and plexor along an area helps to estimate areas of differential tissue density. For example, if tissue of one density surrounds an organ of another density, the examiner outlines the area inside which there are no changes in percussive quality to estimate the size of the organ (e.g., heart, liver, or spleen). In pathologic situations such as fluid accumulations (pleuritic or ascitic), the areas of dullness percussed will help to outline the size of the effusion.

When beginners have difficulty with percussion, it is because of technique. Applying firm pressure with the pleximeter on the body surface is important. Loose application often will cause dampening of the sounds. The second common flaw in technique is not keeping the plexor wrist loose. This enables the plexor finger to rebound better off the pleximeter, creating a better sound quality.

Auscultation

The term *auscultation* literally means the use of hearing to obtain physical findings. In the earliest of times, this was limited to merely listening to sounds emanating from the patient. Then, perhaps, in order to hear better, astute clinicians would place their ear on the surface of the patient. Technology then was developed when clinicians observed that they could hear better when they placed a diaphragm over the structure that would then transmit vibrations with less extraneous interference through a solid tube placed near the observer's ear (monaural stethoscope). Later, binaural stethoscopes, with flexible tubing, the staple of today's physician, made life easier for clinicians. Technology at present has gone beyond the stethoscope with the advent of electronic stethoscopes that project sounds through an amplifier (used often for teaching purposes). Moreover, Doppler sonography has been a significant advance in the use of sound to produce clinical information. However, for the purposes of primary care clinicians, we will emphasize the use of the stethoscope.

FIGURE 2–1 illustrates the basic Sprague stethoscope. The chest piece contains both a diaphragm, whose vibrations transmit preferentially high-pitched sounds, and a bell, which transmits preferentially lower-pitched sounds. The stethoscope does not amplify sound, but rather, it filters extraneous tones. The clinician places it relatively firmly on the patient's skin (never the clothing!) to create a good seal. He or she faces the challenge of selecting various sizes for the bell or diaphragm. It is more difficult to localize sounds in small children, especially with larger bells and diaphragms. However, less surface contact and inadequate seals with smaller bells and diaphragms render poorer filtration of extraneous sounds. It is important to check the stethoscope's chest piece periodically for cracks in the diaphragm, as well as irregularities in the rubber or plastic rim around the bell. The rubber or plastic earpieces of the stethoscope should fit the examiner with a good seal. The clinician should check the earpieces regularly for cracks, tears, and cerumen accumulation.

Since each examiner perceives sounds in his or her own way, experience will help to develop a system to codify the incoming stimuli. The stethoscope detects sounds from the thorax (heart and lungs). The quality of the heartbeat may be sharp or muffled. Timing and location are also important. Are there any extraneous sounds (i.e., murmurs, rubs, clicks, or gallops)? How are the breath sounds? Is inspiration and expiration proportional? Are there wheezes (high-pitch squeaks), rales (crinkling sounds), or rubs? Where are they located? What does the abdomen sound like? Are the bowel sounds normal, increased, or diminished? Are there adventitious sounds such as bruits? One may apply the stethoscope to any part of the body. Are there adventitious cranial sounds (bruits)? We emphasize the use of the stethoscope in further detail in the ensuing chapters.

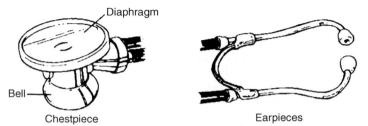

FIGURE 2–1 The Sprague Stethoscope. *The chest piece combines the bell and diaphragm, with a valve to direct the air through either. The earpieces are connected by a spring that holds them in place. (From* DeGowin's Diagnostic Examination, *8th ed. New York: McGraw-Hill, 2004, Fig. 3.2, p. 46.)*

Physical Examination

General Comments

A physical examination may be a full or a diagnostic examination depending on the circumstances of the visit. In this section we will go through screening exams for infants, children, and adolescents, noting which areas to emphasize in which age groups. A diagnostic examination will use the patient history as a guide to which parts of the general examination to emphasize.

Full examinations in infants, children, and adolescents are usually well-child examinations (routine checkups) but may be abbreviated in the form of a screening preoperative or sports physical examination. Preoperative evaluation searches for potential surgical or anesthetic problems and therefore would put more emphasis on any history of previous complications with surgery and anesthesia, allergies, and cardiorespiratory problems and on examinations of the mouth, oropharynx, and cardiovascular and respiratory systems. Sports physical examinations focus more on past history of trauma, fractures, brain or spinal cord injury, and overuse problems, as well as on cardiovascular, respiratory, and musculoskeletal systems. This is also a time to discuss use of supplements in sports.

The first order of business is to do whatever it takes to put the patient at ease. We will discuss techniques unique to the different age groups below. An exam room should be as comfortable as possible for the patient. The patient, wearing a thin gown, should feel satisfied with the room temperature. The walls should contain educational material for parents and older children. Ideally, certain rooms should be set aside specifically for children or adolescents with age-appropriate wall hangings. An exam room should be equipped properly and include examination gowns, stethoscope, pneumatic otoscope, ophthalmoscope, sphygmomanometer, penlight, tongue depressors, reflex hammer, tuning fork, pin and monofilament for testing sensation, tape measure, gloves (preferably nonlatex), lubricant, equipment for pelvic examination, sterile swabs (both plain and in transport culture medium), nasopharyngeal swabs, and bandages.

The physical examination should be systematic and well organized. The physician should "examine by region but think by system." The order of the regions examined will depend on the age of the patient and the situation. Clinicians often like to start at the top, the head, and work down to the feet. Young children, ages 15 months to 3 years, find physicians in white coats approaching their heads with instruments very anxiety provoking. An early examination of the oropharynx with a tongue depressor will put a quick end to any trust in the physician. It is often necessary to "think fast" and examine parts to which the patient may be more amenable at that given time.

Generally, the standard examination starts with a statement of *gestalt,* assessing overall physical development (morphology), nourishment,

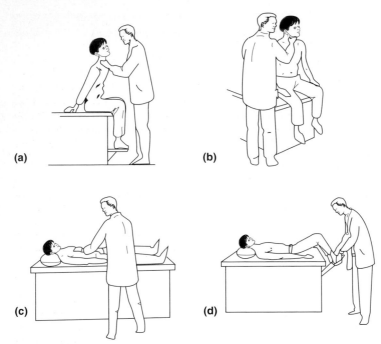

(a)   **(b)**

(c)   **(d)**

FIGURE 2–2 ***The Office Screening Examination.*** *A. Patient draped and sitting (physician facing). B. Patient draped and sitting (physician to the right and back). C. Patient draped and supine (physician to the right). Place the patient in the left lateral decubitus position to listen at the cardiac apex. D. Female pelvic exam. Patient draped and supine, knees and hips flexed (physician at foot). (From* DeGowin's Diagnostic Examination, *8th ed. New York: McGraw-Hill, 2004, Fig. 3.3, p. 49.)*

activity, alertness, demeanor, hydration, and level and type of distress. Record the vital signs. Children and adolescents, like adults, can be examined in four basic positions (FIGURE 2–2). Examine the patient from his or her right side. Typically, from head to foot, it begins with the patient in the sitting position with the physician viewing first head-on and then from the right side and the back. Evaluate the skin, head, eyes, ears, nose, throat, neck, breasts, and thorax in this position. Then place the patient in the supine position or possibly the lateral decubitus position and assess the lungs, heart, and abdomen. Finally, perform rectal and genital exams in the supine position with the knees bent. The table for a female pelvic examination, if necessary, should have stirrups. Note that this sequence minimizes the number of position changes during an evaluation. This allows for less patient discomfort and more efficiency.

Infants, Ages 1 Month to 2 Years

General Considerations

Most nonpediatricians would state that an infant exam is the most difficult of all because infants do not communicate well. Nor do they dissemble, thus making simple observation an easy tool with which to read them. But there are disadvantages that one must overcome. It is more difficult to examine infants in a systematic way because they are often agitated and uncooperative. The physician should be seated in a calm manner with the infant placed in the mother's lap. It may be helpful for the physician to get below eye level of the patient so that he or she does not appear big and threatening. Depending on the infant's level of stranger anxiety, he or she may sit calmly but react poorly to an examination. Infants are distractible, so the physician may take advantage of this by offering up a toy or a magazine. Playing games such as "give and take" or simply smiling may help to ease tension. It is helpful to encourage the mother to remain in the infant's line of sight at all times for reassurance. It is often helpful to accustom the infant to the equipment by allowing him or her to play with it first. Since infants often become tachypneic and tachycardic when anxious, it is best to take vital signs when they are at ease.

If possible, perform a systematic exam as illustrated earlier, although it may be necessary to make exceptions to capitalize on a quiet moment to hear heart tones or respiratory sounds. For purposes of this discussion, we will assume a fully cooperative patient and perform a systematic regional exam. Also, we will discuss what parts of the examination to emphasize in which age group. Please consult subsequent chapters for further details and techniques for the examination, as well as for elicitation and interpretation of specific findings.

The Examination

GESTALT

Do not forget to employ all your senses. Check for alertness, demeanor (playfulness, fussiness), morphology, nourishment, and hydration. Does your subjective assessment of the infant's pain correlate with the parent's? One must be careful using certain terms such as *irritable* or *lethargic*. Irritability may be multifactorial, from bacterial meningitis to general annoyance at strangers and their unwanted attention. Lethargy may bespeak increased intracranial pressure but also may indicate the mere need for a nap. Therefore, the evaluator must qualify these statements by whether the irritable patient is always in this state or consolable. It is important to determine whether the lethargic patient does respond appropriately to stimuli. A febrile child is a "frequent flyer" in a physician's office, and it is incumbent on the examiner to recognize a "toxic" infant. Does he or she make eye contact? Often such children appear sad or uncomfortable, with their eyebrows in the typical "omega" position. They may be pale, listless, slightly tachypneic, or perhaps grunt with respirations. A sick patient may smell of acetone owing to accelerated fatty acid breakdown.

VITAL SIGNS

Take at least four vital signs at each office visit. These may include temperature, pulse, respiration, blood pressure, pulse oximetry, length, or weight. Plot all vital signs on the appropriate chart graphs. We address further interpretation in a separate chapter. The initial assessment will triage for patients in need of immediate attention, such as basic life support or urgent or routine priority.

HEAD

Check the overall size (macro/microcephaly) and shape of the head. What is the size and shape of the fontanelle? Is it flat, sunken, or bulging? Are the sutures closing prematurely? The head may be narrowed in the bitemporal dimension owing to premature closure of the sagittal suture (dolicocephaly or scaphocephaly) or narrow in the anteroposterior dimension owing to premature closure of the coronal sutures (brachycephaly) or premature closure of the metopic suture (trigoncephaly). The head may be transiently flattened at the occiput from the "back to sleep" positioning now used in infancy. Examine the head for any signs trauma (e.g., bruising, swelling, abrasion, or laceration).

EYES

Are there any striking abnormalities? How are the eyes set? If they are too close together, they are *hypoteloric;* if they are too far apart, they are *hyperteloric.* Do they slant in any direction? Are there inner canthal folds? Are they protuberant, either primarily or owing to relative midfacial hypoplasia? Are the irises aligned properly, or are they nasally (isotropia) or temporally (esotropia) located? Assess this by placing a penlight in front of the patient to check the position of the corneal light reflex, which should be central in each pupil. Always check the retina for red reflex with an ophthalmoscope. White or silver reflections often have serious ramifications. Do the eyes have full range of motion? Are there any abnormal movements? Are the pupils of normal and equal size, and do they react to light and accommodation? Are the corneas clear? Are they of normal size? Is there any discoloration (yellow, blue) or bleeding of the sclera? Are the conjunctivae red or swollen from acute inflammation? Is there a "sandpaper" or "cobblestone" appearance of chronic inflammation? Always examine the eyelids and lashes for swelling, discoloration, discharge, or crustiness.

EARS

Because the ear canal is the one place on the body where skin is directly on bone, it is very sensitive to touch. Make every effort to minimize the child's discomfort. Use one hand to apply gentle traction to the pinna to straighten the canal while the other hand holds the otoscope between two fingers, allowing it to pivot with the child's movements. The hand with the otoscope should rest on the child's head so that movement of the head will result in simultaneous movement with the otoscope. Is the pinna well formed and normally set? Are there any abnormal skin tags? Are the canals well formed? They tend to be narrow and S-shaped, and it may be difficult to get through to the tympanic membrane. The tympanic membrane examination is the most frequent evaluation a pediatrician will ever perform, and it always must include adequate lighting and a pneumatic head to assess motion. The ear canals often are partially or completely obstructed with cerumen. The decision to remove cerumen with a spatula or irrigation will depend on the importance of the exam.

Nose, mouth, and throat

Are there any obvious malformations? Is there any obstruction to airflow? Assess the nares for abnormal movements (flaring) and the size and color of the nasal turbinates. Are there any clefts of the lip or palate? It is important to examine the palate visually as well as digitally to detect bony clefts with and without an intact mucosa. Evaluate the tonsils for size, erythema, and exudate. Is the uvula of normal size and midline? Are the teeth in good condition? What is the status of dentition (primary versus secondary teeth)? Adenoids, located behind the palate, are not seen directly, but enlargement may be suspected if the patient uses open-mouth breathing at all times.

Tips to examine the mouth and throat in infants and toddlers

Ideally, the examiner will win the child over, and he or she will either willingly "open wide" or allow an examination during a smile or a yawn. An oral exam with a tongue depressor is a truly noxious experience for a child. Moreover, a child will not forget a previous bad encounter. It is important to be able to check "moving targets" very quickly. Sometime it is necessary, as unpleasant as it may be, to quickly advance a tongue depressor between clenched teeth and apply gentle but consistent backward pressure.

Neck

Are there any masses, clefts, or dimples? Are they located midline or laterally? Is the neck supple with full range of motion? Does the infant hold his or her neck straight, or does he or she prefer one side (torticollis)?

Thorax

Are there any malformations, bony or muscular? Are the nipples of normal size and placement? Are there supernumerary nipples?

Lungs

Observe for breathing pattern. Is it fast or labored, shallow or deep? Are there any adventitious sounds with respiration, such as stertor, wheezing, or grunting? Percuss the chest, especially in a focused examination for any respiratory problems. Auscultation will be of help with sounds that may not be audible with distant observation, particularly with fine crinkly sounding rales, squeaky rubs, or soft wheezes. A stethoscope detects prolonged inspiration or expiration easily.

Heart

Can you visualize or palpate any heartbeats? Are there any abnormal vibrations such as thrills? Where does the examiner feel the impulse of the heartbeat? Auscultation is the crux of the cardiac evaluation. What is the heart rate? Are the heart tones strong or weak? Are the sounds single or split? Are there any adventitious sounds such as murmurs, rubs, clicks, or gallops? Where are the sounds located? In what part of the cardiac cycle do they occur?

ABDOMEN

Visualize the shape. Is it protuberant or scaphoid? Are there any obvious findings such as vessels, striae (stretchmarks), abnormal vasculature, or discolorations such as bruising? Palpation may be most revealing. Is it soft? Is there is any hardness to palpation? Where is it located? If there is any guarding on examination, is it under the patient's control? Attempt to use all techniques of distraction to make this determination. Does palpation of the abdomen elicit any pain? Are there any masses, and are the liver and spleen of normal size? Percussion will reveal size and location by density of masses and solid organs such as the liver or spleen. A stomach dilated with air will sound tympanitic to the observer. It is important to assess the quality of bowel sounds with the stethoscope. Are they normoactive, hypoactive, or hyperactive? What is their pitch and quality?

MUSCULOSKELETAL

Are the extremities well formed? It is critical to perform a Barlow and Ortolani maneuver at each well-child examination during the first year (see Chapter 11) to evaluate for developmental dysplasia of the hip. Are the pulses strong and equal? Is there any swelling or discoloration?

GENITALIA

Are they well formed and not ambiguous? If the patient is male, is he circumcised, and does the penis have its meatus placed properly? Are his testes bilaterally palpable and descended? If the patient is female, are the genitalia well formed? Is the hymen intact yet perforate? Is the urethral opening located properly and visible? Is there any redness or discharge?

INTEGUMENT

Are there any discolorations? Is the overall color cyanotic or jaundiced? How is the texture, temperature, and moistness? Are there any rashes? Describe them as macular, papular, or maculopapular or vesicular. Does a rash blanch when the examiner applies pressure? What is the distribution of the rash? Are there any signs of trauma (e.g., bruising, petechiae, and purpura)? Hair and nails are part of this evaluation. Is there hair loss or discoloration? What is the distribution? Are the nails normally sized and shaped? Is there any thickening, discoloration, or clubbing?

LYMPHATIC

Are there enlarged, palpable lymph nodes? Where are they located? Are they tender? Describe their shape (well circumscribed, round, or irregular). Are they mobile? Are they soft, firm, or hard?

NEUROLOGIC

This examination may be more difficult on an infant because patient cooperation is necessary. Simple observation and play are sufficient for most of this exam. Evaluate cerebral function based on observing developmental landmarks, specifically the patient's gross and fine motor capabilities, speech and language, and adaptive and personal-social behavior. Assess overall tone. Is the infant hypo- or hypertonic? Is the gait normal? Are there any signs of weakness or spasticity? Assess cerebellar function mainly by gait and overall coordination. Deep tendon reflexes should be symmetric and normoactive. In smaller infants, neonatal reflexes should not persist much beyond 2 months of age. Strength should be symmetric. Cranial nerves may be difficult to evaluate in an uncooperative infant, but note obvious findings such as poor or nonexistent eye contact, strabismus, and nystagmus. Is the face symmetric? Does the patient turn toward sound? Is his or her speech and language age-appropriate? Observe gag reflexes and tongue symmetry.

Children, Ages 2 to 12 Years

General Considerations

Children are more cooperative than infants during a physical examination and will answer questions readily. Older children will be more independent and may be more willing to undergo examination on the table without holding onto a parent. However, the examiner must use discretion. If a child is particularly frightened for any reason, it may be necessary to have the parent console him or her.

It is important for the examiner to engage the child to develop rapport. After arriving, ask the child what he or she likes to do and be prepared to discuss the subject. Although it becomes more difficult for an older physician to keep up with current-day music, sports, TV shows, and video games, it is necessary to do what it takes to maintain credibility. A "cool" examiner gets better information.

The examiner should have a firm grounding in child development in order to appreciate the various cognitive, linguistic, and thinking processes at given ages. Moreover, levels of advancement may be different for children of the same age. Thus tailor questions to individuals.

We will not emphasize congenital malformations or illnesses in the assessment of children because we discussed them during the infant examination.

The Examination

GESTALT

What is your first impression of the patient? Have you been able to engage him or her? What is the level of alertness and responsiveness? What is the patient's affect? Does the child appear toxic or in any distress? What is the state of nourishment and hydration? Assessment of pain is an integral part of an initial evaluation, and it is important to correlate the patient's or the parent's assessment of pain with how the patient appears. As with infants, use all your senses. Does the odor of bacterial infection emanate from the nose or throat? Does the patient smell of acetone?

VITAL SIGNS

Measure and record temperature, pulse, blood pressure, and weight at each visit. These vital signs should be reviewable as a sequence as well as a point in time. As with infants, the vital signs should be used for triage purposes, although it behooves the examiner to determine whether the vital sign measured correlates with the appearance of the patient. If a height or weight measurement shows a marked inconsistency with previous assessments, repeat it.

HEAD

As with infants, evaluate the size and shape of the head, although congenital malformations most likely have been addressed earlier. Are their signs of trauma?

EYES

Examine the eyes for visual acuity. A cooperative child will perform reliably on the standard Snellen eye chart. Do the eyes protrude normally from their sockets? As with infants, examine the pupils for size, shape, and reactivity. Is there full range of motion? Are the conjunctivae inflamed or with exudates? Evaluate the sclerae and corneas for clarity, bleeding, discoloration, and abnormal markings. Does light bother the child's eyes? Look carefully at the anterior chamber for blood, especially when evaluating for eye trauma. Also, fluorescein dye examination is an integral part of evaluation for eye trauma.

EARS

Children are more cooperative than infants and thus may report pain or discomfort with otoscopic examination. It behooves any examiner of a child to be well versed in the use of the pneumatic otoscope. Examine the ear canal for redness or exudates. Audiometry and tympanometry always must be available and used freely in a pediatric office or clinic. Since children often accumulate cerumen in their ear canals, it is important to remove all wax in order to perform a reliable evaluation. Examiners should be skilled in the use of a curette and irrigation. Are the ear canals clear, or are they red, or do they contain exudates? What is the color and shape of the eardrum? Is it bulging or retracted? Are the light reflexes normal? Does the drum appear retracted or dull? Is it mobile?

Important points about pneumatic otoscopy are as follows: Good tympanic membrane motion trumps morphologic findings when ruling out a middle ear effusion. A good seal is essential because an eardrum will not move if there is air leakage. Often a child or infant may be crying and, in so doing, will perform a Valsalva maneuver, thus increasing pressure in the middle ear and inhibiting mobility of the tympanic membrane. It is helpful to insufflate while the crying patient is drawing in his or her breath because this is the time when middle ear pressure will be at its lowest.

NOSE, THROAT, AND MOUTH

Look for nasal deformity, most likely associated with trauma in this age group. Is there discoloration of the nose? Looking in the nostrils, is there evidence of obstruction? Does it originate with the septum or the turbinates? What is the color (red, blue) and texture (hard, boggy) of the obstruction? Is there clear or purulent nasal discharge? Is it malodorous? As with infants, evaluate the palate and uvula for size and orientation. Are the tonsils enlarged or inflamed? If they are, is there concomitant bulging of the soft palate? Examine the teeth because dental caries are prevalent in this age group. Does tapping on a tooth elicit severe pain? How are the teeth aligned?

NECK

Are there any masses? Where are they located? Are they hard or soft? Are they mobile or tender? If there is pain or tenderness, is it located in the midline or laterally? Is the neck supple? Is there any pain on flex-ion or extension? Does the patient report any other symptoms with movement of the neck (e.g., pain, numbness, or tingling)? Does the patient hold his or her neck straight while sitting?

THORAX

Check for malformations. In the event of trauma, place your hands circumferentially around the thoracic cage and squeeze firmly but gently to elicit any pain or tenderness.

LUNGS

Use your skills in observation, palpation, and percussion and auscultation to determine the location of any densities in the chest and to evaluate heart size. Observe for respiratory rate as well as any difficulty or discomfort with breathing (retracting, splinting). Dullness and tympani of the chest will assess for air or fluid content as well. Auscultation will reveal whether there are any rales, rubs, wheezes, or rhonchi. Have the patient inhale and exhale as deeply as possible in order to assess for prolonged inspiration or expiration. Breath sounds traversing a wider airway surrounded by fluid may have a "tubular" quality. Egophony (the sound of a voice like a goat) is helpful in assessing the extent of a pleural effusion. All these findings will be discussed in further detail in Chapter 8.

HEART

Observe for chest movements associated with heartbeats in a thinner patient. Is the patient in any visible respiratory distress, coughing or wheezing? Is there any cyanosis? Is the patient active or listless? Feel the chest wall. Are there any palpable thrills? Where is the point of maximal intensity? Percussion is also helpful to delineate cardiac size. Use the stethoscope to assess heart sounds and murmurs. Are the heartbeats strong, or do they sound muffled? Are the sounds single or split? Does the interval between the splits vary? Where do you hear a murmur at its loudest? Where in the cardiac cycle does it occur, systole or diastole? Is it in early or late systole or diastole? How loud is the murmur? Describe the quality of the murmur. Is it coarse, low- or high-pitched, variable or consistent in intensity throughout? Are there any rubs or gallops? Refer to Chapter 9 for further detail.

ABDOMEN

Observe for overall size and shape. Is the abdomen flat or distended? Are there any abnormal skin markings, bruises, vessels, or striae? Evaluate for liver and spleen size. Keep in mind that in children a normal liver and spleen may be palpable 1 to 2 cm below the costal margins. Check for abdominal masses. Try to describe a mass. How big is it? Does it feel well encapsulated, or is it irregular? Does it cross the midline of the abdomen, or could it be bilateral? Look for tenderness or guarding. In which part of the abdomen is this most pronounced? Is there rebound tenderness? Percussion is helpful for delineating abdominal masses and evaluating liver and spleen size. It also may help to determine if the fingers are overlying solid tissue, air-filled tissue, or just the air space of a dilated stomach. Auscultation will determine if bowel sounds are normal, hyperactive, or hypoactive. Assess the quality of the bowel sounds for pitch and volume. Evaluate costovertebral angle tenderness to assess for renal disease.

MUSCULOSKELETAL

Check range of motion of the joints. Is there any redness, tenderness, heat, swelling, or stiffness? Is the muscle mass appropriate for age? Is the back straight? Is there lateral deviation (scoliosis) or anteroposterior deviation (kyphosis or lordosis)? Evaluate this by having the patient bend over and touch his or her toes.

GENITALIA

The examination is similar to that of an infant. Check for signs of puberty.

INTEGUMENT

The evaluation of skin, hair, and nails is similar for infants and children.

LYMPHATIC

The evaluation is also similar to that of infants.

NEUROLOGIC

Children will be more cooperative than infants, so more information is obtainable. Does the child appear to be neurodevelopmentally appropriate for age? Check for cerebral function by determining orientation to name, location, and time or administer a "mini-mental status exam" if appropriate. Evaluate cerebellar function by testing for overall coordination. Look for ataxia of both lower and upper extremities. At times, ataxia can be confused with weakness, so testing without gravitational forces is necessary. Check for finger-to-nose coordination, rapid alternating movements, and Romberg sign. Does the patient's speech sound normal, or is it scanning? Evaluate all extremities for strength, and record the results using a standard scale. Test deep tendon reflexes for both upper and lower extremities. Examine cranial nerves carefully with particular attention to the ocular fundi for vascularity and sharpness of the optic disc. This is particularly important while evaluating patients with head trauma. Check the optic cup for enlargement. Test other cranial nerves. Evaluate the oculomotor (III), trochlear (IV), and abducent (VI) nerves via range of ocular motion. The olfactory (I) nerve serves the sense of smell. The trigeminal (V) nerve is involved in facial sensation and strength of the jaw muscles. Test the facial (VII) nerve for facial motor function and taste of the anterior two-thirds of the tongue. The eighth cranial nerve, the auditory nerve, transmits sound to the brain for further interpretation. The glossopharyngeal (IX) nerve and the vagus (X) nerve serve palatal sensation and are involved in taste of the posterior third of the tongue, the gag reflex, and other autonomic functions serving heart rate and respiration. The spinal accessory (IX) nerve supplies motor function to the trapezius and sternocleidomastoid muscles, and the cranial (XII) nerve (hypoglossal) serves tongue movement. Please consult Chapter 12 for further detail.

Adolescents, Ages 12 to 21 Years

General Considerations

As is the case with taking a medical history in the adolescent patient, performing a physical exam requires sensitivity to varying stages of personal and social development, privacy, modesty, and socially charged topics. It is important to assure patients that you respect their privacy and modesty. The adolescent may be fully dressed or gowned sequentially, exposing and re-covering areas as necessary for examination.

It is generally a good idea to continue the flow of conversation during the exam to put the patient at ease. The physician simply may narrate what he or she is doing or talk about the latest music or TV shows. The examiner should be conscious of his or her own facial reactions and comments made during and regarding the exam because they can have a lasting impact on the patient's perception of himself or herself and his or her health.

During adolescence, the frequency of common childhood infections decline, and almost all congenital abnormalities have surfaced, whereas the frequency of psychological and social problems increases. The examiner should be alert to signs of depression and other psychiatric problems, substance abuse, self-inflicted injury, eating disorders, abuse and violence, and sexually transmitted diseases.

The Examination

GESTALT

Observe posture, mood, eye contact, dress, piercings, and tattoos, but take them with a grain of salt. There are many cultural aspects of Western society that result in the appearance of an adolescent being incongruent with whom they truly are. Antisocial dressing styles that on the surface may appear to be pathologic actually may represent fitting in with a peer group and being a well-adjusted adolescent. Body posture in the office that projects an image of disinterest in the visit really may represent a normal adolescent behavior of acting too busy to be there. On the other hand, body habitus, grooming, and scars from violence or self-inflicted wounds are significant.

SKIN

The examiner should become familiar with common dermatologic problems in adolescence, including varying degrees of acne, which typically is found on the face but also commonly is found on the chest, back, and arms. The examiner should inquire about the origin of scars found on exam. Look for the hyperpigmented, velvety-appearing acanthosis nigricans on the back of the neck and in the axillary region in overweight patients, which often bespeaks insulin resistance.

HEAD

Examine the head and scalp. Common findings include areas of alopecia, scaling of the scalp, infestation with lice and nits, and pre- and postauricular and suboccipital lymphadenopathy. Examine areas of alopecia closely to see if stubs of hair remain (traction alopecia and tinea capitis) or if it is completely devoid of hair (alopecia areata).

EYES

The eye exam, especially the funduscopic exam, is probably never easier than it is in an adolescent patient. The patient is old enough to be completely cooperative yet young enough that he or she usually does not have disorders of the cornea, lens, or iris that could make the exam difficult. For this reason, we recommend that young physicians regularly examine the fundus of their adolescent patients both for practice and to familiarize themselves with normal exam findings. The screening eye exam also should include visual inspection of the lids, palpebral and bulbar conjunctivae, sclerae, and corneas. Examine extraoccular movements for conjugate or disconjugate gaze. Examine pupils to ensure that they are equal and appropriate in size for the level of lighting and are round and reactive to both light and accommodation. Visual field examination to confrontation is not usually part of the screening exam, but it is performed if necessary. Assessing visual acuity using a Snellen chart or other device should be routine in all patients.

FUNDUSCOPIC EXAM TECHNIQUE

Examiners with long hair should pull it back to keep it away from the patient's face during the exam. Perform the funduscopic exam in a darkened room. Since the iris may take a few minutes to dilate fully, it is often worthwhile to darken the room and spend a few minutes clarifying history or obtaining more ophthalmologic history before beginning the exam. Bright light and a wide beam from the ophthalmoscope will cause papillary constriction and make the exam difficult. The examiner should dim the light and narrow the beam to the minimum necessary to see the fundus. The examiner should hold the ophthalmoscope in the right hand and use the right eye to examine the patient's right eye and the left hand to examine the left eye to avoid directly facing the patient at an uncomfortably close range. The examiner should begin the exam by finding the red reflex from 1 to 2 feet away from the patient. The free hand should be placed on the patient's forehead with the thumb applying gentle upward traction to the eyebrow. This will help the patient keep the lid open and will serve as reference point as the examiner moves for a closer exam. Hold the ophthalmoscope with the pad resting on the examiner's own eyebrow. Ideally, the examiner should keep the red reflex in view through the ophthalmoscope as he or she approaches the patient, getting as close as 1 inch from the patient's cornea. The thumb on the eyebrow prevents the examiner from bumping into the patient. Locate and examine the optic disc. Examine the remaining portions of the retina by following each of the major vessels from the disc to the periphery. Finally, examine the macula by asking the patient to look briefly at the light.

EARS

As with younger children, the examiner should note the presence or absence of cerumen or discharge that may be in the canal and swelling or erythema of the canal wall. Examine the tympanic membrane for bony landmarks, a normal cone-shaped light reflex inferiorly, and color and mobility. Patches of white scarring may occur in patients who have had recurrent middle ear infections. Estimate the percentage of the tympanic membrane that is scarred. Note the color and clarity of the effusion through a translucent tympanic membrane. Observe for mobility of the tympanic membrane with insufflation.

NOSE

Note the presence of nasal congestion and the color and presence of swelling of the nasal mucosa. Pale, boggy mucosa with clear rhinorrhea is consistent with allergies, whereas a purulent discharge and thin, erythematous mucosa are more likely to be an upper respiratory infection. Mucosal ulcerations often are consistant with cocaine abuse.

MOUTH AND THROAT

Dental caries becomes more prevalent in adolescents. The tonsils should be decreasing in size compared with younger children but may become very large with infectious mononucleosis or streptococcal pharyngitis. Note the presence of exudates on the tonsils. Examine the teeth for erosions of the enamel, which may be secondary to frequent vomiting.

NECK

Check for range of motion, lymphadenopathy, tracheal position, and thyromegaly. Lymphomas are at increased incidence at this age. Note the consistency of any nodes found in the neck.

CHEST AND LUNGS

Note normal resting breathing pattern, including the approximate ratio of inspiratory time to expiratory time. Note whether chest expansion is equal or asymmetric from splinting. Examine for tactile fremitus if there are other findings or a history suggestive of pneumothorax, but this is not part of a routine examination. Perform percussion in any patient who has respiratory symptoms or abnormal findings on inspection or auscultatory exam. Auscultate each area of the chest. Listen anteriorly, posteriorly, and between the posterior and anterior axillary lines bilaterally. When warranted, auscultate the apices using the bell of the stethoscope above the clavicles.

HEART

Ideally, perform this in a quiet room to hear all findings. The ventilation system heard in most rooms with the stethoscope on is louder than the diastolic murmur of mitral stenosis. The examiner should listen carefully to each sound until it can be determined whether it is normal or abnormal. Listen to S_1 for volume and splitting. Listen to S_2 for volume and splitting. Splitting of S_2 is normal in adolescents. It should vary with inspiration and should be wider in the later portions of the inspiratory phase. Paradoxic splitting in the late portion of expiratory phase and fixed splitting indicate pathology and warrant further evaluation. Each component of S_2 should be evaluated. The aortic component should be heard throughout the precordium, whereas the pulmonary component, because of lower pressures, should be heard only at the base. Splitting of S_2 heard at the apex then is abnormal because the pulmonary component should not be heard there and indicates pulmonary hypertension. Note the characteristics of any murmurs, including timing (systolic versus diastolic), quality (blowing, harsh, or musical), shape (diamond or holosystolic), location, grade, and radiation. Systolic murmurs can be subdivided based on timing within systole. Refer to the Chapter 9 for more detail.

BREASTS
Note the Tanner stage (FIGURES 13-2 through 13-4).

ABDOMEN
Is the abdomen scaphoid, flat, or protruberant? Bowel sounds in any area of the abdomen are audible in any quadrant. There is no need to listen for them in all quadrants; however, the physician may want to listen in more than one location for bruits such as at the renal arteries. Percuss to assess the size of the liver, spleen, bladder, and any other masses. In general, the spleen is located posteriorly and superiorly. As a result, it must be approximately three times normal size to be palpable. This will appear as any dullness in Traube's space (normally tympanitic over the gastric bubble) during deep inspiration when it is only twice normal size. Perform light palpation in all four quadrants and include assessment for rebound tenderness before proceeding to deep palpation. Deep palpation should be deep. Look for hydronephrosis and intraabdomenal and retroperitoneal masses. The examiner may palpate kidneys in an adolescent, although this is more difficult than in a small child.

GENITALS
Since adolescents of the same age may be in different stages of physical development and sexual experience, they also may have different levels of comfort with the genital exam. Always ensure privacy and modesty. The examiner should wear gloves for all portions of the genital exam (see FIGURES 13–2 through 13–4 for Tanner staging).

MALE PATIENTS
It is generally easier to perform an accurate genital exam on adolescent males with the patient standing. Note Tanner staging. Examine the genitals for evidence of sexually transmitted diseases, including urethral pain, irritation, or discharge; ulcerations or vesicles of the penile shaft, glans, or meatus; and veruccae and infestation of the pubic hair with lice. Palapte the testes for Tanner staging and evidence of atrophy or masses and the epididymis for evidence of swelling and tenderness. Place the finger into the scrotum and move upward toward the inguinal canal while the patient coughs or performs a Valsalva maneuver to check for abdominal wall weaknesses or hernias.

FEMALE PATIENT
Examination of the adolescent female will be covered in detail in Chapter 21.

BACK
Scoliosis that was mild in childhood may increase during adolescence. Ideally, this should be identified in late childhood or early adolescence because there is a narrow window of time to intervene. Perform the forward bending test with or without a scoliometer.

EXTREMITIES

Look for staining from nicotine, cutting, and injection tracks. Look for markings on the proximal phalanx of the first two digits, suggesting self-induced vomiting.

NEUROLOGIC

A systematic screening exam is easy and quick in adolescents. Check for mental status, cranial nerve function, motor tone and strength, sensation, cerebellar function, Romberg test, and deep tendon reflexes as described in Chapter 12.

3 Vital Signs

Vinay N. Reddy

The first quantitative findings obtained on physical examination are the patient's vital signs (i.e., temperature, heart rate or "pulse," respiratory rate, and arterial blood pressure) and basic anthropometric measurements (i.e., weight, height, and head circumference). These are important as stand-alone measurements, but trends in these values, over the short or long term, are also important diagnostic signs. To detect and interpret trends, one must obtain and record vital signs and anthropometric measurements consistently.

Consistency: Accuracy, Precision, and Repeatability*

To be consistent, a particular measurement must be accurate, must be precise, and must be repeatable. These terms are not synonymous. *Accuracy* is a measure of how close a measurement system comes to yielding a true value of the *measurand* (what we are measuring). The accuracy of a measurement system, whether an instrument, an examiner, or a combination of an instrument and an examiner, compares a measured value with a known quantity for that measurement (*gold standard*). A high-accuracy instrument has a low measurement error, or difference between the measured and true values. Often accuracy is expressed as a percentage: the absolute measurement error (the absolute value of the difference between the true and measured values of the measurand) as a percentage of a given true value or of the "full scale," or maximum, value that the instrument can measure. Keep in mind that the accuracy can vary with the true value of the measurand or with other factors.

Precision refers to the smallest difference between two quantities that the instrument (and examiner) can detect. Taking a scale as an example, a low-precision instrument may be able to show that there is a 1-g difference in weight between two objects, whereas a higher-precision instrument may be able to show a 1.01-g difference between the same two

---

*Portions of this section are taken from Chapter 4, "Transducers," in Vinay N. Reddy, *Principles of Medical Instrumentation*. St. Louis: St. Louis University School of Medicine, copyright 1984, Vinay N. Reddy, and are used by permission of the author.

objects. High precision is necessary for high accuracy because a low measurement error is achievable only if small differences in value are detectible. However, a measurement can be extremely precise and still highly inaccurate, such as the examination room scale that tells you that your teenage patient weighs 5.83484 kg just after your examination table collapsed under him.

Numeric values for one physiologic measurement may vary depending on the measurement technique. Heisenberg's Uncertainly Principle states that it is impossible to make several measurements on a system without variation of the process itself. Fortunately, the effect of the measurement process is not great enough to matter in most clinical situations *as long as each measurement uses as close to the same process as possible*. This is the principle of *repeatability*: measuring a particular quantity more than once should yield the same value or as close to the same value as the accuracy and precision of the measurement system allow. Repeatability often depends on the technique used in measurement and therefore on the person making the measurement. As an example, the measurement of a child's head circumference may vary with technique but can be more consistent if the same examiner were to have made all measurements.

Vital Signs

The classic vital signs are temperature, pulse (heart rate), respiratory rate, and peripheral blood pressure. The term *vital* comes from the Latin *vitae* ("life"); the vital signs are a rough indicator of life. A nonliving person has a heart rate, respiratory rate, and systolic and diastolic blood pressures of zero and a temperature at or steadily approaching that of the environment. Until relatively recently, a heart rate of zero was a major criterion for the determination of death.

Temperature

Internal, or core, temperature is closely regulated in all warm-blooded species, including humans. Normal temperature varies with time of day and level of consciousness. A person's temperature falls somewhat when he or she is asleep. Peripheral temperature varies to a greater degree than does core temperature, and physiologic mechanisms conserve heat in cold environments and disperse heat in warm environments. The hypothalamus mainly exerts temperature control as a "thermostat." Excess heat dissipates primarily by conduction, radiation, and convection from the body surface as a result of sweating and evaporation of sweat, warming and humidification of cool inhaled air and exhalation of warmed air, and excretion of urine and stool that are at or near core temperature at the time of excretion. Surface losses and sweat depend on peripheral tissue perfusion. Reduced peripheral circulation conserves heat, whereas increased peripheral circulation, along with increased respiratory rate and tidal volume, promotes heat loss. A person who cannot sweat, whether from dehydration, heat stroke, or genetic abnormalities (e.g., hypohidrotic ectodermal dysplasia, a congenital absence of sweat glands), will not lose excess heat as well as a normal person and is at risk for severe hyperthermia and its sequelae. Both surface losses and sweating are functions of body surface area, as is heat absorption from the environment, whereas internal heat production is more a function of body volume and weight. A small person such as an infant has more body surface area relative to weight than an adult or larger child and therefore has more difficulty maintaining constant core temperature; infants thus have wider normal temperature ranges than do older children and adults, and premature infants are at particular risk for heat loss.

Thus it is most useful to measure a patient's core temperature with a thermometer or temperature probe placed in the rectum, esophagus, or stomach. The latter two sites are not practical for routine temperature measurements, and rectal temperature measurement carries a risk of trauma, especially in infants and in very active small children. Oral temperature measurement with the probe placed under the tongue is common in adults and older children but requires patient cooperation. Increased respiration or recent Popsicle or coffee intake may vary the result.

Commonly, a probe placed deeply into the axillary fossa as possible while holding the upper arm tightly against the upper chest to prevent factitious low temperature from exposure of the probe to ambient air measures axillary temperature. Axillary temperatures are used widely in pediatrics but have limitations. One important problem is that axillary and core temperatures are not consistently related and depend on age, size, and peripheral perfusion (the latter because the axilla and shoulder are not quite part of the body core). The common practice of adding 1 to the axillary temperature (or subtracting 1 from the rectal temperature) to obtain the oral temperature is inaccurate and can lead to inappropriate diagnoses or procedures. When reporting temperatures, caregivers, patients, and parents should relate the actual number displayed on the thermometer and the anatomic location used for measurement.

The type of thermometer is also important. Ideally, the thermometer probe should be small, both for patient comfort and to allow rapid measurement. Temperature measurement with a mercury-filled glass thermometer can take as long as 3 to 4 minutes because the mercury needs to warm to the patient's temperature. However, mercury thermometers are no longer in use owing to environmental and toxicologic concerns. Alcohol-filled glass thermometers respond somewhat faster than mercury thermometers. Most professional and home patient thermometers are now electronic, using an electric sensor to measure temperature, and some can yield a reading in a few seconds.

Ear thermometers are also popular in pediatrics. These use an infrared sensor to measure the temperature of the tympanic membrane, which should represent core temperature even better than does rectal temperature. Unfortunately, this depends on the sensor having an unrestricted "line of sight" to the eardrum. Obtaining an accurate tympanic temperature can be difficult in small infants, who tend to have narrow and somewhat convoluted ear canals, or in patients with large accumulations of cerumen.

S KEY SIGN
▼ **Fever**   The definition of fever is a core temperature of 38.0°C (100.4°F) or higher. There is a tendency among laypeople to call any temperature above 37.0°C (98.6°F) a fever. This often leads to inappropriate treatment with antipyretics and can result in inappropriate diagnostic procedures.

Fever can result from any insult that affects the hypothalamic "thermostat." The most common causes of fever in pediatrics are infections; these result from direct effects of the infectious agent or from pyrogens released by the agent either in its normal metabolism (e.g., bacterial toxins) or in its destruction (e.g., products of bacteriolysis). Such exogenous pyrogens induce production of endogenous pyrogens such as interleukin-1 (IL-1), IL-6, interferon-γ (IFN-γ), and tumor necrosis factor (TNF) and may be the first or only physical sign of an occult abscess. Endogenous pyrogens also can be present as a result of autoimmune processes (such as systemic lupus erythematosis or juvenile rheumatoid arthritis), immune reactions to other exogenous agents, or malignancies (such as leukemia or lymphoma).

Fever in an infant younger than 60 days is of particular concern because elevated temperature may be the only early sign of sepsis or meningitis. (These patients are not able to report headaches or neck pain, and physical signs of meningitis such as nuchal rigidity and Brudzinski and Kernig signs are unreliable in this age group.)

In older children in whom physical signs can be more reliable, the workup can fit more closely to the patient's findings. If fever is the only presenting sign, with no abnormal physical findings, frequent causes include urinary tract infection (3 to 6 percent of febrile children younger than age 2 years without other signs; higher in girls and in uncircumcised boys under 1 year of age) and occult bacteremia (about 3 percent in children younger than age 3 years with a temperature of 39°C or higher).

S KEY SIGN
▼ **Hyperthermia**   Hyperthermia is elevated temperature resulting from unregulated overproduction of heat or impaired heat-shedding mechanisms as opposed to fever, where a pathophysiologic process changes the regulatory set point. Severe fever does not necessarily lead to hyperthermia unless there is disruption of the physiologic compensatory mechanisms. The most common causes of hyperthermia are environmental, behavioral, and toxin-mediated.

Environmental hypothermia is elevated ambient temperature with impaired heat shedding. The latter may be due to dehydration, leading to decreased sweat production, or to decreased sweat evaporation because of high ambient humidity or improper clothing. Often all these factors are at work. An unfortunately common example is heat stroke in a football player practicing or playing in full uniform in hot, humid weather.

The problem becomes worse in persons with disorders that impair sweating, such as hypohidrotic ectodermal dysplasia, who may develop hyperthermia after even moderate exercise. Even if the sweat glands are intact, dysfunction of the neurologic pathways that control sweating (including anticholinergic agents and sympathectomy) may impair heat loss and result in hyperthermia.

Behavioral hypothermia is mainly a matter of poor judgment on the part of patients and caregivers, as in the example of the football player mentioned earlier. This may manifest as improper clothing for the environment or as unavailability of or failure to drink extra fluids such as water.

S KEY SYNDROME

▼ **Malignant Hyperthermia** *Malignant hyperthermia* is an inherited disorder of muscular sarcoplasmic reticulum in which sustained muscle contraction and heat production occur after administration of succinylcholine or certain inhalation anesthetic agents. In addition to hyperthermia, patients develop rigidity, rhabdomyolysis, metabolic acidosis, and hemodynamic instability.

S KEY SYNDROME

▼ **Heat Cramps** *Heat cramps* are forceful, painful muscle contractions, usually in large muscle groups such as the posterior lower leg muscles (gastrocnemius and hamstrings). These commonly occur after exercise and appear to be due to electrolyte imbalance because of replacement of fluid losses from sweat with relatively hypotonic fluids such as water.

S KEY SYNDROME

▼ **Heat Exhaustion** *Heat exhaustion* is fatigue, malaise, headache, dizziness, hypotension, tachycardia, nausea, and vomiting, usually resulting from intravascular volume depletion owing to sweat losses. Body temperature may be normal or mildly elevated, but sweating is profuse; the patient's mentation is normal.

S KEY SYNDROME

▼ **Heat Stroke** *Heat stroke* is elevated temperature (sometimes >40.0°C) along with mental status changes ranging from confusion to coma. Classically, cessation of sweating occurs in heat stroke, resulting in the classic sign of hot, dry skin, but some patients have continued to sweat profusely even with elevated temperature and mental status changes. Heat stroke may be a result of exertion, as in athletes, but also may be seen without exertion, as in infants who remain too long in a parked car on a hot, sunny day. Inadequate fluid intake contributes to heat stroke, which develops more rapidly along with exertion and its associated increase in fluid losses.

S KEY SIGN

▼ **Hypothermia** The definition of *hypothermia* is not as precise as that of fever, but a temperature of less than 35.5°C (96.0°F), or less than 36.0°C (96.8°F) in an infant, should raise most pediatricians' eyebrows. Hypothermia can be the result of a problem with the hypothalamic thermostat, just as fever. Practically, a child, especially an infant, who is hypothermic in a warm environment should have an evaluation for infections, particularly bacterial or viral sepsis. Other noninfectious causes of hypothermia include hypothyroidism, brain neoplasms, strokes, hypoglycemia, and chronic malnutrition. However, since heat loss is much greater in small children owing to their high surface-area-to-weight ratio, cold environments and improper protection from the elements are more common causes of hypothermia. Hypothermia is protective against tissue ischemia, and cold-water drowning with immersion hypothermia is often more survivable than warm-water drowning.

Heart Rate and Rhythm

Often an examiner will assess heart rate and rhythm with a stethoscope. However, one can obtain a great deal of information with no equipment other than one's fingers by assessing a patient's peripheral pulses.

The palpable arterial pulse results from the quick rise in arterial pressure during left ventricular contraction. Mechanically, the arterial tree is a capacitance that tends to delay and dampen the pressure wave. The degree of delay and dampening, and thus the volume and contour of the palpated pressure wave, depends on the size and flexibility of the arterial segments through which the wave flows. The regularity of the pulse is a function of the heart's pacemaker and conduction mechanisms.

The most accessible peripheral pulses are over the common carotid, brachial, radial, femoral, dorsalis pedis, and posterior tibial arteries. In addition, pulses are palpable in the popliteal fossae, although the popliteal arteries usually are not superficial enough to appreciate pulse contours and volumes. Traditionally, the pulse is palpated over one of the radial arteries, especially in older children and adults. However, palpating both radial (or brachial) arteries and both femoral (or dorsalis pedis or posterior tibial) arteries and comparing pulse volume, contour, and arrival time may lead to a preliminary diagnosis of coarctation of the aorta. Measuring blood pressure in all four limbs will confirm or deny this.

▼ KEY FINDING
◤ Sinus Arrhythmia *Sinus arrhythmia* is a change in the heart rate with respiration, with increased rate during inspiration and decreased rate during expiration. *This is normal in children* and becomes less prominent with advancing age, although many adults exhibit sinus arrhythmia.

▼ KEY FINDING
◤ Tachycardia *Tachycardia* is a heart rate above the normal range for age. This may be due to excitement or fear—simply induced in young children merely by mentioning vaccinations—and is a normal response to exercise or to pain. However, tachycardia also may occur with fever,

anemia, hyperthyroidism, drug toxicity (e.g., anticholinergics such as atropine and diphenhydramine, adrenergics such as over-the-counter decongestants, psychostimulants such as methylphenidate and other amphetamines, and cocaine), and many acute and chronic illnesses. Tachycardia with normal blood pressure but with peripheral hypoperfusion may represent early shock in children, whose cardiovascular systems are much more capable of maintaining blood pressure in the face of intravascular hypovolemia than those of adults. Hypotension in the pediatric patient with shock is a late and ominous sign.

▼ KEY FINDING

◥ Bradycardia *Bradycardia* is a heart rate below the normal range for age. Some patients, especially well-trained athletes, may have rates lower than the norms owing to conditioning. Pathologic causes of bradycardia include cardiac conduction defects, drug toxicity (including opiates, benzodiazepines, and other sedatives), and severe malnutrition.

▼ KEY FINDING

◥ Heart Rate Lability *Heart rate lability* is changes in the heart rate while the patient is at rest and not explained by other stressors. Causes include drug toxicity and severe malnutrition.

▼ KEY FINDING

◥ Irregular Rhythms *Irregular rhythms* are many and varied, caused by congenital heart disease, innate problems with the conduction system, and metabolic disorders such as hyper/hypokalemia and hyperthyroidism. Consult Chapter 9 for more detail.

Respiratory Rate

Measure the respiratory rate by counting the number of respirations in *1 full minute*. This may not be strictly necessary in older children and adolescents with regular breathing. However, infants are *periodic breathers*. They may breathe rapidly for a few seconds and then pause for several seconds before breathing again. The periodic breathing is normal as long as the overall rate (over 1 minute) is not excessive.

▼ KEY FINDING

◥ Apnea The definition of *apnea* is cessation of breathing for more than 20 seconds and/or associated bradycardia, cyanosis, or pallor. Cyanosis is more marked with longer periods of apnea. The apnea may be *central* (caused by an abnormality in the neural control mechanism) or *obstructive* (a mechanical or anatomic blockage of the respiratory tract). Obstructive causes include aspiration following gastroesophageal reflux and anatomic abnormalities such as a tracheoesophageal fistula, bilateral choanal atresia, or the Pierre Robin syndrome in a newborn. Tonsil hypertrophy may result in apnea during sleep in older children, especially the obese. Central apnea may be due to sepsis, metabolic disorders (especially acid-base disorders), drug toxicity (including opiates and benzodiazepines), or congenital defects of respiratory control, including central pontine hypoventilation (Ondine's curse).

▼ KEY FINDING
Tachypnea *Tachypnea* is a respiratory rate above normal range for age (60 respirations per minute in infants, falling to 30 to 40 respirations per minute by age 1 year and to 14 to 20 respirations per minute by adulthood), usually in response to increased oxygen demand or increased carbon dioxide production. Tachypnea is a normal response to exercise; it also may result from fever, pain, and fear. Tachypnea also may occur with sepsis or pneumonia (especially in infants), aspiration, anemia, hyperthyroidism, pneumothorax, pulmonary embolism, or cardiac failure.

▼ **S** KEY SYNDROME
Transient Tachypnea of the Newborn *Transient tachypnea of the newborn* (TTNB) is a period of tachypnea in the first few hours after birth, apparently related to retained amniotic fluid in the lungs, which resolves as postnatal lung expansion continues and the retained fluid is absorbed into the bloodstream. Chest roentgenography may help differentiate TTNB from pneumonia in some cases, but tachypnea with hypoxia in a newborn infant generally is treated as pneumonia until blood cultures have been negative for several days.

▼ KEY FINDING
Bradypnea *Bradypnea* is a respiratory rate below normal range for age. This may be nonpathologic if Pa_{O2} and Pa_{CO2} are normal (a proxy for Pa_{O2} measurement is pulse oximetry, but direct measurement of Pa_{O2} and Pa_{CO2} requires blood gas testing). Hypercapnia (Pa_{CO2} >45 mm Hg) or hypoxia may be a consequence of central nervous system (CNS)–depressant agents (e.g., opiates, benzodiazepines, or alcohol), uremia, or CNS abnormalities, including hydrocephalus and tumors.

Peripheral Blood Pressure

Our ultimate physiologic interest is in central blood pressure and the perfusion pressure in the end organs. However, measuring central arterial blood pressure is impractical even in an operating room or intensive care unit, and it is certainly not feasible in other settings—thus the measurement of peripheral blood pressure in most clinical encounters. One can obtain a rough idea of peripheral arterial pressure by palpating a major artery and assessing the volume and contour of the pulse, as described earlier, but quantifying the pressure is necessary for full interpretation and for monitoring trends.

The most common method of measuring peripheral arterial pressure is sphygmomanometry, or the *Riva-Rocci method*. The examiner places a

I	"A loud clear-cut snapping tone"	$P_{cuff} = P_{systolic}$
II	"A succession of murmurs"	$P_{diastolic} \ll P_{cuff} < P_{systolic}$
III	"The disappearance of the murmurs and the appearance of a tone resembling to a degree the first phase but less well marked"	$P_{diastolic} < P_{cuff} \ll P_{systolic}$
IV	"Muffling" of taps	$P_{diastolic} \leq P_{cuff}$
V	Silence	$P_{diastolic} < P_{cuff}$
II and III may be separated by a period of silence, or auscultatory gap		

FIGURE 3–1 The Korotkoff Sounds. (*Descriptions of the Korotkoff sounds are taken from Goodman, EH and Howell, AA. Further clinical studies in the auscultatory method of determining blood pressure,* Am J Med Sci (1911) 142:334–352, *as quoted by Geddes, LA, In:* The Direct and Indirect Measurement of Blood Pressure, *Chicago: Year Book Medical Publishers, 1970.*)

cuff containing an inflatable bladder around an arm or leg proximal to an accessible artery and connected to a pressure gauge and a source of air pressure, usually a rubber bulb with a pressure-relief valve. While palpating the pulse in the artery distal to the cuff, he or she inflates the cuff, thus increasing pressure around the extremity. When the pulse is no longer palpable, the examiner releases cuff pressure while listening over the artery with the stethoscope bell. As cuff pressure decreases, a sequence of varying sounds (the Korotkoff sounds) become audible (FIGURE 3–1).

The American Heart Association recommends diastolic pressure as the cuff pressure at which Korotkoff sound V (silence) occurs. However, there are cases in which silence never occurs even at a cuff pressure of zero. In such instances, sound IV (muffling) should be the diastolic pressure because a diastolic pressure of zero is not actually possible. The cuff pressure at sound IV (muffling) is often arbitrarily the diastolic pressure regardless of when silence occurs. Many examiners record the pressure at sounds I (for systolic pressure), IV, and V in their notes (e.g., 105/70/65).

Oscillotonometry and Automatic Blood Pressure Measurement

It is possible for a computer to "listen" to the Korotkoff sounds and differentiate between them, thus enabling automatic blood pressure measurement. However, the most widely used method of automatic pressure measurement involves a different phenomenon. When the cuff is inflated to a pressure well above systolic pressure and then slowly deflated, pressure applied to the cuff by the artery will cause small oscillations in the cuff pressure. These oscillations appear when P_{cuff} is roughly at $P_{systolic}$, reach maximum amplitude when $P_{cuff} = P_{mean\ arterial}$, and disappear when P_{cuff} is roughly at $P_{diastolic}$. Most automatic non-invasive blood pressure measuring instruments use this method. *Note that oscillotonometric $P_{systolic}$ and $P_{diastolic}$ are not necessarily the same as those of auscultation.* However, the oscillometric measurement of mean arterial pressure correlates well with the invasive direct measurements that are the gold standard for blood pressure measurement, and oscillotonometry is less examiner-dependent than the Riva-Rocci method.

Important Points

1. It is tempting to listen while applying pressure and taking the cuff pressure at which sounds disappear as the systolic pressure. Unfortunately, the auscultatory gap—the period of silence that sometimes *but not always* occurs between sounds II and III—may result in underestimating systolic pressure or overestimating diastolic pressure. It is safer to palpate the distal (radial or foot) pulse, inflate the cuff to a pressure about 30 mm Hg above that needed to abolish the distal pulse, and *then* listen for Korotkoff sounds.

2. The auscultatory gap is often present in an obese patient's arm and is more likely to be noticeable if venous pooling occurs distal to the cuff (e.g., if the cuff tightens slowly) or if there is second blood pressure measurement immediately after the first measurement. This is often avoidable by having the patient's arm elevated while pressurizing the cuff and by pressurizing rapidly to a pressure above $P_{systolic}$.

3. The actual pressure applied to the artery depends not only on cuff pressure but also on cuff bladder size and placement and on the size of the limb. A narrow cuff will require higher pressure than a larger cuff would to apply the same amount of pressure to the underlying artery. Thus, measuring blood pressure with a cuff that is too narrow will produce an apparent blood pressure higher than the true pressure. Conversely, a cuff that is too large will yield a blood pressure measurement that is lower than the true pressure. The bladder within the cuff should be at least 20 percent wider than the diameter of the limb (whether arm or leg) and should be at least half as long as the circumference of the limb. Apply the cuff snugly to the limb so that the midpoint of the bladder is over the artery proximal to the listening point. If the cuff is loose, the bladder will "puff up" before pressing on the artery, and the "puffed up" bladder will compress the artery over a shorter length than the flat bladder, producing the same effect as a cuff that is too narrow.

4. Owing to hydrostatic effects, the measured blood pressure also varies with the height of the cuff relative to the heart. The measured pressure will be approximately that at the aortic arch if the cuff is at the level of the arch but higher if the cuff is below the arch and lower if the cuff is above the arch; the pressure difference can be predicted by measuring the height difference, but it is much easier to eliminate the difference by holding the arm during measurement so that the cuff is at the same level as the heart.

KEY FINDING
◤ Hypertension Refer to Chapter 14.

KEY FINDING
◤ Hypotension Although some patients, usually trained athletes, have relatively low blood pressure, *hypotension* accompanied by tachycardia and hypoperfusion is pathologic. Causes of hypotension include hypovolemia owing to inadequate fluid intake; increased insensible loss owing to fever, severe vomiting, blood loss, capillary leakage (from anaphylaxis or sepsis), polyuria (from diabetes mellitus, diabetes insipidus, or diuretic use or misuse), excessive and uncompensated sweating (heat exhaustion or heat stroke), and adrenal insufficiency (including abrupt withdrawal of chronic corticosteroid therapy); impaired vascular tone owing to sepsis, drugs (including vasodilators and tricyclic antidepressants), and acute spinal cord injury; and decreased cardiac output.

S KEY SYNDROME
◤ Shock Unlike adults, who become hypotensive early in the course of shock, children are able to preserve their blood pressure until the late stages of *shock*, partly through peripheral vasoconstriction but primarily by increasing their cardiac output through tachycardia. Therefore, tachycardia with normal blood pressure is frequently the presentation of shock. Hypovolemia and hypovolemic shock are usually identifiable in the early stages by tachycardia, but septic shock also can present initially as tachycardia and can, if diagnosed soon enough, be treated with volume resuscitation (in addition to antibiotics).

S KEY SIGN
◤ Orthostatic Changes in Blood Pressure and Heart Rate Since the cardiovascular system must maintain a relatively constant cerebral perfusion pressure, changes in body position and posture must engender compensatory changes in central arterial pressure and in the distribution of blood flow to different parts of the body. Central arterial blood pressure decreases immediately on sitting up or standing up, but heart rate increases almost immediately in response to the pressure drop. As vascular tone changes throughout the body to readjust flow distribution, the heart rate decreases. Ultimately, the heart rate and central arterial pressure return nearly to their levels prior to the position change. Persistent *orthostatic tachycardia* occurs when the vasculature fails to redistribute blood flow, and the heart rate must remain high to maintain cerebral perfusion pressure. In *orthostatic hypotension,* the central pressure does not rise sufficiently to maintain adequate cerebral perfusion; this may occur without symptoms, but lightheadedness and even syncope may follow if orthostatic hypotension is sufficiently severe. Orthostatic hypotension may occur without tachycardia if the heart cannot beat faster owing to pacemaker or conduction defects or to medications with negative chronotropic effects.

Since heart rate and central arterial pressure will vary immediately after changes in position, measurements taken right on position change are almost certain to be abnormal. It is preferable to wait after each position change before the next measurement, as in the following procedure:

1. Have the patient lie supine for at least 5 minutes.
2. Measure heart rate and blood pressure with the patient still supine.
3. Have the patient sit up.
4. *Wait 2 minutes.*
5. Hold the patient's arm so that the cuff is at the level of the heart, and measure the sitting heart rate and blood pressure.
6. Have the patient stand upright.
7. *Wait 2 minutes.*
8. Hold the patient's arm so that the cuff is at the level of the heart, and measure the standing heart rate and blood pressure.

Orthostatic tachycardia and hypotension may occur in a patient who has been at bed rest for a prolonged time. Thus it is important to have the patient sit up as frequently as possible while in bed. Other causes of orthostatic tachycardia and hypotension include hypovolemia, autonomic dysfunction, and chronic malnutrition.

Anthropometrics

Weight and height are a function of genetic factors and of the patient's environment and nutrition, beginning with gestation. Head circumference is a convenient proxy for the measurement of brain volume and also depends on genetic factors, environment, and nutrition. Measure weight and height at every well-child examination and head circumference at every well-child visit until age 2 or until the child's anterior fontanelle has closed. Plot these measurements on standard growth charts published by the National Center for Health Statistics (NCHS). Use special charts instead of the general-population charts for certain populations, such as children with trisomy 21.

Weight

Always use a calibrated scale, either balance-beam or electronic. For consistency between measurements, use the same scale at each visit. Ideally, weigh the patient wearing only a diaper (if in infancy) or an exam gown and underwear; in any event without heavy clothing or shoes. The most consistent weight is a *basal weight* obtained in the morning on awakening, after voiding and stooling and before eating or drinking, but this is only practical for inpatients. Voiding before weighing may be desirable if weight manipulation is in question.

Height

Height in children who can stand is the distance from the floor to the level of the highest point of the scalp. The patient should stand barefoot and erect, with his or her scapulae, buttocks, and heels touching the wall but not the occiput. Compress or separate thick hair so that it is not included in height. Wall-mounted stadiometers help provide consistency and repeatability between measurements.

Measuring a baby's length is more difficult, especially in the newborn period when muscle tone is increased. Obtaining the most consistent measurements is best using a board with a stationary head rest and a sliding foot plate. Place the baby on the board with his or her scalp touching the head rest, and extend the legs gently but firmly as far as possible; then place the foot plate against the soles and read the length from the scale.

Head Circumference

Measure the head circumference with a tape placed around the head and positioned so that it encircles the maximum possible diameter while touching the glabella. In newborns with considerable head molding after vaginal delivery, the tape may have to pass over the tip of the "cone." A common error in newborns is to measure the circumference from glabella to inion. When this measurement is plotted on a growth chart, the child will appear to be relatively microcephalic, but a correct measurement encompassing the "cone" will be more consistent. If possible, the same examiner should measure the head circumference at every examination, including the nursery assessment.

S **KEY SYNDROME**

Failure to Thrive *Failure to thrive* is weight loss or failure to gain weight without obvious cause. Beside frank weight loss, the working definitions include

- Weight less than the 3rd percentile for age (all percentiles are based on the standard National Center for Health Statistics growth chart)
- Weight less than the 5th percentile for height
- Weight less than or equal to 80 percent of "ideal" weight for height
- Triceps skinfold thickness of 5 mm or less
- Growth rate less than 20 g/day from birth to age 3 months or less than 15 g/day from ages 3 to 6 months
- Weight falling through two or more "major percentile" (e.g., 5th, 10th, 25th, 50th, 75th, 90th, and 95th) curves
- Falling off a previously established growth curve

Although systemic disease may prove to be the underlying issue, most cases of failure to thrive turn out to be psychosocial in nature. The most common cause of failure to gain weight is inadequate nutritional intake owing to developmental or psychiatric problems (e.g., autism, mental retardation, or schizophrenia), emotional deprivation, or failure to supply food to the child as active abuse or owing to neglect or economic problems. Organic causes are multisystemic and appear in various chapters in this book.

4 Development of a Differential Diagnosis from the History and Physical Examination

Arthur N. Feinberg and Vinay N. Reddy

Making correct medical diagnoses is a scientific endeavor. Humankind has employed scientific reasoning since ancient times, although it came more to fruition during the Renaissance. Over long years, technology has changed, but this only involves the tools we use. Sadly, we often resort to high-technology "tests" before we perform a complete history and physical examination. Studies have demonstrated that state-of-the-art magnetic resonance imaging may yield diagnoses not consistent with those ultimately found at autopsy. Good clinical evaluation is still essential to developing working hypotheses, which then get "tested." Always remember: Tests test hypotheses, not patients. Good working hypotheses serve two purposes: to guide us to which tests to employ and to guide us in their interpretation.

The basic framework for scientific reasoning has stood the test of time and has not changed. We make observations, make hypotheses, gather data, and analyze them to test (validate or refute) them. Quoting Bertrand Russell (1872–1970): ". . . the framing of hypotheses is the most difficult part of scientific work and the part where great ability is indispensable. So far, no method has been found which would make it possible to invent hypotheses by rule. Usually some hypothesis is a necessary preliminary to the collection of facts, since the selection of facts demands some way of determining relevance. Without something of this kind, the multiplicity of facts is baffling."

Hippocrates (460–377 B.C.) stated: "There are in fact two things, science and opinion; the former begets knowledge, the latter ignorance." In other words, there was, and still is, an ongoing "tug of war" between fact and opinion. Sir William Osler (1849–1919) epitomizes scientific reasoning in his statement: "To carefully observe the phenomena of life in all its phases, normal and perverted, to make perfect that most difficult of all arts, the art of observation, to call to aid the science of experimentation, to cultivate the reasoning faculty, so as to be able to know the true from the false—these are our methods." In order to make the best diagnostic and therapeutic decisions, all data gathered must be correct and timely. Every clinician thinks daily: "What do I want to know, and when do I want to know it?"

Human minds are capable of thinking on one end of the spectrum, scientifically, based solely on cold facts, or thinking, on the other end of the spectrum, religiously, based solely on faith. Historically, medical reasoning has developed along scientific lines. However, we all know that medicine is not a perfect science, and although we strive to gather the most appropriate data and to interpret them correctly, physicians and patients are complex entities whose experiences have profound effects on gathering and interpreting data. Hippocrates knew this when he stated, "It is more important to know what sort of person has a disease than to know what sort of disease a person has." Thus clinicians, although doing their best to apply the scientific method, still find themselves embedded in that "tug of war" between fact and opinion. We must recognize, humbly, that we can gather imperfect data and that we have to make judgments every day. In the section below labeled "The Diagnostic Framework" we apply the scientific method with allowance for uncertainty and judgment, illustrated in its final steps.

The Diagnostic Framework

The human mind always seeks information, sorts it, eliminates what appears to be irrelevant, correlates the data, and then puts together the remainder into a unifying hypothesis. It often repeats this sequence, not necessarily consciously. Thus the time-tested diagnostic framework has evolved out of the scientific method (adapted from De Gowin):

Step 1: Take a history. Elicit symptoms.

Step 2: Develop hypotheses. Generate a mental list of pathophysiologic processes and diseases that might produce these symptoms. Then use processes of sorting, eliminating, and correlating to narrow it down.

Step 3: Perform a physical examination. Look for signs of the physiologic processes and diseases suggested by the history, determine what corroborates it, eliminate further what is irrelevant, and perhaps identify new problems to add to the list.

Step 4: Generate a differential diagnosis. List the most probable hypotheses in the order of their possibility.

Step 5: Test the hypotheses. Select laboratory tests, imaging studies, procedures, and consultations with appropriate likelihood ratios to evaluate your hypotheses. Do this mindful of risk, cost, benefit, and logistics.

Step 6: Modify your differential diagnosis. Use the results of the tests to evaluate your hypotheses, perhaps eliminating some and adding others and adjusting the probabilities.

Step 7: Repeat steps 1 to 6. Reiterate your process until you have reached a diagnosis or have decided that a definite diagnosis is neither likely nor necessary.

Step 8: Make the diagnosis or diagnoses. When the tests of your hypothesis are of sufficient certainty that they meet your stopping rule, you have reached a diagnosis.

Step 9: If uncertain, consider a provisional diagnosis or watchful waiting. Decide whether more investigation (return to step 1), consultation, treatment, or watchful observation is the best course based on the severity of the illness, the process, and comorbidities. If the diagnosis remains obscure, retain a problem list of the unexplained symptoms and signs, as well as the laboratory and imaging findings; assess the urgency for further evaluation; and schedule regular follow-up visits.

Medical Reasoning within the Diagnostic Framework

Step 1: Take a history (gather data).

Comments: First, allow the patient to tell the story in his or her own words. Listen carefully, and do not interrupt. Only knowledge, training, and experience will enable us to "fill in the blanks" with relevant questions. Some patients are more articulate than others. As an example, if a patient states only that he has a "bellyache," only experience and training will allow us to ask, "Have you ever had this before?" "Do you have fever?" "Is it steady or does it come and go?" "What part of your belly hurts?" "Is there nausea or vomiting?" "Is there jaundice?" etc. Although it is important to take as complete a history as possible, we realize, consciously or not, that it would not be necessary to delve into past history of fractures at this time. However, as the story unfolds, although we might not have thought initially of asking about school performance, this may become relevant. Thus we are now gathering, sorting, eliminating, and reassessing data.

Step 2: Develop hypotheses.

Comments: Generate a list of possible diagnoses. This may be quite large. However, we are still sorting and reassessing. Using our patient with a "bellyache" as an example, the fact that he is Caucasian would safely eliminate sickle cell crisis as a possibility. If the pain is intermittent and not localized, appendicitis becomes less likely at this time. However, based on knowledge, experience, and common sense, it is unlikely that the patient's race will change in the next few hours, but there is still the possibility that this abdominal symptom may evolve into a constellation of symptoms and signs that speaks more toward appendicitis. One may make further eliminations using other historical points, such as timing or severity. For example, if the patient in question has had these same symptoms for 3 years, an acute abdomen or a malignancy may be less likely, but one should consider chronic conditions such as inflammatory bowel disease. If the patient is having severe acute abdominal pain and distension and appears lethargic, this would point more toward a surgical diagnosis such as volvulus or intussusception.

Step 3: Perform a physical examination.

Comments: At this point we are gathering more data. With more facts, our minds are not only sorting and eliminating but also correlating.

The human mind uses several means to correlate. One example is pattern recognition. The German idiom *augenblick* ("blink of the eye") illustrates this. Every examiner brings with him or her a lifetime's experience. Moreover, observers may have had similar experiences but have incorporated them differently. To illustrate this, there is the old story of two men walking down the street at the same time a woman is walking on the opposite side. One of the men notices her and says to the other, "Look at that elderly woman. She seems to be in her early seventies, has gray hair, walks with a mild limp, holds her left arm and wrist slightly flexed, but speaks quite fluently with what seems to be a middle-European accent." The second man replies, "Oh, that's my mother." Thus we all look at things in the aggregate or in its parts based on our own personal experience.

With less experience, the learner is more likely to use a systematic approach, whereas the more experienced physician may be more likely to use the *augenblick* approach. However, it is important to realize that no matter how much experience a physician may have, if the *augenblick* approach does not render a comfortable feeling with the diagnosis, it is necessary to fall back on the systematic approach. Thus it is incumbent on all of us not to forget how to use a systematic approach.

Another means of correlating data involves matching hypotheses. Match the patient's symptoms and signs with those of the hypothesized diseases. Suppose that the patient's history and physical examination, after all the appropriate elimination and pattern recognition is completed, does not produce any perfectly clearcut answer. Now it may be necessary to employ a matching system, a more conscious effort than *augenblick*. Look at the constellation of history and physical findings, and list all the clues. At this time, say, we have five clues: a, d, e, k, and n. We then draw on our training, knowledge, and experience, as well as our references, to determine which diagnoses have any of these five clues. Thus, if diagnosis W includes clues a, d, f, j, and l; diagnosis X includes clues d, k, m, r, and t; diagnosis Y contains clues a, b, d, e, and k; and diagnosis Z contains clues a, d, e, f, and n, we see that choices Y or Z have the highest probability of being the correct diagnosis.

Sometimes, additional clues from the physical examination may not corroborate the historical points and, furthermore, may lead to diagnoses of other diseases with varying degrees of relatedness. This leads to *branching hypotheses,* which may enlarge the differential diagnosis.

Step 4: Generate a differential diagnosis.

Comments: Depending on the historical and physical findings, there may be one or more diagnostic possibilities. One may now employ different schemes to help narrow diagnoses further. A system may be amenable to one or more schemes, examples of which are

- *Anatomic.* A careful history and physical examination may be amenable to narrow diagnoses by region (e.g., esophagus, stomach, duodenum, small bowel, large bowel, liver, and pancreas). Seizures may be analyzed by region, specifically frontal, parietal, temporal, occipital, etc. Diagnosis may be morphology-driven, specifically, size, shape, feel, and distribution.

- *Etiologic.* The classic scheme used in pediatrics consists of breaking down diagnoses into the following categories: congenital/genetic, infectious/inflammatory, nutritional/metabolic/toxic, traumatic, neoplastic, vascular, and psychological. This may be applied for each involved region that a careful history and physical examination has demonstrated.
- *Physiologic.* Each individual system has its unique physiology. As an example, once a genitourinary problem has been narrowed down to the kidney, is the problem glomerular or tubular? A firm grounding in cardiovascular physiology is often necessary to determine if a diagnosis is a result of cardiac failure or arrhythmia? What is the mechanism of a patient's cyanosis?
- *Epidemiologic.* Since infants, children, and adolescents are distinctly different; certain diagnoses may have a higher incidence or prevalence in one particular age group.

In succeeding chapters we have used one or more of these schemes in developing differential diagnoses. Because each system is unique, we choose not to employ a "cookie cutter" approach. Hence, after a thorough history and physical examination and hypothesis generation, the contributors of each chapter apply anatomic, etiologic, physiologic, and epidemiologic approaches most relevant to the system. For example, dermatology is an "observation and palpation" art, hence the initial anatomic breakdown (macules, papules, vesicles, etc.) in the summary tables. In the field of neurology, the physical examination will provide significant information pertaining to anatomic location; thus we employ next the "etiologic" breakdown to narrow the diagnoses. However, the reader is encouraged to invoke as many methods as he or she sees fit to narrow down diagnoses in any way possible.

We acknowledge the fact that certain symptoms and physical findings may present as manifestations of problems relevant to different systems. To quote Buttercup from Gilbert and Sullivan's *HMS Pinafore* (1878): "Things are seldom what they seem. Skim milk masquerades as cream. . . ." The clinician must keep an open mind as to what system the diagnosis may belong. TABLE 4–1 illustrates how a given symptom may fit into more than one system. It is incumbent on both primary care clinicians and specialists to "think outside the box" when necessary. For example, a child below the third percentile in height may have an endocrinologic or renal explanation for this. Thus each chapter acknowledges this and encourages the reader to keep his or her mind open to several different systems.

At this point we must switch from a data-gathering/eliminating/correlating mode and enter the age-old battlefield of fact versus opinion and prepare to make judgments. It may be possible to settle on a diagnosis at this point. If our patient with the "bellyache" has mild pain, mild diarrhea with no blood or mucus, diffuse mild abdominal tenderness, no guarding or rebound tenderness, and normal to increased bowel sounds, we may feel comfortable making a tentative diagnosis of gastroenteritis. However, if the patient had mild pain, no diarrhea,

TABLE 4-1 Conditions Ostensibly from One System That May Be Caused or Mimicked by Other Systems

System	Problem	Other Causes
GI	Jaundice	Heme: hemolytic anemia; metabolic: carotenemia
	Vomiting	CNS: ↑ICP, renal: uremia; endo: hypoadrenalism; ENT: labyrinthitis; psych: eating disorders
	Diarrhea	Endo: hyperthyroid, psychogenic
	Constipation	Endo: hypothyroid, psychogenic; CNS: cord lesions, CP; GU: UTI
	Abdominal pain	Pulm: pneumonia; GU: stones, UTI, PID, hematocolpos, hydronephrosis; endo:↑Ca^{2+}, DKA, Addison's, psychogenic
	Hematemesis	Heme: bleeding diathesis; ENT: epistaxis
Pulmonary	Stridor	Endo: ↓Ca^{2+}; CNS: brain injury with vocal cord paralysis
	Cough	Cardiac: CHF; ENT: FB in ear; toxic: drug side effects; psychogenic: drug abuse ("huffing"), marijuana, habit cough, allergy; CNS: chronic aspiration
	Wheeze	Cardiac: CHF; endo: Addison's, allergy; GI: GERD; psych: vocal cord dysfunction
Pulmonary/ cardiac	Chest pain	Musculoskeletal: costochondritis, slipped rib; GI: pancreatitis, subphrenic abscess, GERD
	Cyanosis	Hepatogenic cyanosis; metabolic: methemoglobinemia; CNS: central hypoventilation, neuromuscular disease
	Tachypnea	Metabolic acidosis, psychogenic hyperventilation
	Hypertension	Renal disease (hyperaldosteronism); endo: hyperthyroid, Cushing's, hyperaldosteronism
	Hypotension	Endo: Addison's, hypothyroidism, congenital adrenal hyperplasia
	Bradycardia	Endo: hypothyroidism
	Tachycardia	Endo: hyperthyroidism; psych: anxiety

Renal/GU	Polyuria/freq	Endo: diabetes mellitus; CNS: central diabetes insipidus, spinal cord pathology, MS; psych: diuretic abuse, polydipsia, sexual abuse
	Oliguria/retention	Pulmonary and CNS: SIADH; CNS: spinal cord injury, demyelinating disease
	Hematuria	Hematol: bleeding diathesis, anticancer drugs; psych: factitious
CNS	Headache	Renal: hypertension; ENT: sinusitis, psychogenic
	Seizure	Metabolic: hypoglycemia, hyper-/hypoelectrolytemias, hypocalcemia, inborn errors of metabolism; renal: uremia; psych: syncope, hyperventilation, narcolepsy; cardiac: arrhythmia; GI: GERD (Sandifer syndrome)
	Altered consciousness (lethargy, agitation)	Renal: uremia; hepatic: liver failure; endo: hypoadrenalism, DKA, hypoparathyroidism, hyperthyroidism; metabolic/toxic: Wilson disease, poisoning; pulmonary: CO_2 narcosis
	Focal weakness	Ortho: bone pain (Parrott's paralysis owing to injury, tumor, rickets, scurvy)
Psych	Psychosis	GI: Liver failure; GU: uremia; heme: porphyria lupus erythematosis; metab: Wilson disease
	Anxiety	Endo: hyperthyroidism, catecholamine excess, hypoparathyroidism; pulm: hypoxia; toxic: medications (steroids, catecholamines)
Endo	Poor linear growth	Renal, infectious, cardiac, pulmonary: chronic conditions of almost any kind
	Late puberty	GI: IBD; psych: eating disorders; CNS: craniopharyngioma; heme-onc: late effects of cancer treatment

Abbreviations: CNS = central nervous system; DKA = diabetic ketoacidosis; GERD = gastroesophageal reflux disease; GI = gastrointestinal; GU = genitourinary; SIADH = syndrome of inappropriate antidiuretic hormone secretion; UTI = urinary tract infection; ENT = ear, nose, throat; PID = pelvic inflammatory disease; ICP = intra-cranial pressure.

right lower quadrant tenderness, no guarding or rebound tenderness, and decreased bowel sounds, we may hypothesize a diagnosis of appendicitis and feel the need to look further into the matter.

Step 5: Test the hypotheses.

Comments: It is possible that our patient may be experiencing an early stage of appendicitis. Now invoke laboratory and imaging.

Step 6: Modify your differential diagnosis.

Comments: If a complete blood count reveals a normal white blood cell count, and the urinalysis is normal, we may decide on a diagnosis of gastroenteritis based on the preponderance of evidence. However, if the white blood cell count is elevated, this may militate more toward a diagnosis of appendicitis, although it is by no means an absolute certainty at this point. Always keep in mind that if a laboratory test result is not consistent with the clinical picture, repeat it. Mistakes in specimen handling and procedure do occur.

Step 7: Repeat steps 1 to 6.

Comment: Have we forgotten something? Have we left out any historical points? Do we have a travel history? Are there any pets in the home? Are there any other possible exposures? Did the patient have a rectal examination? Although one may not perform a rectal examination on every patient, it seems necessary to perform one now.

Step 8: Make the diagnosis or diagnoses.

Comment: If the answer is certain, stop at this point. As for our patient with the possible diagnosis of appendicitis, where do we go from here?

Step 9: If uncertain, consider a provisional diagnosis or watchful waiting.

Comments: We are still in the battlefield of fact versus opinion. We do not have enough facts to make a definitive diagnosis at this time. Now is the time to ask the questions: "How much uncertainty can I tolerate?" and "What do I want to know, and when do I want to know it?" There are options. One may decide to reexamine the patient to determine if there are any changes that would indicate that the diagnosis of appendicitis is declaring itself clinically. Are we running the risk of a rupture if we wait too long? Is it logistically possible for both doctor and patient to meet again in 4 hours? Another choice would be to obtain a CT scan of the abdomen. Can we schedule this on short notice? Does the patient have coverage to pay for this more expensive study? Will we save any more time than repeating an examination in 4 hours? Another option is to call for a surgical consultation. Does the community have a pediatric surgeon? Are we prepared to have our patient operated on now?

Sometimes there remains not a questionable diagnosis but rather several possibilities. After answering the question "What do I want to know, and when do I want to know it?" and feeling comfortable that deferring one or more of the diagnoses will not carry dire consequences, one may make further attempts to narrow the possibilities by applying the *principle of parsimony*. This is known as *Occam's razor* or *lumping* as opposed to *splitting*. This approach is often more helpful in younger patients than in the elderly, who are more likely to have multiple problems. Another tool for prioritizing diagnoses is to place them in their order of probability. The old saw that "common things occur commonly" is helpful, but one must decide to pursue rarer diagnoses in a timely fashion, if necessary.

This exercise illustrates both the objectivity and subjectivity involved in making medical diagnoses. Although we strive to use the scientific method, there is still much uncertainty in our professional lives. Education, experience, and knowledge will lessen but never eradicate uncertainty. In summary, to quote Sir William Osler: "The practice of medicine is an art, based on science."

Computers in Differential Diagnosis

Most of the steps in the diagnostic framework require the knowledge and experience of a trained human eye (and ear and hand and sometimes a nose). Certainly the physical examination cannot be delegated to an untrained person—and definitely not to a machine. It is the province of the physician to take the steps involving judgment and reasoning. However, it is possible to automate some of these steps, especially those involving correlation of information and generation of potential differential diagnoses. The present-day ubiquity of computers allows us to automate these steps.

In the simplest terms, a computer is a calculating machine that performs its calculations in a predefined sequence (a *program*) and that can run different parts of the program based on decisions (Is *A* less than, equal to, greater than, or not equal to *B*?). We humans can do this, too, and we are much more flexible in our thinking than are computers, but computers can calculate much faster than we can. The computers used to write this book perform well over 1 billion operations each second.

Computers have no inherent ability to reason. Their "reasoning ability" comes from their (human-designed) programming. Their main benefit to us is in the speed with which they can process information and make their "decisions." The best-known benefit of high-speed computing is management and use of the medical literature, which is now far too extensive to be manageable without computers. Evidence-based medicine as we now use it would be impossible without Internet-based literature search tools, and the mere act of searching the literature for information is useful to correlate and compare candidate differential diagnoses. However, physicians and medical informaticians have developed and continue to refine programs that can give clinicians more specific and helpful aids to diagnosis. These tools may suggest differential diagnoses or recommend additional diagnostic studies beyond those the clinician has already obtained. For example, such a program, when "told" that an adolescent girl has palatal lacerations, dental erosion, and abrasions over the dorsal knuckles of her right hand, will suggest obtaining amylase, lipase, and potassium levels.

Some will even suggest therapies, as well as recommend-against therapies that may be harmful (such as checking medication lists for agents to which a patient has allergies). Computerized physician order entry

(CPOE) systems take this one step further by suggesting additional orders (usually based on clinical pathways or protocols) or flagging possibly inappropriate orders.

Some well-written decision-support programs have yielded "correct" diagnoses at a higher rate than physicians in comparative trials, but this result may be misleading because even experienced and expert physicians may consider the same patient's case and not come to the same diagnostic conclusion. Remember that it is the physician who creates the program—the computer merely memorizes and sorts data very efficiently. These programs are not to override the physician's clinical judgment—the physician remains professionally and legally responsible for the patient's care—but they may be a useful adjunct to the diagnostic process, especially with the exponential growth of medical knowledge.

Arthur N. Feinberg

Although the neonatal period is defined as the first 4 weeks of life, we limit this chapter to evaluation in the term newborn nursery. Our goals include

1. To develop a prenatal history encompassing early, middle, and late pregnancy and delivery. We will emphasize maternal medical, family, and social history; monitoring for prenatal diagnosis; and fetal monitoring at labor and delivery.
2. To review a thorough healthy newborn assessment. We examine by region and evaluate each for inspection, palpation, percussion, and auscultation where applicable.
3. Since newborns cannot provide histories, we will assess in lieu of symptoms key postnatal problems as reported by a caretaker or a health professional.
4. To assess pathologic signs and, in conjunction with prenatal history, physical examination, and laboratory and imaging studies, to synthesize diagnoses.

We will develop a clinical approach to the most common problems that a neonatal nurse will report: growth problems, large-for-gestational age (LGA) and small for gestational age (SGA), temperature instability (hyper/hypothermia), tachypnea and apnea, vomiting, lethargy/poor feeding, irritability/jitteriness, seizures, pallor/plethora, cyanosis, heart murmurs, jaundice, and dermatologic conditions. Please refer to Chapter 6 for discussion of dysmorphology.

Prenatal History

KEY MATERNAL PROBLEM

■ **Infectious** Gather a thorough history on any maternal infectious illness during the pregnancy. Most likely the mother was screened for *group B streptococcal infection.* If she was positive, was she treated adequately with antibiotics during labor (doses every 4 hours, with last dose within 4 hours of delivery)? Were there any exposures to other bacteria, such as *Escherichia coli* (maternal urinary tract infection), *Listeria,* or *Mycobacterium tuberculosis*? Did the mother have any sexually transmitted infections such as *syphilis, gonorrhea, human immune-deficiency virus*

(HIV), *Chlamydia,* or *Ureaplasma*? Viral infections during early pregnancy such as *rubella, cytomegalovirus,* and *varicella* will cause fetal malformations. *Hepatitis B and C* will cause disease in newborns owing to maternal transmission. *Herpes simplex types 1 and 2* may produce a sepsis-like picture and can be overwhelming and devastating. Also, *Enterovirus* will cause a sepsis-like picture with jaundice, myocarditis, or meningitis. *Parasitic infestations,* specifically *toxoplasmosis,* also will cause fetal anomalies. A careful travel history will help to elucidate possible exposures to other parasites.

KEY MATERNAL PROBLEM
Noninfectious Maternal medical history is important. Ask about common conditions such as *diabetes mellitus, hypertension,* endocrinologic disorders such as *hypo/hyperthyroidism,* and maternal immunologic disorders that predispose to antibody transmission across the placenta (*immune thrombocytopenic purpura, myasthenia gravis, collagen-vascular disorders,* etc.) because they have profound effects on newborns. Maternal pulmonary, cardiac, renal, hematologic/oncologic, and neurologic disorders may play a role in newborn outcome, as will many of the medications used to treat these conditions. Are there any potentially inheritable conditions?

TABLE 5-1 *Noninfectious Maternal Conditions Affecting the Newborn*

Maternal Condition	Newborn Findings
Congenital heart disease	Intrauterine growth retardation (IUGR)
Diabetes mellitus	Hypoglycemia, hypocalcemia, polycythemia, large for gestational age (LGA), microcolon, asymmetric septal hypertrophy, caudal regression syndrome
Hypertension	IUGR
Obesity	Macrosomia, hypoglycemia
Hyperthyroidism	Transient neonatal thyrotoxicosis
Hypothyroidism	Neonatal hypothyroidism
Hyperparathyroidism	Neonatal hypocalcemia
Immune thrombocytopenic purpura	Neonatal thrombocytopenia
Myasthenia gravis	Transient weakness
Malignancy	Metastasis, fetal effects of treatment
Sickle cell anemia	IUGR
Systemic lupus erythematosus	Rash, anemia, thrombocytopenia, neutropenia, third-degree heart block IUGR
Renal failure	Fetal effects of medications (see TABLE 5–3)
Seizure disorder	

Adapted from Stoll BJ, Kliegman RM (eds.): *Nelson Textbook of Pediatrics,* 17th ed. Philadelphia: Elsevier/Saunders, 2004: p. 533, with permission from Elsevier.

It is critical to obtain a full environmental and social history. Is the fetus at risk because of homelessness or unsanitary surroundings? Does the mother have a history of substance abuse, including tobacco, alcohol, and/or street drugs? Was there exposure to environmental hazards such as chemicals or pesticides? Evaluate any medication the mother took during the pregnancy for any effect on the fetus or newborn, either teratogenic or symptomatic. TABLES 5–1 through 5–3 list maternal conditions and fetal exposures that may be problematic.

TABLE 5–2 *Infectious Maternal Conditions and Their Fetal Effects*

Maternal Condition	Newborn Findings
Bacterial	
Group B streptococcus	Sepsis, pneumonia, meningitis
E. coli	Sepsis, pneumonia, meningitis
Klebsiella, Proteus, Pseudomonas	Sepsis, pneumonia, meningitis
Neisseria gonorrhoeae	Sepsis, pneumonia, meningitis, conjunctivitis (ophthalmia)
Mycoplasma pneumoniae	Pneumonia
Chlamydia trachomatis	Conjunctivitis
Syphilis	Snuffles, rhagades, saddle-nose deformity, metaphysitis, jaundice, hepatosplenomegaly (HSM)
Viral	
Rubella	IUGR, cataracts, microphthalmia, HSM, pulmonic stenosis, patent ductus, deafness, "blueberry muffin" skin (thrombocytopenia)
Varicella embryopathy	Cicatrix scarring, poor limb development, multiple eye, brain, and spinal cord abnormalities
Perinatal disease	Severe chickenpox, pneumonia, hepatitis, encephalitis
Cytomegalovirus (CMV) embryopathy	IUGR, HSM, jaundice, purpura, microcephaly, cerebral calcifications, chorioretinitis, deafness
Perinatal disease	Pneumonia, sepsislike picture
Herpes Hominis	SEM (skin-eye-mucous membrane), encephalitis, systemic (hepatic)
Hepatitis B, C	Neonatal hepatitis B, C infection
Parvovirus B-19	Anemia, fetal hydrops
Enterovirus (echo-coxsakie)	Sepsis picture, jaundice, myocarditis, meningitis
Parasitic toxoplasmosis (embryopathy)	Similar to CMV + hydrocephalus

Adapted from Stoll BJ, Kliegman RM (eds.): *Nelson Textbook of Pediatrics*, 17th ed. Philadelphia: Elsevier/Saunders, 2004: p. 534, with permission from Elsevier.

TABLE 5-3 *Teratogenic Effects of Maternal Exposures during Pregnancy*

Agent	Effect
Anticancer drugs	Fetal loss, malformations (aminopterin, cytoxan, azathioprine, 6MP)
Busulfan	IUGR, cleft palate, multiple endocrine gland abnormalities
Antibiotics	
Aminoglycosides	Deafness
Tetracyclines	Hypoplastic teeth, cataract, limb malformations
Chloroquine	Hearing loss
Quinine	Abortion, thrombocytopenia, deafness
Nitrofurantoin	Hemolytic anemia in patients with G6PD deficiency
Cephalosporins	Direct + Coombs' test
Sulfonamides	Interfere with bilirubin protein binding, hemolysis in G6PD deficiency patients
Antiseizure medications	
Carbamazepine	Spina bifida
Phenytoin	↑Fontanel, hypertelorism, facial cleft, hypoplastic nails, low hairline
Valproate	Midface hypopolasia, narrow bifrontal diameter, cardiac lesions, hyperconvex nails
Trimethadione	Midface hypoplasia, prominent forehead, up-slanted eyebrows, short up-turned nose, midline cardiac defects, genital anomalies
Phenobarbital	Vitamin K deficiency, sedation
Anti-inflammatory drugs	
Salicylates	Bleeding, prolonged gestation
Ibuprofen	Oligohydramnios, pulmonary hypertension
Indomethacin	Oliguria, oligohydramnios, pulmonary hypertension, intestinal perforation
Antihypertensive drugs	
Atenolol	IUGR, hypoglycemia
Propranolol	Hypoglycemia, bradycardia, apnea
Reserpine	Stuffy nose, drowsiness, hypo/hyperthermia
Captopril	Oligohydramnios, ↓renal function
Steroid medications	
Progesterones, anabolic steroids	Fetal masculinization
Prednisone	Oral clefts

(Continued)

TABLE 5-3 *Teratogenic Effects of Maternal Exposures during Pregnancy (Continued)*

Agent	Effect
Thyroid medications	
Iodide	Goiter
Methimazole, propylthiouracil	Goiter, hypothyroidism
Diuretics	
Acetazolamide	Metabolic acidosis
Thiazides	Thrombocytopenia
Vitamin D	Hypercalcemia, supravalvular aortic stenosis
Isotretinoin (Accutane)	Multiple facial, skeletal, and cardiac anomalies
Psychotropic drugs	
Thalidomide	Phocomelia, deafness
Lithium	Ebstein anomaly
Haloperidol	Withdrawal
Imipramine	Withdrawal
Fluoxetine	Withdrawal, hypertonicity
Environmental toxins	
Hyperthermia	Spina bifida
Mercury	Deafness, blindness, peripheral neuropathy (Minamata disease)
Polychlorinated biphenyls (PCB)	IUGR, skin lesions
Anticoagulant	
Coumadin	Vitamin K deficiency, bleeding, hypoplastic nose, bone stippling, seizures
Drugs of abuse	
Cocaine	IUGR, microcephaly, gastroschisis, seizures
	Congenital heart lesions, withdrawal syndrome
Amphetamines	Withdrawal syndrome
Opiates	IUGR, sudden infant death syndrome
Tobacco	
Medications used during labor	
Dexamethasone	Periventricular leukomalacia
Oxytocin	Jaundice, hyponatremia
Magnesium sulfate, sympathomimetic tocolytics	Respiratory depression, lethargy, meconium plug, tachycardia

Adapted from Stoll BJ, Kliegman RM (eds.): *Nelson Textbook of Pediatrics*, 17th ed. Philadelphia: Elsevier/Saunders, 2004: p. 541, with permission from Elsevier.

Prenatal Examination

Prenatal Testing Modern prenatal care involves monitoring for many potential problems. By time of delivery, maternal blood type, *group B streptococcus, rubella, hepatitis,* and *possibly HIV status* are documented on the chart, all of with which the pediatrician should be familiar. *Alpha-fetoprotein* levels will be elevated in *neural tube defects, gastroschisis/omphalocele, cystic hygroma, multiple gestation,* and *congenital nephrosis;* it will be diminished in *trisomies* and *intrauterine growth retardation* (IUGR). All pregnant women are monitored for any conditions they may have (e.g., anemia or diabetes) in order to allow for best fetal outcomes.

Ultrasonography has become routine for almost all pregnancies and is most helpful in prenatal diagnosis. It is most helpful for monitoring fetal growth. Normal intrauterine growth patterns are well established and appear in FIGURE 5–1. *Oligohydramnios* and *polyhydramnios* have many serious implications for a fetus, and ultrasound easily identifies them (TABLE 5–4). Many anatomic defects detected before birth allow for appropriate anticipation on the part of both family and physician and, in many cases, prenatal therapy. Detectable anatomic conditions are *spina bifida, hydrocephalus, agenesis of the corpus callosum, Dandy-Walker malformation, hydronephrosis, omphalocele/gastroschisis, gastrointestinal obstruction, and diaphragmatic hernia.* Nuchal pad thickening occurs in *Turner syndrome and trisomies 21 and 18.* Measuring the distance from the skull to the uterine wall determines scalp edema that may be present in *fetal hydrops.*

Fetal cardiac monitoring may reveal potentially treatable arrhythmias such as *supraventricular tachycardia* and *heart block.*

Amniocentesis has many helpful applications during gestation, specifically to evaluate chromosomes of a fetus in high-risk situations such as family history or advanced maternal age. Assays for amino acids, organic acids, hormones, and enzymes are helpful for diagnosing metabolic disorders and will allow for prenatal diagnosis. Amniotic fluid is helpful for following pregnancies with *Rh isoimmunization* (measurement of optical density to assess amount of bilirubin) and for determining fetal lung maturity (lecithin:sphingomyelin ratio). Cordocentesis obtains fetal blood to provide information regarding hematologic and infectious conditions.

Monitoring Pregnancy, Labor, and Delivery It is important to assess and maintain placental sufficiency during gestation. Nonstress tests (NSTs), contraction stress tests (CSTs), and biophysical profiles (BFPs) measure fetal well-being, a reflection of placental sufficiency. NSTs assess fetal heart rate increases associated with normal movement. CSTs assess the fetal heart rate during uterine contractions, either spontaneous or induced by nipple massage or oxytocin

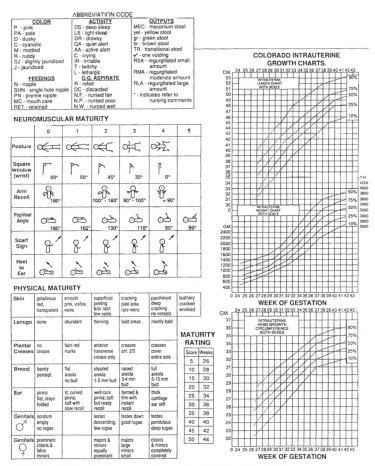

FIGURE 5–1 *Evaluation of Length, Weight, Head Circumference, and Gestational Age.*

administration. The BFP measures fetal heart rate, breathing, tone, and movement, along with amniotic fluid volume.

During labor, fetal monitoring assesses changes in heart rate associated with uterine contractions. Early decelerations are due to head compression and are common and benign. Variable decelerations are a consequence of cord compression and may be ominous. Late decelerations result from fetal hypoxia owing to uterine vessel spasm and indicate the need for immediate delivery. Beat-to-beat variability is also an indicator of fetal well-being, the loss of which is worrisome. A steady, unvarying heart rate usually indicates catecholamine production as a consequence of significant fetal hypoxia and distress. The pediatrician should be aware of any abnormalities of these studies in their newborns, particularly if they are attending a delivery.

TABLE 5–4 *Etiologies of Oligohydramnios and Polyhydramnios*

Oligohydramnios	Polyhydramnios
IUGR	Anencephaly-hydranencephaly-hydrocephaly
Amniotic fluid leak	Upper GI obstruction (duodenal atresia, etc.)
Anuria (renal agenesis,	Diaphragmatic hernia
obstruction)	Cystic adenomatoid malformation of lung
Twin-twin transfusion	
Meds (ACE inhibitors,	Trisomies
indomethacin)	TORCH infections
	Fetal hydrops immune, nonimmune
	Maternal diabetes, twin-twin transfusion
	(recipient), polyuria, chylothorax, teratoma

Adapted from Stoll BJ, Kliegman RM (eds.): *Nelson Textbook of Pediatrics*, 17th ed. Philadelphia: Elsevier/Saunders, 2004: p. 534, with permission from Elsevier.

The Newborn Assessment

General Considerations

Gestalt

Initial impression can be most useful in determining which infants need extra attention. Assess overall state of arousal by evaluating whether the newborn is asleep (deeply or lightly), awake with small amount of movement, or awake with significant movement or crying. Is the cry lusty, or is it weak or high-pitched? Is the baby consolable? Assess newborn color and respiratory effort. Is the baby blue or pink? Is the breathing comfortable? If it is rapid, is it quiet or noisy? Is the breathing rate too slow, or are there periods of apnea? How is the infant's posture? Normally, a term newborn will assume flexion of all extremities, except for the thighs, which abduct (FIGURE 5–2). Are there any obvious malformations on immediate observation? Refer to Chapter 6 for more details.

Apgar Score

Immediately on delivery, assess the newborn by the standard Apgar score, as illustrated in TABLE 5–5. Usually, hospital personnel will perform this evaluation at age 1 minute and at age 5 minutes. If the score is less than 7, the evaluation is repeated every 5 minutes for up to 20 minutes or until two scores of 7 or greater are achieved, whichever comes first. If heart rates and respirations are extremely low, it will be necessary to perform appropriate neonatal resuscitation.

Transition

Newborn transition from fetal to neonatal life usually takes a few hours and manifests as changes in color, pulse, respiration, alertness, and activity, similar to the Apgar score. A normal newborn may appear slate blue initially but will become pink to ruddy during the transition period. Also,

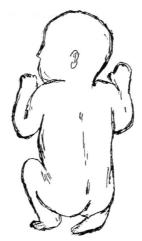

FIGURE 5-2 *Normal Newborn Posture.*

tachypnea to levels of 60 to 100 breaths/min will occur during the first hour, possibly owing to amniotic fluid accumulated in the lung or as a correction for initial metabolic acidosis. Normally, a newborn is awake and active with good tone during the first 60 minutes of life and then may sleep afterwards.

Measurements

For a term newborn, small for gestational age falls 2 standard deviations below the mean of 3175 g (7 lb) at 2500 g (5 lb, 8 oz), and large for gestational age falls 2 standard deviations above the mean at 4000 g (8 lb, 13 oz). Neonatal length, weight, and head circumference are plotted in FIGURE 5–1. Although these are the standard measurements, take others if clinically necessary. Some of these are head measurements, such as occipital/frontal diameter and fontanelle size; ocular measurements, such as outer and inner canthal distance, palpebral fissure slant, and

TABLE 5-5 *Apgar Score for Newborn Assessment*

Score	0	1	2
Heart rate	Absent	<100 beats/min	>100 beats/min
Respirations	Absent	Weak cry, hypoventilation	
Muscle tone	Limp	Some flexion	Active motion
Reflexirritability	No response	Grimace	Cough or sneeze
Color	Blue or pale	Pink, acrocyanosis	Completely pink

From Fletcher, MA. *Physical Diagnosis in Neonatology*. Philadelphia: Lippincott-Raven, 1998.

corneal diameter; ear measurements, such as position, rotation, and size; mouth measurements, such as columella and philtrum; chest measurements, such as thoracic circumference, internipple distance, and sternal length; and perineal measurements, such as anal placement, penile length, and testicular volume.

Gestational Age

The standard Dubowitz examination assesses gestational age (see FIGURE 5–1). Large for gestational age (LGA) babies often have immediate problems to address, such as birth injury (*ecchymosis, intracranial hemorrhage, clavicle fracture,* and *diaphragmatic* and *brachial plexus paralysis*). Metabolic problems may include jaundice, hypoglycemia, *hyperviscosity syndrome, renal vein thrombosis,* and *seizures.* Etiologies for LGA babies include maternal diabetes, obesity, and chromosomal syndromes such as Beckwith-Weidemann and cerebral gigantism (*Sotos syndrome*). Small for gestational age (SGA) babies are usually secondary to *placental insufficiency* from infection, infarction malformation, tumor, or twin-to-twin transfusion. Maternal conditions such as hypertension (*toxemia, placental abruption,* or *HELLP syndrome*), renal disease, malnutrition, and lack of prenatal care contribute to poor fetal growth. Primary fetal conditions, most commonly chromosomal disorders, congenital anomalies, infection, and immunodeficiency, are causes of poor intrauterine growth. SGA infants often will have problems with *hypoxia, acidosis, hypoglycemia,* and *polycythemia.*

Complete Physical Examination

Examine a healthy newborn by anatomic region. It may be practical first to examine areas that require auscultation if the infant is quiet. Since infants may be somewhat irritable in early transition, undressing them or moving them around may be disruptive. In a seemingly healthy newborn, most of the information is structural and may anticipate future problems. FIGURE 5–3 shows a standard newborn assessment hospital form.

▼ KEY FINDING

■ Head   The average head circumference for a term newborn is approximately 34 cm. Observe the size and shape of the head. Transillumination should be available in a newborn nursery and is a helpful observation tool. Macrocephaly may be familial and benign but also may be associated with *Beckwith-Wiedemann syndrome, Sotos syndrome, neurocutaneous syndromes,* and *chromosomal disorders* such as *fragile X* or *Klinefelter syndrome.* Macrocephaly associated with an enlarged, bulging fontanelle should bring to mind obstruction to cerebrospinal fluid (CSF) flow often in posterior fossa abnormalities such as *Dandy-Walker* and *Arnold Chiari syndromes* and *cystic malformations.* Are there areas that transilluminate, indicating abnormal collections of CSF in the subdural, subarachnoid, intraventricular, or posterior fossa regions? Microcephaly may be familial or genetic but also may be associated with congenital infection (TORCH), *maternal abuse of alcohol and cocaine, or intrauterine cerebrovascular accidents.* Are there any obvious malformations

Infant Name:		MRN#

Maternal History

Mom's Name _____ Age _____ Type/RH _____ HBSA: ☐ Pos ☐ Neg

OB. Doctor _____ G ____ P ____ AB ____ LC ____ RPR: ☐ Pos ☐ Neg

Prenatal History _____ EDC _____ Rubella: ☐ Immune ☐ Non Immune

AROM/SROM ____ Date/Time _____ Hrs. _____ HIV: ☐ Pos ☐ Neg ☐ Declined ☐ Pending

GBBS: ☐ Pos ☐ Neg ☐ Unknown Treated in Labor greater than 4 hours ☐ Yes ☐ No ☐ Antibiotic:_____

Complications: During Labor _____

During Delivery _____

Type of Delivery: Mods Prior to Delivery:_____

☐ Vaginal ☐ C-Section _____ Physician:_____

Infant History

Birthdate _____ Time _____ Apgars: 1 min _____ 5 min. _____ Physician After Discharge: _____

Delivery Complications _____

Sex ☐ M ☐ F Wt. _____ LBS _____ OZ _____ GMS. _____ % TILE LENGTH: _____ IN _____ CM _____ %TILE

E.G.A.: BY DATES: _____ WKS. By DUBOWITZ: _____ WKS. HC: _____ IN _____ CM _____ %TILE

☐ Breast ☐ Bottle

PHYSICIAN ADMITTING AND DISCHARGE PHYSICAL

ADM. PHYSICAL DATA	DISCHARGE PHYSICAL DATA
(Code: ☑ = No abnormalities ⊙ = Abnormalities present)	(Code: ☑ = No abnormalities ⊙ = Abnormalities present)

ADM. PHYSICAL DATA			DISCHARGE PHYSICAL DATA		
1 ☐ Reflexes	7 ☐ Lungs	12 ☐ Anus	1 ☐ Reflexes	7 ☐ Lungs	12 ☐ Anus
2 ☐ Skin: color, lesions	8 ☐ Heart	13 ☐ Trunk/Spine	2 ☐ Skin: color, lesions	8 ☐ Heart	13 ☐ Trunk/spine
3 ☐ Head/Neck	9 ☐ Abdomen	14 ☐ Extremities/Joints	3 ☐ Head/Neck	9 ☐ Abdomen	14 ☐ Extremities/Joints
4 ☐ Eyes	10 ☐ Umbilicus	15 ☐ Tone/Appearance	4 ☐ Eyes	10 ☐ Umbilicus	15 ☐ Tone/Appearance
5 ☐ ENT	11 ☐ Genitals	16 ☐ Femoral pulses	5 ☐ ENT	11 ☐ Genitals	16 ☐ Femoral pulses
6 ☐ Thorax			6 ☐ Thorax		
			☐ EARLY DISCHARGE/SINGLE EXAM PERFORMED		

DESCRIPTION OF ABNORMAL FINDINGS (if any)	DISCHARGE SUMMARY	☐ Normal Course ☐ Other:
	Wt. _____	HEAD CIRCUM _____
DATE Signature:	DATE Signature:	

Hepatitis B vaccine: ☐ NOT GIVEN ☐ GIVEN Nurse:_____

If given: Date _____ Time _____ IM Site _____ Dose _____ Lot # _____

Hearing Screen Date: _____ OAE: L _____ R _____

PROGRESS NOTES

9000158 (10/05)   NEWBORN ASSESSMENT   (White - Chart   Yellow - physician)

FIGURE 5–3 *Standard Neonatal Assessment Form.*

or protrusions such as an encephalocele? Is the skull oddly shaped? Are there swellings and discolorations, blisters, and ulcerations possibly secondary to trauma of delivery or fetal monitoring? Palpate the head. Skull bones are mobile to the point of overriding each other while passing through the birth canal. There also may be skull molding (familiarly the "cone head"). The initial head circumference may be small but will increase over the first few days as the molding and overriding resolve. Trauma of delivery may produce a *cephalohematoma,* actually a linear skull fracture, or a *caput succedaneum,* diffuse scalp edema that crosses a suture line. Check the sutures for premature closure, which will present as a sharp ridge along the suture line. This may not be apparent in the immediate newborn period. Occipital plagiocephaly occurs commonly today because of babies being placed in the "back to sleep" position and may be asymmetric if the baby has torticollis or a strong tonic neck reflex. Check the scalp for hair distribution. Are there any visible lesions or defects such as pits or areas of hair loss? Are there scalp abnormalities under the areas of hair loss (nevi, scars)? Note their location.

▼

▼ **Eyes** The neonatal eye examination is chiefly observational but can be difficult if the infant is agitated. Check general anatomy of the eye by assessing size, shape, and position. Are they large (*macrophthalmos*), small (*microphthalmos*), slanted upward or downward, or too close (*hypotelorism*) or too far apart (*hypertelorism*). If these findings are immediately obvious, it is important to check for other congenital anomalies and consider chromosomal disorders or other syndromic conditions. The most extreme form of hypotelorism is *cyclopia* with single midline facial structures, and this is invariably associated with midline brain abnormality (*holoprosencephaly*). Check the eyelids for edema and anatomic defects such as *coloboma* (cleft) and *ectropion* (exposed palpebral conjunctivae). Eyelid edema is common in a healthy newborn and is usually associated with eye prophylaxis or depends on lymphatic flow from the recumbent position. Obvious abnormalities of eyelashes or eyebrows, very long lashes, high-arched brows, and single brow (*synophrys*) are associated with genetic abnormalities. The nasolacrimal duct system is frequently obstructed (*dacryostenosis*), producing excess tearing. Drying tears may be yellow and crusty. Infection, *dacryocystitis,* has far more profuse exudates with a deeper yellow or more greenish hue. However, it is important to rule out other extrinsic causes, such as cysts of the tear duct (*dacryocystocele*), *encephaloceles,* which may enter through the nasolacrimal system, appearing as a mass in the inner canthal region, and *hemangiomas.*

Examine the sclerae, corneas and conjunctivae, and irides and lenses. Are the sclerae white, or are they yellow (jaundice) or blue (*osteogenesis imperfecta*)? Often the pressure of delivery will produce *scleral hemorrhages* that form around the lateral limbi and are benign and self-limiting. Corneal enlargement (>10 mm in diameter) may be *congenital glaucoma* and merits immediate ophthalmologic referral, especially if associated with corneal opacity, tearing, and photophobia. Refer patients with corneal opacities owing to cataracts or malformations (*keratoconus, cornea plana*) early. The conjunctivae may show redness or discharge from neonatal prophylaxis. Evaluate the irides and lenses with an ophthalmoscope. Although a good view of the ocular fundus in an awake newborn is virtually impossible, examination for red reflex (FIGURE 5–4) may demonstrate *leukocoria* (cat's eye or white reflex), which carries a large differential diagnosis, *including retinoblastoma, cataracts, Coats' disease, persistent hyperplastic primary vitreous, retinal dysplasia* and *detachment, congenital infection,* and others, meriting immediate referral. The ophthalmoscope will reveal malformation of the iris such as *aniridia* (absence, often associated with *hemihypertrophy* and *Wilm's tumor*), pigmentary defects, colobomata, and Brushfield spots in *Down syndrome.* Most newborn irides are gray in color, and the answer to the common question "What color are my baby's eyes" should be "Wait until age 4 months when the color will be apparent." Dislocation of the lens may be associated with *Marfan syndrome* or *homocystinuria.* Normal newborns have vision, albeit highly myopic.

Many normal newborns will make eye contact or track and react to light by blinking or pupillary response (*miosis*). Lack of these responses

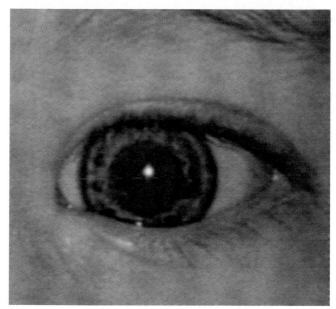

FIGURE 5–4 *Normal Red Reflex.*

may raise suspicion of severe visual problems. Also, *searching nystagmus* may be a sign of *cortical blindness* in a newborn. It is normal to have dysconjugate pupils at times up to age 6 months. However, if the pupils are always in an esotropic (toward the inner canthus) or *exotropic* (outer canthus) position, early referral is appropriate.

KEY FINDING

Ears Inspect the morphology of the ears for size, shape, and position. Is the external auditory meatus patent? Are there any abnormalities approximating the ear such as preauricular pits or skin appendages? Otoscopy in the newborn is difficult because of the accumulation of vernix. Also, a small neonatal ear has a narrow S-shaped curve to the canal that is often difficult to negotiate. Detecting tympanic membrane mobility is often difficult owing to the softness of the ear canal, which will move easily, creating the figure-ground illusion that the drum is moving. Most newborns undergo state-mandated auditory screening by otoacoustic emissions. Failure of this test should generate an immediate referral for further audiologic and otologic evaluation.

Enlarged ears (*macrotia*) or small ears (*microtia*) as an isolated finding may be hereditary or sporadic and is not significant. Enlarged ears should bring to mind chromosomal or syndromic conditions such as *fragile X syndrome, Cohen syndrome,* and others. Small or atretic ears, similarly, may bespeak chromosomal or syndromic abnormalities such as *Goldenhar syndrome, Treacher-Collins syndrome,* and *trisomies 13, 18,* and *21,* among others. See Chapter 6 for more detail. Any atretic ear is deaf, and early audiologic evaluation is necessary to prove otherwise.

Ears may be low set or malrotated. Draw an imaginary line that originates at the outer canthus to the ipsilateral ear, running with the slope of the eye. If the ear falls below this line, it is low set. To assess rotation, the angle made by intersecting lines of the vertical axis of the head and the long axis of the pinna should be less than 20 degrees. Preauricular sinuses and pits, unless associated with other anomalies, are usually autosomally dominantly inherited traits and are benign. Many ears whose helices are over- or underfolded (cup-ears) are either positional owing to uterine placement or sporadic and are of no clinical significance.

◢ Nose Inspect the nose for any malformations. Since all newborns should have immediate suctioning at birth, failure of the De Lee catheter to pass through the nares may indicate *choanal atresia.* There may be congenital *clefts* or *dimples.* There may be deviation, often positional in nature. An excessively broad or narrow nose may be associated with chromosomal or syndromic conditions and with other midline defects such as *Crouzon syndrome, Treacher-Collins syndrome,* or *holoprosencephaly.* Nasal masses may be extrinsic and are associated with *gliomas, encephaloceles, dermoids,* and *hemangiomas.* Nasal obstruction can be a difficult problem for newborns because they breathe through their noses and have difficulty adapting to mouth breathing. Other than genetic, syndromic, and traumatic etiologies for nasal obstruction, consider inflammations and infections such as *congenital syphilis, Chlamydia, rhinitis medicamentosa* (maternal medication), and *polyhydramnios.*

◢ Mouth, Tongue, and Throat Check for any obvious malformations, including the palate, gingivae, and lips. Is there symmetry? Are there any *clefts* of the lip or palate? It is most important to palpate the palate for the possibility of a *submucous cleft. Mucosal cysts* occur commonly on the palate (*Epstein's pearls*), the gingivae, and the buccal mucosa. *Natal teeth* may occur and are often loose. Remove them to prevent aspiration. They may be the primary teeth but sometimes are a third set. Is the philtrum well formed? If it is too flat, consider *fetal alcohol syndrome,* especially if it is associated with cleft palate and IUGR. Does the mouth droop? If this occurs while crying, there could be absence of the depressor anguli oris muscle. If the mouth droops at all times with or without concomitant eyelid droop, consider cranial nerve palsies or obstetric injury. Check the tongue for size. Enlarged tongues should bring to mind *hypothyroidism, Beckwith-Wiedemann syndrome,* or, rarely, *storage diseases.* The tongue may fall back (*glossoptosis*), causing airway obstruction, associated with retrognathia, indicative of *Pierre Robin syndrome*. Look for *ankyloglossia* (tongue tie) and *ranulas* (salivary gland cysts below the tongue). Ankyloglossia, unless extreme, usually does not require intervention, but refer all ranulas for removal. Observe and auscultate carefully for any obstruction to respiration as a consequence of any of these lesions.

KEY FINDING

Neck Most newborn necks are quite short, but if they are abnormally so or not mobile, this may be a result of bony abnormalities as in *Klippel-Feil syndrome*. Check the neck for sinuses and tags in the postauricular region and along the anterior sternocleidomastoid border. A mass in the body of the sternocleidomastoid muscle indicates a possible bleed and may produce subsequent torticollis. Midline masses should bring to mind thyroid disorders such as *thyroglossal duct cyst*. Neck masses may compromise respiration and require immediate evaluation, and may be *dermoid cysts, hemangiomas, cystic hygromas, teratomas,* or *reactive lymph nodes*. Webbed necks should bring to mind *Turner syndrome,* sometimes associated with generalized edema, or other collagen disorders that cause skin laxity such as *Ehlers-Danlos syndrome*. Observe and auscultate carefully to localize areas of upper airway compromise as a result of any of these lesions.

KEY FINDING

Thorax This area is conducive to inspection, palpation, percussion, and auscultation.

Inspection

Look for any obvious malformations. Is the chest symmetric? Is the diameter enlarged (*air trapping, intrathoracic masses, diaphragmatic hernia*). Or is the diameter too narrow (positional owing to *oligohydramnios, uterine positioning, skeletal dysplasia, absence of pectoralis muscle, Jeune thoracodystrophy,* or *muscle weakness such as spinal muscular atrophy*)? Is the baby breathing comfortably and at a normal rate (40 to 60 breaths/min)? Normal term newborns will breathe periodically, that is, slow or absent respirations for about 5 seconds, followed by rapid respirations. During pathologic breathing, one may observe nasal flaring, chest retractions, head bobbing, and/or grunting. Note that suprasternal or sternal retractions indicate upper airway problems, whereas intercostal and subcostal retractions indicate smaller airway problems. Asymmetric breathing patterns should bring to mind *diaphragmatic* or *brachial palsy, pleural effusion,* or *hemo-, chylo-,* or *pneumothorax*. Are there any external dermatologic abnormalities such as nipples that are supernumerary, small, or abnormally spaced? Think of *Down syndrome* (hypoplastic and narrow spaced) or *Turner syndrome* (shield-like chest, widely spaced). Look for skin color changes such as cyanosis or jaundice. As an adjunct to direct observation, transillumination may be helpful to evaluate the contents of the chest cavity (air, bowel, fluid).

Palpation

Palpate the clavicular areas for crepitus of fractures or for ascent of air from a pneumomediastinum. Pain over the ribs indicates that there may be a fracture. Palpation may demonstrate tactile fremitus, as seen in pneumonia, or decreased fremitus, as in effusions. Feel the cardiac area for point of maximal intensity, hyperactive precordium, or thrills. These may indicate significant congenital heart disease. Palpate breast tissue in the newborn. It is considered normal, secondary to maternal hormones, and may accompany milk secretion (*witch's milk*). If there is erythema and tenderness, consider mastitis as a diagnosis.

Percussion

Small newborns make it difficult to localize by percussion.

Auscultation

Listen to the newborn with and without a stethoscope. The cry may be indicative. Is it lusty, weak, hoarse, or high-pitched? Weak cries are nonspecific and indicate many abnormalities (see section below on lethargy as a symptom in the newborn). Hoarse cries bespeak *hypothyroidism*, and high-pitch cries should bring to mind neurologic damage, kernicterus, or chromosomal abnormalities (especially *cri-du-chat syndrome*). If the infant is tachypneic, is it noisy or quiet? Noisy tachypnea usually indicates upper airway involvement (rhonchi or stridor due to intrinsic or extrinsic airway obstruction) or lower airway involvement (grunting or wheezing), whereas quiet tachypnea usually has a CNS origin or can be from a respiratory compensation for a *metabolic acidosis*. *Cardiac failure* in the newborn may present with tachypnea and grunting or wheezing, along with sweating and easy fatigability.

The stethoscope is an important tool for diagnosing cardiac or respiratory problems. Listen for sounds that may confirm what we hear without the stethoscope such as rhonchi. The stethoscope may help to localize the sounds to the pharynx, trachea, or bronchi. Listen for rales and wheezing. Listen for heart tones and their intensity, rhythm, and the different components of the first and second cardiac sounds and adventitial sounds such as murmurs, rubs, or gallops. This may be quite difficult in an infant whose heart rate averages about 140 beats/min. Keep in mind that a newborn with severe congenital heart disease may demonstrate no cardiac murmur until the differential pressures have developed between the left and right sides of the heart during the first several days of life.

KEY FINDING

Abdomen

Inspection

The newborn abdomen is proportionally larger and rounder than that of an adult. Furthermore, as the baby swallows air and food after birth, the abdominal girth increases. Does the abdomen appear distended? If so, does it originate from high or low intestinal obstruction, *Hirschsprung's disease* (aganglionic megacolon), or extraintestinal pathology such as *meconium peritonitis, ascites, hemoperitoneum,* or *pneumoperitoneum*? Observe the abdominal skin for discoloration such as jaundice or cyanosis (central). Venous markings are normal on a newborn abdomen but should not be tortuous or distended. Check the umbilical area for hernias. Large hernias may indicate *hypothyroidism*. Very large umbilical protrusions may be *omphaloceles,* necessitating immediate repair. Abdominal contents may protrude through the abdominal, more often to the right of the umbilicus in *gastroschisis,* also requiring immediate attention. Count the umbilical vessels, which should consist of one vein and two arteries. If there is only one artery, is it an isolated finding, or are there other congenital anomalies present? If there is leakage from the umbilicus, think of urine through a *patent urachus* or stool through a patent *omphalomesenteric duct*. Separation of the rectus abdominis muscles with some bulging is normal for a newborn (*diastasis recti*). A flat (scaphoid) abdomen should bring to mind *diaphragmatic hernia*. Loose, floppy abdominal skin may indicate underdevelopment of the abdominal wall, as in the *Eagle-Barrett (prune-belly) syndrome* also associated with genital abnormalities.

Palpation

Check for abdominal masses. The most common cause for a palpable abdominal mass in a newborn is *cystic dysplasia of the kidney*. Other renal causes include *polycystic kidneys* (autosomal recessive or dominant), *ureteropelvic obstruction, renal vein thrombosis, Wilms' tumor, bladder obstruction,* and *neurogenic bladder*. Adrenal causes include hemorrhage, neuroblastoma, and others. Gastrointestinal causes are *duplications, cysts,* and *lymphangiomas*. Liver enlargement may be caused by *hematomas, tumors* (benign or malignant), or metastatic disease, especially from *neuroblastoma*. Biliary causes for abdominal masses include *choledochal cysts* and *hydrops of the gallbladder*. Genital tract problems include ovarian cyst or tumor and *hydrometrocolpos,* usually from an *imperforate hymen*.

Percussion

Although it is difficult to localize pathology by this technique, it is helpful to outline organ margins to determine if there is excess air, either extra- or intraintestinal.

Auscultation

Newborns often have less active bowel sounds until feeding is well established. However, overactive bowel sounds may be indicative of an intestinal obstruction, and absent bowel sounds for several minutes may indicate peritonitis.

◤ The Perineum

Female Genitalia

A normal female newborn may demonstrate edema of the labia, especially with a breech presentation, and this resolves spontaneously. A
creamy vaginal discharge, sometimes streaked with blood, is due to
maternal hormones and is also within normal limits. Hymenal anatomy
has many normal variants, including clefts, cysts, crescents, and ridges.
However, an *imperforate hymen* (bluish bulge) causes *hematometrocolpos*
and requires immediate attention. Also, a septate hymen may indicate
duplications higher in the genital tract. Virilized female genitalia present with clitoromegaly and labial fusion. Causes for this include fetal
congenital adrenal hyperplasia and *virilizing tumors of the ovary or adrenal
glands* and maternal *tumors with hormone production affecting the fetus,
exogenous: progestogens, stilbestrol,* and androgens. Consult Chapter 13 for
further discussion.

Male Genitalia

The normal penis should be longer than 2.5 cm. Often it is buried in a
preputial fat pad and appears deceptively small. Pressure on the mons
pubis region with penile stretching usually will reveal a normal penile
length. A true micropenis should bring to mind *hypopituitarism*, often
accompanied by *hypoglycemia*. *Hypoadrenalism* and other *genetic syndromes* also may cause micropenis. Make certain that the penile opening is located close to the tip. Sometimes it is located ventrally, often
associated with incomplete foreskin and chordee (ventral shortening)
and requires surgical repair. With more severe forms of *hypospadias*, the
meatus is located on the penile shaft, at the penoscrotal junction, or on
the scrotum. These require immediate attention. *Epispadias* is insufficient closure of the dorsal aspect of the penis and is sometimes associated with *exstrophy of the bladder*. Check the scrotum for size and contour. *Bifid scrotum* and *hooded scrotum* may be normal variants if not
associated with other anomalies. An enlarged scrotum may be due to
normal edema after delivery (especially breech) and resolves spontaneously. *Hydrocele* is the most common cause of an enlarged scrotum, is
not associated with discomfort, and transilluminates easily. Neonatal
hernias may appear as a hydrocele but do not transilluminate. These
should be referred for repair, whereas most hydroceles will resolve with
no intervention. Infections and *torsions* are associated with discomfort
and require immediate attention. Tumors are rare in newborns. Make
certain that the testes are palpable bilaterally and are descended. Normal testicular volume for a newborn is more than 1.1 ml. Testes may
be high in the scrotum or in the inguinal canal, and one must follow
them for eventual descent. If the testes are nonpalpable, and if there are
any other genital abnormalities, consider *congenital adrenal hyperplasia*
(3β-hydroxysteroid dehydrogenase deficiency), *hermaphroditism, androgen
deficiency,* or *resistance* or *syndromic conditions*. Consult Chapter 13 for
further detail.

Ambiguous Genitalia

Sometimes it is difficult to determine the gender of a newborn immediately at birth. Consult Chapter 13 for further discussion.

KEY FINDING

The Back Inspect the back for obvious masses or deformities. *Spina bifida* may present either covered with skin or open. Other causes of midline masses include *sacrococcygeal teratomas* and *lipomas*. Check the entire posterior midline for dimples or sinuses. If they occur further than 2 cm away from the anus, they may well communicate with the central nervous system (CNS); refer them immediately. Abnormal tufts of hair in the sacral region may bespeak *spina bifida, tethered cord*, or other CNS abnormalities. *Pilonidal sinuses* and *cysts* occur within 2 cm of the anus and are benign if the examiner sees the floor of the dimple. If not, ultrasound may be necessary to delineate the anatomy. Check the anus for patency. Ninety-nine percent of normal newborns should pass meconium within the first 48 hours of life. Congenital *scoliosis* is not normal, and it is necessary to image the spine for abnormalities.

KEY FINDING

Extremities

Upper

Check the arms, hands, and fingers for obvious deformities such as hypoplasia and amputation phocomelia. Are there fractures? This may indicate *osteogenesis imperfecta.* Are the extremities stiff and malformed, as in *arthrogryposis?* Count fingers. Isolated *syndactyly* or *polydactyly*, especially with an extra fifth finger located proximally, is usually a benign autosomally dominant condition. However, polydactyly may be associated with many other genetic and syndromic conditions. Check where the fingers are set, especially the thumb. Consult Chapter 6 for further detail. Are there any signs of brachial palsy, *Erb syndrome* with weakness of shoulder abduction and external rotation and weakness of elbow flexion and wrist extension (*Porter's tip syndrome*), or *Klumpke syndrome* with clawing of the involved hand (FIGURES 5–5 and 5–6).

Lower Extremity

Inspect the legs for obvious deformities, the same as with the upper extremity examination. An extreme form of lower limb dysplasia may be a consequence of the caudal regression syndrome seen in infants of diabetic mothers. Evaluate the lower extremity from the hips down to the toes. *Developmental dysplasia of the hip* may appear in more severe cases as a shortened, medially rotated leg with asymmetric gluteal folds and a positive Galeazzi sign with unequal knee height (FIGURE 5–7). Always perform a Barlow maneuver (with the hips adducted, grab femur encircling the knee, and push posteriorly), and follow with the Ortolani maneuver (abduct the hips). The Barlow maneuver will force

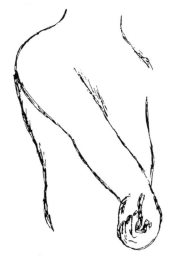

FIGURE 5–5 *Erb Palsy.*

the hip out of the socket, and the Ortolani maneuver will relocate it with a "klunk" sensation (FIGURES 5–8 and 5–9).

Femoral anteversion or *retroversion* and *internal tibial torsion* or in-curved feet (*metatarsus adductus*) may be normal in newborns as a result of fetal positioning, especially if the limbs are flexible and easily manipulated into a normal position. If the foot is permanently in the equinovarus position (forefoot supination, varus angulation, and medi-ally facing soles), this is a *club foot* and must be referred immediately for

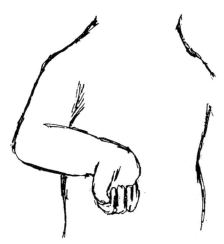

FIGURE 5–6 *Klumpke's Palsy.*

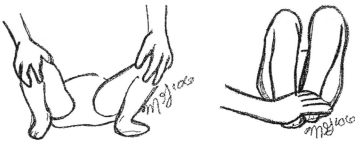

FIGURE 5-7 *Galeazzi Sign.*

casting. With any extremity malformation, always check for any spinal abnormality that may be a cause.

KEY FINDING
Neurologic Examination A term newborn examination must take into consideration cerebral, cranial nerve, sensory, and motor functioning.

Cerebral

Although they cannot answer our questions, newborns demonstrate varying levels of consciousness and alertness. Objective scales assess newborn states, ranging from coma to fully awakened state. Soon after birth some newborns may show preference for their mothers or other

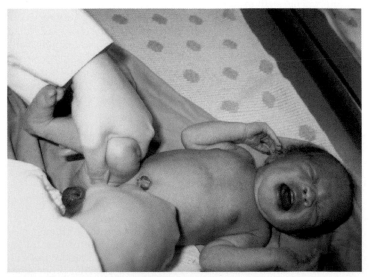

FIGURE 5-8 *Barlow Maneuver.*

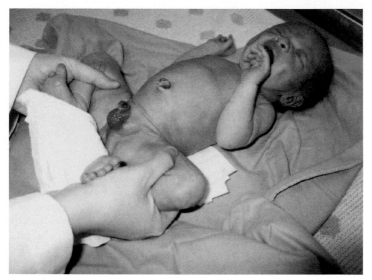

FIGURE 5-9 *Ortolani Maneuver.*

familiar faces by making more prolonged and intense eye contact. Some may orient toward sound. Is the baby alert or sleepy, active or lethargic, tense or relaxed, or quiet, fussy, or tremulous? Are there any abnormal movements such as *athetosis* (writhing)? If the baby is fussy, is he or she consolable? Does he or she seem to respond to cuddling at any time? Remember that a normal newborn's state of alertness will fluctuate, so it may be necessary to do prolonged or several evaluations. Some newborns are capable of making seemingly purposeful defensive maneuvers. For example, they will be able to bat at a cloth if put over their faces. Some will extend their necks while being held for assessment of a retinal light reflex, thus making it even more difficult for the examiner.

Cranial Nerve

Refer to Chapter 12.

Sensory

Newborns see, albeit myopically, and hear. Many newborns can make eye contact and can follow around the midline, the presence of which may be reassuring to the examiner. Newborn hearing screening measuring otoacoustic emissions is routine in every state. Immediate follow-up of an abnormal screen is important. Newborns definitely feel pain and discomfort and will withdraw reflexively and cry. Thus proper anesthesia or analgesia is mandatory for all procedures.

Motor

As in any neurologic examination, evaluate general tone (normal, hypotonic, or hypertonic) and posture (normal, opisthotonic, decorticate, or decerebrate). Newborns generally maintain a mildly flexed position of all four extremities. Posture may be asymmetric with preference to one side, but tone should be normal. Look carefully for any evidence of focal weakness, unilateral or bilateral. Refer to Chapter 12 for further detail.

Reflexes

Newborns are more reflexive than at any other stage of their lives. It is not entirely clear why newborns have them, but there are some anthropologic explanations, such as primitive survival or instinctive preparation for fright/flight. Newborn reflexes are helpful for assessing spinal function, both sensory and motor, but may be present and normal in newborns with anencephaly and thus are not helpful for assessing cerebral damage. There have been more than 80 newborn reflexes described. We will illustrate some of the more commonly used ones often described as *active reflexes*. Abnormalities usually present with overreaction, underreaction, or asymmetry.

Suck. The baby will suck automatically if a finger or pacifier is placed in his or her mouth.

Moro. After gently lifting the baby by the arms with the head still on the mattress, release your grip so the baby's back falls to the underlying surface. The baby will have a double response—first, arm abduction and elbow extension and then arm adduction, elbow flexion, and finger curling (FIGURE 5–10).

Startle. Often confused with the Moro reflex, elicit it similarly, but the baby will flex the arms only and have a generalized startle. Repetition will habituate this response.

Grasp. The baby will automatically grasp onto anything placed in his or her hand.

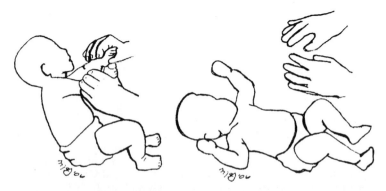

FIGURE 5–10 *Moro Response.*

Tonic neck. When the infant is relaxed, turn the head to one side. The
   infant will assume the *en garde* position with the arm that would
   hold the sword on the same side the head faces and the other arm
   flexed and held up straight (FIGURE 5–11).

Traction. Place fingers in the infant's palms. As he or she grasps, lifting the baby will elicit elbow and neck flexion. Similarly, pulling
   the infant to a sitting position or raising the infant from the
   supine position from the shoulders also will elicit neck flexion
   (FIGURE 5–12).

Perez response. Hold the infant in the prone position, grasping under the
   abdomen. Gentle rubbing up the spine will elicit flexion of the
   extremities and extension of the neck. Similarly, elicit the Vollmer
   response by rubbing down the spine, which will cause flexion of the
   lower extremities and extension of the back.

Galant response. Hold infant in the prone position as in the Perez
   response, and rub lightly along the flank. The baby will move his
   or her buttocks toward the ipsilateral side. This reflex is particularly
   amusing to older siblings (FIGURE 5–13).

Magnet response. Grasp both heels and press the thumbs on balls of
   infant's feet, thus dorsiflexing them. The baby will extend the legs
   (FIGURE 5–14)

Supporting reaction. Hold the infant upright with both hands around the
   thorax, and then gently place both feet on the surface. The infant
   will attempt to extend both legs and straighten the trunk.

Placing response. Similar to the supporting reaction, have the infant rub
   the dorsum of the foot under the edge of a bassinet or a table top.

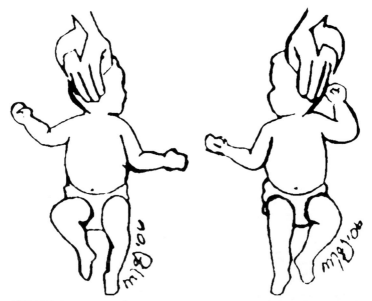

FIGURE 5–11 *Tonic Neck Reflex.*

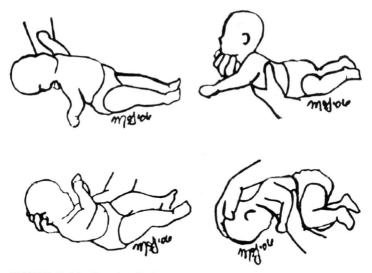

FIGURE 5–12 *Traction Reflex.*

The infant will bring his or her foot up on the surface in a walking-like manner (FIGURE 5–15).

Stepping. Hold the infant upright with both feet on the surface of a table. Move the infant from side to side to elicit stepping movements. This is the second-best reflex for an older sibling's amusement (FIGURE 5–16).

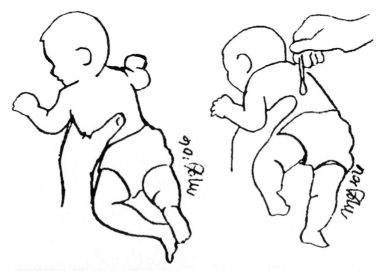

FIGURE 5–13 *Galant Response.*

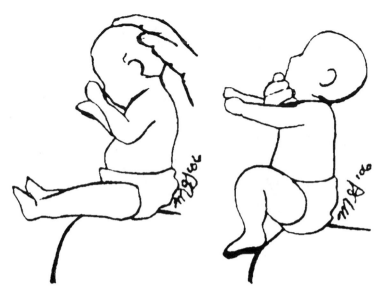

FIGURE 5–14 Magnet Response.

Crossed extension reflex. With the infant lying supine, straighten out one
   leg at the knee, and stroke the plantar surface of that foot with your
   other hand. The opposite leg should first flex and then abduct, the
   toes will fan, and then the leg will extend and abduct, pointing its
   foot toward the foot that was stroked.

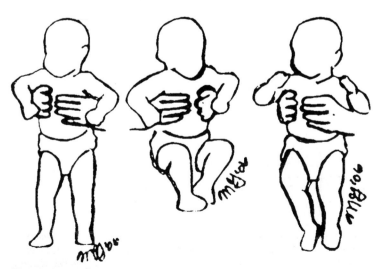

Figure 5–15 Placing Response.

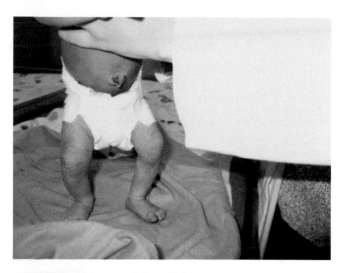

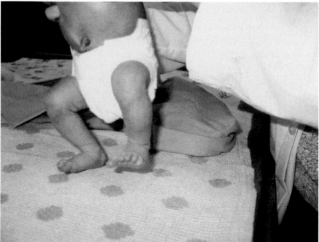

FIGURE 5-16 Stepping Movements.

Babinski reflex. Scratching the lateral aspect of the foot will elicit dorsiflexion of the big toe and fanning of all the others.

Ankle clonus. Abruptly press your thumb on the ball of a foot to produce
sudden dorsiflexion. Normally, there should be fewer than five beats
of clonus.

Also note that there are many tests for muscle tone that are passive.
Examples are the scarf sign, the heel-to-ear maneuver, the popliteal
angle, and the wrist window. They also assess tone in gestational age
assessment (see FIGURE 5–1).

Common Problems in a Term Newborn

Growth Problems

Small for Gestational Age

Small for gestational age is defined as more than 2 standard deviations below the mean. In full-term newborns this is 2500 g or less. Maternal, fetal, or placental problems may contribute to this. Obtain a maternal history, asking about hypoxia (cardiac or pulmonary disease), hypertension, sickle cell anemia, advanced diabetes mellitus, malnutrition, and drug abuse, including tobacco. Gross and microscopic examination of the placenta will be helpful to assess for scarring, infarction, infection, tumor, or insufficient size or surface area. Newborn causes are *chromosomal* or *syndromic disorders, multiple gestation, congenital infection* (TORCH), and *insulin deficiency.*

Large for Gestational Age

Large for gestational age is defined as more than 2 standard deviations above the mean, or 4000 g, in a term newborn. Is the mother diabetic? Infants of diabetic mothers are long and "jowly" appearing owing to the action of their own excess production of insulin as a response to maternal hyperglycemia. Check for many other anatomic problems associated with *infants of diabetic mothers,* such as polyhydramnios, *microcolon* (abdominal distension), *congenital heart disease* (asymmetric septal hypertrophy, conotruncal anomalies), and *caudal regression syndrome.* Syndromic causes of large for gestational age babies include *Beckwith-Wiedemann syndrome* (omphalocele, large tongue, and organomegaly) and *Sotos syndrome* (cerebral gigantism associated with large head circumference in a newborn).

Temperature Instability
Newborns, especially small ones, have difficulty maintaining their temperature owing to a lack of fat and immaturity of the hypothalamic thermostat.

Hyperthermia

Any report from a neonatal nurse regarding fever in a newborn merits immediate attention. The febrile newborn is septic unless proven otherwise, and the physician should have a low threshold for pursuing an evaluation. Always review prenatal history, especially maternal carriage of group *B streptococcus* and appropriateness of antibiotic prophylaxis. Most nurseries have protocols for immediate newborn evaluation for all mothers who are colonized. *Neonatal sepsis* is protean in manifestation and may appear as hypothermia, lethargy, poor feeding, vomiting, abdominal distension, and jaundice. If clinical suspicion for sepsis is high, a full evaluation should be conducted including a complete blood count (CBC), urinalysis, chest x-ray, and cultures of blood, CSF, and urine. C-reactive protein (CRP) determination is a nonspecific test of inflammation and should not be used in the initial evaluation, although levels over 4 mg may point toward the diagnosis. There are nonpathologic causes for hyperthermia, including overwrapping and maternal epidural anesthesia, but do not attribute fever to these alone unless the newborn is otherwise asymptomatic and free of risk criteria for sepsis. Keep in mind that sepsis is not relegated to bacteria, and it is important to consider viral infections, especially *Herpes hominis*.

Hypothermia

Hypothermia may result from inadequate swaddling but also, in conjunction with other symptoms, as mentioned above under "Hyperthermia," may indicate *sepsis* and may be a more ominous sign than hyperthermia. Lower neonatal reserves of glycogen and fat often result in *hypoglycemia,* but consider *inborn errors of metabolism* when it is associated with vomiting and lethargy.

● KEY PROBLEM

■ **Tachypnea** Neonatal tachypnea has many anatomic origins, including respiratory, cardiac, and neurologic. There also may be many origins, including *infectious* and *metabolic*. When confronted with a tachypneic newborn, always ask further questions as to the time of onset (birth or later). Is the tachypnea deep or shallow? Is it symmetric? Is the patient comfortable or not? Check the progression (static, worsening) and degree of distress (grunting, flaring, or retracting). Is there accompanying cyanosis or pallor? Is the newborn alert and vigorous or irritable or lethargic? Is there fever or vomiting? Is there a peculiar odor to the baby?

Always review the prenatal and delivery history for any clue pointing to infection or trauma. Examine the newborn carefully for any signs of upper airway obstruction (stridor), absence or asymmetry of breath sounds, rhonchi, rales, or wheezes. Do a complete cardiac examination, listening for heart rate, murmurs, intensity of heart tones, and peripheral pulses.

It is important to prioritize the evaluation of the tachypneic newborn depending on the suspected diagnosis and severity of the illness. Pursue pulmonary, cardiac, or neurologic causes if the history and physical examination lead to them. Vomiting, lethargy, irritability, and temperature instability are nonspecific and should prompt evaluation for infectious, metabolic, or neurologic etiologies. We outline diagnostic considerations below:

Respiratory

Is there evidence of upper airway blockage? Consider *choanal atresia,* nasal trauma, or any congenital malformation or compression of the tracheobronchial tree (*stenosis* or *aberrant vessels or aortic arch remnants compressing the area*). Always have a low threshold for ordering a chest x-ray on a tachypneic newborn. It is rapid and economical and provides much valuable information. Consider *aspiration syndromes* (vernix, stomach contents, and meconium), pneumonia, extrapulmonary accumulation of air (*pneumothorax*), blood (*hemothorax*), or lymph (*chylothorax*). Congenital abnormalities of lung formation may include emphysema and cystic adenomatoid malformation. If a newborn remains cyanotic despite O_2 administration (hyperoxia test), think of persistent fetal circulation (*pulmonary hypertension*). *Hyaline membrane disease* is very rare in a term newborn but may be associated with polyhydramnios or cesarean section delivery and has a higher incidence in *infants of diabetic mothers.*

More commonly, a newborn will be tachypneic owing to slow evacuation of lung fluid. The symptoms occur immediately after birth. There may be flaring and retracting, but the infants do not appear very ill. This is *transient tachypnea of the newborn* and is benign and self-limiting.

Cardiac

It is important to note that absence of a heart murmur in a tachypneic newborn does not eliminate the possibility of severe cardiac disease. Many murmurs depend on a differential pressure between the left and right circuits, which has not developed as yet. If cyanosis is present, perform a hyperoxia test, and if the newborn is unable to improve the O_2 saturation, *cyanotic heart disease* is a definite possibility. It is important to pursue a cardiac evaluation in a timely fashion and to administer prostaglandins to maintain patency of the ductus arteriosus pending definitive treatment. The most common cyanotic lesions are the *five T's: transposition, tetralogy of Fallot* (less likely in the immediate newborn period), *tricuspid atresia, truncus arteriosus,* and *total anomalous pulmonary venous return.* Other lesions such as pulmonary atresia also may cause cyanosis. Another significant ductal-dependent lesion is *hypoplastic left heart syndrome,* which also requires prostaglandins and rapid diagnosis. All newborns with cyanotic heart disease merit immediate evaluation by a pediatric cardiologist.

Cardiac failure is very rare in the term newborn nursery and is due most commonly to critical aortic stenosis. It will manifest as lethargy, poor feeding, pallor, and diaphoresis. If a newborn has an apparent chromosomal syndrome, always look carefully for congenital heart disease. This is especially true for newborns with *Down syndrome.* Evaluate them immediately for *endocardial cushion* (AV communis) defect regardless of any physical findings. Consult Chapter 9 for more detail.

Neurologic

Tachypnea of neurologic origin is notably quiet. Sometimes the normal stress of delivery will cause a temporary metabolic acidosis for which the newborn compensates by tachypnea. This is benign and self-limiting. However, serious neurologic injury, e.g., *intracranial hemorrhage,* often will present as tachypnea, lethargy, or irritability. Similarly, *neonatal meningitis* presents as such and must be diagnosed and treated immediately.

Infectious

Tachypnea may be less specific than hyperthermia, especially if isolated. Raise suspicion for sepsis if there are predisposing risk factors or if the infant appears even slightly ill. If clinical suspicion is relatively low, some experts suggest a "modified" sepsis workup, leaving out a lumbar puncture because of the low risk for meningitis in a newborn that is not strongly symptomatic. Others suggest a full evaluation because of differences in management between sepsis and meningitis. As with hyperthermia, do not forget to include viruses, especially *herpes*.

Metabolic

Tachypnea may be a nonspecific indicator of general stress and may be secondary to *hypoglycemia* or abnormal electrolytes, including *calcium* and *magnesium*. Always consider *inborn errors of metabolism,* especially in newborns that are lethargic or vomiting or have a distinct odor to them. In these instances, tachypnea is a respiratory compensation for severe metabolic acidosis. Consult Chapter 12 for an approach to these patients.

● KEY PROBLEM

◼ Apnea Apnea in a term healthy newborn is relatively rare. It is defined as a period of more than 20 seconds and should not be confused with normal periodic breathing owing to relative immaturity of CO_2 receptor centers in the medulla. Consider respiratory causes as outlined under "Tachypnea" and hypoxia and neurologic causes such as *seizures, intracranial hemorrhage, herniation, infarction, neuromuscular disease, phrenic nerve paralysis, toxins,* and *medications. Infectious* causes include sepsis of all etiologies. *Metabolic* causes as discussed earlier, as well as *hypothermia,* are considerations. Gastrointestinal etiologies include straining at stool and *gastroesophageal reflux* (GER).

● KEY PROBLEM

◼ Poor Feeding, Vomiting, and Constipation

Poor Feeding/Lethargy

This is usually a nonspecific finding and may have multiple causes, including infectious, metabolic, cardiac, and neurologic, as discussed earlier. Pathology of the gastrointestinal (GI) tract is relatively rare as a cause.

Vomiting

This occurs frequently in a newborn and is important to assess in order to develop a sensible diagnostic plan. On what day of life did it start? Does it occur immediately after feeding? Is it projectile? Is there any blood, bile, or stool? Is the baby ill-appearing? We outline causes of vomiting below:

Upper gastrointestinal. It is best to break down gastrointestinal etiologies of vomiting into upper and lower causes. If vomiting occurs right after feeding, consider the upper GI tract. A common cause is *tracheoesophageal fistula,* the most common type of which is a blind esophageal pouch, where immediately at birth a De Lee suction catheter will not pass. Consider *GER* and *motility disorders* such as *achalasia* and *hiatal hernia.* Gastric causes of vomiting include congenital abnormalities such as *pyloric atresia, volvulus, duplication,* and *antral webs.* These are often suspected because of abdominal distention associated with *polyhydramnios* and an excessive amount of amniotic fluid suctioned from the stomach at birth. *Hypertrophic pyloric stenosis* is very rare in the term newborn nursery but may occur in the neonatal period, especially with a history of macrolide administration. *Duodenal atresia* is a significant cause of vomiting in the newborn and, like the preceding gastric causes, will present with abdominal distension as well. Other causes of duodenal obstruction include *annular pancreas* and *Ladd bands.* Bilious vomiting may be due to obstruction at or below the sphincter of Oddi and merits immediate investigation.

Middle gastrointestinal. Think of *ileal* or *jejunal atresias,* as well as *Ladd bands, malrotation, volvulus,* and *intestinal duplications. Intussusception* occurs very rarely in the immediate newborn period.

Lower gastrointestinal. Vomiting may not occur until day 3 of life and may be feculent in nature. Absence of stool or constipation often occurs. Ninety-nine percent of normal term newborns should pass stool within 48 hours. Stooling patterns are variable, ranging from once every other day to eight times per day. Consistency is also variable, with breast-fed babies having mushier stools. Always perform at least a visual examination of the anus for patency. Colonic obstruction may be due to *stenosis, atresia,* or *duplications,* and external obstruction may result from *Ladd bands, malrotation,* and *volvulus.* Aganglionic megacolon (*Hirschsprung disease*) and *meconium ileus* (cystic fibrosis) are always considerations. Sometimes newborns appear obstructed from a hard meconium plug, and removal by enema administration of Gastrografin will produce immediate relief. This condition is not associated with cystic fibrosis.

Nongastrointestinal. Keep in mind that vomiting can be nonspecific and is associated with infectious, neurologic, or metabolic disorders, as discussed earlier. Constipation can have metabolic causes such as *hypothyroidism.*

KEY PROBLEM

◤ **Irritability/Jitteriness**   Irritability or jitteriness in the newborn may be normal in a small, thin baby. Often the trauma of a normal delivery may leave a newborn slightly irritable as they make the adjustment to extrauterine life. More severe or protracted symptoms should bring to mind *metabolic/toxic* (*hypoglycemia, hypo/hypernatremia, hypocalcemia,* or *drug-withdrawal*) or *neurologic* disorders (*congenital malformation, trauma,* or *infection*). Consider causes of hypoglycemia such as *hyperinsulinism* (*infant of diabetic mother, nesidioblastosis,* or *Beckwith-Wiedemann syndrome*), depleted glycogen stores, endocrine (*hyperinsulinism, hypopituitarism,* or *hypoadrenalism*), and metabolic disorders (*gluconeogenesis* or *fatty acid breakdown*). *Neonatal seizures* (see below) are often subtle in nature and may appear as hyperirritability. Severely jaundiced newborns may manifest kernicterus as irritability, high-pitch cry, deafness, sunset eyes, and chorioathetosis. *Hypocalcemia* may be secondary to *low birth weight, phosphate overload, hypoparathyroidism* (consider *Di George syndrome*), or *renal failure.* Consult Chapters 12, 13, and 14 for more detail.

KEY PROBLEM
Seizures
Neonatal seizures, as in older children, may be tonic, clonic, or myoclonic but also may be subtle in presentation and appear as irritability and stereotyped movements such as lip-smacking, blinking, or bicycling. Because of deficiency of myelination in the newborn, symptoms and electroencephalographic (EEG) changes may be quite variable. The most common cause of neonatal seizures is *hypoxic-ischemic encephalopathy.* Consider *congenital malformations, CNS trauma* (*intracranial hemorrhage*), *infection* (*sepsis, meningitis,* or *viral infection such as TORCH*), and *metabolic* conditions such those discussed earlier under "Irritability/jitteriness," as well as inborn errors of metabolism (see Chapter 12 for further detail). Of particular interest in the neonatal period is *pyridoxine deficiency,* which will respond dramatically to pyridoxine administration. After ruling out the preceding causes, neonatal seizures may be benign, as in familial seizures (autosomal dominant and self-limited to about 6 months), and "fifth-day fits," which last for about 1 day and are without sequelae.

KEY PROBLEM
Pallor or Plethora
Newborns are normally plethoric and have hemoglobin values around 17 mg/dl. Often delayed cord clamping or positioning of the newborn too low or high relative to the placenta will cause plethora or pallor. *Twin-to-twin transfusions* will cause plethora in the recipient and pallor in the donor. Plethora may be present in *infants of diabetic mothers* and those with *Beckwith-Wiedemann syndrome, adrenogenital syndrome,* or *thyroid disorders.* Pallor is usually due to blood loss (including placental), but it is also important to consider sepsis and severe *congenital heart disease* (heart failure). Congenital anemia not from blood loss is relatively rare, but one must consider *dyserythropoiesis, Diamond-Blackfan syndrome, neonatal parvovirus B-19 infection,* and *hemolytic disease* (alloimmune or autoimmune). Anemia in its severest form may be associated with severe edema (*hydrops fetalis*) as a consequence of high-output cardiac failure.

KEY PROBLEM
Cyanosis
Cyanosis in the newborn is usually cardiac or respiratory in origin. See previous discussions for respiratory and cardiac causes of tachypnea, as well as Chapters 8 and 9 of this book. *Polycythemia and methemoglobinemia* will appear as cyanosis and often are mistaken for cardiopulmonary conditions. Cyanosis may be *factitious* (acrocyanosis with concomitant falsely low pulse oximetry readings owing to poor circulation).

KEY PROBLEM

Heart Murmurs As discussed earlier, absence of a heart murmur does not rule out severe congenital heart disease. Soft upper sternal border murmurs frequently are due to a patent ductus arteriosus, which is benign and self-limiting. Administration of oxygen (hyperoxia test) will cause the murmur to disappear owing to spasm of the ductus in response to O_2. If a newborn is symptomatic (tachypnea and cyanosis), heart murmurs merit immediate attention with pediatric cardiac consultation. Observe an asymptomatic newborn with a heart murmur, evaluate, and refer as needed. See Chapter 9 for more details.

KEY PROBLEM

Jaundice Neonatal jaundice is extremely common and usually is benign and self-limiting, such as physiologic (third day) jaundice and breast-milk or *breast-feeding jaundice*. We will discuss causes of jaundice requiring intervention, with emphasis on when to suspect and how to identify them. As a general rule, clinically apparent jaundice within the first 24 hours of life merits closer scrutiny. Also, jaundice appearing after the third day may be significant. If a newborn has other signs, including but not limited to fever, tachypnea, pallor, lethargy, vomiting, and distension, immediate evaluation is necessary. Usually unconjugated hyperbilirubinemia (see below) will appear with a yellow or orange tinge, whereas conjugated hyperbilirubinemia will appear with a greenish hue.

Simplistically, jaundice is intrahepatic, hepatic, or posthepatic. A normal red blood cell has a lifespan of 120 days, hemolyzes, and releases unconjugated bilirubin, which is then circulated through the liver for conjugation to a water-soluble diglucuronide (see Chapter 10 for further detail). Thus prehepatic jaundice will be unconjugated hyperbilirubinemia, and intrahepatic jaundice may be conjugated, unconjugated, or both, depending on whether the disorder occurs before or after conjugation. Posthepatic jaundice occurs after conjugation, involves the biliary system from the canaliculi to the larger ducts, and is conjugated hyperbilirubinemia.

Prehepatic Jaundice

This reflects the excessive breakdown of red blood cells (RBCs), releasing unconjugated bilirubin into the bloodstream. Consider hemolytic causes of excessive RBC breakdown such as innate membrane defects (*spherocytosis, elliptocytosis, pyknocytosis,* and *stomatocytosis*). A normal RBC membrane may be vulnerable to breakdown by abnormal enzymes, as seen in *glucose-6-phosphate dehydrogenase* (G6PD) and *pyruvate kinase deficiency*. Note that hemoglobinopathies such as sickle cell disease do not cause jaundice in the newborn because of the protective effect of fetal hemoglobin. It is important to consider immunologic causes, alloimmune such as *Rh, ABO,* and *other minor blood group incompatibilities,* as well as, more rarely, autoimmunity. In maternal autoimmune disease, antibodies may cross the placenta, causing temporary symptoms in a newborn. Also, bleeding into an enclosed space, as in *cephalohematoma* or *intracranial* or *intramuscular hemorrhage,* will cause more rapid

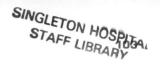

breakdown and release of RBCs. If a newborn is polycythemic, the excess volume of RBC breakdown will predispose to unconjugated hyperbilirubinemia. Sometimes inadequate intake will prevent passage of bilirubin through the urine and stool. Bilirubin may reoxidize to the unconjugated form (bilirubin oxidase) and cause jaundice. Infants with *Down syndrome, prematurity,* and *hypothyroidism,* as well as *Asian infants,* are more susceptible to prolonged unconjugated hyperbilirubinemia.

Intrahepatic Jaundice

This type of jaundice refers to malfunction at the carrier-protein step, during which time bilirubin transfers into the hepatocyte; the conjugation step, during which time UDP-diglucuronosyl transferase polarizes the bilirubin molecule to the water-soluble form; and the step that releases conjugated bilirubin into the bile canaliculi. *Gilbert syndrome* will affect carrier-protein function and is associated with higher neonatal bilirubin levels. Absence of conjugating enzyme may be partial in the autosomal dominant form or complete in the lethal autosomal recessive form of *Crigler-Najjar syndrome. Breast-milk jaundice* is presumably due to a steroid compound inhibitor of conjugation, in contrast to *breastfeeding jaundice,* which is most likely due to diminished intake as maternal milk supply builds up during the first 3 days of life. *Infection,* bacterial, viral, or fungal, will have an impact on hepatic structure and function. Damaged hepatocytes, especially when *disseminated intravascular coagulation* is present, will produce conjugating enzyme deficiency. Note that intrahepatic jaundice may contain conjugated bilirubin because infection often will damage bile canaliculi as well. *Rotor* and *Dubin-Johnson* (black-pigmented liver) *syndromes* are due to inability of the hepatocyte to release conjugated bilirubin.

Posthepatic Jaundice

Disorders of biliary drainage through the smaller ducts up to the common bile duct, cystic duct, and gall bladder cause conjugated hyperbilirubinemia. Typically, the jaundice persists and may produce a more greenish color to the skin. Other findings, such as acholic stools and hepatomegaly, may be present. It is critical to address the possibility of *biliary atresia* first because prompt diagnosis and early intervention with the Kasai procedure will produce better long-term results. Other causes of conjugated hyperbilirubinemia include *congenital paucity of bile ducts, Byler syndrome, inspissated bile syndrome, choledocal cyst, congenital infection (TORCH), bacterial sepsis, neonatal hepatitis,* and *metabolic diseases such as alpha$_1$-antitrypsin deficiency, tyrosinemia,* and *galactosemia* and *meconium ileus* secondary to *cystic fibrosis.*

KEY PROBLEM

■ **Dermatologic Conditions** Neonatal dermatology is a textbook unto itself, so we will limit our discussion to well term infants in the newborn nursery. We will emphasize: common benign transient conditions, developmental abnormalities, skin peeling, pigment disorders, hemangiomas, and hamartomas.

Common Benign Transient Conditions

Newborns often will have transient color changes usually owing to vasomotor instability. They may be mottled (*cutis marmorata*) or have acrocyanosis or have erythema over half the body that lies dependent (*harlequin color change*). Newborns normally will have peeled skin, particularly if born after the projected date. If not excessive, this will resolve spontaneously.

Papules are very common in the newborn and are most often *inclusion cysts* containing keratin. *Sebaceous hyperplasia* is pinpoint papules usually located on the nose. This is not to be confused with milia, larger white papules found over the face. Inclusion cysts are located most often on mucosal surfaces. Midline palate cysts are *Epstein's pearls,* and alveolar cysts are *Bohn nodules.* Newborns may develop tiny pinpoint lesions (*miliaria*), which are due to obstruction of the eccrine duct (sweat gland). They are often a consequence of overheating and *appear in the form of miliaria crystallina (clear fluid)* or *miliaria rubra (inflammation).* *Erythema toxicum* consists of macular or papular lesions with a surrounding wheal. These lesions appear in the newborn nursery, will come and go, and may last up to 3 weeks. They may be mistaken for pustules, but pustules are not fleeting and contain a more whitish core. If in doubt, a Gram stain will differentiate between the two, with pustules containing polymorphonuclear granulocytes (PMNs) and erythema toxicum containing eosinophils.

Noninfectious pustular lesions are common in newborns. *Neonatal acne* may be inflammatory but never consists of comedones. It is self-limiting and does not reflect any development of acne in later life. *Transient neonatal pustular melanosis* is common in darker-pigmented individuals and appears in three stages: (1) pustules, (2) resolving pustule with surrounding scale, and (3) pigment deposit. Sometimes the earlier stages occur in utero, so a newborn may appear with pigmented lesions only.

Developmental Abnormalities

There are many developmental anomalies such as *supernumerary nipples, preauricular sinuses,* and *skin tags, branchial cleft remnants* seen on the lateral neck. They are generally benign and may require removal if they become infected or if cosmetics are an issue. Midline lesions may be of more concern. Median raphe cysts are often in the perineal scrotal area in newborn males and are benign. However, image any midline cyst, dimple, or protrusion of any kind (*tail, hemangioma, lipoma,* or *tuft of hair*) for the possibility of CNS communication. Defects in hair formation on the scalp, especially with abnormal underlying skin, should raise suspicion for *aplasia cutis.* The umbilicus is a location for developmental abnormalities. *Granulomas* occur commonly, but any secretions from them should raise suspicion for a *patent urachal or omphalomesenteric duct remnant. Amniotic bands,* acquired from premature rupture of the amnion sac, will leave constriction bands and in more severe cases frank clefts and amputations.

Skin Peeling

As discussed earlier, this may be a normal variant. However, if it is more severe, it may indicate *ichthyosis*. Ichthyosis may appear as diffuse erythema with severe scaling, or *lamellar ichthyosis,* and often is associated with the *collodion baby syndrome.* Other forms of ichthyosis, such as ichthyosis vulgaris and the X-linked recessive type, are not common in the newborn nursery.

Pigment Disorders

Hypopigmentation in the newborn may be general or local. *Albinism,* with its many types, is associated with generalized depigmentation and associated ocular findings. Check for platelet function in the *Hermansky-Pudlak syndrome.* Partial albinism may represent *Chediak-Higashi syndrome* and is associated with recurrent pyogenic infection and white blood cell (WBC) abnormalities. *Metabolic* disorders such as *phenylketonuria* (PKU) and others that involve synthesis of melanin from phenylalanine and tyrosine also create generalized hypopigmentation. Examples of localized hypopigmentation are sometimes *genetic,* as in *hypomelanosis of Ito* with the pattern following Blaschko lines or *piebaldism,* which demonstrates sharp demarcations of extensive depigmentation following a symmetric pattern. A white patch may be the earliest detectable sign of *tuberous sclerosis*; it is often oval-shaped (ash-leaf) and more apparent with a Wood's lamp.

Hyperpigmentation

Mongolian spots are the most common form of hyperpigmentation, seen in darker-complected newborns. They are always blue in color and are sometimes mistaken for bruises or child abuse. They are self-limiting but may last through childhood. Diffuse hyperpigmentation characterizes *hypoadrenalism,* often with accentuation on the palms, soles, and mucus membranes. Most individuals who develop *lentigines* (freckles) do not manifest them in the newborn period; however, those who do often have *syndromic* conditions (*LEOPARD, Carney, McCune-Albright,* and *Peutz-Jeghers syndromes, etc.*). Consult a textbook of neonatal dermatology for more detail. Consider many other *genetic* conditions associated with hyperpigmentation, such as *incontinentia pigmenti,* which starts as vesicular and follows Blaschko lines; *xeroderma pigmentosum* (chromosomal breakages); and other phakomatoses. Café-au-lait spots of *neurofibromatosis* may appear in newborns. *Melanocytic nevi* are of varying size, shape, and pigment distribution. Observe them for potential malignant degeneration starting at birth.

Hemangiomas and Hamartomas

Hemangiomas are either vascular malformations (dysplastic vessels) or tumors (cellular overgrowth). *Vascular malformations* may be of capillaries as in the common salmon patch (angel kiss on forehead, stork bite on nape of neck), which are benign and usually self-limiting, although they may remain on the nape of the neck. Larger port-wine stains do not regress and grow with the child. They may be associated with deeper, larger vascular malformations and are of particular concern in *Sturge-Weber syndrome* (unilateral facial distribution and sharply demarcated midline border) with associated cerebral arteriovenous (AV) malformations and ocular involvement or in *Klippel-Trenaunay syndrome* with incapacitating hemihypertrophy. Vascular malformations may be located along the midline dorsal spinal column but are of no concern for CNS abnormalities unless there are other findings such as cutaneous swelling or dimples. Vascular malformations may be telangiectatic as in *ataxia telangiectasia* or *Weber Osler-Rendu syndrome*, but the skin lesions usually appear after the newborn period. Venous malformations are usually blue in color, and lymphatic malformations are clear and cystic (hygroma). Arteriovenous malformations can be located superficially or deep and may be invasive, disfiguring, and cause severe complications such as external compression of vital structures or platelet trapping (*Kasabach-Merritt syndrome*). Several *syndromic* conditions are associated with vascular malformations. Consult a textbook for these.

Hamartomas are a collection of one or more tissue structures at varying states of maturity. A common epidermal nevus is the *sebaceous nevus of Jadassohn*, which is a waxy, cobblestone, oblong lesion most often located on the scalp or face. They are associated with malignant degeneration and should be observed for changes and removed during adolescence. *Sebaceous nevi* may appear in other patterns, such as linear, verrucous, or comedonal, and may have extra cutaneous findings involving the CNS, eye, skeleton, heart, and genitourinary (GU) tract. Other hamartomas may consist of eccrine, smooth muscle, or connective or fatty tissue.

Confirmatory Laboratory Tests and Imaging

Screening is an integral part of care for all newborns. All screening tests should be sensitive and cost efficient, have a beneficial intervention, and have reliable backup tests for positive results. Every state in the union plus Washington, DC, has its own panel of metabolic screening tests; thus there is no uniformity. In the year 2002, states ranged from doing 3 screens to doing as many as 36. At that time, the most commonly screened metabolic conditions were phenylketonuria (PKU) (51), hypothyroidism (51), galactosemia (50), hemoglobinopathies (44), congenital adrenal hyperplasia (CAH) (32), maple syrup urine disease (MSUD) (24), biotinidase deficiency (24), and homocystinuria (17). Others were medium-chain acyl-CoA dehydrogenase deficiency (MCAD) (5), tyrosinemia (3), and cystic fibrosis (CF) (4). Only three states (MA, NC, and WI) used an expanded newborn screen consisting of 30, 36, and 21 conditions, respectively. Each state other than those three averaged six tests per newborn. Recently, 29 states have added an expanded screen. As of January 1, 2006, universal screening for CAH, homocystinuria, biotinidase, MCAD, tyrosinemia, and CF has increased to 42, 39, 37, 36, 36, 27, and 12 states, respectively. At present, 32 state screens include additional fatty acid, organic acid, and amino acid disorders. It is incumbent on the primary care physician to act immediately on any abnormal newborn screen.

Most newborn nurseries screen all newborns at age 24 hours for serum bilirubin. Established normative values are helpful to determine which newborns will merit closer scrutiny for neonatal jaundice.

All states now have universal hearing screening (28 mandatory and 23 universally offered) by an otoacoustic emissions screening test. These, too, should be followed up immediately with a repeat screen and more definitive testing if necessary. We outline laboratory and imaging studies to corroborate diagnostic suspicions based on prenatal history, physical examination, and abnormal clinical signs in TABLES 5–6 through 5–8.

TABLE 5–6 *Summary of Initial Laboratory and Imaging Based on Prenatal History*

Prenatal History	Laboratory	Imaging
Maternal infections		
Group B strep	CBC, cultures, urinalysis	Chest x-ray (CXR)
Hepatitis B	Hepatitis panel	Head CT if micro/ macrocephaly
TORCH infections	TORCH titers, urine CMV culture	
HIV infection	ELISA studies, Western blot	
Herpes hominis	Culture (eye, throat, rectal), LFTs	MRI of head
Maternal noninfectious		
Diabetes	Glucose, Hgb, Ca^{2+}	
ITP (idiopathic thrombocytopenic purpura)	Platelet count	
Hyper/ hypothyroidism	T_4, TSH	
Drug abuse	Drug screen of blood, urine, or meconium	
Oligohydramnios	Urinalysis, BUN, creatinine	GU ultrasound
Polyhyramnios	Glucose Hgb, Ca^{2+} (calcium)	Head CT, CXR, Abd flat plate, especially if symptomatic
Abnormal prenatal ultrasound	Chromosomes if multiple abnormalities	Repeat ultrasound + CT or MRI to better delineate abnormality
Fetal bradycardia	ECG, lupus antigens if third-degree block	
Fetal tachycardia	ECG, T4, TSH	

Abbreviations: TORCH = toxoplasmosis, other agents, rubella, cytomegalovirus, and herpes simplex; BUN = blood urea nitrogen; ELISA = enzyme-linked immunosorbent assay.

TABLE 5-7 Summary of Appropriate Laboratory and Imaging Based on Initial Physical Assessment

Physical Finding	Laboratory	Imaging
Large for gestational age	Glucose, Hemoglobin, Calcium	X-ray clavicle if suspect fracture
Small for gestational age	Glucose, TORCH titers, chromosomes (if dysmorphic)	CT of head if suspect TORCH
Dysmorphic features	Chromosome studies	Echocardiogram if suspect Down syndrome
Macrocephaly	Chromosomes, toxoplasmosis titer	CT if suspect hydrocephalus
Microcephaly	Chromosomes, TORCH titers	CT if >2 SD below mean
Hyper/hypotelorism	Chromosomes if dysmorphic	MRI of head
Blue sclerae		Bone series for fractures
Enlarged, simple, low-set, atretic ears	Chromosomal studies	
Obstructed nares	O_2 saturation (pulse oximetry)	CT of choanal region
Cleft palate	Chromosomes if dysmorphic	Swallow study, if necessary
Short neck severe torticollis		X-ray of cervical spines
Web neck	Chromosomes for Turner syndrome	
Heart murmur	Pulse oximeter, hyperoxia test	ECG, echocardiogram
Cyanosis	Pulse oximeter, blood gas, hyperoxia test	CXR, ECG, echocardiogram

Finding	Labs	Imaging
Jaundice	Bilirubin (total and direct), type and Coombs', CBC, reticulocytes, TSH if severe and persistent, sweat Cl-, alpha$_1$-antitrypsin, galactose, and tyrosine, if conjugated	HIDA scan if ↑direct bilirubin
Scaphoid abdomen	Basic metabolic panel (BMP)	CXR, Abd flat plate
Abdominal distension	BMP (glucose, electrolytes BUN)	Abd flat plate, ultrasound, or CT
Abdominal mass		Abdominal ultrasound → CT
Two-vessel umbilical cord		Abd ultrasound if dysmorphic
Enlarged testicle		Consider ultrasound
Enlarged, painful testicle		Immediate ultrasound
Hypospadias		GU ultrasound for anomalies
Hypogonadism	BMP, chromosomes	Pelvic ultrasound or MRI
Micropenis or ambiguous genitalia	BMP, chromosomes, DHEA and androstenedione level, cortisol level, FSH, LH, human growth hormone, prolactin	Pelvic ultrasound or MRI
Virilization	BMP, chromosomes, 17-OH progesterone, ACTH, DOC levels, androgens, estrogen levels in females	
Limb deformities	Chromosomes if dysmorphic	X-rays

TABLE 5–8 *Summary of Laboratory and Imaging Studies Based on Key Signs*

Key Sign	Laboratory	Imaging
Hyperthermia	CBC, U/A, CRP, urine and blood cultures, LP if ill-appearing (sepsis evaluation) HSV evaluation (see TABLE 5–6)	CXR CXR CXR
Hypothermia if symptomatic	As in hyperthermia + glucose, lytes, pH, and NH$_3$ if ill-appearing	
Tachypnea	As in hypothermia	CXR, echocardiogram if suspect cardiac disease, head CT if suspect CNS disease
Apnea	As in tachypnea + toxicology studies if suspicious	CXR, head CT if suspect CNS disease
Vomiting	As in hypothermia	Abd x-ray (air-fluid levels, no gas in rectum, double-bubble of duodenal obstruction)
Irritability/ jitteriness	Lytes, BUN, creatinine, glucose, Ca^{2+}, PO$_4$, bilirubin if jaundice, parathyroid hormone, chromosome 22 eval if ↓ Ca^{2+}	Ultrasound, CT if necessary Head CT if suspect CNS prob,
Seizures	As in irritability/jitteriness, pH, NH$_3$, TORCH titers; consider sepsis/ meningitis evaluation if febrile or ill-appearing	Cranial ultrasound, head CT, EEG
Cyanosis, heart murmur, jaundice	As in TABLE 5–7	As in TABLE 5–7
Pallor, plethora	CBC	

Abbreviations: CBC = complete blood count; CA = Calcium; CNS = central nervous system; CRP = C-reactive protein; CXR = chest x-ray; HSV = herpes simplex virus; lytes = electrolytes; LP = lumbar puncture; NH$_3$ = ammonia; PO$_4$ = Phosphate; U/A = urinalysis.

6

The Pediatric Dysmorphology Diagnostic Examination

Bryan D. Hall and Helga V. Toriello

Dysmorphology is the study of human congenital anomalies. This term was coined over 40 years ago by Dr. David W. Smith. Congenital anomalies can affect any part of the body and can range in severity from negligible, to having cosmetic significance, to being incompatible with life. Approximately 3 percent of all newborns have a significant congenital anomaly that can interfere with normal body function. Anomalies can occur in isolation or as part of a pattern. The importance of making a dysmorphologic diagnosis includes determining prognosis, managing medical concerns, and counseling families about recurrence risk.

The goals of this chapter include

1. Outline of the steps in making age-specific diagnoses
2. Description of a range of possible anomalies
3. Review of diagnostic methods for the more common conditions of dysmorphology

Glossary of Terms

The examiner must have some idea of how to classify or categorize the observed physical features, and the following definitions are helpful:

Anomaly. This is synonymous with *birth defect.* An anomaly can occur as a result of various pathogenic mechanisms. These include

- *Malformation.* Caused by faulty development of a particular structure during embryogenesis. A malformation is an intrinsic defect of development. Examples include *cleft lip, anophthalmia,* and *bladder exstrophy.*
- *Deformation.* The result of a secondary effect of compression, restraint, or biomechanical distortion of an already formed body part, which usually occurs anytime after 10 fetal weeks (or even postnatally!). Examples include *clubbed feet,* a *bowed limb,* and *plagiocephaly.*
- *Disruption.* A secondary defect in which an extrinsic agent causes tissue destruction and cell death to the point where the resulting

defect looks like an anomaly. Examples include *amniotic band amputations, cleft palate* owing to *glossoptosis,* and *webbed neck* owing to nuchal *edema.*

- *Dysplasia.* This refers to abnormal development of a specific tissue. For example, an intrinsic abnormality of ectodermal development leads to one of the many forms of *ectodermal dysplasia* with effects on skin, hair, teeth, and nails.

Major anomaly. A basic alteration that is severe enough to require intervention and that has potential for long-term impact medically, surgically, and/or psychologically. Examples include *spina bifida, bilateral cleft lip/palate,* and *omphalocele.*

Minor anomaly. A defect that either requires no treatment or can be totally or mostly corrected. Examples include *metopic ridge, low-set ears, accessory nipple,* and *absent fifth finger flexion crease.* Minor anomalies can have cosmetic significance but do not generally require surgical or medical intervention.

Minor variant (in some references also called *common variant*). A low-frequency congenital feature that can occur in the normal population. It is often familial but also can be an integral part of a multiple congenital anomaly syndrome (e.g., *epicanthal folds* and *clinodactyly*).

The terminology sometimes can be confusing. Some authors use the term *minor abnormalities* and subdivide it into three groups: *minor congenital malformations, minor variants,* and *transient developmental disorders.* Others use the term *minor congenital anomalies* and subdivide it into *mild malformations* and *minor anomalies.* Yet others subdivide the term *minor variants* into *minor anomalies* and *spectrum variants.* And finally, others divide *minor variants* into *minor anomalies* and *common variants,* with the distinction being frequency and implication. Minor anomalies have a frequency of 4 percent or less, and common variants have a prevalence of greater than 4 percent. In addition, the presence of three or more minor anomalies is associated with an increased risk for the presence of one or more major anomalies. No matter the nomenclature, the presence of several minor variants (minor anomalies, etc.) should spur a search for one or more major anomalies.

In addition to single anomalies, multiple anomalies may have various terms, such as

Syndrome. A recurring pattern of anomalies (e.g., malformations, deformations, and disruptions) that allows for a secure diagnosis. The combination of features most likely represents a specific etiology.

Sequence. A situation where a single event, usually undefined, leads to a single anomaly that has a cascading effect of causing local and/or distant deformations and/or disruptions. The best example is that of *Potter sequence* secondary to whatever caused the severe, prolonged oligohydramnios with secondary *lung hypoplasia,* abnormal face with prominent infraorbital folds, and large, cartilage-deficient ears.

Association. An exclusion diagnosis in which a nonrandom occurrence of multiple anomalies cannot be explained by chance alone and that has no consistent etiology. Core features usually number six to eight; however, they rarely occur all together. At least three to four of the core features must be present to consider an "association" diagnosis. *VATER/VACTERL* association with its *v*ertebral defects, *a*nal atresia, *c*ardiac defects, *t*racheoesophageal fistula, *e*sophageal atresia, *r*enal defects, and radial *l*imb defects is a good example.

Field defect. A single (monotropic) developmental defect in an embryologic area where an error causes a major anomaly that disturbs contiguous developing structures. Most single-field defects involve midline structures such as *holoprosencephaly* with *hypotelorism* and *median cleft lip* or *exstrophy of the bladder* with *omphalocele, genital defects,* and *lumbosacral spina bifida,* as in *OEIS* complex.

Finally, although most of the preceding terms pertain to congenital findings, some individuals can have *acquired dysmorphisms.* This term indicates that the individual was phenotypically normal at birth and for some period postnatally but then started to look different and develop new external features. Metabolic disorders such as *Hurler syndrome* and *progeria* are examples. Always review photographs of the patient from birth to confirm the acquired nature of the dysmorphism. This is also true of presumed prenatal dysmorphism.

History

General Comment

In addition to obtaining historical information from infancy, childhood, and adolescence for individuals with malformations and genetic disorders, it is necessary to include a genetic family history, gestational history, and neonatal history. In no other area of medicine is such an expansive history required to optimize the opportunity for a diagnosis.

KEY HISTORY

Family The family history has equal importance at all ages. To maximize the practical value of a family history, it must be thorough and detailed. This requires time and patience. Minimally, obtain a three-generation history. It may be necessary to go further back to find similarly affected relatives. A general question asking if anyone in more remote generations had any genetic disorders or birth defects of any kind is a good initiator. Additionally, if your basic three-generation history suggests a linear inheritance pattern such as X-linked or autosomal dominant inheritance, you are obligated to ask questions about the side of the family that has potential obligate affected individuals, nonexpressing individuals, and carriers, their offspring, and *their* offsprings' offspring.

Consanguinity is important to consider because its presence increases the risk of autosomal recessive disorders. However, this clearly can be a sensitive issue. It is easiest to ask if the parents were blood-related before the marriage, are cousins, or have last names on both sides of the family that are the same. If a positive response is forthcoming, much more detail is necessary. Sometimes older relatives such as a grandmother or a great aunt may be able to give specific details. Do not routinely take the response "we're distant cousins" at face value because people are usually much more closely related than they think. Although one would like specific answers to these types of questions, some historians will balk because they think you want an *exact* answer. At this point, the questioner needs to be creative. If a family member does not know the height of a first cousin, then give him or her an alternative choice: "Is he or she as tall as you or me?" Frequently, the family member can provide a better estimate of the cousin's height in this manner.

Directive questions may be necessary to guide the interview. Mothers or primary caretakers often inadvertently state important and dynamic developmental milestones inaccurately. For instance, a hypotonic child's mother may say that he sat up at 8 months, and you know that this is not likely. You can then ask if the child had to be placed into a sitting position or if he could get there himself. If the mother says, "He couldn't get into a sitting position by himself," the child does not meet the true definition of sitting alone, which should occur between 6 and 8 months of age.

In instances of facial dysmorphism, it is critical to establish whether the child's facial features represent primary facial anomalies/ abnormalities or are familial traits. Almost invariably, the parent will say that the child looks like a relative, or when an individual trait is the issue, "he has the Jones' nose" or the "Smith's ears." This may be true, but it must be verified by either seeing those relatives or reviewing photographs of them. It is important, when possible, to have photographs of the relative at the same age as the child. Additionally, reviewing photographs of close relatives at different ages may reveal unsuspected similarities. If the patient is older, it is helpful to document through family photographs his or her facial phenotype at different ages.

When obtaining a family history, basic information includes (1) ages and/or birth dates, (2) height/weight as appropriate, (3) development (motor and intellectual) plus behavior issues, (4) general health, with emphasis on chronic illnesses, premature deaths, and cancer, (5) past surgeries and/or hospitalizations, (6) genetic disorders/ birth defects, (7) parental consanguinity, and (8) phenotype similarities. Additionally document and verify any testing of relatives if possible. This is particularly true for chromosome studies, molecular tests, metabolic evaluations, and radiologic examinations such as skeletal x-rays, CT scans/MRIs, echocardiograms, ultrasounds, and renal scans. Reports of evaluations of relatives with potentially related problems by geneticists, neurologists, ophthalmologists, orthopedists, cardiologists, nephrologists, gastroenterologists, dermatologists, developmentalists, psychiatrists/ psychologists, plastic surgeons, and neurosurgeons can be extremely useful.

▼ KEY HISTORY
▼ Gestational Before dealing with the present pregnancy involving the patient (propositus), establish the outcome of any previous pregnancies (e.g., liveborn, miscarriage, abortion, or stillbirth). Were any of

these abnormal? How? A number of malformation syndromes are associated with recurring pregnancy loss (e.g., *trisomy 18* and *Roberts' syndrome*), and some have an increased risk of occurring in future pregnancies.

The gestation involving the propositus requires all the preceding as well as documenting the maternal and paternal ages at the time of the delivery. Older maternal age (35 years and over) has a dramatically increased risk for *Down syndrome*. Older paternal age has an increased incidence of new mutations for disorders such as *achondroplasia* and *Apert syndrome*. Did the mother have any prenatal testing or procedures such as amniocentesis, chorionic villus sampling (CVS), ultrasound, and/or maternal serum screening (alpha-fetoprotein)? Did the mother have any concomitant *infectious* illness such as viral infections (e.g., cytomegalovirus), hypertension, heart problems, diabetes mellitus, seizures, or neuromuscular disorder? Drug and *toxic* environmental exposures such as prescription medicine, social drugs (e.g., tobacco or alcohol), illicit drugs (e.g., cocaine), chemicals (e.g., mercury or solvents), and metals (e.g., lead) can potentially be teratogenic. It is necessary to identify not only exposures but also the time and duration of the exposures. Most teratogens cause anomalies primarily before the tenth gestational week.

Abnormal amounts of amniotic fluid may explain abnormal findings. *Oligohydramnios* (i.e., deficient fluid) is always present with lack of urine production (e.g., *renal agenesis/Potter sequence*) or when produced urine cannot escape into the amniotic fluid (e.g., *urethral obstruction/cystic dysplastic kidneys*). *Polyhydramnios* (e.g., excessive fluid) occurs primarily when swallowed amniotic fluid cannot get to the gut for absorption (e.g., *esophageal atresia*) or when the fetus has poor swallowing (e.g., *holoprosencephaly*). It is important to note the degree of fetal activity and when it first occurred. Mothers who have had previous liveborns usually can tell you accurately if the present baby moved normally or at least at the same as in the previous pregnancies. First-time mothers have more difficulty. If you ask a primigravida about fetal activity and she is not sure, then ask if the baby's movement hurt. This usually would mean strong and/or normal fetal activity. If the mother could hardly feel any movements, this would mean diminished fetal activity in hypotonic conditions such as *Down, Prader-Willi*, and *Zellweger syndromes*. Fetal activity is usually detectable at between 4 and 5 months; consequently, any reduction in or lack of activity after 5 months is of concern (e.g., *arthrogryposis*).

Because of the common use of diagnostic ultrasounds during pregnancies, the family usually has an estimate of baby size prior to delivery. This information may contribute to a diagnosis. Complications of labor and delivery are important information because they may have an impact on or even cause a newborn's difficulties. The fetal position, particularly breech, has a high association with intrauterine hypotonia. Knowing a fetus was "fixed" in the same intrauterine position for more than 2 months may explain asymmetry of the skull as in *plagiocephaly*.

Unfortunately, all too often pregnancy and gestational events give no clues to the anomalies present at birth.

Neonatal (Birth to 30 Days) The weight, height, and head circumference are the critical birth parameters to document. Compare these data with those of siblings and parents. Asking about the child's neurologic status, particularly alertness/consciousness and degree of physical activity, will give some indication of central nervous system (CNS) function. Were there any seizures, and what was the developmental progress in the first month? If posture and muscle strength (e.g., tone) are abnormal, the child is often "bent" and/or "floppy." Be suspicious if the newborn's tone is "really good" or if he or she has "good head control" in the first week.

One should ask questions concerning the cardiorespiratory system. Was there tachypnea, apnea, labored respirations, or cyanosis? Did the child have a murmur, heart defect, or echocardiogram?

Assess alimentary function. How well did the child suck and swallow, and how much time was required to complete a feeding? Did the child have any problems with vomiting or with bowel movements? Was there surgery to repair an *esophageal atresia, duodenal atresia, imperforate anus,* or *diaphragmatic hernia*?

If any birth defects were present, where were they located, and specifically how did the medical personnel describe them? Many parents have trouble accurately describing the anomalies, so it may be necessary to review the medical records or talk to the child's physician.

Ask questions regarding hematologic abnormalities (e.g., anemia, polycythemia, or thrombocytopenia), metabolic problems (e.g., acidosis, hypoglycemia, hypo/hypercalcemia, etc.). Check if the newborn metabolic screen and hearing test results are available.

Finally, if any problems were detected in the newborn, what transpired during the first month of life, and did any new problems surface? After discharge, were there any follow-up consultations or readmissions?

Infants (Ages 1 Month to 2 Years) Obtain the present and past weights, heights, and head circumferences. Plot them on the Centers for Disease Control and Prevention (CDC) growth curves. If they are abnormal, refer to the newborn birth weight and length to determine if child had been appropriate for gestational age (AGA), large for gestational age (LGA), or small for gestational age (SGA). If the child is only postnatally growth-deficient, one can assume that there is an ongoing medical problem, or it is part of the genetic influence of the accompanying syndrome.

Document developmental milestones. If there are delays, try to determine if it is intellectual (cognitive), motor, or both. Speech development and behavior are very important additional information. Is the child receiving special services such as physical, occupational, and speech therapy? Has the patient had any formal developmental testing?

Have there been any new illnesses or surgeries? Chronic or unusual illnesses may indicate a specific disorder. Surgical interventions not anticipated during the neonatal period may be clues to an overall condition or identify an organ or cellular tissue as a component of a particular syndrome. The status of the child's hearing and vision needs repeat assessments.

If there is an ongoing diagnosis, then new findings potentially can help treatment and/or prognostication. For an unknown diagnosis, newly recognized features may improve the chances for making a specific diagnosis.

Ask which specialist/subspecialists have seen the child since the neonatal period (see listing under "Family History") because information from evaluations by specialists is extremely helpful. However, families often do not receive reports from these evaluations, so obtain consent forms for release of medical information. Establish the pattern and time of follow-up specialist visits, and do not hesitate to call a specialist for updating of recent visits.

Update all laboratory results and any new details regarding family history. An unanticipated laboratory test may give you the clue as to a specific diagnosis. Also, families represent a dynamic continuum with new babies, deaths, and intrafamilial communications, which can be most helpful. Be careful not to assume that dissimilar birth defects in a new baby are not etiologically related. Familial translocations in chromosome disorders can have two different phenotypes depending on whether the translocation carrier(s) gave the deletion or duplication.

KEY HISTORY
Childhood (Ages 2 to 12 Years) Continue to document weight and height. Have growth patterns changed? Are previously normal growth parameters now abnormal? Has the child had any workup for growth disturbance? Have there been any signs of puberty?

By 2 to 4 years of age, most children's psychomotor development will appear as normal or abnormal except in instances of mild delay or when physical factors limit the child's ability to respond accurately. Obtain copies of any formal developmental testing. Document school performance and grade level (e.g., special classes). Inquire about behavior problems such as attention deficit hyperactivity disorder (ADHD; this may suggest *neurofibromatosis type I*), autism (associated with *fragile X syndrome*), tics (suggestive of *Tourette syndrome*), sleep disturbance (consider *Smith-Magenis syndrome*), and temper tantrums (common in *Prader-Willi syndrome*).

Is the child having any new or persisting neurologic or neuromuscular difficulties such as seizures, tight "heel" cords (e.g., spasticity), high arches (e.g., as in *Charcot-Marie-Tooth syndrome*), or trouble walking up steps (e.g., as in *Duchenne muscular dystrophy*)? Are there any unexplained signs/symptoms such as headaches, loss or regression of skills, limb weakness, tremors, etc.?

Always reevaluate hearing and vision. If the child has a hearing loss, it will be necessary to find out if it is conductive (e.g., as in *Goldenhar syndrome*), sensorineural (e.g., as in *Waardenburg syndrome*), or mixed (e.g., as in *Treacher Collins syndrome*). Occasionally, a family will say that loud sounds cause their child to scream (*hyperacusis*). This is common to *Williams syndrome*. Question further any vision problems that require glasses or surgery. Always check for the presence of cataracts, glaucoma, myopia (particularly if severe), ocular palsies, and structural eye defects.

Newly recognized features and/or anomalies continue to present in childhood. They are usually cryptic and include anomalies such as pulmonary stenosis (e.g., as in *Noonan syndrome*) or supravalvular aortic stenosis (e.g., as in *Williams syndrome*), unilateral renal agenesis (e.g., as in *Klippel-Feil syndrome*), horseshoe kidney (e.g., as in *Turner syndrome*), submucous cleft palate (e.g., as in *velocardiofacial syndrome*), and agenesis of the corpus callosum (e.g., as in *acrocallosal syndrome*). Their presence may raise the possibility of a previously undiagnosed syndrome.

As before, it is necessary to review all new evaluations, laboratory studies, and family changes.

KEY HISTORY

▼Adolescents (12 to 21 Years) Document puberty and growth rate. Establishing the parents' onset and extent of their puberties and growth patterns may aid in diagnosis. Abnormalities in puberty and growth almost always occur in sex chromosome disorders such as *Turner* and *Klinefelter syndromes* but are also common in multiple congenital anomaly syndromes.

Intellectual status is generally clear by now. If mental retardation is present, it is necessary to determine if it is mild, moderate, or severe. Behavior issues such as autism, ADHD, and violent reactions and psychiatric problems such as bipolar disorder, obsessive-compulsive disorder, and schizophrenia may accompany some disorders.

New illnesses or surgeries may lack specificity but occasionally can reveal cryptic clues toward a diagnosis. For patients with diagnosed conditions, they may affect prognosis or indicate further study is needed.

The recognition of new clinical features or anomalies is less common in this group; however, you are dependent on the experience and astuteness of past observers, and caregivers may not see some of the patients in this age group regularly.

Review of the adolescent's hearing and visual status, ongoing or past evaluations (specialists or otherwise), family history changes, and results of laboratory studies continues to be important. If this is the first evaluation for a genetic and/or malformation problem, a detailed history from neonatal through adolescence is mandatory.

A good history tweaks the observer's mind and eyes, maximizing the accuracy of the physical examination and, ultimately, the potential diagnosis.

Physical Examination

General Comment

A genetic or dysmorphologic physical examination is unlike any other. Features are often subtle and require assimilation (e.g., pattern recognition) for correct categorization or diagnosis. Frequently, it is necessary to measure body areas or structures to establish if they are of normal size or of normal distance separation. Mandatory measurements are weight, height, and head circumference. Important common measurements are diagonal ear diameter, chest circumference, internipple spacing, inner canthal distance, interpupillary distance, palpebral fissure length, and total hand length (third finger and palm length). Occasional measurements would include anterior fontanel size, corneal diameter, arm span, upper segment–lower segment ratio, foot length, testicular size, and penis length. If there are normative data for the specific item in question, you should perform the measurement and avoid making a clinical judgment by intuition.

Never examine the part(s) you consider abnormal first. Stand back and observe the child before beginning the physical part of the examination. Observe the cry/voice, color, breathing pattern, posture, proportions, symmetry, and contours, as well as the child's recognition of his or her environment. Carefully examine the face. Dissect the face visually into geographic sections (FIGURE 6–1), which include (1) forehead, (2) eyes, (3) nose, (4) malar/maxillary/philtrum, (5) mouth, (6) mandible, (7) ears, (8) neck, and (9) overall appearance (gestalt). Each of these areas has sizes, proportions, and predictable positions relative to each other that can be visually and measurably comparable with family facial features and population norms. Consider ethnic and racial backgrounds when determining whether facial features are truly abnormal. See TABLE 6–1 for abnormal facial features and conditions most often associated with them.

The physical examination will vary with the age groupings (e.g., neonates, infants, children, and adolescents) and will follow the sequence of categories of general, growth, neurologic findings, cranium, face, chest/abdomen/back (i.e., trunk), genitalia, limbs (e.g., long bones, hands, and feet), and ectoderm (e.g., skin/hair).

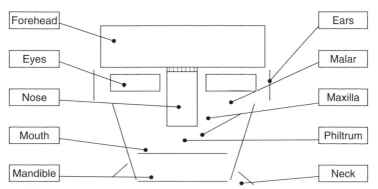

FIGURE 6–1 *Example as to How to Divide the Face into Geographic* ***Sections.*** *Each section (e.g., forehead, nose) should be examined separately for certain basic features and then related to adjacent segments. Only then should the sections be "gestalted" as a whole. The hatched area where the nasal bridge meets the forehead is the glabella.*

TABLE 6-1 *Facial Features That May Be Helpful Diagnostic Clues*

Forehead	Contributing Factors	Ex/Disorder
High/wide	Bilateral coronal synostosis	Apert syndrome
Prominent	Sagittal synostosis, macrocephaly	Neurofibromatosis
Short	Microcephaly	Seckel syndrome
Recessed	Frontal microcephaly	Holoprosencephaly

Eyes	Contributing Factors	Ex/Disorder
Up-slanted	Hypotelorism	Down syndrome
Down-slanted hypoplasia	Hypertelorism/malar Collins	Apert, Treacher
Hypotelorism	Anterior brain hypoplasia	Holoprosencephaly
Hypertelorism	? Abn./incomplete medial migration	Frontonasal dysplasia
Epicanthal folds	Unknown/?flat nasal bridge	Down syndrome
Dystopia canthorum	Unknown	Waardenburg I syndrome
Ptosis	Neurologic/muscle abnormality	Noonan syndrome
Short palpebral fisures	? Poor eye growth	Fetal alcohol syndrome (FAS)
Coloboma (iris/lid)	Failure of fusion	Isodicentric 22, Treacher Collins, Crouzon syndromes
Proptosis	Shallow orbits	Crouzon

Nose	Contributing Factors	Ex/Disorder
High bridge	Unknown	Marfan syndrome
Flat bridge	Cartilage hypoplasia	Achondroplasia
High-set nose	Missing middle third	de Lange, Williams syndromes
Parallel nose	Unknown, ? neurologic	Moebius syndrome
Prominent tip	Unknown	Velocardiofacial (VCF) syndrome
Bulbous tip	Unknown	Trichorhinophalangeal syndrome
Wide/separated nares	Incomplete facial migration	Frontonasal dysplasia

(Continued)

TABLE 6-1 *Facial Features That May Be Helpful Diagnostic Clues*
(Continued)

Malar/Maxilla	Contributing Factors	Ex/Disorder and Philtrum
Malar hypoplasia	Unknown	Treacher Collins syndrome
Maxillary hypoplasia	Craniosynostosis	Apert syndrome
Midface hypoplasia	? Skeletal dysplasia/ dysostosis	Conradi syndrome
Short philtrum	Growth deficiency	FAS, VCF
Simple philtrum	Growth disturbance	FAS
Recessed philtrum	Maxillary hypoplasia	Reiger syndrome
Prominent philtrum	Unknown	Trisomy-13 (without cleft)

Mouth	Contributing Factors	Ex/Disorder
Large mouth	Macroglossia, unknown	Beckwith-Wiedemann, Williams syndromes
Small mouth	Growth disturbance	Trisomy-18
Thin upper lip	? Growth disturbance	FAS, de Lange syndrome
Large lips	Unknown	Coffin-Lowry syndrome
Downturned corners	Unknown	Russell-Silver syndrome
Lip pits	Unknown	Van der Woude syndrome

Mandible	Contributing Factors	Ex/Disorder
Small (micrognathia)	? Vascular deficiency	Pierre Robin syndrome
Large	Hyperostosis	Craniometaphyseal syndrome
Prognathic	Fibrous dysplasia	Cherubism

Ears	Contributing Factors	Ex/Disorder
Small (not microtic)	? Growth deficiency	Down, Meier-Gorlin syndromes
Microtia	Unknown, unilateral facial microsomia	Hemifacial microsomia
Laterally protrude	Cartilage deficiency	Fragile-X syndrome
Tag/pits	Assoc. with microtia	Treacher Collins syndrome
Uplifted lobules	Nuchal edema	Turner syndrome
Attached lobules	Unknown	Roberts syndrome

(Continued)

TABLE 6–1   *Facial Features That May Be Helpful Diagnostic Clues*
(Continued)

Neck	Contributing Factors	Ex/Disorder
Short	Fused/flat vertebrae	Klippel-Feil syndrome
Web	Nuchal edema	Turner, Noonan syndromes
Low hairline	Short neck	Klippel-Feil syndrome
Clefts	Unknown	Branchio-otorenal syndrome

General	Contributing Factors	Ex/Disorder
Triangular face	? Growth aberration	Sotos, Russell-Silver syndromes
Broad/square face	Unknown, hyperostosis	Cherubism
Narrow face	Unknown, ? small facial bones	Marfan syndrome
Retracted face	Midface hypoplasia	Smith-Magenis syndrome
Expressionless	Cranial nerve abnormality	Moebius syndrome

KEY FINDING

Neonates (Birth to 1 Month)

General

Newborn infants present unique phenotypic issues. Their faces are swollen, and they have excess subcutaneous "baby fat." Interpretation of observed features must include these confounding factors. Additionally, the limbs are relatively shorter and more bowed at this age.

Growth

The birth weight and length define whether the child is too small [i.e., *intrauterine growth retardation* (IUGR)] or too large (i.e., *macrosomic*). The presence of other features in IUGR newborns such as normal head circumference, small triangular face, and short fifth fingers (e.g., *Russell-Silver syndrome*) or in macrosomic newborns with large triangular face, hypotonia, and myopathic face (e.g., *Sotos cerebral gigantism*) help to identify a syndrome etiology. *Infants of diabetic mothers* can be macrosomic, but head circumference is usually normal. Syndromic intrauterine growth aberrations can have asymmetry (e.g., hemiatrophy/hemihypoplasia of *Russell-Silver syndrome*) or hemihypertrophy (e.g., *Beckwith-Wiedemann syndrome*). Comparison of limb length, hand/foot sizes, labial size, and buttock mass and facial symmetry can show subtle differences in size. Adjacent semicircular leg creases that don't match and are not secondary to hip dislocation suggest a growth problem. Children with congenital *Marfan syndrome* and intrauterine *hyperthyroidism* have excessive lengths but low weights.

Neurologic

Muscle tone is the most important feature to evaluate in the neonate. Reduced tone (hypotonia) or increased tone (hypertonia) appears, respectively, as flaccid hyperextension or overly flexed position. In hypotonia, resistance to extension or abduction at the joints is poor. Palpate muscle mass if hypotonia is suspected because it is often reduced. Hypertonic neonates, although a rarity, will have hard, tight muscles with hyperactive reflexes and fisted hands. The loose or hypermobile joints seen in connective tissue disorders such as *Ehlers-Danlos syndrome* can mimic hypotonia. Tone abnormalities often relate to CNS dysfunction, and this mandates investigation. Tone also can change because some brain-damaged children, as well as some with syndromes (e.g., *tetrasomy 12p*), may be hypotonic initially but later become hypertonic and spastic.

A normal cry, good facial movement, good suck, alertness, and normal physical movement constitute an excellent prognosis for a normal neurologic state. High-pitched or weak cries suggest CNS problems. Poor facial movement can indicate muscular problems (e.g., *myotonic dystrophy*) or paralysis (e.g., *Moebius syndrome*). Weak suck often is associated with hypotonia (e.g., *Prader-Willi syndrome*) and decreased physical movement. Irritability can indicate brain damage and/or dysfunction or drug withdrawal.

Cranium

The most important aspects of the neonatal cranium are size (occipitofrontal head circumference), configuration (e.g., *plagiocephaly, acrocephaly, brachycephaly,* and *scaphocephaly),* fontanels, and sutures. *Microcephaly* is usually associated with a short, posteriorly recessed forehead and small fontanels. *Macrocephaly* is usually associated with a prominent and/or high/wide forehead and large fontanels. *Plagiocephaly* is an asymmetric skull with a prominence of one side of the forehead and its contralateral occiput that most often results from abnormal intrauterine position. *Acrocephaly* is a high skull associated with coronal suture fusion, and brachycephaly is a short skull with a flat occiput. Scaphocephaly is a long skull with a prominent occiput and forehead that is often associated with sagittal suture fusion and/or macrocephaly. The two major fontanels are the larger anterior fontanel at the juncture of the coronal, sagittal, and metopic sutures and the posterior fontanel at the juncture of the posterior sagittal and lambdoidal sutures. Too large a fontanel is common in macrocephalic states such as *hydrocephalus, craniosynostosis* (e.g., *Apert syndrome*), *osteogenesis imperfecta,* and *achondroplasia.* Small or absent fontanels are typical for all classes of microcephaly. Identify premature fusion of the sutures by running a fingertip over the suture. Fusion is a ridge that is palpable or borders that are flush and rigid. Overlapped suture edges can mimic fused sutures. However, they are not fused if one side of the suture is higher with the fingertip dropping downward or upward as it crosses the suture. Sutures that are too wide indicate increased CNS pressure or some space-occupying lesion. Usually, sutures are abnormally wide if a fifth fingertip can fit between the suture edges.

Face

The examination of the face will be discussed in greater detail under infancy (1 month to 2 years) because of the many confounding factors mentioned previously. Any gross defects such as cleft lip or anophthalmia will be evident immediately. Other neonatal features such as *micrognathia, microtia, hypo/hypertelorism, facial hemangioma,* or *bifid nasal tip* call for closer evaluation. However, many patients lack such obvious defects, but more subtle features appear unusual on general examination. Document each feature of concern (e.g., epicanthal folds, upslanted eyes, thin upper lip, or flat malar bones) and compare it with familial features. If nonfacial abnormalities are present (e.g., *hypertonia, hypoplastic thumb,* or *heart defect*), then odd facial features may well represent a component of a syndrome. More detailed examination of the fac*e should include an eye examination* (e.g., *coloboma* or *cataract*), *patency of the nares* (e.g., *CHARGE/choanal atresia*), and intraoral structures such as gingiva, frenulae, tongue, and palate. Compare the child's facial features with those in his or her parental background.

Chest/Back/Abdomen

The chest size and configuration are the two most important features to observe. Measure the chest circumference by placing a tape measure around the chest at the nipple level. A concomitant measure is the internipple distance straight across from the medial borders of the areola. A small chest is frequently a feature of skeletal dysplasias (e.g., *Jeune thoracic dystrophy*). Wide-spaced nipples are rare and are not truly a feature of *Turner syndrome* or conditions with chest deformities. Note the chest symmetry by the nipple placement, and palpate the pectoralis major muscles for hypo/aplasia (e.g., *Poland anomaly*). Chest indentations (e.g., pectus excavatum) and prominence (e.g., pectus carinatum) are common in some syndromes such as *Noonan* and *Coffin-Lowry syndromes*, respectively, but also occur in normal individuals. Defects in sternal fusion can be part of *pentalogy of Cantrell* (lower sternum) and in *PHACE syndrome* (upper sternum). Descriptions for overall chest configuration include tubular (e.g., *Ellis-van Creveld syndrome*), bell-shaped (e.g., *campomelic dysplasia*), and barrel-shaped (e.g., *achondrogenesis*). A flared lower rib cage may be normal, part of a skeletal dysplasia, or represent rib anomalies. Evaluation of the back is less informative in the neonate except for midline defects such as spina bifida, sinuses, hemangiomas, skin tags, and hair tufts. Any midline defect should instigate a search for abnormal neural tube closure and the effects of denervation. Spinal curvatures are hard to detect in the neonate unless they are severe. *Scoliosis, kyphosis, lordosis,* or a mixture thereof frequently occurs with abnormal vertebral formation (e.g., *Klippel-Feil, VACTERL,* and *Goldenhar syndromes*), particularly when *dyssegmentation, hemivertebra,* and *multiple fusions* have occurred. Vertebral malformations often cause shortening of the spine, but patients with skeletal dysplasias with *platyspondyly* also have short spines. Absence or hypoplasia of the sacrum can be palpable and is common in *infants of diabetic mothers.* Palpation of the spineous processes will give accurate indication of the presence of vertebral bodies.

Abdominal defects in the neonate also primarily involve the midline. Syndromic abdominal defects often include *umbilical hernias, omphalocele, gastroschisis,* and *bladder exstrophy.* Umbilical placement is usually about midway between the xyphoid and pubis. It is low set in bladder exstrophy (e.g., *OEIS complex*) or high set in omphaloceles associated with lower sternal defects. The umbilical hernia is common as an isolated defect but can occur in omphalocele-related conditions such as *Beckwith-Wiedemann syndrome.* It can be "pouty" (e.g., *Aarskog syndrome*) or raised on a mound of skin (e.g., *Beare-Stevenson syndrome*). Gastroschisis is usually not syndrome-related and is off the midline. Peritoneum does not cover the extruded abdominal contents as in an omphalocele.

Genitalia

We discuss only malformations or features associated with syndromes (not due to endocrine or sex chromosome disorders). *Hypospadias* is the most common genital malformation in syndromes such as *Smith-Lemli-Opitz syndrome, G/BBB syndrome,* and *Mowat-Wilson syndrome. Epispadias* is displacement of the urethral opening on the dorsal surface of the penis. It is always present in exstrophy of the bladder whether isolated or part of a field defect (e.g., *OEIS complex*). *Cryptorchidism* is common in many syndromes (e.g., *Noonan syndrome*), as are small testes. Large testes (macroorchidism) occur primarily in *fragile-X syndrome* but usually not until late childhood or adolescence. Scrotal hypoplasia is usually secondary to cryptorchidism and/or small testes. The small scrotum usually has poorly formed rugae. An overriding scrotum (*shawl scrotum*) is one in which the upper scrotal skin rises over the base of the penis and is a typical finding in *Aarskog syndrome. Micropenis* is associated with syndromes (e.g., *Prader-Willi syndrome*) or in association with CNS anomalies (e.g., holoprosencephaly). *Macropenis* is rare and is primarily the result of urethral atresia (e.g., *prune-belly syndrome*). Rarely, the penis displaces inferiorly into or below the scrotum (e.g., *penoscrotal transposition*). This can be associated with cloacal defects or *VACTERL*-like conditions, and some are associated with chromosome anomalies (e.g., *deletion of 13q*).

Limbs

The limbs consist of the long bones, hands, and feet divided into three segments: *rhizomelic* (proximal), which includes the humerus and femur; *mesomelic* (middle), which includes the ulna, radius, tibia, and fibula; and *acromelic,* which consists of hands and feet. When examining the limbs, the major points of concern are length, size, proportion, contour, symmetry, and mobility.

In neonates and infants, the hands (fingertips) fall between the midpelvis and the lower pelvis when the arms extend downward along the side of the body. If the hands fall above this point, the limb is short, assuming that the spine is of normal length. A number of skeletal dysplasias have flat (*platyspondyly*) vertebrae. Frequently, in disproportionate dwarfing conditions, two or more segments are short, but one is more shortened, as is the case in the *rhizomelic* shortening of achondroplasia.

Naming skeletal dysplasias such as *Langer mesomelia* and *acrodysostosis* (acromelia) derives from the segment that is the shortest. The majority of short limbs are bowed, with those having the more severe bowing also having medial flexion creases/skin folds and skin dimples over the point of maximum convexity. Reduced joint mobility presents in the knee as a contracture and in the elbows as restricted extension and supination.

Overgrowth of the limb and/or digits is rare but can occur in neurofibromatosis, *Proteus syndrome,* and *Klippel-Trenaunay syndrome.* Undergrowth is much more frequent and is a common component of proportional short stature conditions. Small hands and fingers, which are otherwise structurally normal, occur in *Russell-Silver* and *Prader-Willi syndromes.* Measure hand length by adding the palm length (distance from wrist to the base of the third finger) and third finger length (distance from the base of the third finger to the fingertip). *Brachydactyly* means "short digits" but in common usage implies short and broad digits. Most individuals with brachydactyly will have a skeletal dysplasia or dysostosis. The type of brachydactyly is determined by the pattern of phalanges that are short (types A to E), and confirmation requires x-rays. Certain nonclassic skeletal disorders such as pseudohypoparathyroidism and *Turner syndrome* have 4-5 metacarpal shortening, which is evident clinically by the corresponding knuckles sinking down with the hand fisted.

If there are an abnormal number of digits, determine which ones are involved? Polydactyly and oligodactyly can be postaxial (fifth finger side), preaxial (thumb side), or central (midline of hand). The same classification applies to the feet. Postaxial polydactyly is the most common type (e.g., as in *Bardet-Biedl syndrome*). Preaxial polydactyly is the next most common type (e.g., in *infants of diabetic mothers* and in *Townes-Brocks syndrome*). Central polydactyly is rare (e.g., *oral-facial-digital syndrome type VI* and *Pallister-Hall syndrome*). *Oligodactyly* is most common on the preaxial side but only on the hand (e.g., as in *Fanconi anemia*), and it is often associated with radial hypo/agenesis. Generally, there is a reduction of thenar mass with even mild thumb hypoplasia. *Postaxial oligodactyly* usually involves primarily the fifth finger, which is rarely missing but is hypoplastic or short (e.g., *Feingold syndrome, ulna-mammary syndrome*). *Central oligodactyly* occurs primarily in split hand–split foot (*lobster claw, ectrodactyly*) syndrome and at least involves the area of the third and fourth digits with a residual cleft. Occasionally, all digits can be missing.

Syndactyly (webbing) of the second and third toes is very common among otherwise normal individuals, as well as in those with certain syndromes (e.g., *Smith-Lemli-Opitz syndrome,* in which the frequency of 2-3 syndactyly is over 90 percent). In the hand, various patterns of syndactyly (e.g., 2-3, 3-4, 4-5, and 1-2 in order of frequency) can occur as regular patterns in specific syndromes. More fingers (2-4 and 3-5) can be syndactylous, and in Apert syndrome all fingers may be webbed (mitten type). The main difference with the toes is that 1-2 syndactylies are more common than 1-2 finger syndactylies.

Nail abnormalities (hypoplasia, absence), camptodactyly (bent, flexed fingers), *arthrogryposis* (multiple joint contractures), and flexion/extension creases are other conditions requiring evaluation. Consult a text for more detail.

Skin

In the neonate, one is mostly interested in gross anomalies involving skin color, pigment, vessels, texture, edema, and hair. Besides observing the skin from a distance, run the underside of your fingers across the child's skin to get a feel for the texture. Most gross skin anomalies would be in the form of scalp defects (e.g., trisomy 13), cutis aplasia elsewhere on the body, tags, bullae (e.g., epidermolysis bullosa), scars (e.g., amniotic bands), and pits/dimples. Excessive redness of the skin could be due to polycythemia (e.g., Down syndrome). Hypopigmentation (e.g., *albinism*), hyperpigmentation (e.g., *incontinentia pigmenti* or *giant hairy nevus*), and localized hemangiomas (e.g., *Sturge-Weber syndrome*) are usually obvious in the newborn period. Very thick, scaly skin suggests some sort of *ichthyosis,* and very smooth skin, a connective tissue disorder. Localized nuchal and pedal edema is common in *Turner syndrome,* and generalized leg and hand/foot edema is typical for *Milroy disease.* Hypotrichosis (sparse hair) of the scalp, eyebrows, and eyelashes suggests *X-linked hypohidrotic ectodermal dysplasia,* and *generalized hypertrichosis* (excessive amount and abnormal location of hair) is a major feature of *Cornelia de Lange syndrome.*

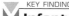
KEY FINDING

Infants (Ages 1 Month to 2 Years)

Growth

Repeat procedures under "Neonatal History." Pay closer attention to rate of growth when plotting the growth curves. There are curves specific for growth rate available. In the absence of a nutritional intake problem, a dropoff or flat-lining of weight gain or height suggests an endocrine problem. Excessive edema, particularly around the eyes, plus increased lethargy, might suggest hypothyroidism. Truncal obesity and a high-pitched voice could represent pituitary and growth hormone deficiency. Note body proportions.

Neurologic

Developmental milestone abnormalities indicate potential neurologic problems. Reflexes and intraocular examination are now practical and more accurate. In particular, observe cranial contour and size plus suture and fontanel status. Tone and muscle mass need constant reevaluation. Always check coordination/balance in the ambulatory infant. Alertness and recognition of the environment may identify potential problems. Volume and quality of speech are especially important to establish.

Face

The face, if abnormal, offers the quickest and most accurate avenue to a diagnosis. It is during infancy that facial features become more representative of the child's ultimate facial features. It is also during this period that the skin thickens, hair patterns and color become better defined, and permanent eye color emerges.

FIGURE 6–1 divides the face into previously mentioned segments, each with the most common and/or pertinent features noted in dysmorphologic examinations. When possible, subsequent illustrations include contributing factors that set the stage for that feature's presence. It is very important to remember that most of these listed individual features are present as normal variants in the general population and that they represent abnormalities only by differing from their normal family background. *Treacher Collins syndrome* (FIGURE 6–2) demonstrates malar hypoplasia, down-slanted eyes, lower lid coloboma, and microtia. *Velocardiofacial* syndrome (FIGURE 6–3) illustrates high nasal bridge, short philtrum, abnormal nasal tip, and small mouth. *Conradi syndrome* (FIGURE 6–4) shows flat nasal bridge, high-set nose, and long philtrum. *Sotos* syndrome and *Russell-Silver syndrome* (FIGURE 6–5) reveal triangular face (both), thin upper lip (Russell-Silver), and laterally protruding ears (both).

Chest/Back/Abdomen

With less subcutaneous fat, the true size of the chest and its configuration become more obvious; however, the examination remains similar to that of the neonate. Sometimes pectus deformities develop that were not present before. Note absence or hypoplasia of the clavicles (*cleidocranial dysplasia*), which allows the shoulders to droop and rotate anteriorly, making the upper chest look narrow. *Accessory (supernumerary)*

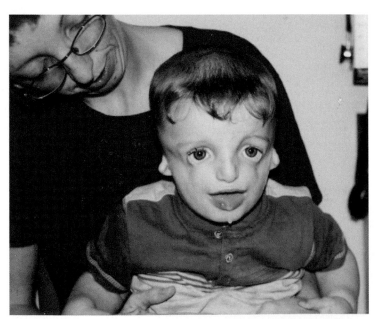

FIGURE 6–2 A Boy with Treacher Collins Syndrome. *Note (1) triangular face, (2) high, wide forehead, (3) high nasal bridge, (4) down-slanted eyes and droopy lower eyelids secondary to malar hypoplasia, (5) prominent nasal tip, (6) thin upper lip, (7) everted lower lip, and (8) microtia.*

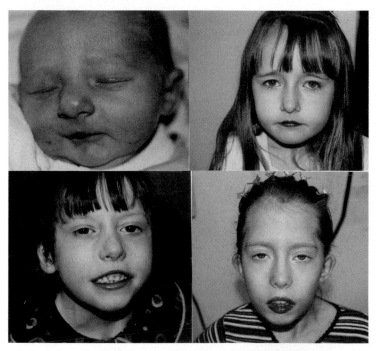

FIGURE 6–3 *Four Children with Velocardial Facial (VCF) Syndrome.*
Upper left: (1) High nasal bridge, (2) full nasal tip and small jaw (micrognathia),
and (3) slight cupid bow mouth contour. Upper right: (1) Prominent nasal tip,
(2) parallel nasal contour from high nasal bridge to nasal tip, and (3) slight
cupid bow mouth contour. Lower left: (1) High nasal bridge, (2) prominent and
full nasal tip, (3) short, simple philtrum, and (4) inverted V-shaped mouth con-
tour. Lower right: (1) Mild ptosis, (2) high nasal bridge, (3) prominent nasal
tip, (4) short, simple philtrum, (5) small mouth, and (6) small ears (microtia).

nipples, which occur normally in 5 percent of the general population, are
visible along the mammary line as dark gray spots with a thin central
crease.

The back examination is similar to that at other ages, but curvature
is easier to see. Look carefully for a localized but more extreme form of
kyphosis in the lower thoracic and upper lumbar region. This is a *gibbus* deformity and occurs with vertebral defects in that region or with
metabolic storage disorders such as *Hurler* and *Hunter syndromes.* Defects
of the vertebral bodies of the cervical spine can be a consequence of *Sprengel deformity,* in which a poorly anchored scapula displaces superiorly.
Small/hypoplastic scapulae occur in campomelic dysplasia. Recheck
midline dimples and pits for drainage.

Except for the possibility of a developing umbilical or inguinal hernia,
the abdominal examination does not change much from the neonatal

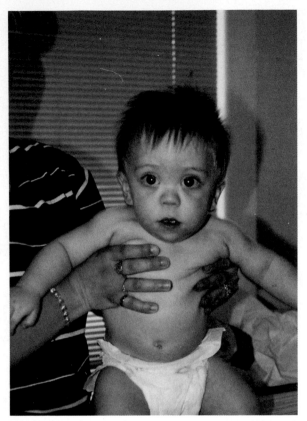

FIGURE 6–4 *A Young Infant with Conradi Syndrome (chondrodysplasia punctata).* Note (1) high, wide forehead, (2) very flat nasal bridge, (3) high-set nose with secondarily long philtrum, (4) epicanthal folds, (5) upslanted right eye, (6) small mouth, and (7) micrognathia.

examination. Reevaluation of the abdomen for visceromegaly and masses is mandatory.

Genitalia

There should be no major changes since infancy. It is always important to check for testicular descent.

Limbs

Proportions are now easier to judge as the child thins out and begins to attain adult proportions. Previous bowing needs some quantitation to determine any changes. Assess joint mobility at each visit. Are the Achilles tendons tight, and has the foot position worsened, as in secondary pes cavus and/or equinovarus? Reevaluate muscle mass and

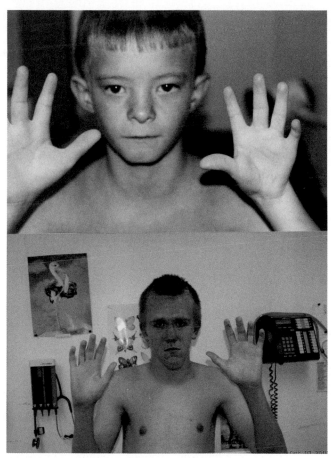

FIGURE 6–5 Two Boys with Triangular Facies. *(Above) A child with Russell-Silver dwarfism. Note (1) triangular small face, (2) simple philtrum, and (3) thin upper lip. (Below) A large male with Sotos syndrome (cerebral gigantism). Note (1) large triangular face, (2) high nasal bridge, and (3) large mandible (prognathism).*

tone. Palpate for the presence and size of the patella (e.g., absent patella in the *nail-patella syndrome*). Look at the digits for flexion (*camptodactyly*) or deviation (*clinodactyly*) plus discrepancy in length and abnormal dorsal and ventral flexion and extension creases. Subtle webs or syndactyly may be more evident.

Ectoderm (Skin)

The skin is continually changing. Wrinkles and creases may appear (e.g., *cutis laxa, Ehlers-Danlos syndrome, DeBarsy geroderma osteodysplastica*), suggesting premature aging. Thinning of the skin can suggest collagen defects (e.g., *Ehlers-Danlos syndrome, type 4*) and allows subcutaneous blood vessels to become readily visible. Thick skin can suggest storage diseases, edema, or hyperkeratosis. Tight skin (e.g., as in *mandibuloacral dysplasia*) is most unusual and deserves attention. Raised or pedunculated skin lesions (neurofibromas) may indicate *neurofibromatosis*. Increasing nevi and café-au-lait spots also suggest *neurofibromatosis*. Hypopigmented streaks along the lines of Blaschko (e.g., *hypomelanosis of Ito*) and a similar distribution of hyperpigmented streaks (e.g., *incontinentia pigmenti*) are of concern. Raised, rough, and linear brownish yellow streaks are likely to represent linear sebaceous nevus syndrome. Pigment located in unusual places such as the penis (e.g., *Bannayan-Riley-Ruvalcaba syndrome*) or axilla (e.g., *Rabson-Mendenhall syndrome*) is always important to pursue. Observe any new rashes, such as facial telangiectatic spots (e.g., *Bloom syndrome*), facial "butterfly distribution" of a red rash (e.g., *tuberous sclerosis* or *lupus*), or a mottled red rash (e.g., *Rothmund-Thomson syndrome*) on the face and body. Changes in the amount of scalp, eyebrow/eyelash, and body hair suggest an ongoing process that may alter the phenotype dramatically.

▼ KEY FINDING
M Children (2 to 12 Years) No major changes in examination. Growth, development, and maturation continue to be dynamic changes that demand regular scrutiny.

▼ KEY FINDING
M Adolescents (12 to 20 Years) No major changes in examination. Increased facial bone growth, particularly in the mandible; facial hair growth and thicker skin alter the male's facial gestalt tremendously. Obesity may alter the appearance of both males and females. Puberty and the development of secondary sexual characteristics dominate this period. Inadequate breast development plus short stature would suggest *Turner syndrome*. Small testes in the presence of tall or normal stature and truncal obesity are typical of *Klinefelter syndrome*. Large testes in a boy with laterally protruding ears, triangular face, and mental retardation suggest the need for a workup of *fragile-X syndrome*.

Summary of Findings

Determine what features are primary (anomalies) and which are secondary (deformation, disruption). If one of the anomalous features is very rare and/or unique, consult a text for associated syndromes. After that, add the other primary features and see if the pattern matches any of the associated syndromes. Often, a rare feature is not present, and you must evaluate all features as an overall pattern to see if it matches a known syndrome or condition. Occasionally, deformational or disrupted features, when added to the anomalies, can be the pivotal factor in establishing a recognizable pattern (see additional reading list for excellent resources to complete this approach successfully). Diagnostic computer programs that are excellent include the London Database and

POSSUM. Initial examination does not reveal a diagnosis in up to 33 percent of children with multiple congenital anomalies. Repeated follow-up evaluation remains the best aid to the diagnostician.

Confirmatory Laboratory Evaluation

Various tests are available to either determine the cause of a child's anomalies or to confirm a suspected diagnosis. Investigative testing includes chromosome analysis, subtelomere *fluorescent in situ hybridization* (FISH) probes, metabolic screening, and a newer technique called *comparative genomic hybridization* (CGH). In the case of a suspected diagnosis, specific tests include FISH probes, mutation analysis, skeletal radiographs, biochemical studies, and others. See TABLE 6–2 for a list of some of the most common syndromes and confirmatory diagnostic testing.

When to Refer

There are two major indications for referral: diagnostic and educational. Refer to a dysmorphologist (generally a clinical geneticist) if a diagnosis is not apparent after repeated examinations and routine diagnostic testing. In this case, a referral to a dysmorphologist (generally a clinical geneticist) may be helpful in achieving a diagnosis. The dysmorphologist often has resources not readily available to the general pediatrician. After definitive diagnosis, referral to a genetics center for counseling about recurrence risks, prognosis, information about participation in research studies, etc. is especially helpful to the family.

TABLE 6-2 *Common Conditions and Appropriate Testing, If Any*

Condition	Diagnostic Testing	Comment
Down syndrome	Karyotype	Diagnosis based on clinical manifestations
VACTERL association	No testing available	
Fetal alcohol syndrome	No testing available	Significant maternal alcohol consumption necessary
Fragile-X syndrome	Molecular testing to determine CGG repeat number	>99% have a CGG expansion in the gene; <1% have a point mutation or other alteration
Klinefelter syndrome	Karyotype	
Fetal hydantoin syndrome	No testing available	Maternal ingestion of hydantoin
Noonan syndrome	*PTPN11, KRAS* gene testing	50% have a detectable mutation in *PTPN11*; 10% have a detectable mutation in *KRAS*
Velocardiofacial syndrome	FISH probe for 22q11	>95% of those with clinical manifestations of this syndrome have a detectable deletion
Diabetic embryopathy	No testing available	Maternal diabetes during pregnancy
Neurofibromatosis I	NF1 molecular testing	Protein truncation testing identifies ~80% of mutations; sequence analysis identifies ~90% of mutations
Turner syndrome	Karyotype	
Goldenhar syndrome	No testing available	Likely heterogeneous
Trisomy-18	Karyotype	
Marfan syndrome	*Fibrillin 1* mutation analysis	Mutations found in 70–93% of those with Marfan syndrome; however, *fibrillin 1* mutations also cause numerous other conditions, so may not be helpful as a diagnostic test; mutations in *TGFBR1* and *TGFBR2* cause conditions that resemble Marfan syndrome

Stickler syndrome	Mutation analysis of *COL2A1*, *COL11A1*, or *COL11A2*	In those with a Stickler syndrome phenotype, a mutation in one of these three genes is found in 70–80%.
Trisomy-13	Karyotype	
Cornelia de Lange syndrome	*NIPBL* mutation analysis	50% have a detectable mutation
Ehlers-Danlos syndrome (EDS)	Biochemical or molecular testing of collagen, depending on the type of EDS	Detection rate depends on the type of EDS; mutations found in 30–50% of those with EDS I or II; biochemical analysis identifies collagen abnormalities in >95% of those with EDS IV
Sotos syndrome	*NSD1* mutation analysis	80–90%
Beckwith-Wiedemann syndrome	Molecular genetic testing, but various causes including UPD, methylation abnormalities, gene mutations	Detection rate depends on testing that is done. *Note:* A karyotype will identify a chromosome 11 abnormality in 1% or fewer of those with BWS.
Osteogenesis imperfecta	Radiographs, collagen testing	Mutations found in 100% of those with OI I, 98% of those with OI II, 60–70% of those with OI III, and 70–80% of those with OI IV
Prader-Willi syndrome	Methylation studies of 15q	>99% detection rate
Achondroplasia	Skeletal radiographs, mutation analysis of *FGFR3*	Radiographs will make the diagnosis in most; if mutation analysis is done, >99% will have an identifiable mutation

(Continued)

TABLE 6-2 *Common Conditions and Appropriate Testing, If Any (Continued)*

Condition	Diagnostic Testing	Comment
Saethre-Chotzen syndrome	Mutation analysis of *TWIST1*	46–80% have an identifiable mutation
Tuberous sclerosis	Mutation analysis of *TSC1* and *TSC2*	70–80% will have an identifiable mutation in either gene; 20–30% will have no mutations identified
Angelman syndrome	Methylation studies of 15q; *UBE3A* mutation analysis if methylation studies negative	78% will have an abnormality of methylation; 11% have detectable mutations of *UBE3A*
CHARGE syndrome	*CHD7* gene testing	~70% of those with clinical features of CHARGE syndrome have an identifiable mutation
Williams syndrome	FISH probe of 7q	Deletions found in >99% with a clinical diagnosis of Williams syndrome
Smith-Lemli-Opitz syndrome	Serum 7-dehydrocholesterol determination	>99% will have elevated levels of 7-DHC
Rett syndrome	*MECP2* gene testing, either via mutation analysis or quantitative PCR	80% have an identifiable mutation; 16% have an identifiable deletion
Kabuki syndrome	No testing available	
Smith-Magenis syndrome	FISH probe of 17p11.2, mutation analysis of *RAI1* if FISH probe negative	90% have an identifiable deletion; 5% or fewer have a mutation of *RAI1*

The Eyes, Ears, Nose, Throat, Neck, and Oral Examination

Elyssa R. Peters, Monte Del Monte, Jonathan Gold, Ashir Kumar, and Joseph A. D'Ambrosio

EYE EXAMINATION

The goals of this section are

1. To outline the physiology, mechanics, and pathophysiology that produce signs and symptoms of diseases of the eye and visual system in childhood
2. To outline the functional anatomy as it relates to these signs and symptoms
3. To catalogue the key problems, signs, and symptoms in infants, children, and adolescents and discuss important similarities and differences
4. To learn the key examination techniques to complete a physical examination related to the eye and ocular adnexa
5. To create a list of ocular diagnoses in a table and to compare their occurrence in each age group
6. To outline confirmatory laboratory, imaging, procedures, and referral criteria

Physiology and Mechanics

The ocular system in infants and children is a combination of the brain and, as its extension, the eyes. Infants are not born with normal vision or binocular vision. They develop it by a normal process of complex communication and feedback from the brain as the eye interprets the world. This requires an interaction of cranial nerves and the autonomic nervous system with the brain to allow a properly focused clear single image to fall on the retina and then be transmitted to the appropriate areas of the brain. Understanding the normal development of this interaction is important in order to recognize ocular disease and dysfunction.

Six of the 12 cranial nerves are involved in ocular physiology and mechanics. Cranial nerve II, the optic nerve, allows afferent input for visual stimuli, as well as pupillomotor activity. Electrical impulses from the retina travel via cranial nerve II through the optic chiasm, the temporal and parietal lobes of the brain, and ultimately, to the occipital cortex to begin the process of translation into vision. Cranial nerve III, the oculomotor nerve, innervates the medial, superior, and inferior rectus muscles, as well as the inferior oblique muscle, and the levator palpebrae superioris elevates the upper eyelid. Additionally, cranial nerve III carries the parasympathetic afferent input of the pupillomotor muscle fibers in the iris, which dilate the pupil. Cranial nerve IV, the trochlear nerve, innervates the superior oblique muscle. Because of its long, unprotected course from the superior brain stem along the side to exit the cranial vault inferior to the brain stem, this is the most likely nerve affected by trauma. Cranial nerve V, the trigeminal nerve, is responsible for sensory input from the cornea and eyelids. The sympathetic nerve supply to the eye, involved in vasomotor and pupillomotor function, travels via the trigeminal nerve. Cranial nerve VI, the abducens nerve, provides innervation to the lateral rectus muscle. It also has a long course beneath the brain stem along the floor of the cranium, which makes it vulnerable to ischemic injury and palsy caused by brain swelling after a closed-head injury. Lastly, cranial nerve VII, the facial nerve, has both motor and sensory functions. These nerves, as well as the afferent limb of the corneal sensory reflex, supply the eyelid orbicularis muscles, which close the eyes.

Functional Anatomy

The most external portion of the ocular system is the eyelid. The muscular component of the eyelid includes the orbicularis muscles, Muller's muscle, and the levator palpebrae superioris. These muscles all act in opening and closing the eyelid. Proper closure of the eyelid is important to protect the anterior external structure of the eye, including the cornea and conjunctiva. Additionally, these muscles act as a "lacrimal pump" in tear drainage via the nasolacrimal system. Improper position of the eyelid also can provide clues to potential problems with these muscles and the nerves that supply them, as well as the sympathetic and parasympathetic nervous system.

The eyelids cover the sclera, conjunctiva, and cornea. The sclera acts as a rigid framework for the globe. The cornea is a clear five-layer structure (corneal epithelium, Bowman's membrane, stroma, Descemet's membrane, and endothelium) that allows for the entry and refraction of light to focus an image onto the retina. In fact, the corneal surface, not the lens, provides the major refractive power of the eye, accounting for over two-thirds. In conjunction with the eyelids, goblet cells in the conjunctiva, which cover the sclerae (bulbar) as well as line the inner eyelid (palpebral), help to provide the proper moistening and lubricating composition of the tear film. The anterior chamber boundaries are the posterior aspect of the cornea, the aqueous drainage system in the anterior chamber angle, and the anterior aspect of the iris and lens. The anterior chamber consists of aqueous humor, a product of the ciliary epithelium in the posterior chamber. It flows through the pupil into the anterior chamber and drains out via the trabecular meshwork into Schlem's canal. This aqueous humor provides nourishment for the cornea and lens, and the relationship between its production and drainage is responsible for maintaining the normal intraocular pressure in the eye (FIGURE 7–1A–C). Increased production (rare) or, more commonly, reduced outflow (drainage) of aqueous humor from the eye causes the elevated intraocular pressure that leads to glaucoma.

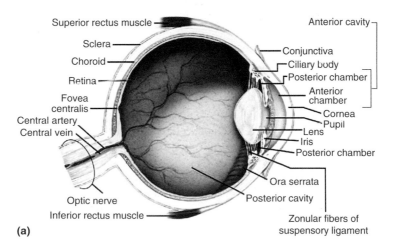

(a)

Labels: Superior rectus muscle, Sclera, Choroid, Retina, Fovea centralis, Central artery, Central vein, Optic nerve, Inferior rectus muscle, Anterior cavity, Conjunctiva, Ciliary body, Posterior chamber, Anterior chamber, Cornea, Pupil, Lens, Iris, Posterior chamber, Ora serrata, Posterior cavity, Zonular fibers of suspensory ligament

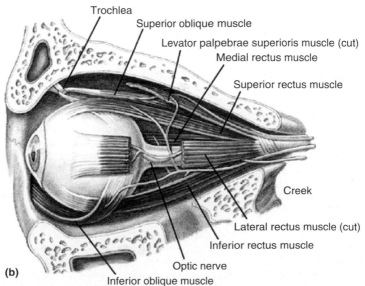

(b)

Labels: Trochlea, Superior oblique muscle, Levator palpebrae superioris muscle (cut), Medial rectus muscle, Superior rectus muscle, Creek, Lateral rectus muscle (cut), Inferior rectus muscle, Optic nerve, Inferior oblique muscle

FIGURE 7–1 *A. Anatomy of the Eye. B. External Eye Muscles. C. Neural Pathways for Vision.*

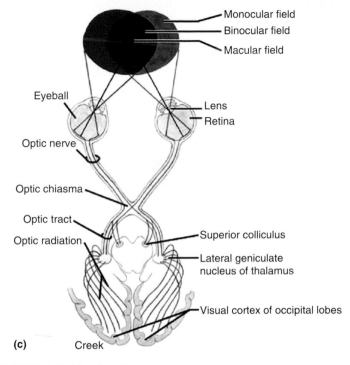

FIGURE 7–1 *(Continued)*

The lens, lens zonules, and ciliary body divide the eye into anterior and posterior portions or segments. The lens functions to further refract light, so its clarity is of utmost importance for clear vision. Additionally, the lens is able to change shape to provide *accommodation*, i.e., focus images at different distances clearly on the retina. Posterior to the lens is the posterior segment of the eye, made up of the ciliary body, the vitreous, the retina, and the optic nerve. The ciliary body, as mentioned previously, secretes aqueous humor and, in addition, contains the ciliary muscle that contracts to change the shape of the lens, allowing for focus and accommodation.

TABLE 7–1 *Actions of the Extraocular Muscles*

Muscle	Primary	Secondary	Tertiary
Medial rectus	Adduction		
Lateral rectus	Abduction		
Inferior rectus	Depression	Extorsion	Adduction
Superior rectus	Elevation	Intorsion	Adduction
Inferior oblique	Extorsion	Elevation	Abduction
Superior oblique	Intorsion	Depression	Abduction

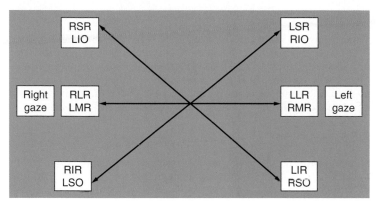

FIGURE 7-2 *Major Field of Action of the Extraocular Muscles.*

The vitreous gel provides a structural framework for the posterior segment of the globe. The posterior sclera is lined by the choroid and retina, where translation of visual images to neural impulses occurs, which then are transported to the brain. The retina is composed of 10 neural and structural layers. In order for visual information to pass through the retina from the photoreceptors of the outermost layer to the ganglion cells of the inner layer to the optic nerve, all 10 layers must be intact and functioning well. The optic nerve provides the connection of the eye to the brain, which interprets and translates information.

The extraocular muscles are of special importance to the pediatrician examining the eye. There are seven extraocular muscles, including the medial, inferior, lateral, and superior rectus muscles (MR, IR, LR, and SR), the superior and inferior oblique muscles (SO, IO), and the levator palpebrae superioris (discussed earlier). TABLE 7–1 shows the actions of each of these muscles.

Each muscle has a yoke muscle in the opposite eye that provides conjugate movements of both eyes to a specific gaze position, maintaining alignment and binocular vision (FIGURE 7–2). Note that this figure demonstrates a functional approach (visual fields) in contradistinction to the purely anatomic approach (ocular positioning) illustrated in Chapter 12. Disruption or imbalance of any of the extraocular muscles by palsy or mechanical restriction can lead to diplopia, strabismus, and amblyopia.

Taking a History

The key details of the history for the ocular system vary depending on the age of the patient. Infants and younger children require that the parents report much of the history. However, as children mature, they often can report key details of their own ocular history.

Infants

When obtaining history from the parents regarding the ocular system, the first question, as with any medical evaluation, is the chief complaint or reason for the visit. Once this is determined, obtain the basic historical details, including age at onset and duration of the problem. Birth, past medical, and family histories are important to obtain by detailed specific questioning because they may affect the diagnosis and treatment.

Children

Similar historical clues are obtainable from the parents for younger children who are unable to communicate the problem. However, as the child becomes able to verbalize, he or she is often quite adept at describing symptoms.

Adolescents

Adolescents most often can describe their problems, but it is essential to continue to allow the parent to add any significant history deemed relevant.

Key Problems

Infants

KEY PROBLEM

Poor Tracking Parents often bring their infant to the office because they believe the child is not fixing on or following objects. Very young infants may be too sleepy to fix and follow much of the time, but most normal infants will fix and follow briskly when alert, even from the first week of life. Poor tracking may be an indication of poor vision from any number of causes, such as cataracts, retinal dystrophy, intraocular tumors, and optic nerve problems. However, another cause of decreased visual function during the first 4 to 6 months of life is delayed visual maturation. This uncommon condition demonstrates very poor or nonexistent visual behavior in a generally otherwise healthy infant that resolves spontaneously by 9 to 12 months of age, with normal visual development thereafter. If a detailed ophthalmic or systemic examination does not detect an ocular abnormality, then watchful waiting for spontaneous resolution is appropriate for the first year.

KEY PROBLEM

Tearing Excess tearing is a common problem among infants, present in up to 5 to 7 percent of normal newborns. It may be due to ocular allergies. It is also frequently a product of *congenital nasolacrimal duct obstruction,* which often resolves by 6 to 12 months of age spontaneously or with conservative lacrimal sac massage. If tearing from this condition persists beyond this time, then nasolacrimal duct probing in the office or under light anesthesia is curative in 90 percent of patients. However, tearing also can be a sign of *congenital glaucoma,* a more serious and urgent ocular condition. Associated signs of corneal enlargement, corneal clouding, or photophobia suggest a diagnosis of infantile glaucoma, which requires urgent referral to a pediatric ophthalmologist for further diagnostic evaluation and treatment to prevent permanent visual loss or blindness.

KEY PROBLEM
Ocular Misalignment Many newborn infants will have mild small-angle intermittent *esotropia* or *exotropia* that will resolve with visual system maturation by 4 to 6 weeks of age. However, true strabismus, such as congenital esotropia, generally presents between 4 and 6 months of age. Additionally, pathologic strabismus may develop from congenital cranial nerve palsy or as part of a systemic or genetic disorder. In fact, ocular misalignment accompanying neurologic symptoms may be a sign of an intracranial process or malignant intraocular tumor such as retinoblastoma, requiring prompt further evaluation to prevent serious injury or death.

KEY PROBLEM
"Pink Eye" An infant presenting with a "pink eye" lends to a wide differential diagnosis. Viral, mild bacterial, and allergic *conjunctivitis* all can present with the nonspecific sign of "pink eye." Consider etiologic agents such as *Neisseria gonorrhoeae* and *Chlamydia trachomatis.* A number of more worrisome diagnoses also must be considered, including *uveitis, orbital cellulitis, endophthalmitis, foreign body, retinoblastoma,* and *leukemia.*

KEY PROBLEM
Corneal Clouding This is a serious problem in infancy that requires immediate attention. A full list of diagnostic possibilities is beyond the scope of this section, but it is important to consider *congenital/genetic* (e.g., *trisomies; Marfan, Alport,* and *Lowe syndromes;* and many others), *metabolic* (e.g., *galactosemia, glycogen storage disease, mucopolysaccharidoses, steroid exposure,* etc.), *infectious* (e.g., TORCH) etiologies.

KEY PROBLEM
White Pupil *Leukocoria,* or white pupil, also has a wide differential diagnosis. It may be a sign of *cataract, Coats disease,* severe *uveitis, intraocular toxacariasis, retinal detachment,* or *intraocular tumor*—the most worrisome of which is *retinoblastoma.* A family history is essential when considering the possibility of retinoblastoma; however, the majority of cases are sporadic. Because of diagnoses that are serious, proper evaluation of leukocoria requires urgent referral to an ophthalmologist who has the specialized skills and equipment to make a diagnosis quickly and accurately and to plan treatment.

● KEY PROBLEM
Abnormal Eye Movements
Abnormal eye movements include wandering or searching eye and nystagmus. The most common cause of horizontal nystagmus is *idiopathic congenital nystagmus*. Very poor vision from any cause, present during the first 3 months of life, can lead to *sensory* or *searching nystagmus*. Nystagmus, often with characteristic patterns, in the presence of good vision can indicate a systemic illness such as *neuroblastoma* (opsoclonus) or an intracranial process such as *chiasmal glioma* or *Arnold-Chiari malformation* (down-beating nystagmus).

● KEY PROBLEM
Difference in Pupil Size
Anisocoria is a difference in pupil size between the two eyes. It could be simply physiologic or could be evidence for systemic disease. It is important to know if this has been present since birth or acquired. If acquired, was there an inciting event, or was it spontaneous? In a patient with physiologic anisocoria, the pupil difference is the same in bright light as it is in dark illumination.

● KEY PROBLEM
Ocular Trauma
Trauma, blunt or penetrating, can affect all parts of the eye. When obtaining a specific history, one always must consider nonaccidental injury in *child abuse* and evaluate further.

● KEY PROBLEM
Orbital Tumor/Mass
Many orbital tumors may present in infancy. The differential diagnosis includes *hemangioma, lymphangioma, eyelid* or *orbital dermoid, neurofibroma, preseptal* or *orbital cellulitis*, and *optic nerve glioma*. Obstruction of the nasolacrimal duct (mucocele) or infection will cause swelling in the inner canthal area. Each has a specific presentation and characteristic appearance that will lead to the diagnosis.

● KEY PROBLEM
Anomalous Head Posture
A head tilt (*torticollis*) or head turn can be due to muscular or neurologic disorders. However, it is important to identify ocular causes of torticollis because they require specific treatment. These include certain strabismus syndromes (*Duane syndrome, Brown syndrome, Möbius syndrome*, others), *third, fourth, and sixth cranial nerve palsy, ptosis,* and *null-point nystagmus*.

Children

● KEY PROBLEM
Poor Vision
Poor vision in children has many etiologies. Simple decreased vision is often due to a *refractive error*. *Amblyopia* is poor vision in one or both eyes from disuse, without an organic origin. Amblyopia can be due to strabismus, anisometropia, or visual deprivation from cataract or other visual axis anomalies that block the formation of a clear image in one or both eyes during the critical period of vision

development. Factitious visual loss begins to present in this age group. Thorough questioning concerning recent stresses involving school performance, social difficulties, family changes, or recent acquisition of new glasses by family or close friends may suggest the diagnosis. Specialized techniques to distract or "trick" the child into demonstrating better visual performance than initially suspected are the key to clinching the proper diagnosis and avoiding expensive and risky workups. Additionally, a full ocular examination is important to rule out other diseases within the ocular system, including corneal disease, *cataract*, and retinal or optic nerve disorders.

KEY PROBLEM

Ocular Misalignment Any type of *strabismus* can occur in children. Children often present with accommodative, or refractive, *esotropia* from 1 to 4 years of age. The onset of intermittent exotropia is also common in this age group. A unique entity to consider is acute-onset benign esotropia caused by a postviral sixth nerve palsy, which can distinguish itself by history and resolution over the course of 6 to 12 weeks. See further discussions of strabismus below.

KEY PROBLEM

"Pink Eye" The "pink eye" in older children can be due to any cause of mild *conjunctivitis,* including bacterial or viral *infection* or allergic reaction. However, conditions that are more serious also may present as a "pink eye" in this age group, including *uveitis,* corneal *foreign body,* or *traumatic abrasion.* These require a more thorough examination if suspected.

KEY PROBLEM

Eye Pain Eye pain in a child accompanies many problems, including *corneal abrasion,* severe *conjunctivitis, uveitis, pediatric migraine,* and *sinus disease.* A good history will give the clinician an idea of the inciting factors, previous trauma or headache, other systemic symptoms, *juvenile rheumatoid arthritis,* or prior exposure to *infective* conjunctivitis. It is important to note the type of pain. Sharp pain or foreign-body sensation may be associated with corneal abrasion or conjunctivitis, whereas a dull, aching pain suggests *migraine* headache or referred sinus pain. Photophobia associated with eye pain suggests *iritis.*

KEY PROBLEM

Headache Children often present with the complaint of frequent headaches. While most childhood headaches are probably due to tension or stress, one must consider pediatric *migraines* in this age group. Pediatric migraine is associated (more frequently than adult migraine is) with nausea, vomiting, and a positive family history. Visual symptoms, including an aura, visual distortion, and photopsia (perceived flashes of light), are also frequent. Sinus disease or uveitis may refer pain to the eye, and careful questioning may elicit the appropriate etiology. It is important to remember that except as noted earlier, ocular or visual problems such as refractive error, convergence, or accommodative insufficiency only rarely cause headache in children. One must consider ominous diagnoses, such as intracranial tumor or increased intracranial pressure, if headache is associated with other neurologic signs, such as cranial nerve palsy or papilledema.

KEY PROBLEM

■ Difference in Pupil Size The finding of *anisocoria* in children suggests similar etiologies to those previously discussed in infants. Physiologic anisocoria is probably most common but is a diagnosis of exclusion. Again, acquired *Horner syndrome,* with its more serious differential diagnosis list, is a consideration. If the pupillary size difference is very small, a congenital Horner syndrome may have been missed previously because the infant pupil is often quite small and dilates poorly in the dark. *Traumatic* mydriasis (excess pupil dilatation) is an important cause of anisocoria, especially in boys, and a proper history is important. Third nerve palsy, either from *trauma* or *congenital* or vascular anomaly, also causes a pupil that is larger on the affected side.

KEY PROBLEM

■ Ocular Trauma As children become more active, they are the group most prone to ocular *trauma,* ranging from a superficial eyelid abrasion to a ruptured or perforated globe. In severe orbital and head trauma, the neurologic status must be stable prior to ocular treatment. Nonaccidental injury is an important consideration.

KEY PROBLEM

■ Eyelid Lesions Orbital and eyelid lesions in childhood include many of those of infancy. Location, size, onset, and duration all are clues that lead to the correct diagnosis. Other lesions commonly seen in this age group are the *chalazion* or *stye (hordeolum).* See further discussion below. These are isolated or multiple lumps on either the lower or upper eyelids and may be unilateral or bilateral. Initial description will be of an acute inflamed isolated area of redness and swelling near or just posterior to the lid margin. They often persist for months in a subacute form without much discomfort or cosmetic deformity.

Adolescents

KEY PROBLEM

■ Poor Vision New-onset poor vision in an adolescent aged 10 to 15 years usually is due to new or progressing *refractive error,* most often *myopia,* accompanied by a complaint of difficulty seeing the board during school. Think of *amblyopia, cataract,* or other causes when the poor vision is unilateral. Factitious visual loss is also more of a possibility in this age group. Association with any neurologic signs or symptoms may warrant further workup.

KEY PROBLEM

Ocular Misalignment Any type of strabismus can develop or become manifest in the adolescent. Latent or intermittent *strabismus,* horizontal of vertical, is often present during infancy or childhood but remains unnoticed until fusion breaks down or deviation increases during the teen years. Again, an acute ocular misalignment merits careful evaluation, especially if accompanied by headaches or other localizing symptoms.

KEY PROBLEM

"Pink Eye" Any type of *conjunctivitis* can cause a "pink eye" in adolescents, as in younger children. Dry eyes, *corneal abrasions, eyelash lice,* and *chronic blepharitis* (eyelid inflammation) also can cause "pink eye" in adolescents. Specific symptoms of severe tearing and pain are more likely a result of contagious viral, especially adenoviral, conjunctivitis. Thick discharge and matting of the eyelid may suggest a *bacterial conjunctivitis.* Itching, rubbing, or stringy, watery discharge suggests an allergic etiology. Foreign-body sensation can indicate dry eye, foreign body, or corneal abrasion, as well as a number of nonspecific problems.

KEY PROBLEM

Eye Pain and Headache Causes of these are similar to those in children. Because of the turmoil of adolescence, *tension headaches* become more prominent. Adolescents are more likely to experience *cluster headaches* with notably severe eye pain, reaching crescendo peaks before subsiding. They also will report ipsilateral tearing and redness.

Eye pain is a nonspecific symptom. Pain following *trauma* can indicate a corneal abrasion or deeper injury. Photophobia may be a symptom of *uveitis,* either idiopathic or part of a systemic *inflammatory* condition such as *rheumatoid arthritis, ankylosing spondylitis,* or *Reiter syndrome* or *infectious* conditions such as *Lyme disease* or *toxoplasmosis.*

KEY PROBLEM

Anisocoria, Trauma, Eyelid Lesions Causes are similar to those in children. See further discussion below.

The Eye Examination

The basic components of an eye examination for all ages are visual acuity, visual fields, external examination, pupillary examination, motility and alignment examination, and ophthalmoscopy. These examinations can be challenging, particularly in uncooperative infants and children. Primary care facilities should have near-vision eye cards and vision charts (Snellen eye chart and its various adaptations for children, such as the Allen picture chart, the tumbling E chart, the picture chart, or the H, O, T, V chart to match letters [FIGURE 7–3]). In addition, basic

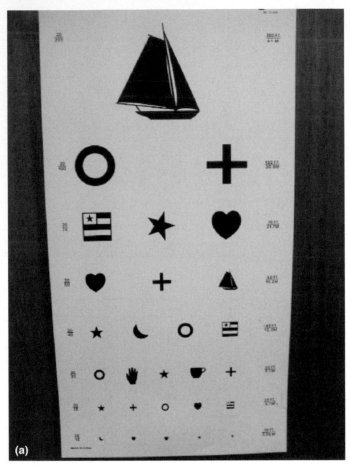

FIGURE 7-3 *A. The Picture Eye Chart. B. Standard Snellen Eye Chart (Letters).*

equipment for an "eye tray" include a penlight, a cobalt blue light, fluorescein strips, Q-Tips, and cycloplegic eye drops (FIGURE 7–4). Q-Tips are useful to evert the eyelid when searching for a conjunctival foreign body. The cobalt light and fluorescein paper are useful in bringing out corneal lesions owing to trauma, foreign body, or infection. Many commercially available machines will evaluate acuity, stereoacuity, binocular and color vision, and alignment but, although very sensitive, will have a very high false-positive yield, resulting in many unnecessary referrals to the optometrist or ophthalmologist.

Infants

By 2 to 3 months of age, infants will follow objects. It is difficult to assess visual acuity in infants because they will follow larger objects even

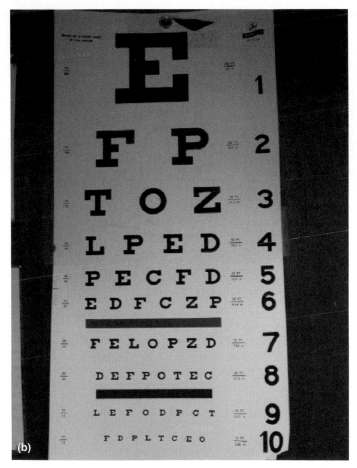

FIGURE 7-3 *(Continued)*

if they have poor vision. Certain "red flags" indicating poor or absent vision in infants include spontaneous nystagmus, often of the "searching" variety. The examiner may glean clues from the other aspects of the visual examination, such as notably severe strabismus (transient malalignment is considered normal in infants up to 6 months of age), lack of pupillary response to darkening a room, corneal clouding, and obvious malformations of the eye, including but not limited to coloboma and microphthalmia, often associated with other congenital malformations. Infants with poor or absent vision may not demonstrate optokinetic nystagmus when viewing moving stripes or dots. If vision is impaired in one eye, frequently an infant will become very agitated if the examiner places his or her hand over the "good eye." Eye alignment may be difficult to evaluate in an infant, but if the examiner can get the baby's

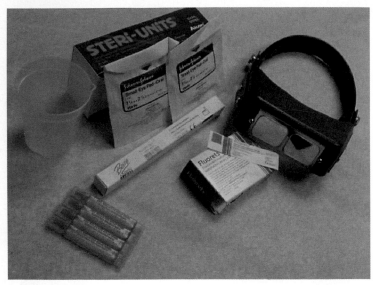

FIGURE 7–4 The Standard "Eye Tray."

attention, shining a pen light 2 to 3 feet directly in front of the infant should demonstrate a reflection of the light bilaterally in midpupil (Hirschberg test). Commonly used terminology for eye alignment includes

Strabismus—misalignment of the eyes
Esotropia—constant inward turning of the eye
Exotropia—constant outward turning of the eye
Esophoria—tendency to turn the eye inward, usually with fatigue or stress
Exophoria—tendency to turn the eye outward, usually with fatigue or stress
Amblyopia—loss of vision, either unilateral or bilateral. Visual loss may be a result of a refractive error in one eye (ametropic) or both eyes (anisometropic) or visual suppression owing to primary strabismus (strabismic). It also may be due to lesions that block vision (deprivation).

Often infants have inner canthal folds that will make the eyes appear esotropic, but the light will reflect normally, thus indicating pseudostrabismus. *Exotropia* refers to outward turning of the eye. All infants should have ophthalmoscopic evaluations on a regular basis to check for abnormalities in the red reflex.

Children

Children should undergo an evaluation similar to that of infants. Strabismus, both esotropia and exotropia, will become more apparent by age $2^1/_2$. Malalignment of the eyes would cause diplopia (double vision) were it not for the brain's capacity to suppress vision in the "wandering" eye (amblyopia). If the wandering eye has no pathology that would cause blindness, performing the "cover test" (covering the normal eye FIGURE 7–5) will realign the wandering eye, which then takes over visual function.

Verbal children will cooperate with a Snellen chart. Perform this test with the patient 20 ft away in a well-lit area. Test vision unilaterally and then bilaterally. The terminology 20/20 refers to normal vision, i.e., visible at 20 ft. Thus 20/40 would mean that the patient with normal vision would be able to read this slightly larger line at 40 ft. If a patient can only see the 20/40 line at 20 ft, this means that he or she can see at 20 ft. what a person with normal vision would see at 40 ft. If vision is more acute than normal, this patient will see the smaller 20/10 line at 20 ft. The patient with normal vision will only be able to see the 20/10 line at 10 ft.

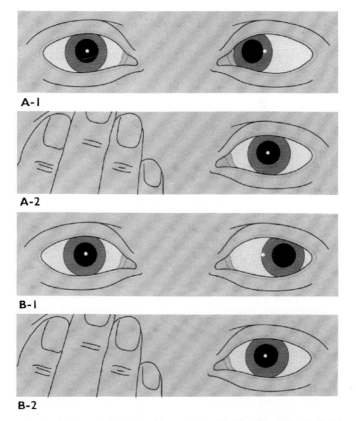

FIGURE 7–5 **The Cover Test.** *(From: Trobe JS:* The Physician's Guide to Eye Care. *Washington: American Academy of Ophthalmology, 2001.)*

Refractive errors become the most common visual problem in this age group. *Myopia* refers to focusing of a visual object in front of the retina, usually owing to increased anteroposterior diameter of the globe, but it also may be due to greater lens refractive power or posterior dislocation of the lens. Most myopias in children are physiologic and not due to pathologic changes in the globe or the lens. Such children will have difficulty with distant vision; thus their vision will be 20/40 or greater. This is rare in infants but does occur in retinopathy of prematurity (ROP), which is becoming more common with better survival rates of premature infants. Other genetic/metabolic causes include ectopia lentis of *Marfan syndrome* or *homocystinuria, keratoconus,* and *Stickler syndrome. Hyperopia* is due to focusing of the visual object behind the retina. Causes are the opposite to those of myopia, and such patients' distant vision may be 20/10 or better. Of interest is the ability of the lens to accommodate to hyperopia by relaxation of the ciliary muscles to thicken the lens, thus "autoprescribing" for this condition. As part of this ciliary response, the eyes also become esotropic. Sometimes, if severe, this condition can lead to fatigue, eyestrain, and blurred vision.

Astigmatism becomes apparent in this age group. This results from irregular curvatures in the cornea and sometimes the lens. Often the patients will squint to select a narrower "pinhole" area that may focus better on the retina.

The external examination will reveal abnormalities such as exophthalmos, enophthalmos, ptosis, lesions of the lid or canthus, abnormalities of tearing (dry or wet), and pupillary abnormalities (loss of consensual light reflex, lack of accommodation, abnormality of shape, asymmetry, dilatation with light, or *Marcus Gunn pupil*). Evaluate the lens for position (ectopia) and for clouding (*cataracts*). Test all gaze positions (FIGURE 7–2). Ocular motility abnormalities could be due to neurologic, muscular, or ophthalmic manifestations of several disorders (e.g., *Graves' disease* or *albinism*). Corneal abnormalities such as abrasions, foreign bodies, clouding, and crystal deposits are apparent on visual inspection, but the use of fluorescein dye and cobalt blue light will augment the examination.

Funduscopic examination becomes easier in children because they are more cooperative. Evaluate the optic disc (sharpness, pallor, or cupping), vessels (profusion, pulsations, engorgement, or nicking), retina (abnormal pigmentation, striping, scarring, hemorrhages, exudates, and lesions), and macula for abnormal coloring, bleeding, scarring, and exudates.

Adolescents

Eye examination of the adolescent is similar to that of children. By this age, one has identified most congenital and metabolic problems, and the funduscopic examination now becomes more important. Thus considerations in adolescents are increased intracranial pressure, benign or otherwise, and more chronic conditions such as *diabetic, hypertensive* and *sickle cell retinopathy.*

Synthesizing a Diagnosis

Since many presenting problems in ophthalmology present as a finding, usually by a caregiver, we expand on our differential diagnoses in the context of key problems.

● KEY PROBLEM

◤ **Lid Ptosis** *Ptosis,* or a drooping of the eyelid, can be *congenital* or acquired, unilateral or bilateral. Determine the age of onset, and evaluate for other ocular abnormalities. Monitor isolated congenital ptosis because it can lead to amblyopia from irregular astigmatism or deprivation. Another type of congenital ptosis is *Marcus Gunn jaw winking,* in which there is a synkinesis between the third and fifth cranial nerves. The ptotic lid will tend to elevate with certain movements of the jaw. Often the parents will note changes in lid position while feeding the infant. As discussed earlier, ptosis can accompany a third nerve palsy and *Horner syndrome.*

Acquired ptosis can result from myasthenia gravis, chronic progressive external ophthalmoplegia (CPEO), or any type of *myotonia* or *muscular dystrophy.* It is important to keep CPEO in mind because it can be associated with potentially life-threatening heart block. Symptoms of myasthenia vary depending on the time of day, and myotonia and muscular dystrophies are progressive and are associated with other muscular symptoms.

● KEY PROBLEM

◤ **Lid Swelling and Canthal Abnormalities** *Lid swelling* could represent either a diffuse or discrete lid problem. Time of onset and course of the swelling are important questions to ask. An isolated lid mass may be a simple *chalazion* or *stye (hordeolum).* Chalazia are due to obstruction of meibomian gland orifices with development of an erythematous lump near the lid margin. The lump may swell, become infected, or rupture. Hordeola are due to obstruction of the apocrine glands of the eyelid. These often need surgical incision and drainage if they do not resolve with conservative medical treatment of warm compresses, eyelid margin scrubs, and topical antibiotic/steroid ointment. Also consider *preseptal* or *orbital cellulitis.* Preseptal cellulitis is generally a more diffuse acute swelling and may be associated with a sinus or superficial skin infection. This is an important entity to recognize because it could progress to an orbital cellulitis, which is vision-threatening. Orbital cellulitis is *infection* of the orbit posterior to the orbital septum. Infection could progress to an abscess or become severe enough to compress the optic nerve and cause visual loss. Other signs of orbital cellulitis are restricted extraocular movements, afferent pupillary defect, and decreased vision. Orbital cellulitis needs urgent treatment with intravenous antibiotics.

Other orbital tumors that may cause lid swelling include *hemangioma, lymphangioma, neurofibroma,* and *rhabdomyosarcoma.* Rhabdomyosarcoma presents acutely as a rapidly growing lid swelling. Consider evaluation for malignancy in any acute, rapidly growing lid tumor not associated with infection. Early diagnosis and treatment have proven quite successful for a good prognosis with rhabdomyosarcoma. Other nonmalignant lid tumors are equally important to identify and treat to avoid *amblyopia* and allow the best possible visual outcome.

Newborns commonly will have nasolacrimal duct swelling, usually an obstruction (*dacryostenosis*) but also possibly *infection* (*dacryocystitis*). In addition, if there is a double obstruction of the nasolacrimal duct, the cyst will have a bluish discoloration.

KEY PROBLEM

Irregular Pupil Aside from anisocoria, an irregular pupil can be a sign of an ocular abnormality. *Congenital* pupillary abnormalities can represent a spectrum of ocular disorders including inherited anterior segment diseases or *colobomata*. Often there is a family history of ocular diseases. In addition, suspect *CHARGE syndrome* (*c*oloboma, *h*eart, *a*tresia choanae, *r*etardation [growth and mental], *g*enital, and *e*ar) in any patient with a coloboma. Acquired pupillary abnormalities also can represent significant intraocular disease. Trauma can lead to pupillary abnormalities by causing iris damage or posterior lens adhesions. A history of eye pain and photophobia might indicate uveitis.

KEY PROBLEM

Anisocoria Although most cases are benign, *traumatic*, or *infectious*, *iritis* can lead to *anisocoria*, generally with the affected pupil being slightly larger. A history of eye pain, systemic disease such as juvenile rheumatoid arthritis, and/or eye trauma may help to establish the correct diagnosis. Evaluation of the pupil difference in dark and bright light is also important for the diagnosis because one needs to establish which eye is affected, the one with the smaller or the larger pupil. If the anisocoria is greater in light, this means that the affected larger pupil is not constricting properly. This may be an indication of partial or complete third nerve palsy. Associated signs include ptosis and inability to fully adduct, elevate, or depress the affected eye. If the anisocoria is greater in the dark, then the affected pupil is the one not dilating properly. This could be a sign of Horner syndrome, a problem in the sympathetic chain. *Horner syndrome* can be *congenital* and often goes with heterochromia, ptosis, and dyshidrosis of the ipsilateral side. Acquired Horner syndrome often indicates a tumor along the sympathetic chain, specifically *neuroblastoma.*

KEY PROBLEM

White Pupil The differential diagnosis for a *white pupil* (*leukocoria*) is quite broad (see under infancy above). The first and most life-threatening condition to consider is *retinoblastoma*. Key questions include family history; however, retinoblastoma is often sporadic, and the key to diagnosis is a thorough dilated fundus examination. Other considerations include *congenital/metabolic* diseases (*dystrophies*), *infectious toxoplasmosis,* and *retinal* diseases. Inquire about *infectious* exposure and overall systemic health to glean clues to a more specific diagnosis.

KEY PROBLEM

Cloudy Cornea A cloudy cornea is a sign that appears usually during infancy and very early childhood. The clouding results from an immature cornea taking on fluid and becoming edematous. The most urgent cause of corneal clouding is *congenital glaucoma*. Associated signs are an enlarged cornea, photophobia, and tearing. Other causes of a cloudy cornea are *congenital* corneal dystrophies or *traumatic* corneal edema secondary to forceps injury at the time of delivery. Congenital glaucoma and some dystrophies can be hereditary; therefore, family history is important. *Peters anomaly* is a congenital corneal opacity probably of embryogenic origin that often is associated with other congenital eye anomalies.

Corneal infections usually demonstrate severe pain and photophobia and are significant. *Keratitis* can occur with *congenital syphilis* as well as be an aftermath of *infectious epidemic conjunctivitis* (adenoviral). *Dendritic keratitis* is associated with herpes simplex infection. Corneal ulcers are a result of serious *infections* such as *Pseudomonas aeruginosa* and *N. gonorrhoeae* and require emergent antibiotic treatment. Corneal ulcers also may result from a sensory or autonomic defect of the eye causing dryness or inability to feel the need to lubricate the eye by blinking.

KEY PROBLEM

Lens Abnormalities As discussed earlier, the causes of *cataracts* are many, a complete list of which is beyond the scope of this section. Other anomalies detectable by ophthalmoscopic examination are *ectopia lentis*—or dislocation. This typically occurs upward in *Marfan syndrome* and downward in *homocystinuria* and may be associated with other ocular anomalies, *infections, tumors,* and *congenital* conditions.

KEY PROBLEM

Funduscopic Abnormalities A complete discussion of pathologic conditions of the retina, vessels, macula, and optic disk is well beyond the scope of this section. We limit this section to conditions that occur more commonly in pediatric practice and are detectable by routine ophthalmoscopy. The primary physician frequently has to evaluate a patient for *papilledema*. Earlier stages consist of venodilatation with loss of pulsations. The disc margin then will become blurred and as the edema progresses will become raised and eventually develop small hemorrhages. It is important to identify retinal hemorrhages in suspected cases of *child abuse* (shaken baby). In adolescents, manifestations of diabetic retinopathy include venous dilatation, microaneurysms, retinal hemorrhage, and exudates. In worse cases, there may be neovascularization. *Hypertensive retinopathy* will demonstrate arteriolar narrowing and arteriovenous nicking in earlier stages, followed by hemorrhages, "cotton wool" exudates, and papilledema with further progression. Evaluate for retinal pigmentation in suspected cases of *chorioretinitis* (*TORCH diseases*) and *retinitis pigmentosa* of *metabolic* and *genetic* etiology. Evaluate the optic disk for pallor (optic atrophy) and for cupping (optic atrophy or childhood *glaucoma*). Examine the macula (when the patient looks into the light) for degeneration or for the "cherry red" spot of *lipid storage diseases*.

KEY PROBLEM

■ Nystagmus and Opsoclonus

Nystagmus is a rhythmic oscillation of one or both eyes. It may be horizontal, vertical, or circular. It can be congenital, and parents will report this. This presents with horizontal pendular or jerk nystagmus that remains horizontal in upgaze and damps on convergence. *Congenital* horizontal nystagmus is often a solitary finding, but pendular nystagmus may accompany *albinism,* ocular anomalies, and severe visual loss for any reason, e.g., *cataract, glaucoma, tumor, retinal disease,* etc. Most patients with congenital nystagmus have stable vision in the 20/50 to 20/200 range, although some have vision as good as 20/25. Acquired nystagmus may be of serious significance (possible *tumor*) and merits neurologic as well as ophthalmologic evaluation. Other types of nystagmus include downbeat nystagmus, which can indicate a congenital *Chiari malformation,* and seesaw nystagmus, a sign of a *craniopharyngioma.* Abnormal spontaneous nonrhythmic and chaotic eye movements represent opsoclonus and must bring to mind *neuroblastoma.*

KEY PROBLEM

■ Strabismus

Strabismus is present in 2 to 2.5 percent of the population and can be broken down into many different categories based on age of onset and type. A detailed history is very important. When did the strabismus begin, and what has been the time course? Congenital third, fourth, and sixth nerve palsies or mechanical restriction of muscles or orbital tissues can present with strabismus in infancy. Examples are *Möbius syndrome,* congenital facial paresis with abduction weakness, *Duane syndrome*, retraction of the globe on abduction, and *Brown syndrome,* restricted or absent elevation of the eye in the adducted position. Associated ptosis and head tilt may occur with strabismus. If an infant is otherwise healthy, these can be isolated findings. Infantile esotropia does not usually have other systemic associations; however, at times, exotropia can be associated with other neurologic problems. Perform a thorough review of systems on these infants. Increased intracranial pressure or postviral cranial nerve palsies can lead to strabismus, and a thorough history regarding prior illness, headaches, and neurologic signs and symptoms is very important.

KEY PROBLEM

■ Red Eye

The red eye can be a sign of different problems in different areas of the eye. Most commonly, the red eye in children is *infectious* (viral, bacterial) or *allergic conjunctivitis.* This is associated with itching and discomfort. *Viral conjunctivitis* is often associated with prior exposure or recent upper respiratory tract infection and may have a mild, watery discharge. Bacterial conjunctivitis demonstrates greater injection and very profuse purulent exudates. The etiology in the younger child tends to be bacterial, whereas in the older child a viral cause is more common. Allergy is another cause of conjunctivitis and pink eye. The clues to allergy are itching, lack of exudates, a cobblestone pattern, its seasonal nature, and other associated seasonal allergic symptoms.

Ocular *trauma* with resulting corneal abrasions, *hyphema* (blood in the anterior chamber), or traumatic *iritis* can cause a red eye, and the history

TABLE 7-2 *Laboratory and Imaging Aids*

Sign or Symptom	Conformational Study	Ruling Out
Leukocoria	CT scan	Retinoblastoma
Sudden lid swelling	CT scan	Rhabdomyosarcoma
Anisocoria		
Horners	MRI neck/thorax	Neuroblastoma
Third nerve palsy	MRI/MRA brain	Aneurysm/AVM
Red eye with joint pain	ANA	JRA
Uveitis	Lyme, *Toxoplasma, Toxocara*, RPR	Infectious uveitides
Hyphema after trauma	CT scan	Ruptured globe/orbital fracture
Asymmetic nystagmus	MRI brain/orbits	Optic glioma
Opsoclonus/irregular eye movements	MRI neck/thorax Abdominal imaging	Neuroblastoma Paraneoplastic syndrome
New-onset VIth nerve palsy	CT, LP	Increased ICP
New-onset variable ptosis	Anti-ACh rec. antibody	Myasthenia gravis
Ptosis with EOM palsy	ECG	Kearns sayre
Coloboma	Cardiovascular, hearing, genitourinary	CHARGE syndrome workup if indicated

Abbreviations: AVM = arteriovenous malformation; EOM = extraocular muscle; ICP = intracranial pressure; LP = lumbar puncture; rec. = receptor; RPR = rapid plasma reagin.

should correspond. Iritis in children, especially in juvenile *rheumatoid arthritis* (JRA), can present silently even if systemic symptoms are present. Without injection, this "white iritis" requires slit-lamp examination for diagnosis. TABLE 7-2 outlines useful laboratory and imaging aids in evaluating ophthalmologic problems.

When to Refer

Referring to the pediatric ophthalmologist is necessary for specialized ophthalmologic testing. The ophthalmologist has the tools to evaluate refractive error as well as examine the eye with a slit lamp and perform a dilated fundus examination. Generally, refer a patient presenting with anything requiring specialty testing. Decreased vision deserves a refraction and evaluation for any other ocular problems. Strabismus of any type needs specialist evaluation for refractive or surgical treatment.

Other eye problems such as conjunctivitis, corneal abrasion, chalazion, and allergy that are nonresolving after initial treatment should have a referral. Slit-lamp examination may demonstrate another problem other than that diagnosed initially. Refer anything that may need a slit-lamp examination for corneal, iris, or lens problems.

Refer anything that may necessitate a dilated examination because only the ophthalmologist has the tools to evaluate the posterior segment fully. Refer patients with suspected posterior segment tumor, optic nerve problem, glaucoma, or retinal problem. The specialist can perform a dilated examination and use direct and indirect ophthalmoscopy to examine the posterior segment.

In summary, referral is necessary for the use of specialized equipment or treatment. That includes slit-lamp examination, dilated examination, refraction, strabismus evaluation and treatment, and other complicated ocular problems needing specialized continuous eye care.

EARS, NOSE, THROAT, NECK, AND ORAL EXAMINATION

Of the entire general pediatric examination, the ears, nose, head, and neck are universal and yield the most information. Unfortunately, this is the also the portion of the examination that many children resist with the greatest vehemence. It is therefore crucial to develop a technique to examine this area of the body systematically, rapidly, and effectively, as well as to have a thorough knowledge of the signs and symptoms in the area. The goals of this section are

1. Review physiology, anatomy, and embryology of the ear, oropharynx, and neck.
2. Enumerate and analyze problems and findings in these areas.
3. Summarize diagnoses by their anatomic location, problems, findings, and age incidence.
4. Discuss further testing as necessary.
5. Discuss indications for referral if necessary.

Physiology and Mechanics

Ear

The ear is divided into three components—the external ear, the middle ear, and the inner ear. The external ear is composed of the auricle, or pinna, and the external auditory canal. Its principal function is to amplify sound from an external source toward the middle ear. The size and shape of these structures are such that they amplify sound with the greatest sensitivity when it is between 500 and 3000 Hz, which is also the usual frequency for human speech.

The middle ear consists of the tympanic membrane, the middle ear space, or tympanic cavity, and the ossicles. It further amplifies sound captured by the external ear by translating small vibrations and, through mechanical action, passes the vibrations on to the oval window and the fluid of the inner ear. The middle ear space is connected to the nasopharynx via the eustachian, or auditory, tube, which acts to equalize pressure between the middle ear space and the ambient air.

The inner ear serves two main functions. The cochlea is the auditory portion of the inner ear. Vibrations on the oval window act via the endolymphatic fluid on the hair cells within the cochlea to transduce sound into electrical activity passed via the auditory nerve (cranial nerve VIII) into the brain. The semicircular canals, the utricle, and the saccule are all part of the vestibular system. The three semicircular canals, oriented at right angles to each other, detect the movement of hair cells associated with turning of the head and convert this into information regarding *angular* motion of the body. The utricle and saccule, on the other hand, contain otoliths composed of calcium carbonate that move with gravity and thus detect *linear* motion of the body.

Mouth and Oropharynx

The oral cavity serves as the most proximal structure in both the gastrointestinal and respiratory systems. Its functions are to (1) lubricate and initiate digestion of food boluses with salivary secretions, (2) mechanically tear and grind solids into digestible and functional pieces via the teeth and jaws, (3) propel food boluses into the posterior oral pharynx and thus into the esophagus (the tongue), (4) provide phonation for speech, and (5) warm and humidify air.

Neck

The neck contains components of the respiratory system (larynx), digestive system (esophagus), endocrine system (thyroid and parathyroid glands), circulatory system (carotid arteries and jugular veins), lymphatic system (cervical lymph nodes), nervous system (cervical spine and cervical plexus), and musculoskeletal system (cervical vertebrae and supporting musculature) all in very close proximity. Problems of the neck require a broad differential diagnosis.

Developmental and Functional Anatomy

Ear

The formation of the ear occurs early in embryogenesis. By about 6 weeks of gestation, the auricle begins to form from the first and second branchial arches, and it appears adult in form by 20 weeks. The ossicles are of adult size by 16 weeks, and the middle ear space is developing. The external auditory canal forms around 28 weeks of gestation. The inner ear is derived from the otocyst at about 6 weeks and is of adult size and shape by 24 weeks. Major malformations of the ear therefore suggest a problem early in embryonic development.

The external ear is composed of the auricle (or pinna) and the external auditory canal. The auricle is a cartilaginous structure that is floppy in young infants but becomes firm by several months of age. Its outermost fold is the helix, and just interior to that is the antihelix. The external acoustic meatus opens into the canal and borders the tragus anteriorly and the concha posteriorly (FIGURE 7–6). There are many normal variations in the anatomy of the auricle.

The S-shaped external auditory canal in infants and young children requires gentle lateral traction to visualize the tympanic membrane. The lateral portion of the canal contains cerumen-secreting glands. Cerumen acts to protect and acidify the canal, thus preventing bacterial colonization. However, excessive cerumen often obscures a view of the tympanic membrane, and one must remove it for an adequate examination (see examination section below).

The tympanic membrane sits at the end of the canal. The tympanic membrane runs on an angle so that the inferior portion is tilting away from the examiner. In infants, this angle is even more severe, making the bony landmarks of the middle ear space difficult to appreciate.

The *manubrium,* or long arm of the malleus, attaches to the medial wall of the tympanic membrane. Viewed from the outside, it courses from the anterosuperior portion of the membrane toward its center and ends at the *umbo,* from which a cone of light sometimes can radiate and spread inferiorly. The lateral process, or short arm of the malleus, appears as a small bulge in the membrane at the upper edge of the manubrium, heading toward the examiner and slightly anterior. The

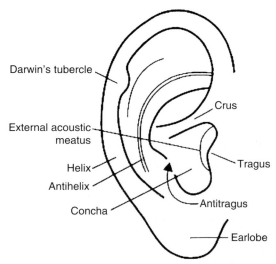

FIGURE 7–6 External Ear. *(From LeBlond RF, DeGowin RL, Brown DD: DeGowin's Diagnostic Examination. New York: McGraw-Hill, 2004, Fig 7.2, p. 194.)*

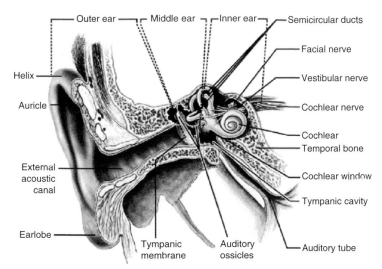

FIGURE 7-7 Ear Anatomy. *(From Van de Graaf KM:* Human Anatomy. *New York: McGraw-Hill, 2002, Fig. 15.28, p. 517.)*

only other ossicle visualized through a translucent tympanic membrane is the *incus,* a portion of which runs posterior and parallel to the long arm of the malleus. The area of the tympanic membrane inferior to the short arm of the malleus is the *pars tensa.* The area superior to the short arm between the malleolar folds is looser and is the *pars flaccida.* It is in the pars flaccida that retraction pockets and cholesteotomas can develop. FIGURES 7–7 and 7–8 illustrate middle and inner ear anatomy

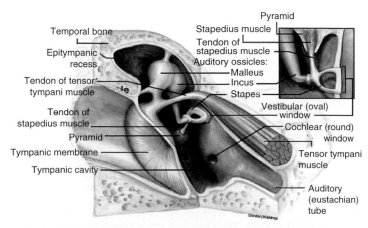

FIGURE 7-8 Anatomy: Inner Ear. *(From Van de Graaf KM:* Human Anatomy. *New York: McGraw-Hill, 2002, Fig. 15.31, p. 518.)*

Mouth and Oropharynx

The mouth forms from an invagination of ectoderm toward the embryonic foregut. By 4 weeks of gestation, these structures have fused, forming a single alimentary canal. The major structures of the mouth form from the branchial arches, which are mesodermal structures in the lateral cervical area of the embryo separating the branchial clefts externally from the branchial pouches internally. The hard palate forms from the medial growth of the lateral palatine processes of the maxilla and generally fuses by 10 to 12 weeks of gestation. Derivatives of the branchial and pharyngeal arches are summarized in FIGURE 7–9 and TABLE 7–3.

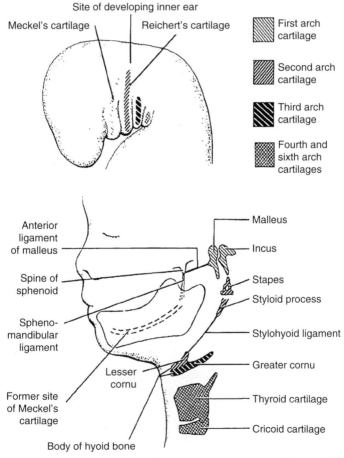

FIGURE 7–9 *Anatomy and Embryology of the Pharyngeal Arches. (From Moore KL, Persaud TVN:* The Developing Human: Clinically Oriented Embryology, *7th ed. Philadelphia: Saunders, 2003.)*

TABLE 7-3 *Structures Derived from Branchial or Pharyngeal Arch Components*

Arch	Nerve	Muscles	Skeletal Structures	Ligaments
First (mandibular)	Trigeminal (V)	Muscles of mastication Mylohyoid and anterior belly of digastric Tensor tympani Tensor veli palatini	Malleus Incus	Anterior ligament of malleus Sphenomandibular ligament
Second (hyoid)	Facial (VII)	Muscles of facial expressions Stapedius Stylohyoid Posterior belly of digastric	Stapes Styloid process Lesser cornu of hyoid Upper part of body of the hyoid bone	Stylohyoid ligament
Third	Glossopharyngeal (IX)	Stylopharyngeus	Greater cornu of hyoid Lower part of body of the hyoid bone	
Fourth and sixth	Superior laryngeal branch of vagus (X) Recurrent laryngeal branch of vagus (X)	Cricothyroid Levator veli palatine Constrictors of pharynx Intrinsic muscles of larynx Striated muscles of the esophagus	Thyroid cartilage Cricoid cartilage Arytenoid cartilage Corniculate cartilage Cuneiform cartilage	

Source: From Moore KL, Persaud TVN: *The Developing Human: Clinically Oriented Embryology.* Philadelphia: WB Saunders, 2003

The lips separate from the skin of the face by the vermilion border. The philtrum is a groove visible in the midline of the face from the nasal septum to the vermilion border of the upper lip. Each lip attaches to the gum by a midline frenulum. The teeth, if present, embed in alveolar ridges. The area between the lip and the alveolar ridge is the vestibule.

The palate arches up and back from the alveolar ridge toward the pharynx, separating the nasal cavity from the mouth. The anterior portion of the palate is bony, whereas the posterior, or soft, palate is muscular and ends in the uvula, a midline structure that hangs freely in front of the posterior wall of the pharynx.

The tongue sits within the bowl created by the mandible. The ventral surface of the tongue attaches to the floor of the mouth by a midline lingual frenulum. Wharton's ducts (which drain the submandibular glands) and several sublingual ducts are visible on either side of the lingual frenulum. The dorsum of the tongue extends backward to the epiglottis. Papillae cover the anterior two-thirds of the tongue. The sulcus terminalis is a V-shaped structure that separates the anterior portion of the tongue (and the mouth) from the posterior portion (and the oropharynx). In the midline, the sulcus terminalis forms the foramen cecum, an embryologic remnant of the thyroid gland. An undescended lingual thyroid may be at this location. The vallate papillae are just anterior to the sulcus terminalis, whereas the fungiform papillae are among the smaller filiform papillae across the tongue's surface. The dorsum of the normal tongue has filiform papillae on the anterior two-thirds. A V-shaped line of fungiform papillae marks the junction between the anterior two-thirds and the posterior third of the tongue, and inexperienced viewers often misconstrue these papillae for lesions (FIGURE 7–10).

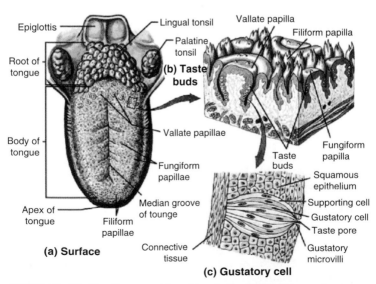

FIGURE 7–10 The Tongue. *(From Van de Graaf KM:* Human Anatomy. *New York: McGraw-Hill, 2002, Fig. 15.6, p. 497.)*

The primary dentition consists of 20 teeth (5 in each quadrant of the mouth), and eruption usually begins at about 6 months of age with the mandibular central incisors (TABLE 7–4 and FIGURE 7–11). The age of tooth eruption is highly variable and familial. In general, tooth eruption is earlier in girls than in boys and in African-Americans than in Caucasians. Missing primary teeth are a relatively uncommon finding, but this occurs more commonly in the permanent dentition.

The parotid gland sits along the lateral surface of the mandibular ramus and is detectable anterior and inferior to the ear when enlarged. It empties into the mouth via Stensen's duct, which opens on the upper portion of the buccal mucosa lateral to the second molar when present. The submaxillary gland lies medial to the anterior portion of the mandible and empties as described earlier.

The palatine tonsils (commonly referred to as *tonsils*) sit in between the tonsillar pillars formed by the lateral portions of the soft palate. The lingual tonsil is invisible with the naked eye but sits at the base of the tongue.

Neck

The larynx occupies the anterior portion of the neck. Its most superior structure is the epiglottis, which protects the airway during swallowing. Its anterior border is formed by the hyoid bone superiorly, the thyroid cartilage and the cricoid cartilage inferiorly, and membranes between each of these structures. The hyoid bone and thyroid cartilage are U-shaped with the open portion posterior. The cricoid cartilage is a ring that sits on top of the trachea. The glottis, or vocal cords, and associated structures sit on top of the cricoid cartilage. In infants and young children, the cricoid cartilage is narrower than the trachea, making the subglottic area a common site of upper airway obstruction. Unlike in adults, the larynx in infants sits very high in the neck, and the thyroid cartilage is often not palpable on examination (see FIGURE 7–9).

The thyroid gland consists of two lobes that lie anterior to the larynx just lateral to and below the thyroid cartilage and an isthmus that crosses the midline anterior to the trachea just below the cricoid cartilage. Embryologically, the thyroid gland descends from the anterior pharynx in the midline via the thyroglossal duct. Remnants of the thyroid gland or duct can appear occasionally in the midline of the neck during childhood. The four parathyroid glands lie embedded in the posterior portion of the thyroid gland lobes.

The superficial cervical lymph nodes are the major lymphatic structures of the face and neck (FIGURE 7–12). Knowledge of the various sites of these nodes and which areas they drain can aid immeasurably in diagnosis. For example, submental nodes (1) typically drain the teeth, mouth, and face. The submandibular nodes (2) drain the upper respiratory tract and oropharynx. The supraclavicular nodes (4) drain the anterior chest and mediastinum. The posterior cervical chain (5) and postauricular (6) and occipital nodes (8) drain the scalp. The preauricular nodes (7) drain the external ear.

TABLE 7-4 *Dentition*

	Tooth	Beginning of Enamel and Dentin Formation	Enamel Completed	Tooth Eruption
Primary	Upper: Central incisor	4 mos. in utero	1.5 mos.	7.5 mos.
	Lateral incisor	4.5 mos. in utero	2.5 mos.	9 mos.
	Canine	5 mos. in utero	9 mos.	18 mos.
	First molar	5 mos. in utero	6 mos.	14 mos.
	Second molar	6 mos. in utero	11 mos.	24 mos.
	Lower: Central incisor	4.5 mos. in utero	2.5 mos.	6 mos.
	Lateral incisor	4.5 mos. in utero	3 mos.	7 mos.
	Canine	5 mos. in utero	9 mos.	16 mos.
	First molar	5 mos. in utero	5.5 mos.	12 mos.
	Second molar	6 mos. in utero	10 mos.	20 mos.
Permanent	Upper: Central incisor	3–4 mos.	4–5 years	7–8 years
	Lateral incisor	10–12 mos.	4–5 years	8–9 years
	Canine	4–5 mos.	6–7 years	11–12 years
	First premolar	18–21 mos.	5–6 years	10–11 years
	Second premolar	24–28 mos.	6–7 years	10–12 years
	First molar	At birth	2.5–3 years	6–7 years
	Second molar	30–36 mos.	7–8 years	12–13 years
	Third molar	7–9 years	12–16 years	17–21 years
	Lower: Central incisor	3–4 mos.	4–5 years	6–7 years
	Lateral incisor	3–4 mos.	4–5 years	6–8 years
	Canine	4–5 mos	6–7 years	9–10 years
	First premolar	21–24 mos	5–6 years	10–12 years
	Second premolar	27–30 mos.	6–7 years	11–12 years
	First molar	At birth	2.5–3 years	6–7 years
	Second molar	30–36 mos.	7–8 years	11–13 years
	Third molar	8–10 years	12–16 years	17–21 years

Source: Adapted from Anderson CL, van Norman Langton C: *Orban's Oral Histology and Embryology,* 6th ed. St. Louis, MO: Mosby-Year Book Inc., 1970.

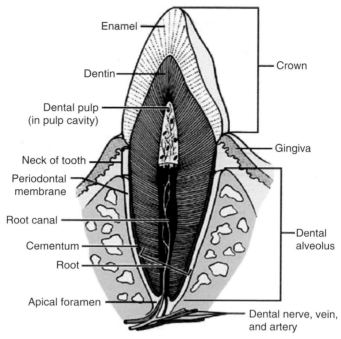

FIGURE 7–11 *The Tooth.* *(From Van de Graaf KM:* Human Anatomy. *New York: McGraw-Hill, 2002, Fig. 18.10, p. 645.)*

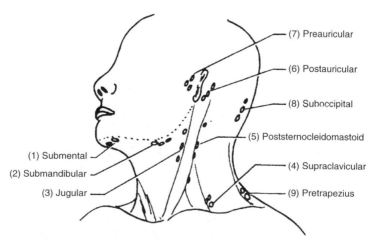

FIGURE 7–12 *Lymphatic System.* *(From LeBlond RF, DeGowin RL, Brown DD:* DeGowin's Diagnostic Examination. *New York: McGraw-Hill, 2004, Fig. 5–1, p. 105.)*

Key Problems

Ear

While some symptoms can be attributed easily to the ear (e.g., ear pain, ear discharge, and hearing loss), other symptoms that are nonspecific (e.g., fever, ear tugging, and irritability) are often associated with ear problems, especially in young children. A good history therefore will take into account the entire clinical picture. A useful framework is to think of the anatomy of the ear and related structures when evaluating key problems.

KEY PROBLEM
Otalgia (Ear Pain)

Auricle

Examination of the auricle should reveal signs of *infection* or *inflammation* from *cellulitis, thermal injury, insect bites, eczema, impetigo,* or *perichondritis*. Perichondritis distinguishes itself from cellulitis by the fact that it does not involve the earlobe. *Herpes* virus can cause a vesicular rash on the auricle. *Trauma* to the auricle is generally obvious (e.g., *hematomas, ecchymoses,* and *bite marks*). Displacement of the auricle away from the skull can be a sign of acute coalescent *mastoiditis* and requires emergency intervention.

Canal

Otitis externa (a.k.a. swimmer's ear) is generally *infection* with *Pseudomonas, Staphylococcus epidermidis,* or fungi and results from canal *trauma* (e.g., from Q-Tips) or excessive moisture. It is associated with canal edema, redness, and discharge, along with exquisite tenderness on manipulation of the auricle or direct pressure on the tragus. *Furunculosis* also can cause canal swelling but localizes to one portion of the canal. *Herpes zoster* can cause a vesicular rash on the posterior wall of the canal. With facial paralysis, this is *Ramsay-Hunt syndrome.* Foreign bodies in the canal include but are certainly not limited to beads, paper, and insects.

Middle Ear

Inquire if the pain is severe. Is it constant or variable? *Eustacean tube dysfunction* produces variable pain owing to changes in middle ear pressure. Acute *otitis media* often results from upper respiratory *infections* and is usually constant. *Perforation* of the tympanic membrane secondary to severe acute otitis can lead to resolution of pain. *Traumatic* perforation of the tympanic membrane can result from blast injury or direct injury from a Q-Tip. Barotrauma can cause ear pain in the setting of rapid changes in pressure (e.g., airplanes or scuba diving) and *eustachian tube dysfunction.*

Referred Pain

Pain in the area anterior to the tragus may result from *infection* of the external auditory meatus (ear canal) but also may stem from derangement of the temporomandibular joint (*TMJ dysfunction* or *TMJD*). This is especially common in older children and adolescents who have severe malocclusion or who are undergoing orthodontic tooth movement. Deviation of the mandible to one side on opening with or without TMJ "click" or pain is highly suggestive of TMJD. *Trismus*, the inability to fully open the mouth, may reflect problems in the TMJ as well as neuromuscular disease.

KEY PROBLEM
Otorrhea (Ear Discharge)

Canal

Otitis externa can cause ear discharge when severe. *Foreign bodies* can generate a localized reaction and cause a purulent discharge. Bloody discharge can occur with direct *trauma* to the canal.

Middle Ear

Discharge can occur with acute *otitis media* in the setting of perforation. Tympanostomy tubes are associated with *otorrhea* in 30 percent of patients. *Chronic suppurative otitis media* can cause recurrent foul-smelling discharge in the setting of either chronic perforation or *cholesteatoma*. Bloody ear discharge or *CSF otorrhea* can be a consequence of *basilar skull fractures.*

KEY PROBLEM
Hearing Loss
Hearing loss may *be conductive* or *sensorineural. Congenital* causes of hearing loss are often sensorineural, although craniofacial abnormalities are also associated with conductive hearing loss. A good history will include information on congenital infections (i.e., *TORCH syndrome;* see Chapter 5), *severe neonatal jaundice, prematurity, craniofacial abnormalities, exposure to ototoxic medications* (e.g., aminoglycosides or loop diuretics), *perinatal asphyxia, bacterial meningitis, prolonged mechanical ventilation, known genetic syndromes*, and *family history* of deafness or hearing loss. Refer to the examination section for information on distinguishing conductive from sensorineural hearing loss.

Canal

Canal atresia or stenosis, foreign body, excessive cerumen, and *otitis externa* all can block transmission of sound from the environment to the middle ear.

Middle Ear

Middle ear *effusion* is the most common cause of conductive hearing loss in children. In young children, hearing may appear intact, but speech discrimination may be impaired. Perforation of the tympanic membrane, *cholesteatoma*, and *otosclerosis* also can impair sound conduction. Traumatic disruption of the ossicles is a rare cause.

Inner Ear

Cochlear agenesis, *ototoxic agents*, damage to the hair cells from loud noise, or invasive tumors all can cause sensorineural hearing loss. Congenital hearing loss may have onset at birth or later in life and can be associated with various *congenital* syndromes.

Other

Tumors or *demyelinating disease* can affect the auditory pathway in the brain, causing hearing loss.

KEY PROBLEM

Vertigo *Vertigo* is a subjective sensation of motion (usually spinning), whereas *dizziness* is a general term referring to a sense of altered orientation to the environment. Young children may have difficulty describing their symptoms and may present with nonspecific signs such as *clumsiness, nystagmus,* or *vomiting.* Vertigo is a rare complaint in children.

Middle Ear

Eustachian tube dysfunction with or without effusion can cause vertigo or dizziness.

Inner Ear

Acute *infectious* (usually viral) *labyrinthitis, perilymphatic fistula,* and *vestibular neuronitis* and *trauma* (labyrinthine concussion) and *Meniere disease* (endolymphatic hydrops) are all rare causes of vertigo in children.

Other

Benign paroxysmal vertigo most commonly causes recurrent vertigo in children and may be a migraine variant. Rare CNS causes of vertigo include *seizures, meningitis, encephalitis, brain abscesses,* and *tumors.*

KEY PROBLEM

Tinnitus *Tinnitus* is abnormal noise heard in the ears and is common in children. Its pathophysiology is obscure. Persistent tinnitus can be associated with any *middle ear dysfunction* or *sensorineural hearing loss* (see above).

Mouth and Oropharynx

We shall treat the mouth and oropharynx together because many conditions can affect both simultaneously. Again, an anatomic approach is helpful in evaluating symptoms, validated by physical examination.

KEY PROBLEM

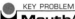**Mouth/Throat Pain**

Lips and Tongue

Infectious causes such as *herpes simplex virus* (HSV) *stomatitis* generally presents with vesicles and ulcers on the lips and anterior palate, unlike *herpangina,* which presents on the posterior palate, tonsils, and pharynx. *Cheilitis* (cracked, scaly lips) is generally due to *contact dermatitis* or irritation from drying. *Nutritional vitamin deficiencies* rarely can cause cheilitis at the angles of the mouth.

Mouth

The most common causes are *infectious. Aphthous ulcers* (canker sores) are common in children. Recurrent aphthous stomatitis presents with shallow, painful ulcers on the tongue and buccal mucosa, particularly on the inner surfaces of the lips. The etiology is uncertain, but infection most likely does not play a role. *Thrush* is usually a white coating on the tongue, cheek, and soft palate. It is sometimes difficult to differentiate from milk coating on the tongue, but thrush is not easily removed by scraping a tongue blade and is invariably also found on the mucosal surfaces and particularly in the vestibule. Severe thrush may present as an angry, red, bleeding surface, particularly in an immunocompromised patient.

Tooth abscesses or caries can be painful. *Trauma* (from chronic cheek biting, thermal injury, or chemical burns) can cause localized lesions in the mouth. A child's *tooth grinding,* usually primary teeth, is a common complaint that parents will mention during a well-child examination. The observant clinician may note *abrasion* of the occlusal edges of the anterior teeth and cusps of the molars. In severe cases, the enamel may wear completely through to the underlying yellow dentin. This is a common and benign problem but may require intervention by a pediatric dentist to preserve remaining primary tooth structure until exfoliation occurs.

Hand-foot-mouth disease can cause painful ulcers on the tongue and the buccal mucosa, as well as the hands and feet, and is due to a *coxsackie virus. Crohn disease* can cause mouth ulcers that resemble aphthous ulcers along with other gastrointestinal manifestations. *Behçet syndrome* causes painful mouth ulcers along with *genital ulcers* and *uveitis.* Painful mouth ulcers can occur with neutrophil defects (*leukemia, cyclic neutropenia,* and *agranulocytosis*). *Systemic lupus erythematosus* is associated with oral lesions that can be painful. *Erythema multiforme* can cause lesions on the skin as well as the mucous membranes, including the mouth. *Familial Mediterranean fever* presents with oral ulcers, recurrent fever, and serositis. *FAPA syndrome* (*f*ever, *a*phthous ulcers, *p*haryngitis and cervical *a*denopathy) recurs in 4- to 6-week cycles during childhood—the cause is unknown.

Pharynx

Infectious pharyngitis and *tonsillitis* are common in children and adolescents, although rare in infants or very young children. Viral causes are by far the most common, including common respiratory viruses (*influenza, parainfluenza,* and *coronavirus*), *enteroviruses,* and *HSV* (primary infection). *Epstein-Barr virus* (EBV) and *cytomegalovirus* (CMV) can present as *infectious mononucleosis* with splenomegaly, generalized lymphadenopathy, and fatigue. *Adenovirus* can present with pharyngitis and conjunctivitis together, which is *pharyngoconjunctival fever.* Bacterial causes include *group A streptococcus* (the most common bacterial cause), best predicted by fever, tonsillar exudates, and enlarged cervical lymph nodes, as well as the absence of cough. The classic *scarlet fever* rash associated with *group A streptococcal* infections is probably underdiagnosed. *Gonococcal pharyngitis* can occur in sexually active adolescents; suspect abuse if it occurs in prepubertal children. *Diphtheria* presents with a thick white membrane on the pharynx and can occur in unimmunized children. *Peritonsillar abscess* (quinsy) occurs in older children and presents with fever, a "hot potato" voice, dysphagia, and unilateral swelling of the pharynx. *Ludwig angina* is cellulitis of the submandibular space and typically is a result of group A streptococcal or anaerobic infection. *Epiglottitis* is rare in immunized children and presents with fever, stridor, and a very ill child leaning forward on hands (the "tripod" position).

KEY PROBLEM

■ **Dysphagia (Disordered Swallowing)** A coordinated swallow requires cooperation among the mouth (chewing, salivary lubrication), oropharynx (glottal closure to protect the larynx, soft palate elevation to protect the pharynx), and esophagus (peristalsis, opening of the lower esophageal sphincter). Dysphagia in children can occur locally at the level of the mouth and oropharynx, or the esophagus or may reflect generalized pain or a neuromuscular problem. Is the symptom of recent onset? Is there fever?

Mouth

Any cause of *stomatitis* (usually *infectious*) mentioned in the preceding section can impede the ability to swallow effectively. Anatomic problems such as *cleft palate,* whether complete or partial, can create an uncoordinated swallow.

Throat

Pharyngitis can impair swallowing owing to pain, especially when associated with significant tonsillar swelling (*peritonsillar abscess*) or retropharyngeal swelling (*retropharyngeal abscess*). It is important to inquire about any vocal changes (hoarseness or "hot potato" voice). Is there associated fever? Does the patient appear *toxic*? Are there associated symptoms such as headache or abdominal pain?

Esophagus

Congenital obstructions of the esophagus (*webs, strictures,* and *stenoses*) can impair swallowing and sometimes are associated with respiratory problems, especially when in combination with *tracheoesophageal fistulas.* *Esophageal strictures* can occur owing to *trauma* from caustic ingestion, intubation, or severe *gastroesophageal reflux disease* (GERD). *Foreign bodies* can lodge in the esophagus, especially in the toddler or developmentally disabled child. Several *autoimmune diseases* can affect neuromuscular motility of the esophagus in particular (*scleroderma* and *dermatomyositis*). *Esophagitis* can occur as a result of *reflux* of gastric acid, *herpes simplex* viral infections, or *candidal infections.*

Other

Many neuromuscular disorders can affect the swallowing mechanism. *Cerebral palsy* is a common cause of dysphagia in children. *Myasthenia gravis* (*immune*), *botulism,* and *diphtheria* (*infectious*) all can cause generalized weakness that can lead to dysphagia.

Neck

KEY PROBLEM

Hoarseness and Stridor
Stridor is covered in Chapter 8 because it most always is a result of lower or upper airway obstruction. Hoarseness is quite common in children, and vocal abuse is a common cause, sometimes resulting in vocal cord polyps. In the older child, consider *tumors* of the larynx. Of these, *laryngeal papillomas* are the most common. Rarely, extrinsic masses can cause compression of the airway and produce hoarseness and stridor in children. Causes can include vascular rings, esophageal foreign bodies, an *enlarged thyroid gland,* and a *mediastinal mass.* Finally, in cases of persistent stridor with hoarse voice and cough, consider *GERD,* especially in the child with an underlying neuromuscular abnormality.

KEY PROBLEM

Torticollis
Torticollis, or "wry neck," refers to a positional deformity of the neck with the head tilted to one side and the chin pointing in the opposite direction. In infants, the most common cause is muscular *torticollis* associated with fibrosis and restricted movement of the sternocleidomastoid muscle. Rare causes in infants include cervical spinal abnormalities such as *Klippel-Feil syndrome* and *Sprengel deformity* and *GERD.* In the older child, torticollis is usually due to rotatory subluxation of the first two cervical vertebrae, caused by acute *trauma* or *infection* such as *cervical adenitis* or *upper respiratory infection.* Gradual onset of torticollis in the older child should suggest the possibility of a posterior fossa *tumor.* Dystonic movement disorders and *GERD* (*Sandifer syndrome*) may mimic torticollis.

KEY PROBLEM

Neck Masses
As discussed earlier, multiple organ systems dwell in the neck, making the differential diagnosis for neck masses somewhat broad. However, an organized approach with attention to location and anatomy can help to distinguish among the possibilities. A good history should include the timing of appearance of the mass, the rapidity of enlargement, and any associated symptoms, as well as recent infections, bites, scratches, or environmental exposures, including travel and contact with ill individuals or animals.

Midline Neck Masses

Few structures dwell in the midline, making the differential diagnosis easier. A cystic structure in the midline is likely a *thyroglossal duct cyst.* A solid structure can be a goiter if it is in the normal location for the thyroid gland or a thyroid remnant if it is located superior to that. Enlarged submental lymph nodes, usually *infectious,* can present as masses beneath the jaw. A *dermoid cyst* or *teratoma* or other *neoplasia* occasionally can present as a midline neck mass.

Lateral Neck Masses

Benign cervical lymphadenopathy is by far the most common reason for a neck mass in children. As discussed earlier, lymph nodes can enlarge in reaction to *infections* anywhere in the head and neck. In addition, generalized *lymphadenopathy* can occur in reaction to a number of *infections,* including EBV, CMV, *toxoplasmosis,* and *various malignancies.* Cervical lymphadenitis, in contrast, presents with an acutely enlarged, tender, erythematous, occasionally fluctuant or spontaneously draining lymph node. The most common causes are *Staphylococcus* and *Streptococcus* but also include *Mycobacterium* (both *tuberculosis* and *atypical mycobacteria)* and various diseases inoculated by animals, including *Pasteurella, Tularemia,* and *cat-scratch disease. Lymphoma* can present with an enlarged, nontender, very firm or rubbery lymph node with fever, night sweats, and weight loss. Most benign enlarged lymph nodes regress after 2 weeks; persistence should suggest the need for further evaluation.

In infants, *cystic hygromas* can present with a mass anywhere in the neck or axilla. *Congenital branchial cleft remnants* are neck masses mimicking lymph nodes, often with a fistulous connection to the pharynx. Vascular tumors such as *hemangiomas* and *lymphangiomas* are often soft and compressible with indistinct borders. In older children, *parotitis* can mimic lymphadenopathy but distinguishes itself by extension to the preauricular area.

Key Findings

KEY FINDING

Ear In the infant or young child, a good examination of the ear is often a challenging task. Preparation can help to maximize the return on one's effort. Basic equipment for an ear examination should include an otoscope with a bright light source, an appropriately sized ear speculum, and an insufflator to assess tympanic mobility. Disarm frightened young children by showing them the equipment well before the attempted examination, playing games with the equipment or letting them "examine" the parent or physician. A young child often can be examined in the parent's lap, with gentle immobilization of the head and hands provided by the parent. This can be accomplished by holding the child's hands with one hand and the head against the parent's chest. One also may examine an infant or young child lying down on an examination table. When inserting the speculum into the child's ear, be careful to stabilize the otoscope by placing a finger or hand against the child's head or cheek to prevent sudden movements leading to trauma.

As with other areas, examination should begin with a general assessment of the patient. Craniofacial anomalies are commonly associated with disorders of the ear. Look for dysmorphic features such as those of *Down syndrome, Treacher Collins syndrome,* or *craniosynostosis,* all of which can be associated with ear problems. Any disorder that affects growth of the midface, such as *cleft palate,* also can be associated with ear problems.

Auricle

Examine the position of the ear relative to the eye level. Low-set ears (in which the entire auricle sits below the level of a line drawn between the canthi of both eyes) are associated with several *genetic* syndromes. Major defects of the external ear can be associated with underlying hearing loss. Minor malformations are common and benign. *Infections* can occur in *preauricular pits* if they connect to *branchial cleft cysts.* The so-called cauliflower ear is a sequela of *hematomas* to the auricle causing pressure necrosis. Examine the auricle for redness, swelling, or discharge, which can be associated with various causes discussed earlier. Anterior displacement of the auricle can be associated with acute *mastoiditis.* Pull gently on the helix, and press on the tragus—tenderness with either maneuver is associated with *otitis externa.*

Canal

The pneumatic otoscope is the best instrument to examine the canal, tympanic membrane, and middle ear. Choose the largest ear speculum that will fit in the canal in order to obtain a good seal. Often a small piece of rubber tubing around the speculum can improve it. Pull the pinna gently laterally to straighten the canal and improve the view of the tympanic membrane. Inspect the canal as you insert the speculum for foreign bodies, localized findings on the walls (e.g., *furuncles* and *vesicles), edema,* or mucopurulent discharge. Cerumen commonly accumulates in the outer portion of the canal. If it obstructs the view of the tympanic membrane, remove it with gentle warm-water irrigation. If the cerumen is hard and resistant to removal, use various products (3% hydrogen peroxide [Biscodyl]) to soften it. Under direct visualization, a cerumen loop or spoon also can remove wax.

Middle Ear

Locate the borders between canal and tympanic membrane to be sure that you are looking in the right place. The tympanic membrane is best assessed using a combination of factors, including

Position. The membrane is bulging outward in *acute otitis media,* obscuring the bony landmarks of the manubrium; when middle ear pressure is negative, the membrane retracts, and the short process of the manubrium can look more prominent.

Opacity. The normal tympanic membrane is translucent—one can see bony landmarks well. A dull membrane can be associated with acute infection or chronic scarring.

Color. While a classic *acute otitis* presents with a red tympanic membrane, a crying child also will have red ears, reducing the value of this observation. An infected eardrum also can appear yellow or white, whereas some normal translucent eardrums can appear pink.

Mobility. In infants older than 6 months of age, an insufflator introduces both positive and negative pressure to the eardrum. With a good seal, a normal eardrum will deflect equally with positive and negative pressure. Decreased mobility results from an *effusion* (either acute or chronic) or if the membrane retracts at baseline. A retracted membrane with no middle ear fluid may move with negative pressure from the insufflator. Often struggling children will increase middle ear pressure (Valsalva maneuver), but pumping the insufflator rapidly during the inhalation phase of crying will demonstrate tympanic membrane movement if no fluid is present.

Other. Look for an air-fluid level or bubbles behind the tympanic membrane, indicating an effusion. *Bullous myringitis* presents with blebs on the surface of the membrane—this infection is due to the same pathogens as those of *acute otitis*. A *cholesteatoma* may appear as a gray or white mass behind the membrane.

Inner Ear

Perform a rough hearing test by rubbing fingers together near each ear or by whispering and asking for responses. A Weber and Rinne test can distinguish conductive and sensory loss (see Chapter 12). Audiometric tests can help with young children (see below). *Nystagmus* owing to inner ear dysfunction is rare in children but can be due to vestibular dysfunction, especially if it is horizontal and/or rotatory.

KEY FINDING

Mouth and Oropharynx The technique of the oral examination depends on the age of the patient. Examine infants in the supine position, standing either at the infant's head or feet. It is usually advisable to ask the parent to assist by steadying the head. This also serves as a reminder to the examiner to explain what he or she is doing and to demonstrate to the parent any interesting findings.

In the older infant and toddler, the knee-to-knee position is the easiest method for obtaining a thorough examination of the oral cavity. Before the examination, necessary materials should be at easy arm's reach to the examiner: tongue depressors; bright light source; gauze squares, etc. The child may sit in the parent's lap with his or her back to the examiner and then gently be placed in the examiner's lap when ready.

Examine a cooperative child and adolescent with him or her seated on the examining table with the oral cavity about at the level of the examiner's eyes. For a wheelchair-bound child or adolescent, sit behind the wheelchair and then recline the backrest, if possible. This examination position is what one typically sees in a dental office and works extremely well.

Examination of the oral cavity is an integral part of the entire head and neck examination. As noted in the preceding section, this involves first visual inspection of external structures followed by palpation of the temporomandibular joint (TMJ), the mandible and maxillary bones, the skin of the face, and the lips. Using a gloved hand, evert the lips to examine the tissue in the buccal vestibule, the anterior gingiva and teeth (if present), and the lips themselves. Palpate the lips and cheeks between the index finger internally and the thumb externally, looking for any masses or areas of tenderness. Palpate the palate carefully, looking for evidence of a submucous cleft, especially if a cleft lip or uvula is present. The tongue is easy to examine in the infant, but it is frequently necessary to use a tongue depressor to visualize the hard and soft palates and the posterior pharynx. One has to be quick with this maneuver because the infant frequently will gag and regurgitate, obscuring the view. This is a common occurrence, and if the examiner apologizes to the parent beforehand for making the baby gag, the examination usually proceeds more smoothly and pleasantly. To view the posterior tongue and lateral borders, it may be necessary to wrap a gauze pad square around the tip for traction and gently pull forward.

Begin with a general examination of the face and mouth. Is there an obvious asymmetry or defect such as a cleft lip? Is the mandible small (micrognathia) or retracted (retrognathia)? Note any unusual odors—is the breath fetid or sweet-smelling? Halitosis can be a sign of foreign bodies in the nose, *dental* or *tonsillar abscesses,* or *sinusitis.* Acetone on the breath suggests *ketoacidosis* from diabetes or starvation.

Dry, cracked lips can be a sign of dehydration, *inflammatory* disorders such as *Kawasaki disease,* or simply irritation from lip licking. *Congenital labial frenula* are soft-tissue attachments at the middle upper and lower lips that become easily apparent with retraction and eversion of the lip. In infants it is normal for the maxillary frenulum to extend over the alveolar ridge and onto the palate. Persistence of this thick, muscular attachment after tooth eruption may result in a large *diastema,* or space between the central incisors. The lower attachment (lingual frenulum) in older children may extend up to the interdental papilla and can pull on the free gingival margin to result in severe gingival recession and periodontal disease.

Herpes simplex virus has many manifestations. Primary infection frequently presents as herpetic *gingivostomatitis* with diffuse vesicles throughout the oral cavity and extensive edema and bleeding of the gingival margins. This is invariably painful and may result in severe dehydration as a result of decreased oral intake. The vesicles also may cluster on the vermilion border of the lip as in classic herpes labialis *or* cold sores. Recurrent (secondary) herpes infection may occur as a typical "cold sore" on the lip but also may produce herpetic stomatitis with vesicles on the attached gingiva and hard palate. The differential diagnosis of perioral lesions includes *impetigo,* a bacterial infection caused by *Staphylococcus* and *Streptococcus.* The skin lesions of impetigo usually are described as vesiculopustular honey-colored or golden crusts. Herpetic lesions typically recur at the same location, unlike impetigo, which will vary in location. Young infants often will have a central callus or *sucking blister,* which is benign. Examine the inner surface of the lips with the aid of a tongue depressor. Look for *aphthous ulcers* or other findings.

Certain oral lesions commonly occur in both the primary and permanent dentition. Enamel defects and hypoplastic pits appear with interruption of deposition and/or mineralization of enamel matrix. Severe illness, fever, and malnutrition are common causes of enamel hypoplasia, and the age at which the insult occurred is apparent by the particular teeth involved (see TABLE 7–4 for approximate times of enamel formation). Dental caries consists of brown or black discolorations on the occlusal surfaces of the posterior teeth or between the anterior teeth at points of contact. Milk bottle caries is extensive decay of the maxillary anterior (sometimes lower) teeth in infants who sleep on their backs with a bottle of milk or other sugary liquid. In this condition, the teeth may decay down to the gingival margin and become stumps.

A *parulis*, or gum boil, occurs on the gingivae and represents the opening of a fistulous tract from a periapical abscess. This drainage tract usually opens on the facial (buccal) alveolar plate but also may appear on the hard palate in association with the palatal root of a permanent molar tooth or on the thin lingual plate of the mandible. Although devitalization of the dental pulp with abscess is most frequently a result of dental caries, this process also may be a consequence of dental trauma. Maxillary primary incisors frequently are subject to such trauma, and the subsequent bleeding into the pulp chamber may produce a gray discoloration to the crown of the tooth. A dying nerve is often associated with this and emits gases that expand with intake of hot liquids, causing pain. The pain is relieved on contraction of the gases with exposure to cold liquids. *Infection* with *S. mitis* is a definite contributor to dental caries. *Gingival hyperplasia* may be secondary to certain *medications,* including phenytoin and cyclosporine, or rarely owing to *leukemic infiltration.* Ulceration and bleeding of the gingivae can occur in *Vincent gingivitis,* usually in the adolescent or young adult. A common *toxic* cause in children is *chronic lead exposure,* which shows a line of increased pigmentation on the gums. Tapping a tooth with a tongue depressor will elicit exquisite pain if there is an abscess around it. Gingival swelling also may be present.

Examine the tongue. *Fissured tongue* is a developmental anomaly featuring a prominent midline anteroposterior fissure from which smaller fissures radiate laterally. It occurs more frequently in adults than in children but is a common finding in children with *Down syndrome. Ankyloglossia* is a short lingual frenum that attaches the dorsum of the tongue to the floor of the mouth. This condition is rarely severe enough to require surgical intervention unless the infant has difficulty feeding. Absence of both the lingual and mandibular labial frenula is associated with (1) Ehlers-Danlos syndrome and (2) pyloric stenosis. *Inflammatory* conditions such as *Kawasaki disease* or streptococcal infections may cause prominence of the papillae, the so-called strawberry tongue. In contrast, atrophy of the papillae will give the tongue a smooth appearance. When uniform, this is *glossitis. Geographic tongue* demonstrates irregular, pink, slightly depressed areas with elevated white or yellow borders. The lesions represent areas of flattening and desquamation of the filiform papillae and occur on the dorsum and lateral borders of the anterior two-thirds of the tongue. These lesions are typically asymptomatic but may on rare occasion be painful. Geographic tongue is a chronic, recurring disorder in which the pattern continuously changes, creating a "migratory" appearance. The appearance of the tongue reminds the examiner of a bas-relief map of the earth, hence the name *geographic tongue.* The condition is more common in girls than in boys, and reassurance is usually the only necessary treatment.

Next, examine the oral mucosae. Note whether they are moist or dry. The buccal mucosae may be the site of various causes of painful *stomatitis* discussed earlier. They also may demonstrate enanthems, or intraoral manifestations of systemic diseases. For example, Koplik spots are white lesions noted on the buccal mucosae of patients with *measles. Thrush (oral candidiasis)* will appear as thick, white, adherent plaques on the tongue and buccal mucosae. *Mucoceles* are a result of trauma to a minor salivary gland or its duct. Secretions collect in the soft tissues surrounding the gland and in the dilated duct itself. They typically present as painless swellings on the inside of the lower lip (buccal vestibule) and are usually less than 1 cm in diameter, smooth, and bluish or translucent in appearance. This is the most common area of soft-tissue trauma from the teeth or accidental cheek biting. A mucocele of the floor of the mouth associated with the sublingual gland is a *ranula. Fibromas* are one of the most common lesions of the oral cavity that form when chronic irritation results in reactive connective tissue hyperplasia. They may occur on any oral mucosal surface, particularly the palate, tongue, cheek, and lip. They are typically pink, smooth, firm nodules less than 1 cm in diameter and may be either sessile or pedunculated.

Examine the palate. A cleft palate can be unilateral or bilateral and can occur alone or in combination with a cleft lip or micrognathia (the *Pierre-Robin sequence*). A subtle *submucous cleft palate* is often hard to find and can present only with thinning of the midline of the palate or a bifid uvula. A high arched palate is a minor malformation that can occur alone or in association with various *congenital* syndromes. It also may be secondary to *trauma* from prolonged intubation.

Examine the oropharynx using one of the methods described earlier. The tonsils generally are small in infants but become larger during childhood and may be a chronic condition in young children up to age 10. The size of the tonsils may be graded from 1+ to 4+, with 1+ tonsils lying entirely within the pillars and 4+ tonsils touching in the midline. However, gagging a child will cause the tonsils to move toward the midline, and this can lead to an overestimation of tonsillar size. *Infections* of the posterior pharynx can cause erythema of the tonsils, pharynx, and soft palate, as well as exudates on the tonsils. Causes include *group A streptococci, EBV, CMV,* and *adenoviruses* not distinguishable based on appearance of the pharynx alone, although palatal petechieae may point more toward *strep throat and* gray exudates and uvular edema toward *mononucleosis.* Hand, foot, and mouth syndrome is notable for vesicles throughout the oral cavity, along with tender vesicles on the hands, feet, and buttocks. This is caused by several enteroviruses, most commonly the coxsackie family. Vesicles may occur in the oral cavity only (herpangina). A bulging mass obscuring the tonsil and pressing the uvula is a sign of *peritonsillar abscess,* although many of these patients have *trismus* limiting a view of the pharynx. Asymmetric enlargement of the tonsils should raise suspicion of *malignancy* such as *tonsillar lymphoma.* Enlarged posterior pharyngeal lymphoid tissue can cause a "cobblestone" appearance to the posterior pharynx and suggests chronic drainage from allergic rhinitis.

Neck

Begin the neck examination with inspection. Note any unusual position of the head and neck (see torticollis above) or obvious swelling or masses (see neck masses above). Note whether the child moves the neck freely in the anteroposterior plane—this will help to alleviate concerns about *meningismus.*

Examine the cervical lymph nodes in a systematic fashion, touching all areas in FIGURE 7–12. Use the fingertips to evaluate for lymph node size, consistency, tenderness, and mobility. Cervical lymph nodes are rarely palpable in infants. In children, "shotty" lymph nodes (so called because they feel like buckshot) are normal, as are nontender lymph nodes less than 1 cm in diameter. As discussed earlier, persistently enlarged nodes merit further evaluation.

Palpate for the thyroid gland using the laryngeal cartilages as a landmark. Examine the patient from behind or in front and hyperextend the neck. In an older child, have him or her swallow a glass of water during the examination—thyroid tissue will move up with the larynx during swallowing. If a *goiter* (an enlarged thyroid gland) is present, attempt to auscultate it for bruits.

Assess the range of motion of the neck. Look for resistance to lateral motion associated with muscular torticollis. In an older child, flex the neck while supine—if the child flexes the hips, this can be a sign of meningeal irritation (Brudzinski sign). Examine an older child or adolescent for active range of motion, including anterior flexion, extension, lateral flexion (ear to shoulder), and rotation (chin to shoulder).

Synthesizing a Diagnosis

TABLE 7–5 outlines common diagnoses with their problems, findings, and clinical high points.

Confirmatory Laboratory and Imaging

Ear

Tympanometry

The correct diagnosis of acute otitis media and otitis media with effusion is often difficult. Tympanometry is a useful adjunct that is relatively easy to perform. As with pneumatic otoscopy, perform

TABLE 7-5 *Diagnoses with Problems, Findings, and Clinical High Points*

Diagnosis	Occurrence, Comments	Key Problems	Key Findings
Auricle			
Cellulitis	Rare	Otalgia	Swelling (including earlobe)
Perichondritis	Rare	Otalgia	Swelling (sparing earlobe)
Insect bite	Common	Otalgia	Papular rash
HSV infection	Rare, more in adolescents	Otalgia	Vesicular rash
Trauma	Common	Otalgia	Hematoma, ecchymoses
Eczema	Common	Otalgia	Scaly rash
Impetigo	Common, more in children	Otalgia	Scaly rash with yellow crust
Major ear malformations	Rare	Hearing loss	Canal atresia or stenosis, microtia, anotia
Preauricular sinus	Not uncommon	None or pain	None or erythema/swelling
Minor ear malformations	Common	None	Preauricular pits, tags, variations in pinna formation
Canal			
Otitis externa	Common, less in infants	Otalgia, discharge, swimming	Tragus/pinna traction tenderness, canal edema and tenderness
Foreign bodies	Common, more in children	Otalgia, discharge, hearing loss	Direct visualization, canal edema, discharge
Furunculosis	Not uncommon	Otalgia	Localized swelling, tenderness, pustule
Ramsay-Hunt syndrome	Rare, more in adolescents	Facial paralysis	Vesicular rash in ear canal
Trauma	Common	Otalgia, bloody discharge, injury hx	Localized trauma in ear canal
Cerumenosis	Common	Hearing loss	Excessive cerumen

(Continued)

TABLE 7-5 *Diagnoses with Problems, Findings, and Clinical High Points (Continued)*

Diagnosis	Occurrence, Comments	Key Problems	Key Findings
Middle Ear			
Acute otitis media	Common, less in adolescents URI, fever, hearing loss	Otalgia, discharge, previous immobility of TM, occasional perforation	Bulging, dullness, redness
Barotrauma	Rare	Otalgia, discharge, hearing loss	Perforation, ear discharge
Chronic suppurative otitis media	Rare	Discharge	Perforation of TM, sometimes cholesteatoma
Bullous myringitis	Rare	Otalgia	Red bullae on surface of TM
Cholesteatoma	Rare	Hearing loss, discharge	Cholesteatoma seen behind TM
Otitis media with effusion (serous)	Common	Hearing loss, dizziness	Retracted TM, air fluid level, fluid bubbles, decreased mobility
Ossicular disruption	Rare	Hearing loss	Abnormal hearing
Eustachian tube dysfunction	Common	Hearing loss, dizziness	Abnormal mobility of the TM, air fluid levels, fluid bubbles
Inner Ear			
Congenital hearing loss	Common	Hearing loss, speech and language delay	Dysmorphic features, abnormal hearing
Acute labyrinthitis	Rare, more in adolescents and children	Hearing loss, vertigo, nausea, vomiting,	Hearing loss, horizontal or rotatory nystagmus,
Vestibular neuronitis	Rare	Vertigo, nausea, vomiting	Horizontal or rotatory nystagmus

Perilymphatic fistula	Rare	Vertigo	Nystagmus
Labyrinthine concussion	Rare	Vertigo	Nystagmus
Meniere disease	Rare, more in adolescents	Vertigo	Nystagmus
Lips			
HSV stomatitis	Common, acute ↑ in infants and children	Perioral or mouth pain	Grouped vesicles on red base
Impetigo	Common	Perioral pain	Honey-crusted papules
Cheilitis	Common	Lip pain	Contact dermatitis, dryness
Angular cheilitis	Rare	Lip pain	Dryness, vitamin deficiencies
Mouth and Oropharynx			
Aphthous ulcer	Common	Mouth pain	Oral ulcers
Behçet syndrome	Rare, more in adolescents	Mouth Pain	Oral ulcers, uveitis, genital ulcers
Crohn disease	Rare, more in adolescents	Mouth pain, abd pain, weight loss, constipation	Oral ulcers, arthritis, abdominal tenderness, perianal pathology
Erythema multiforme	Not uncommon	Mouth pain	Oral inflammation, skin rash
SLE	Rare, more in adolescents	Mouth pain	Oral ulcers, multisystem disease
Hand-foot-mouth disease	Common, less in infants	Mouth, throat pain	Perioral and mucosal vesicles and ulcers, vesicles on hands, feet, and buttocks
Herpangina	Common	Throat pain	Ulcers on soft palate and pharynx
Neutrophil defects	Rare	Mouth pain	Oral ulcers
Familial Mediterranean Fever	Rare	Mouth pain	Oral ulcers, fever, serositis
FAPA	Rare	Mouth pain	Fever, adenopathy, pharyngitis, oral ulcers

(Continued)

TABLE 7-5 *Diagnoses with Problems, Findings, and Clinical High Points (Continued)*

Diagnosis	Occurrence, Comments	Key Problems	Key Findings
Pharyngitis	Common	Throat pain	Fever, tonsillar hypertrophy, erythema, exudates
Peritonsillar abscess	Not uncommon	Throat pain	Fever, palatal swelling, trismus, "hot potato" voice, deviation of uvula
Ludwig angina	Rare	Mouth pain	Swelling of floor of mouth
Retropharyngeal abscess	Rare	Dysphagia, stridor	Swelling of posterior pharyngeal wall, stiff neck on flexion
Esophageal stricture	Rare	Dysphagia	
Esophageal foreign body	Rare, more in children	Dysphagia, hx of swallowing foreign body, choking, gagging	
Esophageal web	Rare	Dysphagia, regurgitation	
Neuromuscular disease	Rare	Dysphagia	Various depending on cause

tympanometry by inserting an instrument into the canal and creating a sealed space. The instrument measures the acoustic impedance of the tympanic membrane across a range of pressures from −300 to +300 mm H_2O. FIGURE 7–13 shows typical tympanograms. A normal, or type A, tympanogram (FIGURE 7–13A) demonstrates a peak of maximum compliance of the membrane at 0 mm H_2O. A type B tympanogram (FIGURE 7–13B) shows little or no peak and is associated with effusion, which can be purulent (as in acute otitis media) or serous (as in otitis media with effusion). A type C tympanogram (FIGURE 7–13C) has its peak compliance at negative pressures and

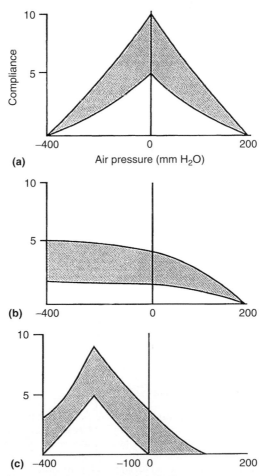

FIGURE 7–13 *A. Tympanogram, type A. B. Tympanogram, type B. C. Tympanogram, type C.* *(From Kliegman, Greenbaum, and Lye:* Pediatric Strategies in Pediatric Diagnosis and Therapy. *New York: Elsevier, 2004.)*

is associated with a retracted eardrum—often seen with chronic otitis media with effusion. A tympanic membrane with a perforation or tympanostomy tube would have a type B tympanogram but would appear to have very large canal volume.

Tympanocentesis

In cases of persistent acute otitis media or otitis media with effusion, aspirating the middle ear space is useful to isolate the offending organisms and determine their antibiotic sensitivities. Perform tympanocentesis by attaching an 18-gauge spinal needle to a syringe and aspirating from the anteroinferior portion of the tympanic membrane under direct visualization with an otoscope. Sedate and immobilize children prior to any such procedure with appropriate informed consent.

Audiometry

For children with suspected hearing loss or those with long-standing effusions, audiometry can help to distinguish the type and severity of the hearing loss. Children 5 years of age or older generally can cooperate with conventional audiometry, which involves measurement of hearing in each ear across a range of frequencies and intensities. Younger children (typically older than 2 years of age) can cooperate with play audiometry, and one can obtain the same kind of information. Visual reinforcement audiometry (VRA) is useful in children older than 5 to 6 months. This test can give information about hearing sensitivity but cannot generate ear-specific information. Otoacoustic emissions (OAEs) and auditory brain response (ABR) screen for hearing loss in newborns. In general, most primary care settings are conducive to conventional audiometry, whereas other forms of audiometry require the assistance of an audiologist.

Other Testing

Common problems of the external and middle ear rarely require laboratory tests or imaging. CT scan or MRI can easily help to diagnose complications of *otitis media* such as *mastoiditis, meningitis,* and *lateral sinus thrombosis.* Lumbar puncture is helpful to evaluate for suspected intracranial infection after ruling out increased intracranial pressure. Vestibular testing can be difficult to perform in children in a primary care setting. Refer this to a specialist.

Mouth and Oropharynx

Laboratory tests can be useful adjuncts in diagnosis for children with *stomatitis* or *pharyngitis.* Rapid assays are widely available and generally reliable for group A *streptococci, influenza, parainfluenza, adenovirus, RSV, HIV,* and *HSV.* Viral and bacterial cultures are available for other infectious causes of *stomatitis* and *pharyngitis.* The heterophil antibody test or "monospot" is reliable in older children and adolescents with *EBV* infection. Order antibody titers when in doubt. Order blood counts and screens for *rheumatologic* conditions as clinically indicated.

Plain x-rays of the neck can be useful in complicated infections of the pharynx and neck, such as *parapharyngeal* and *retropharyngeal abscess.* CT scan can be useful to distinguish *cellulitis* from *abscess* and is more sensitive than roentgenography. Imaging and endoscopy can help to elucidate causes of dysphagia.

Neck

In the setting of potential airway compromise (*epiglottitis, severe croup*), the clinician should first stabilize the airway prior to any testing. Once the airway is stable, auxiliary testing such as plain radiography and/or CT scan can be helpful in some cases of upper airway obstruction such as *croup, epiglottitis,* and *retropharyngeal abscesses.* Foreign bodies are visible on plain film if they are radiopaque. In other cases, these tests may not be helpful. Further testing can include indirect or flexible laryngoscopy or rigid bronchoscopy for direct visualization of the larynx or trachea. Fluoroscopy may be helpful for visualization of external compression of the trachea from vascular or other structures.

In infants with *torticollis,* perform cervical spine x-rays to look for deformities. In older children, MRI may be helpful to examine the posterior fossa for an intracranial process. CT scan may reveal signs of C_1–C_2 *subluxation* in the setting of postviral or traumatic torticollis in the older child.

The *infectious* causes of cervical *lymphadenopathy* and *lymphadenitis* often can be determined based on history and physical examination alone. In cases where the cause is not clear, or when lymphadenopathy persists despite observation or adequate treatment, a number of additional tests may be helpful. Antibody titers to common infectious causes (*EBV, CMV, toxoplasmosis, cat-scratch disease,* etc.) can be helpful in the acute or chronic setting. PPD placement with controls can aid in the diagnosis of *tuberculosis* or *other mycobacterial adenitis.* Check thyroid function tests for a patient with a suspected *goiter.* Finally, biopsy can be helpful with both *infectious* and *malignant* causes of lymphadenopathy.

When to Refer

Ear

Clinical examination alone usually diagnoses problems of the auricle and canal. Examination of the middle ear space can be difficult, especially in those with underlying craniofacial defects. If you are not able to visualize the middle ear satisfactorily, a referral to an otolaryngologist is appropriate. In the setting of persistent *otitis media,* a referral for tympanocentesis is appropriate if you are not equipped to perform this procedure or experienced. Problems of the inner ear, including hearing loss and vertigo, often require additional testing by an audiologist. A neurologist can perform electronystagmography (ENG) to distinguish vestibular from cerebellar causes of *nystagmus.*

Mouth and Oropharynx

Most diagnoses of problems of the mouth and oropharynx should occur in the primary care setting. Dysphagia owing to an impaired oropharyngeal coordination often requires the assistance of a speech pathologist trained in the evaluation of dysphagia. Refer neuromuscular testing such as the Tensilon test for *myasthenia gravis* to a neurologist.

Disorders of the esophagus, on the other hand, often require the assistance of a gastroenterologist who can visualize the structure with the aid of an endoscope and perform additional diagnostic tests as appropriate.

Neck

While the primary care provider can diagnose most cases of *croup*, both congenital and persistent forms of *stridor* generally will require the assistance of an otolaryngologist or a pediatric pulmonologist. An oncologist can help to diagnose *malignant* neck masses, whereas a surgeon generally will perform the biopsy.

8 The Respiratory System

Douglas N. Homnick

The respiratory system consists of structures that start with the nose and end in the terminal lung units, the alveoli, where gas exchange occurs. Like the skin, the respiratory system is in constant contact with the environment and therefore subject to stresses such as temperature, degrees of humidity or dryness, air pollution, and infectious agents. Developmentally, the lung and associated support structures (bony thorax, chest wall musculature, vessels, and nerves) and the conducting airways go through substantial change from infancy through adolescence. The mouth, oropharynx, and nonairway neck are discussed elsewhere (see Chapter 7). In this chapter we will cover other structures that are part of the respiratory system. The goals of this chapter are to

1. Outline the functional anatomy, physiology, mechanics, and pathophysiology that produce signs and symptoms referable to the respiratory tract
2. Understand points of the age-related pulmonary history and physical examination and be able to integrate both in forming plausible differential diagnoses
3. Understand age- and disease-appropriate imaging for evaluation of the respiratory tract and be able to formulate a plan for their use
4. Do the same for laboratory evaluations related to pulmonary disease
5. Understand the difference between restrictive and obstructive pulmonary disease and appropriate age-related pulmonary function evaluation
6. Understand when referral to a pulmonary subspecialist is appropriate

Developmental and Functional Anatomy

Nose, Sinuses, and Larynx

Functionally, the nose consists of the external nose and the internal nose. The lower two-thirds of the central structural portion of the nose is cartilage, and the upper third consists of bone. The term *nares* indicates the openings to the nose, and the nares form the entrance to the anterior chamber or vestibule. The nasal septum divides the nose into two nasal

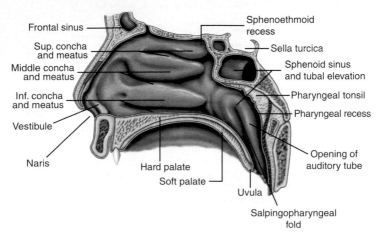

FIGURE 8–1 *Lateral Wall of the Nasal Cavity. (Adapted with permission from Crafts RC:* Textbook of Human Anatomy. *New York: Ronald Press, 1966.)*

fossae, and the lateral wall of the nose consists of four nasal turbinates (supreme, superior, middle, and inferior) or conchae (FIGURE 8–1). The middle meatus, lying under the middle turbinate, is very important because it contains the drainage sites for the maxillary, frontal, and anterior ethmoid sinuses. The nose has two primary functions, olfactory and respiratory. The olfactory region of the nose is located high in the nasal vault, above the superior turbinate, in the cribriform plate. Central axons of sensory hairs in this region travel to the olfactory cortex through the first cranial nerve. Other than the anterior third of the nose, which is lined with nonciliated squamous cell epithelium, the remainder of the nasal and sinus mucosa consists of the same ciliated, pseudostratified columnar epithelium found in the remainder of the respiratory tract. Abundant mucus glands (submucosal glands and goblet cells) provide a mucus layer over the ciliated epithelium, which is essential for mucociliary clearance. The vestibule of the nose also contains numerous hairs or vibrissae. The paranasal sinuses include ethmoid, maxillary, frontal, and sphenoid sinuses (FIGURE 8–2). They are lined with respiratory mucosa and develop as outgrowths or diverticulae of the walls of the nasal cavities. At birth, only the maxillary and ethmoid sinuses are present. Pneumatization of the frontal sinuses does not begin until the first or second year and is not complete until late childhood. The sphenoid sinuses begin to pneumatize in the third year. The larynx and paralaryngeal structures develop from the caudal portion of the laryngotracheal tube that is the primordium of the larynx, trachea, bronchi, and lungs. The cartilage of the larynx derives from the fourth and sixth pairs of branchial arches and the epiglottis from the third and fourth arches. Innervation of the larynx comes from the laryngeal branches of

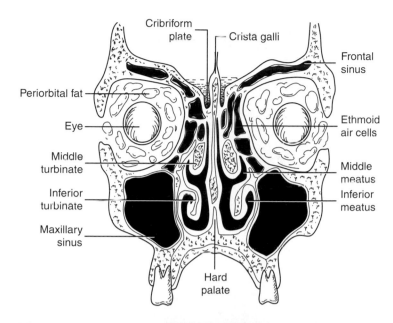

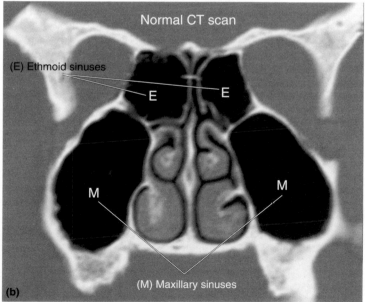

FIGURE 8-2 The Paranasal Sinuses. *Frontal sinuses are not yet developed, as seen in this CT scan of a young child. (Adapted with permission from DeWeese D, Saunders WH:* Testbook of Otolaryngology, *6th ed. St. Louis: Mosby, 1982.)*

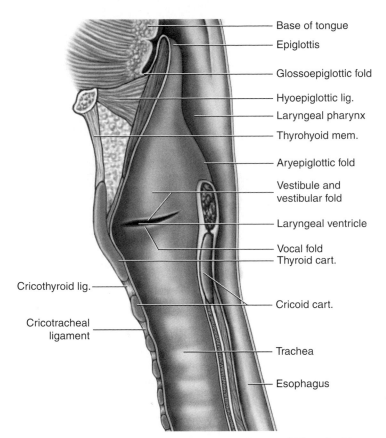

Base of tongue

Epiglottis

Glossoepiglottic fold

Hyoepiglottic lig.

Laryngeal pharynx

Thyrohyoid mem.

Aryepiglottic fold

Vestibule and vestibular fold

Laryngeal ventricle

Vocal fold
Thyroid cart.

Cricothyroid lig.

Cricotracheal ligament

Cricoid cart.

Trachea

Esophagus

FIGURE 8–3 *Anatomic Relationships of the Larynx. (Adapted with permission from Crafts RC:* Textbook of Human Anatomy. *New York: Ronald Press, 1966.)*

the vagus nerve. Its blood supply derives from the superior and inferior thyroid arteries, and lymph drainage is to the middle and upper cervical lymph node chains. The mucosa of the larynx is continuous with the hypopharynx above and the trachea below, which is important to uninterrupted mucociliary clearance. The larynx acts not only as an organ of vocalization but also as an organ of airway protection. Anatomic relationships of the larynx to paralaryngeal structures are discussed in Chapter 7 and shown in FIGURE 8–3. Conditions affecting the nose and paranasal sinuses are listed in TABLE 8–1.

Lung, Intrathoracic Airways, and Thorax

Postnatal lung growth continues at least into adolescence with a tripling of tracheal diameter, an increase in alveolar dimensions by a factor of 4,

TABLE 8-1 *Disorders of the Nose and Sinuses in Infants, Children, and Adolescents*

Key Problem	Differential Diagnosis	Age*	History/Examination	Comments
Nasal obstruction	Choanal atresia	I	Distress with mouth occlusion, unilateral or bilateral	May be evident at birth or later with upper respiratory infection
	Foreign body	C, A	Purulent nasal discharge, often foul-smelling and unilateral.	History and rhinoscopic examination usually reveals diagnosis
	Nasal congestion	I, C, A	Swollen hyperemia with infection or irritation, pale with allergy	Many causes; in infants may be due early to maternal estrogen, later infection
				Allergy in older children and adolescents, vasomotor rhinitis in teens
	Nasal polyps	C, A	May be seen with otoscope speculum as large, shiny, mucus-filled sac	Common in CF and nasal allergy.
Nasal septal defects	Congenital perforation or deviation	I	Visual examination or CT scan	Most commonly occurs secondary to local trauma, e.g., long-dwelling cannula for CPAP, birth trauma, occasionally with infection

(Continued)

TABLE 8-1 Disorders of the Nose and Sinuses in Infants, Children, and Adolescents *(Continued)*

Key Problem	Differential Diagnosis	Age*	History/Examination	Comments
Nasal septal defects	Acquired septal deviation	I, C, A	Visual examination or CT scan	Trauma most common cause
Nasal masses	Hemangiomas, congenital nasolacrimal duct obstruction	I	Direct visualization and CT scan for diagnosis	Polyps very rare in infants
	Polyps, tumors (rhabdomyosarcoma)	C, A		
Epistaxis	Most commonly due to dry air and local trauma	C	Abrasion of the Kiesselbach plexus in the anterior septum	Family history common; worse in winter; rare in infants and decreases in adolescence
	Congenital vascular abnormalities.	I, C	Hemangiomas, hereditary hemorrhagic telangiectasia	Requires subspecialty examination to confirm
	Other: Hypertension, clotting disorders, thrombocytopenia	I, C, A	Often systemic signs	Often history of familial hypertension, renal disease, or clotting disorders
Anosmia	Chronic nasal obstruction (e.g., allergy).	C, A	See above	Most common

			Exam specific to problem	
Other:	Head trauma, CNS tumor, viral or bacterial infections.	C, A		Common with chronic sinusitis, rhinitis, and nasal polyposis
Acute sinusitis	Most often follows an upper respiratory infection, but nasal allergy and second-hand smoke contribute; most often common respiratory bacteria	I, C, A	Facial tenderness and headache are often elicited from children and adolescents but not infants	Probably rarely diagnosed in infants until sinusitis becomes chronic
Chronic sinusitis	Common in conditions involving decreased mucociliary clearance: CF, primary ciliary dyskinesia, immunodeficiency, nasal allergy, GERD with nasal reflux, cleft palate, nasal polyposis, and nasal foreign bodies (e.g., nasotracheal or nasogastric tubes)	I, C, A	Chronic cough, chronic headache, postnasal drip, and other associated chronic respiratory problems (e.g., chronic bronchitis in CF) occur	A high index of suspicion is important to diagnose this in infants; CT scan is necessary to define asymmetric anatomy versus disease

*I = infant; C = child; A = adolescent.

and a tenfold increase in the number of alveoli. Alveolar multiplication continues until late childhood (around age 8 years), and thereafter, increase in lung volume is due to increase in alveolar dimension. A high degree of variability exists in the total number of alveoli at maturity, ranging from about 200 million to 600 million. The reason for this is probably genetic, determining the timing of when alveolar multiplication ceases. Pulmonary arteries parallel the alveolar development during the first couple of years of life, but thereafter, arteries multiply more quickly, reaching a greater artery-to-alveoli ratio by late childhood than in newborn years.

The chest wall consists of both bony structures and striated muscle and changes substantially over time with growth. The thoracic cage consists of 12 pairs of ribs, the 12 thoracic vertebrae, and the sternum. The eleventh and twelfth "vertebral" ribs do not attach to the sternum by cartilage and therefore are "floating." Ossification of the chest wall begins in utero and is not complete until about the twenty-fifth year. As a result, the infant chest wall is very compliant, as evidenced by the pulling in (paradoxical breathing) of the sternum during periods of respiratory distress. This, along with more horizontal placement of the ribs, fewer fatigue-resistant muscle fibers, and higher peripheral airway resistance, leads to a tendency toward early respiratory failure in infants experiencing acute pulmonary disease.

By the end of 16 weeks' gestation, all the conducting airways have formed from the trachea down to the terminal bronchioles. However, there is continuing growth and remodeling of airways throughout childhood and adolescence. Cartilage supports the airways down to the terminal bronchioles, appearing at about 25 weeks' gestation and increasing considerably over the first few months of life. Delayed maturation and absence or extrinsic compression of cartilage can lead to airway compromise. Airway epithelium, found from the posteroinferior nasal turbinate down to terminal bronchioles, plays a very important role in both regulation of inflammation and mucus clearance. Ciliated, pseudostratified, columnar epithelium is essential to the efficient removal of mucus and foreign matter, including microorganisms, from the airway, and disruptions in mucus quantity, viscoelasticity, or cilia can lead to chronic inflammation, infection, and eventual breakdown of the airway wall (bronchiectasis).

Smooth muscle within the airway wall, particularly that of small to medium airway generations, is capable of contracting in response to a variety of stimuli, including chemical, temperature, neurologic stimulation, and emotion. Narrowing of airways, owing to airway inflammation with edema or bronchoconstriction, leads to high airway resistance with increased work of breathing and possible respiratory compromise.

Physiology and Mechanics

The nose serves several important functions. It is the first contact with the outside environment and is the first line of defense against the inhalation of particulate matter. The nose prevents particulates from entering the lower airway through trapping of particulates in nasal mucus associated with the vibrissae and through initiation of sneeze. It is also an air-conditioning organ, providing warmth or cooling and humidity to the lower airway under conditions of normal airflow. The absence of this function, i.e., under conditions of high airflow with mouth breathing (e.g., before exercise), may lead to excess cooling of the airway and the development of bronchospasm. The turbinates increase the surface areas of the internal nose, allowing the transfer of heat and fluid from its vascular surface, thereby increasing the efficiency of temperature regulation and humidification. It is also the organ of olfaction. Not only is this important in recognizing the differences between pleasant and unpleasant odors, but it also provides gustatory sensation as a cofunctioning organ with the taste buds. The sinuses serve to lighten the skull by providing air-filled spaces. The paranasal sinuses are continuous with the upper respiratory tract primarily through the nose and consist of similar epithelium with similar function, i.e., enhancement of mucociliary clearance. Sinus epithelium contains fewer glands than the nose and therefore contributes less to nasal secretions. The larynx serves several functions besides being a connecting airway between the trachea and the hypopharynx. This complex tubular organ functions as a sphincter. Swallowing is a complicated process that requires protection of the airway from the entrance of food and other materials. During swallowing, the arytenoids, the aryepiglottic folds, and the epiglottis fold in to close the trachea and prevent the ingress of foreign material. Without this action, aspiration with subsequent significant respiratory morbidity would occur. The larynx also plays an essential role in the very important protective cough reflex. When foreign material touches the laryngeal mucosa or surrounding structures, this reflex occurs through the vagus nerve. Cough occurs through receptors concentrated at the bifurcations of the lower airways. Increased intrathoracic airway pressure against a closed glottis suddenly releases during coughing, creating airflows high enough to expel foreign material or excess airway secretions. The third role of the larynx is as an organ of phonation. A fine muscular coordination is essential to provide not only the degree of apposition of the vocal cords but also to lengthen them to produce the vibrations necessary for speech. Additional contributory functions to sound and speech include elevation and depression of the larynx itself and actions of the tongue, palate, and lips.

Although the lung has many functions (e.g., defense against infection, acid-base balance, etc.), its prime function is that of gas exchange. Oxygen exchanges for carbon dioxide across the alveolar membrane from pulmonary capillaries. Surfactant produced by specialized (type II) alveolar cells allows for maximum maintenance of lung volume at the end of expiration [functional residual capacity (FRC)]. This allows for continuous gas exchange throughout the respiratory cycle. Defects in surfactant production lead to decreased gas exchange, as evidenced by conditions such as the acute respiratory distress syndrome (ARDS) and the infant respiratory distress syndrome (IRDS, or hyaline membrane disease).

Lung volume and airway caliber relate directly to thoracic volume because elastic tissue supports the lung parenchyma. Lower lung volumes will lead to an overall decrease in airway size and subsequent increased resistance to airflow. This is important when considering the physical examination of young children with airway obstruction or the positioning of older children and adolescents during respiratory distress (see section on the physical examination). Ventilation and perfusion of the lung normally are well matched, except when the lung parenchyma is regionally inflamed, such as in pneumonia, or when obstructed, such as with a foreign body or asthma. Then ventilation-perfusion mismatching leads to hypoxemia.

Normally, the visceral pleura, a thin covering of the lung, is applied without discernible space to the parietal pleura, an envelope of tissue surrounding the lung. The visceral pleura absorb fluid of the parietal pleura and eliminate it through a network of extensive pulmonary lymphatics. Excess fluid produced during states of inflammation (e.g., pneumonitis) or overproduction and/or decreased absorption (e.g., congestive heart failure or disruption of the thoracic duct) leads to collection of fluid between the pleura (effusion) that often leads to increasing respiratory distress. Air within the pleural space (pneumothorax) may occur spontaneously or because of trauma to the airway or lung. When this occurs, the observation that the chest wall moves outward while the lung collapses emphasizes the lung's elastic qualities. The lungs of infants have fewer elastic properties than those of older children and adolescents. This is another reason why airways in the infant lung are less well supported, leading to higher airway resistance and a tendency to develop significant airway obstruction with respiratory decompensation (e.g., with viral bronchiolitis).

The chest wall, including the ribs and respiratory muscles, make up the "pump" of the respiratory system that drives ventilation. Of the respiratory muscles, the diaphragm plays an important role by acting as a piston descending during inspiration and lowering the intrapleural pressure, allowing airflow into the mouth and nose. During its descent, it also increases intraabdominal pressure, which helps to elevate the lower ribs and expand the thoracic cage. This expansion of the thoracic cage allows an increase in lung volume. Dysfunction of the diaphragm owing to a primary defect such as a diaphragmatic hernia or secondary paralysis such as with disruption of one or both phrenic nerves can lead to inefficient ventilation and respiratory compromise. Other important respiratory muscles include the intercostal muscles and the so-called accessory muscles, including the scalenes and the sternocleidomastoids.

History

The discussion of pulmonary history is a supplement to Chapter 1 and is not a substitute for a complete pediatric history. However, the pulmonary history is single-system-directed and must by necessity bring out those relevant influences on its function. As in the general history, determining onset (gradual or acute), duration (chronic = greater than 3 weeks), recurrent (periods of wellness alternating with periods of illness) or persistent, and trigger factors (e.g., viral upper respiratory infection) is essential. The lungs are in contact with the external environment, so environmental history is particularly important. Indoor (e.g., environmental tobacco smoke, wood stoves, pets, etc.) and outdoor exposures (e.g., animals, cold air, industrial, etc.) must be carefully sought. Family history of respiratory illness is also very important because many diseases manifesting in childhood have a genetic basis (e.g., cystic fibrosis or primary ciliary dyskinesia) or genetic predisposition (e.g., asthma). Neonatal history also may indicate a reason for persistent or recurrent respiratory disease, especially in infancy, although even teens may manifest chronic airway obstruction because of neonatal disease such as bronchopulmonary dysplasia (BPD). Key problems commonly encountered as a chief complaint or obtained from the respiratory tract history are discussed by age.

Infants

KEY PROBLEM

Cough Cough in infancy generally arises from irritation of the airways because receptors are concentrated at airway bifurcations. Cough occurs in a phased sequence involving a deep inspiration, closure of the glottis, and relaxation of the diaphragm, along with contraction of the muscles of expiration and sudden opening of the glottis with forceful expired airflow. Causes of cough are acute or chronic depending on duration. Cough continuing beyond 3 weeks is termed *chronic*.

Acute cough in infants is most often due to infection, typically viral. The patient usually produces thin, clear to white mucus, and the cough resolves over a week to 10 days. A brassy, seal-like cough following an upper respiratory tract infection is typical for viral *croup syndrome* (*laryngotracheal bronchitis*). Other causes of acute cough in infants include transient exposure to irritants such as environmental tobacco smoke (ETS). Monitor a cough initially deemed acute, and reevaluate the patient if the cough persists for more than 3 weeks.

Chronic cough in infancy has diverse causes. A *metabolic* reason for cough includes *cystic fibrosis* (CF). Infants with CF presenting with chronic cough often produce yellow mucus, especially in the morning on rising owing to accumulated thick secretions at night. One should seek a history suggestive of intestinal fat malabsorption, including failure to gain weight, large, foul-smelling stools, and ravenous appetite. *Infectious* causes of chronic cough include *Pertussis* (especially in infants with fewer than three vaccinations), marked by severe paroxysms of cough with cyanosis and the classic "whoop" on inspiration; atypical bacterial organisms such as *Chlamydia* and *Mycoplasma* also cause cough paroxysms. Upper respiratory infection symptoms often precede the development of cough in these conditions. Cough of *neurogenic* origin in infants is due primarily to complications of developmental disabilities.

These include chronic aspiration of upper airway secretions and ingested food with tracheal irritation. Onset of wheezing shortly after or during feedings suggests aspiration. *Traumatic* injury to the recurrent laryngeal nerve during surgery or birth leads to laryngeal dysfunction and increases the risk of chronic aspiration. A history of stridor and muffled or hoarse cry suggests this diagnosis and is one of the traumatic reasons for chronic cough. Another traumatic etiology for chronic cough in infants is foreign-body aspiration (usually in those older than 6 months of age). This is consistent with a history of sudden onset of wheeze or stridor while playing with older siblings or crawling on the floor. Residual lung and airway inflammation owing to neonatal lung injury from oxygen and positive-pressure ventilation [*bronchopulmonary dysplasia* (BPD)] can lead to cough of traumatic origin. The perinatal history suggests a risk of BPD. *Toxic* exposures to second-hand smoke and alternative heating sources such as wood and kerosene stoves are causes of chronic respiratory symptom (including chronic cough) in infancy. A good environmental history will assess the risk of toxic exposures. *Immunologic* causes include chronic infection from immune deficiency and hypersensitivity to milk. Unusual infections (e.g., skin) and chronic diarrhea with failure to thrive suggest *immunodeficiency*. Questioning for risk of congenital transmission of the human immunodeficiency virus (HIV) is important. *Allergy* in infancy usually manifests as eczema, but occasionally, postnasal drip from either nasal allergy (rare) or chronic sinusitis can result in chronic cough. Appropriate imaging (sinus CT scan) must corroborate a diagnosis of chronic *sinusitis* in infants. Rarer causes of chronic cough in infants include symptomatic *congenital* lung malformations such as *bronchogenic cyst, cystic adenomatoid malformation,* and *pulmonary sequestration*. Congestive heart failure from congenital heart disease may manifest as cough (*circulatory*).

KEY PROBLEM
Wheezing and Stridor *Wheezing and stridor* are adventitious lung sounds from turbulent airflow through narrowed or obstructed airways. Stridor is a loud, musical, high-pitched wheeze. Wheezing and stridor may occur on inspiration, expiration, or both (biphasic) depending on severity and level of obstruction.

Metabolic causes of wheeze and stridor in infancy are rare. *Hypokalemia* and *hypocalcemia* may cause stridor at this age. Chronic wheezing in infancy from *CF* is a common presenting symptom. Other historical symptoms of CF include large, foul-smelling stools, ravenous appetite, and failure to thrive. *Infectious* etiologies are much more common. Fortunately, *epiglottitis* associated with inspiratory or biphasic stridor and high fever is rare since immunization against type B *Hemophilus influenzae*. Inspiratory stridor following a short prodrome of upper respiratory infection is typical for viral croup. Wheezing from asthma triggered by viral infections is common and is primarily expiratory in nature. Wheezing from viral pneumonia including *respiratory syncitial virus* (RSV) bronchiolitis occurs in early infancy most often during epidemics in middle to late winter and early spring. *Neurogenic* causes of wheeze result in airway inflammation from oral aspiration. This may progress to serious bacterial *pneumonias*. Gagging, choking, and wheezing during or shortly after feedings suggests chronic aspiration. A number of infants with severe disabilities and poor upper airway protective reflexes will aspirate silently, and therefore, a high index of suspicion is necessary. *Gastroesophageal reflux disease* (GERD) is common in children with developmental disabilities, and a history of wheezing following feedings should suggest this diagnosis. Like cough, exposures to environmental *toxins* such as *ETS* may be a cause of chronic wheezing in infants. A history of tracheal intubation in the neonatal period or infancy with subsequent stridor suggests *traumatic* causes, including vocal cord injury or subglottic stenosis.

Allergic causes of stridor are rare in infants. However, a history of wheezing or stridor with hives on exposure to an antigen such as an antibiotic or nonsteroidal anti-inflammatory agent should alert the clinician to potential *anaphylaxis*. *Allergic asthma* occurs later in infancy, particularly in infants with a strong family history of allergy in a primary relative, although in most infants viruses remain the major trigger of asthma.

Congenital causes of wheeze and stridor include delay in development of laryngeal (*laryngomalacia*) and tracheal (*tracheomalacia*) cartilage. Since laryngomalacia and trachomalacia can be isolated or coexist to variable degrees (including *bronchomalacia*), stridor can be quite variable. In typical tracheomalacia, there is a history of persistent, coarse expiratory wheeze from birth or near birth. It does not respond to medications and exacerbates with upper respiratory infections. In laryngomalacia, there is a history of inspiratory stridor, often starting between 2 and 4 weeks of age, increasing in volume over the first few months of life. Biphasic stridor may occur with very severe laryngomalacia, and both severe tracheomalacia and laryngomalacia may cause failure to thrive and require surgical intervention. Stridor also may occur with congenital laryngeal lesions, including *laryngeal webs* and *hemangiomas.* Often the stridor is severe and biphasic and in the case of hemangiomas increases over time with growth of the hemangioma. Patients also may have associated cutaneous hemangiomas. *Circulatory* (and *congenital*) causes of stridor include vascular rings and abnormal vascular anatomy that impinges on airway structures. These include double aortic arch, *aberrant right subclavian artery,* and *pulmonary artery "sling."* The stridor usually is expiratory and persistent with exacerbations during respiratory infection.

KEY PROBLEM
Chest Pain Undoubtedly, infants experience *chest pain* and discomfort as in older children but cannot express their symptoms except through increased irritability. A careful examination will reveal chest wall tenderness on palpation.

KEY PROBLEM
Cyanosis Cyanosis or blue color of mucus membranes (central cyanosis) is usually a sign of serious cardiopulmonary disease. However, peripheral cyanosis, i.e., blue color around the mouth in infants and blueness of cool extremities is most often benign. Cyanosis occurs when reduced hemoglobin reaches 4 to 5 g/dl.

Metabolic causes of cyanosis include CF with significant pulmonary involvement leading to ventilation-perfusion mismatching. The same mechanism occurs with lower airway disease found in *infectious* etiologies, airway obstruction in viral bronchiolitis, and severe *asthma (allergy)*. Consider *neurogenic* causes of cyanosis particularly when there is no historical evidence to support cardiopulmonary disease. Hypoventilation occurring with muscle weakness (*neuromuscular disease*) or because of infant *apnea* and aspiration of foods with *apnea, laryngospasm*, or *pneumonitis* can lead to cyanosis. Infants may not ventilate well during seizures and may become transiently cyanotic. Questioning about tone, level of conciousness, unusual movements, handling of secretions, and feeding behavior helps to point to a specific etiology. *Toxic* causes of cyanosis include *methemoglobinemia* owing to ingestion of water containing high levels of nitrates (*blue baby syndrome*). Methemoglobin exaggerates the "blueness." *Congenital* causes of cyanosis include severe lung malformations such as *congenital lobar emphysema* and *lung hypoplasia.* These conditions will be readily evident in the newborn period. Most other congenital causes of cyanosis are *cardiovascular (circulatory)* in origin and represent the effects of cardiac failure or right-to-left shunt (see Chapter 9). History of cyanosis with crying, without wheeze or cough, suggests a cardiovascular origin. Infants with cardiac failure may present with wheeze, cough, and respiratory distress, as well as failure to thrive. A history of poor feeding with easy fatigability should alert the clinician to possible undiagnosed cardiac disease.

Children

KEY PROBLEM
■ **Cough** Acute causes of cough in children are similar to those in infants in that they are most often a result of infectious agents, particularly viruses. Like infants, children produce thin, clear to white secretions, and there is a history of low-grade or no fever. Resolution occurs in 7 to 10 days, at the most 2 weeks. Cough determined to be continuous beyond 3 weeks is chronic and requires investigation that is more extensive.

Metabolic causes of cough in children mainly occur in those with *CF*. On questioning the parents and child, the cough often will exacerbate with upper respiratory infections and remit very slowly, although incompletely. Cough is more productive in the morning on rising, and sputum is often yellow to green, occasionally gray in color. The history also often will be positive for fat malabsorption with greasy, large, four-smelling stools and slow growth. *Infectious* causes of chronic cough include atypical organisms (*Chlamydia, Mycoplasma*) and, with increasing exposure to more people, *tuberculosis* (TB). As with adolescents and adults, TB can present with acute pneumonia or with a history of cough, night sweats, and weight loss. The risk of disease goes up significantly if the history suggests exposure to individuals with known TB or *acquired immune-deficiency syndrome* (AIDS). *Bronchiectasis*, because of a retained foreign body or *primary ciliary dyskinesia* (PCD), may occur in later childhood and presents with exacerbating and remitting episodes of fever and productive cough often only transiently suppressed with antibiotics. *Pertussis* with a history of chronic and severe paroxysmal cough occurs in a nonimmunized or underimmunized young child. Immunization history is part of the basic pediatric and pulmonary history. *Chronic sinusitis* also may cause chronic cough through both postnasal drip and neurogenic mediated cough from *sinus inflammation.* Increase in cough in the supine position and facial pressure and pain occur. *Neurogenic* causes of chronic cough include *aspiration* of upper airway secretions and food or aspiration of refluxate in children with developmental disabilities and rarely in normal children. Cough occurs during or shortly after feedings. Some older children may be able to relate abdominal or chest symptoms. In older children, psychogenic or habit cough becomes a problem. A careful history, excluding other pulmonary disease, often will provide this diagnosis. Cough of *psychogenic* origin generally is loud, "honking," and often disruptive of social situations. It does not occur during sleep and is not associated with other respiratory symptoms such as wheeze. A *foreign body* in the external auditory canal that stimulates the nerve of Arnold is an unusual cause of chronic cough. The history rarely may lead the clinician to suspect this diagnosis, but more likely the aural foreign body will become evident during the physical examination. *Toxic* causes of chronic cough most commonly result from *ETS* exposure but also, unfortunately, from primary smoking, particularly in the middle school child. Other causes include exposure to alternative heat sources such as a wood stove or irritant chemicals and particulates, as often found in farming environments. The environmental history should help to elucidate a toxic etiology. *Foreign-body aspiration* is still a cause of cough at this age. Usually there is a history of choking on a food or other item (e.g., a pen cap), and the symptoms are acute. However, in the case of a disabled child who constantly puts small objects in the mouth, there is a risk of foreign-body aspiration with a delay in diagnosis unless the index of suspicion is high because of the sudden onset of symptoms. Cough associated with pulmonary infiltration owing to collagen-vascular disease (*lupus erythematosis, rheumatoid arthritis*) and related diseases such as *sarcoidosis* and *Wegener's granulomatosis* begins in childhood. Most often the history will bring out systemic symptoms associated with these conditions. As children progress through the preschool years, *allergic* sensitization to aeroallergens such as pollens becomes more common, resulting in postnasal drip from chronic allergic rhinitis and chronic cough from asthma. A family history of allergy along with a careful review of potential triggers such as exercise, cold air, and seasonal pollen blooms is helpful in determining risk. Asthma may present only as dry, nonproductive or minimally productive cough (cough-variant asthma) that often is worse at night and with exercise, laughing, or cold air exposure. Occasionally, *congenital* lung malformations become evident in later childhood with cough and lung infiltration. A history of recurrence of *pneumonias* in the same lung location should alert the clinician to this possibility. In addition, *H-type tracheoesophageal fistula*, albeit rare, may present later in childhood with cough and wheeze associated with eating, particularly with ingestion of thin liquids. Previously undiagnosed *vascular rings* may be a *circulatory* cause of chronic cough and the use of angiotensin-converting enzyme (ACE) inhibitor drugs. Cough along with chest pain, fever, and sputum production may occur during the *acute chest syndrome of sickle cell disease.*

KEY PROBLEM
Wheezing and Stridor   *Metabolic* causes of *stridor* are rare but include *laryngospasm owing to hypocalcemia. Wheezing* can accompany CF exacerbations because many patients with this disease also manifest reversible airway obstruction similar to asthma. With newborn screening for CF in many states and early recognition of cases through sweat and genetic testing, fewer patients are reaching childhood without a diagnosis. *Infectious* causes of stridor include *viral croup* before about 5 years of age, and the history generally will show a prodromal period of low-grade or no fever with upper respiratory infection symptoms. Stridor and high fever associated with *epiglottitis* are rare with current immunizations; however, history of acute onset of stridor and high fever also should alert the physician to the possibility of *retropharyngeal* or *peritonsillar abscess.* Wheezing associated with respiratory infection is usually a manifestation of asthma in children because wheezing owing to *viral bronchiolitis* generally is limited to infants. Wheezing also may accompany acute exacerbations of *bronchiectasis* from CF or PCD. *Neurogenic* causes of stridor includes *vocal cord dysfunction* (VCD) occasionally encountered in preteens (see discussion in adolescents). Like infants, children with developmental disabilities are prone to aspirate with resulting wheezing. *Toxic* exposures, including caustic or irritating chemicals and smoke, can lead to acute laryngospasm with stridor and wheezing.

Neoplasia also may be a cause of stridor or wheezing if a mediastinal or intrathoracic tumor exerts pressure on the airway or is located within the airway. Large lymph nodes also may impinge on the airway and produce wheeze or stridor, and gastroenteric cysts may compromise the airways. *Traumatic* causes of wheeze or stridor are *toxic inhalation* and *foreign-body aspiration.* The history consists of sudden onset of wheeze or stridor in an otherwise well child. Often there is a history of playing on the floor in the case of small children, or the older child will be able to relate choking on food or another object. Retained foreign body leads to reactive inflammation and eventually infection. Children with BPD often will continue to wheeze well into childhood and beyond.

Allergy, specifically *asthma*, is by far the most common reason for wheezing in childhood. The history often will show a seasonal trend and specific triggers such as viral infections, exercise, and cold air or suggest an environmental antigen such as pollen, grass, etc. There is often a family history of allergy, including allergic rhinitis, eczema, or asthma. Other symptoms include night cough and cough with the triggers mentioned earlier. Other allergic manifestations such as eczema and allergic rhinitis may be present as well. Wheezing in *asthma* may be episodic or persistent. Another manifestation of airway allergy in childhood is *spasmodic croup*. Stridor occurring suddenly, often during the early morning hours, with or without prior respiratory illness can occur repeatedly in older children and lasts from hours to a day or two. These children also may have other allergic symptoms such as asthma or allergic rhinitis. *Congenital* causes of wheeze and stridor often become evident before childhood years, but occasionally, an *H-type tracheoesophageal fistula* will be an exception. A history of cough and wheeze associated with ingestion of foods, particularly thin liquids, will suggest chronic aspiration. *Circulatory* causes of stridor or wheeze, such as vascular rings, may not declare themselves until childhood. *Congestive heart failure* may be an occasional cause of wheeze in older children (see Chapter 9).

KEY PROBLEM
Chest Pain Chest pain is common in children and adolescents. *Metabolic* cause of chest pain is *CF associated with bronchitis and cough.* Pleuritic pain or sharp pain on deep inspiration is common in CF, especially during acute exacerbations of chronic infection. Pleuritic pain or pleurisy is also common in both viral respiratory *infections* such as those with coxsackie B virus (epidemic *pleurodynia*) and with bacterial *pneumonia*. Inflammation of the lung and pleura also may lead to effusions and progress to *empyema*. The history often will reveal cough, fever, and increasing dyspnea prior to the onset of chest pain. Chest pain also may be associated with diaphragmatic irritation owing to *subphrenic abscess* or *pancreatitis*. A history of *foreign-body* aspiration with subsequent fever and chest pain may indicate retention of the foreign body in the airway with subsequent reactive inflammation and infection. *Herpes zoster* presents as a vesicular rash located over the chest wall in a pattern to suggest involvement of a dermatome and is both a *neurogenic* and *infectious* cause of chest pain. Chest discomfort and pain also may occur with *hyperventilation* associated with psychosomatic disease such as panic attack or disorder, although this is more common in teens. *Traumatic* causes of chest pain, besides foreign-body aspiration, include a history of chest trauma (e.g., during sports activities) with localized *contusion*. If severe, consider *rib fracture*. *Costochondritis,* or pain over the sternum at the costochondral junction(s), may follow upper body exercise such as weight lifting or any sports activity using the upper body, although a specific cause may not be readily evident. *Spontaneous pneumothorax* leads to acute chest pain. The risk increases with diseases such as *cystic fibrosis* and *acute asthma,* but it also may occur in healthy children. Pneumothorax and *hemothorax* may occur after significant chest trauma or thoracic surgical procedures. *GERD* with substernal burning is common in children, and inquiry as to timing of pain to ingestion of meals is important. Inhalation of irritants and smoke also may lead to chest pain or discomfort. One should seek a history of inhalation of volatile substances such as organic solvents when suspecting *toxins* as an etiology of acute onset of chest pain and dyspnea in an otherwise healthy child. *Congenital* causes of chest pain include pleurisy and pneumonitis associated with lung malformations such as *lung cyst, cystic adenomatoid malformation,* and *pulmonary sequestration*. A history of recurrence of pneumonia in the same location is a clue to an infected malformation or a retained foreign body.

See Chapter 9 for discussion of *circulatory* causes of chest pain. In patients with sickle cell anemia, acute chest pain associated with crisis or with *acute chest syndrome* occurs commonly. One should ask about prior testing for sickle cell disease and family history of all African-American children presenting with acute chest pain. Children with pulmonary embolus from lower extremity injury, heart disease, or familial coagulopathy such as *factor V Leiden* mutation often have acute chest pain associated with other symptoms such as dyspnea, cyanosis, and hemoptysis.

● KEY PROBLEM

■ **Cyanosis** Central *cyanosis* is a sign of serious disease and represents significant desaturation of hemoglobin. In forming the differential diagnosis systematically, an assessment of intermittent versus persistent cyanosis is important. Only in very severe lung and airway disease is cyanosis persistent. More often it occurs intermittently when respiratory demand exceeds oxygen transport across the lung, when there is significant ventilation-perfusion (V/Q) mismatching, or abnormal hemoglobin. *CF* children with moderate to severe disease rarely display cyanosis at rest but often do during exertion, but with very severe disease, they show it persistently. *Infectious* causes include *viral* or *bacterial pneumonia* sufficient to cause significant V/Q mismatching or atelectasis owing to airway obstruction from secretions. Significant upper airway obstruction owing to *viral croup, pharyngeal abscess,* or *tonsillar abscess* can lead to alveolar hypoventilation, especially with fatigue, and then subsequent hemoglobin desaturation. A history of acute onset of stridor, difficulty swallowing, often with drooling, and fever will suggest *retropharyngeal abscess,* and low-grade fever with acute stridor following upper respiratory infection will suggest viral croup. *Neurogenic* cyanosis is due to alveolar hypoventilation that occurs during seizures or apnea. Acute bronchoconstriction, an autonomic response that responds to beta-adrenergic and anticholinergic drugs with asthma, is also neurogenic. Progressive neuromuscular disease (e.g., *Duchenne muscular dystrophy* or *spinal muscular atrophy*) and *cerebral injury* lead to hypoventilation and eventually to cyanosis. A *toxic* cause of cyanosis is inhalation of smoke or chemicals such as hydrocarbon solvents. This leads to airway and parenchymal inflammation that affects ventilation and perfusion. Although low oxygen saturations occur in methemoglobinemia and carbon monoxide toxicity, color of the skin and pulse oximetry may not reflect the level of oxygen desaturation. *Traumatic* causes of cyanosis owing to accidental or nonaccidental injury become more common in this age group. *Near-drowning* not only may cause cerebral anoxia with subsequent apnea but also may cause secondary pneumonitis and acute respiratory distress syndrome with ventilation-perfusion mismatching and subsequent hypoxemia. *Traumatic* injury to the chest wall can produce pneumothorax, penetrating injury from rib fracture or foreign body, and lung contusion with subsequent pulmonary hemorrhage. *Swallowing dysfunction* and *GERD* associated with developmental disability are common in this age group and lead to traumatic and recurrent and inflammation of the airways and lung. A history of gagging or choking on feedings, prolonged gag, or wheezing immediately after or during feeds should suggest one of these diagnoses. An *allergic* cause of cyanosis at this age is ventilation-perfusion mismatching and/or fatigue associated with increased work of breathing from acute asthma or spasmodic croup. A history of acute exposure to an allergenic food (e.g., peanuts) or bee sting followed by acute onset of stridor, swelling, urticaria, and dizziness or lightheadedness should suggest *anaphylaxis*. *Congential* lesions not associated with neuromuscular or primary cerebral dysfunction such as primary pulmonary lesions (*bronchogenic cyst*, *pulmonary sequestration*, and *lung cyst*) often have a history of recurrent pneumonias in the same location with short intervals of improvement following antibiotic therapy. *Bronchiectasis* as a manifestation of *primary ciliary dyskinesia* begins to manifest later in this age group. A history of chronic sinusitis, rhinitis, and otitis media usually with persistent drainage and sometimes situs inversus (50 percent of patients) suggests this diagnosis. *Pectus excavatum*, unless very severe, is not associated with cyanosis or exercise restriction, nor is *pectus carinatum*. Both are primarily cosmetic and rarely require intervention. Parents and patients often bring these concerns to their primary care provider. *Circulatory* causes of cyanosis at this age include cyanotic congenital heart disease and *acute chest syndrome* or *acute bacterial pneumonia associated with sickle cell crisis*. An adequate general medical history should reveal these problems.

Adolescents

Adolescence is a time of turbulent transition from childhood to adulthood, as well as rapid growth. Psychosomatic symptoms referable to the respiratory tract, injury, concerns over chest wall contour, and the other illnesses seen in later childhood, all can manifest at this age.

KEY PROBLEM

Cough Chronic *cough* is usual in adolescents with *CF* even during periods of relatively wellness. The cough varies with state of infection, becoming more severe and productive during pulmonary exacerbations. A variable history of hemoptysis can occur with increasing cough in this *metabolic* disease. Any lower respiratory tract infection that causes inflammation, particularly of airways or pleura, can cause cough. *Infectious* etiologies are similar to those in children. *Neurogenic* causes of chronic cough includes *psychogenic cough* or *cough tic*. The history will reveal that the cough is not present during sleep and is disruptive of social interaction, including school participation. The cough is hollow and "brassy" in nature and nonproductive, and distraction can cause it to decrease or disappear temporarily. Similar to the situation in younger children, *aspiration* of food in adolescents with developmental delay causes chronic cough. *Toxic* causes of chronic cough increasingly include substance abuse in adolescents. One always should seek a history of inhalation of solvents ("huffing") and smoke (including marijuana, clove cigarettes, ETS, and tobacco). ACE inhibitors for hypertension may result in bothersome chronic cough. A history of exposure to inhaled irritating substances or aspiration of a foreign body may be *traumatic* causes of chronic cough. A history of choking on a *foreign object* prior to the onset of cough is easier to obtain from a teen than from a younger child. Any lesion that exerts pressure on the airway, such as abnormal vascular structure (e.g., vascular ring) or mediastinal *neoplasm* (e.g., *lymphoma, thymoma, teratoma*, etc) may be a cause of chronic cough. Most *circulatory*-related abnormalities such as vascular rings will manifest in earlier childhood. Occasionally, a *congenital* lesion, such as a *bronchogenic cyst*, will present in adolescence as cough. *Asthma* may present with dry, nonproductive cough and little history of wheezing (*cough variant* or *cough-equivalent asthma*). A history of exacerbations of cough with respiratory infection, specific environmental exposure (e.g., pets), exercise, and cold air is common, and nasal *allergy* and eczema often coexist.

KEY PROBLEM
Wheezing and Stridor
Wheezing associated with lung disease in CF is very common, but its persistence with antibiotic treatment should alert the clinician to the possibility of complicating *allergic bronchopulmonary aspergillosis* or *asthma*. *Stridor* may sometimes be due to other *metabolic* causes, including *hypokalemia* and *hypocalcemia*. Viral or bacterial lower airway *infection*, particularly in the adolescent with asthma, is commonly associated with wheezing. Infection leading to *retropharyngeal* or *peritonsillar abscess, laryngitis,* or *epiglottis* may present with stridor in teens. *Neurogenic* causes of wheezing include exacerbations of *asthma* associated with strong emotion, fear, anxiety, and anger. *Vocal cord dysfunction* (VCD) becomes a common cause of episodic stridor in this age group. A typical history of VCD includes acute onset of stridor and inability to talk during exercise or with stressful events. Patients relate a feeling of throat tightness that resolves on the cessation of activity. During a VCD episode, there is no compromise of ventilation. As with children of other ages with developmental disabilities, aspiration of upper airway secretions or refluxate with accompanying laryngospasm or bronchoconstriction can lead to periodic stridor and wheezing. Inhalation of irritant chemicals can be another *traumatic* and *toxic* cause of wheezing and stridor. One usually encounters at younger ages congenital stridor owing to *subglottic stenosis* or other intrinsic or extrinsic laryngeal lesion, although occasionally *neoplasms* of the head and neck may present later with stridor. *Congestive heart failure*, usually in teens with known congenital heart disease, may present with cough and wheezing. Additional *circulatory* causes of stridor and wheeze include *vascular rings* missed in earlier childhood. Recurrent wheezing is the hallmark of *asthma,* and a careful history will reveal the triggers for asthma episodes. Other *allergic* causes of acute stridor include *spasmodic croup* and the occasional episode of subglottic swelling owing to *anaphylaxis*. A careful history may reveal a specific trigger such as *insect sting* or *food exposure*.

KEY PROBLEM
Chest Pain
CF as a *metabolic* disease causes chest pain as a common manifestation of acute exacerbations of chronic *pneumonia* or with *pneumothorax*. Pleuritic pain or pain associated with chest muscle strain, accompanying severe cough, also may be present. This and other *infectious* causes of chest pain occur in adolescence as in childhood.

Coxsackie B acute pleurodynia, as well as pleurisy with other viruses and with bacterial pneumonia, occurs commonly in a teen with increasing cough and respiratory distress. *Subphrenic abscess* and *pancreatitis* may manifest as lower chest pain. *Pneumonia* also may present with a history of abdominal pain. *Neurogenic* causes of chest pain include *herpes zoster* manifesting as a vesicular rash along a chest wall dermatome. Pain derived from *gastritis* and *esophagitis* owing to *GERD* is neurogenic in origin. *Neoplasia* with involvement of the pleura (*mesothelioma* or more often metastases) or with pressure on mediastinal structures may be a cause of chest discomfort and pain. A history of accompanying systemic symptoms such as decreased appetite, dyspepsia, fever, night sweats, and fatigue often accompanies pulmonary and mediastinal neoplasia. *Toxic* causes of chest pain include *inhalation injury* and pneumonitis, as in younger children, although inhalation is more often intentional in adolescents (e.g., glue, gasoline, or hydrocarbons). One should seek a careful history of substance inhalation in the case of acute respiratory symptoms, especially without upper respiratory infection symptoms or fever. Chest wall pain becomes more common in adolescence and in some cases may be *traumatic* (i.e., related to sports injury) but is often *unknown* and likely related to rapid growth. Sometimes trauma to the abdomen bordering on the chest (e.g., liver and spleen) can cause chest pain. However, adolescents are more likely than younger children to complain of pain associated with *GERD*. *Costochondritis* with pain on palpation over the costochondral junction is common. This often relates to activities such as weight lifting or chest trauma from contact during sports. *Tietze syndrome* occurs with a history of painful swelling over the sternal junction. Pain and tenderness over the xyphoid is termed the *xyphoid syndrome.* A history of intermittent costal margin pain often is due to the *slipping rib syndrome.* Stress fractures of the ribs with localized chest pain and tenderness and a history of chest wall pain on inspiration are common with certain sports activities such as rowing, baseball pitching, and golf. Particularly in early adolescence, painful nodules of the breasts (*benign gynecomastia*) can be troubling to both male or female adolescents, and mastitis may occur later in adolescent girls. An unusual syndrome with a history of intermittent acute, sharp chest pain occurring over the precordium and lasting from a few seconds to minutes, sometimes relieved by changing position, occurs commonly in adolescents and is termed the *precordial catch syndrome* (also known as *Texidor's twinge*). The history usually reveals no specific initiating factor. Referred pain from the thoracic spine (e.g., in scoliosis or diskitis) may present as chest wall pain. Acute chest pain with or without chest wall trauma is a presenting symptom of *pneumothorax* in an otherwise healthy teen. Pain from *congenital* lesions is less likely at this age. Occasionally, a lung malformation or congenital *neoplasm* will manifest in teens. *Circulatory* causes of chest pain are the same as in the childhood years, although, occasionally, *coronary artery disease* and *mitral valve prolapse* may cause pain in this age group. In cases of radiating pain or increasing pain with exercise, cardiology referral is appropriate. Anterior chest pain or discomfort can occur with chronic cough, and the historical evaluation of *asthma* and *allergy* should uncover this.

KEY PROBLEM

Cyanosis As in younger children, most cyanosis in teen comes from ventilation-perfusion mismatching from *primary lung disease* or from *hypoventilation*. In *CF,* advanced lung disease with significant airway obstruction and pulmonary fibrosis leads to at first intermittent and then persistent hypoxemia and cyanosis with nighttime waking and dyspnea. A history of nighttime awakening with dyspnea would lead the clinician to suspect the need for oxygen in these patients. Any *infectious* cause of a significant ventilation defect such as severe pneumonia (viral or bacterial) can lead to cyanosis. History of fever, cough, and gradually increasing respiratory distress will lead one in this direction. Infections such as *epiglottitis* or *retropharyngeal* or *tonsillar abscess* can cause sufficient airway obstruction to affect ventilation and produce cyanosis. A history of stridor, fever, and difficulty swallowing often will precede these emergent conditions. Immunocompromised teens are at particular risk of severe infection, often with opportunistic organisms such a *Pneumocystis carinii* that characteristically produce sufficient hypoxemia to cause cyanosis. *Neurogenic* cyanosis includes seizures with *hypoventilation* sufficient to produce significant hypoxemia and *aspiration syndromes* associated with *developmental disabilities*. *GERD,* with aspiration, may promote secondary infection leading to cyanosis and, as with aspiration of food or secretions by mouth, can be both a *neurogenic* and *traumatic* cause of airway obstruction and lung inflammation with intermittent or persistent cyanosis. Inhalation of *toxic* chemicals, such as hydrocarbons, may lead to sufficient lung inflammation to cause cyanosis. One always should seek a history of intentional or accidental exposure to chemicals. Abnormal hemoglobin such as in *methemoglobinemia* may give the appearance of cyanosis. Although most *congenital heart disease* with left-to-right shunt sufficient to produce persistent or intermittent cyanosis is evident by this age, patients with marginal compensation may decompensate with infection, leading to *congestive heart failure* with cyanosis. Consider *circulatory* causes of cyanosis, including *pulmonary hypertension* owing to progressive lung disease with destruction of the pulmonary capillary bed, significant, untreated hypoxemia, or obstruction to pulmonary arterial outflow (e.g., *valvular disease, pulmonary stenosis, cardiac insufficiency with cor pulmonale, etc.*). Refer to the Chapter 9 for discussion of cyanosis owing to congenital and acquired cardiac disease. *Pulmonary embolism,* although rare, can occur with trauma, sickle cell disease, and inherited disorders of coagulation such as *factor V Leiden mutation*. The presence of acute chest pain, with dyspnea, cyanosis, and occasionally hemoptysis, in a patient with any of the preceding conditions or a family history should alert the clinician to this possibility. Cyanosis in *allergic* conditions can occur with acute upper airway obstruction owing to *anaphylaxis* but is more commonly associated with severe *asthma*. Significant ventilation-perfusion mismatching owing to widespread small airway obstruction leads to both hypercarbia and cyanosis. With increased work of breathing, hypoventilation and increasing cyanosis may precede apnea, often heralded by changes in the level of consciousness.

Physical Examination

Respiratory physiology and thoracic and pulmonary anatomy change significantly from infancy to adolescence. The principles of the carefully done physical examination remain the same (inspection, palpation, auscultation, and percussion), but applying them to children of different ages demands patience and well-practiced technique. The passive examination, if an option, is always the best in a young, uncooperative child. Examples of passive manipulation include placing a child supine to bring out wheezing (it lowers lung volume and therefore decreases airway caliber) rather than trying to obtain a forced expiration.

Infants

KEY FINDING

Inspection Observe abnormalities of chest conformation or the thoracic spine on first inspection. Absence of the pectoralis major muscle unilaterally indicates *Poland syndrome* (anomalad). Rib or thoracic vertebral anomalies (e.g., hemivertebrae) lead to chest wall asymmetry. Increased anteroposterior thoracic diameter is present with airway obstruction and early, severe neuromuscular disease (e.g., *type I spinal muscular atrophy*) and may cause a small thoracic cage and diminished intercostal musculature. Pectus deformities of the anterior chest wall (FIGURE 8–4) begin to become evident at this age, but unless severe, they become increasingly more noticeable with age. Observe respiratory rate because increased respiratory rate is often a first sign of pulmonary disease in infants. Observation of rate, rhythm, and respiratory pattern

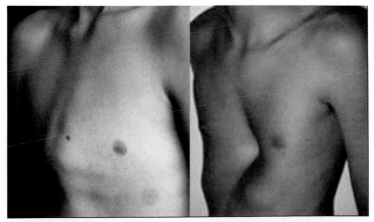

FIGURE 8–4 *Pectus Carinatum (left) and Pectus Excavatum (right).*

is important. Depth of respiration and frequency will change significantly during sleep state and activity, and infants and young children have a particularly wide range of normal values (FIGURE 8–5). Because of this wide range and variation, counting respirations for a full minute on at least a couple of occasions is best practice. *Tachypnea* (abnormally high breathing frequency) is found in metabolic conditions such as fever or acidosis, anemia, and congenital heart disease, as well as viral or bacterial infection. *Hyperpnea* (abnormally deep respirations) may accompany metabolic conditions such as acidosis. *Hypopnea* (abnormally shallow breathing) can occur in CNS disease or in sleep-disordered breathing. Pattern of breathing is important to observe in this age group. Short respiratory pauses of less than 10 seconds occur frequently in infants in the first few months of life. If separated by less than 20 seconds, they are termed *periodic breathing* and are found in normal newborns, older premature infants, and some infants with developmental disabilities stemming from CNS dysfunction (e.g., *perinatal asphyxia*). True *apnea* (pause > 20 seconds), with or without cyanosis and/or bradycardia, is rare but is reason for immediate evaluation and intervention. Because of the highly compliant chest wall and more horizontal orientation of the diaphragm in infants and young children, increasing respiratory effort manifests as inward drawing of the chest wall termed *retractions*. Head bobbing and suprasternal retractions are good indicators of upper

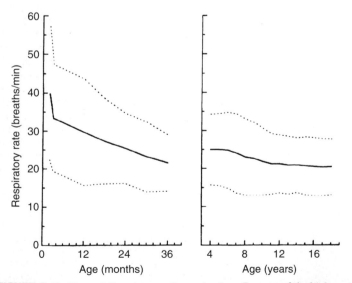

FIGURE 8–5 *Normal Respiratory Rates by Age. Because of the high variability of rates in young infants, it is necessary to count rates for a full minute. (Adapted with permission from Chernick V, Boat TF, Wilmott RW, Bush A (eds):* Kendig's Disorders of the Respiratory Tract in Children, *7th ed. Philadelphia: Saunders-Elsevier, 2006.)*

airway obstruction, and intercostal and subcostal retractions are good indicators of lower airway obstruction. Flaring of the alae nasi (nasal flaring) occurs frequently in newborn and young infants accompanying increased work of breathing and is often present along with retractions and tachypnea. Seesaw respirations, i.e., drawing in of the chest wall with outward motion of the abdomen, occurs during inspiration in young infants with highly compliant chest walls. In any young child, this pattern of paradoxical breathing can be ominous and may indicate impending respiratory failure. Extrathoracic inspection is vital to the complete pulmonary assessment. Concavity of the abdomen may indicate the presence of diaphragmatic hernia, and protruding abdominal masses or weakness in the abdominal musculature may prevent or impede diaphragmatic excursion, leading to respiratory distress. Birth trauma, especially with the use of forceps or with difficult presentation with manual extraction, can lead to unilateral *phrenic nerve trauma* with subsequent asymmetric diaphragmatic excursion. This appears as differential chest wall excursion or paradoxical abdominal movement.

Observe the fingers and toes for evidence of digital clubbing. Clubbing is rare in infancy and generally becomes evident in early childhood, associated with chronic pulmonary, cardiac, or hepatic disease. Since it is a more prominent sign in older children, there is a more intensive discussion in later sections.

KEY FINDING

Palpation *Palpation* often confirms findings on inspection of the head and neck, chest wall, and abdomen and is an essential component of the complete pulmonary examination. Examining the neck for masses and determining correct position of the trachea are important. A finger placed in the suprasternal notch in infants should reveal a normal slightly right deviation of the trachea. Palpation of the thoracic often will reveal rib anomalies as a cause of chest asymmetry. During crying, the transmission of airway vibrations decreases with the presence of significant thoracic masses, fluid accumulations, or consolidation. Evaluate this by placing the hands on each side of the chest wall. Palpation of the abdomen is essential because masses and enlarged organs limit diaphragmatic excursion and lead to respiratory compromise. The absence of palpable upper abdominal organs in the face of a scaphoid abdomen leads the examiner to suspect *herniation* of the abdominal contents into the thorax, requiring emergency intervention.

KEY FINDING

Auscultation Auscultation of the chest and upper airway is an important adjunct to other aspects of the respiratory tract examination. Evaluate respiratory sounds for intensity or amplitude, pitch of lung sounds, and timing during the respiratory cycle. Lung sounds are named by use and convention. They are the same in infants, children, and adolescents and are summarized in TABLE 8–2.

Auscultation of the infant chest is often a challenge owing to limited cooperation and high respiratory rates. Some useful suggestions to

TABLE 8–2 *Characterization of Lung Sounds*

Lung Sound	Name	Location	Pathology
Discontinuous fine, high pitched, low amplitude, short duration	Fine crackles	Small to medium airways	Early airway closure and secretions
Discontinuous coarse, low pitched, high amplitude, long duration	Coarse crackles	Larger airways	Secretions
Continuous high pitched	Wheeze	Central and lower airways	Turbulent airflow through narrowed airways with subsequent wall vibration
Continuous low pitched	Rhonchus	Larger airways	Secretions and abnormal airway distensibility and collapse
Continuous or discontinuous dry crackles heard peripherally	Pleural rub	Pleural space	Inflamed pleura with minimal effusion
Continuous or discontinuous, musical, high pitched over midline chest or neck	Stridor	Large airways and larynx	Abnormal collapsibility of airway or lesion within trachea or upper airway

optimize this effort are listed in TABLE 8–3. A good deal of information comes from simply listening (while observing) without the stethoscope. Much of the time, one can hear *stridor, snoring, grunting,* and *wheezing.* Inspiratory stridor indicates upper airway obstruction and may change with position. In dynamic conditions such as laryngomalacia, the stridor is louder in activity and crying and softer during sleep. Often with a fluttering character, it decreases with gentle traction on the mandible and in a prone position with the neck extended and is louder when supine with the neck flexed. Fixed obstruction owing to vocal cord paralysis or extrathoracic anomalies usually is not positional

TABLE 8–3 *Tips for Performing the Respiratory Examination on Infants and Children*

1. Perform the examination in a warm, well-lit room with a minimum of noise distraction.
2. Do as much of the examination as possible with the child on a parent's lap.
3. Warm instrumentation is essential.
4. Quiet breathing is best heard during feeding or with use of a pacifier.
5. Lung sounds are best heard during the inspiratory portion of a deep breath during crying in infants.
6. Guard the privacy of adolescents with proper draping and gowns, as well performing the examination without parents present.
7. The passive examination is always the best, e.g., decubitus x-rays for foreign-body aspiration, supine positioning to bring out wheezing in infants, examination during sleep, etc.

but increases with activity and crying. A hoarse and muffled cry usually accompanies any vocal cord weakness. Snoring occurs most often in a supine position and in young infants usually accompanies nasal obstruction, although a good pharyngeal examination to rule out hypertrophy of tonsillar tissue or masses (e.g., *thyroglossal duct cyst*) is important. Grunting occurs primarily in premature and very young infants and represents partial closure of the glottis during expiration to maintain positive end-expiratory pressure. This helps to avoid early closure of small, inflamed airways toward the end of expiration and helps to maintain alveolar stability in the case of surfactant deficiency. Wheezing is primarily expiratory and reflects turbulent airflow in tubular structures of the lower (intrathoracic) airway. With increasing airway obstruction, the wheeze may become biphasic, i.e., heard during both inspiration and expiration.

The stethoscope is still a useful tool to assess the location and character of lung sounds. Because of the relatively thin chest wall of small infants, transmission of airway sounds can occur widely and may be somewhat more difficult to localize. Use of the diaphragm of a stethoscope head that is able to fit between the ribs over the intercostal muscles can help in this effort. Deep inspirations are important to assess local lung sounds. In young infants, these occur during the deep breaths taken during crying. Position may affect differential lung sounds, and a straight posture is important. It is best to examine young children on the mother's lap, although the supine position may bring out wheezing better than the upright position. Symmetric auscultation of all lung segments to assess for the presence of crackles, as well as decreased intensity and change of pitch (often during crying), will help to localize areas of consolidation. Coarse central expiratory (or biphasic) wheeze usually reflects airway lesions such as tracheomalacia, and peripheral and diffuse wheeze indicates small airways disease (e.g., asthma or bronchiolitis). Asymmetric wheeze always should alert the examiner to the possibility of a foreign-body aspiration at any age. Auscultation over the head and neck can be useful in localizing upper airway obstruction.

KEY FINDING

◤ Percussion   *Percussion* of the chest wall assesses acoustic response to a vibratory force applied to lung tissue. The technique requires practice and consists of tapping of the middle finger of one hand with the middle finger of the other while it is applied to the chest wall. It is essential that one does this symmetrically and that the response is assessed for resonance (hollowness) and dullness (flatness). This is often not useful in young infants and frequently will elicit poor cooperation and crying. The technique is of more use in older children.

Children

Children's level of cooperation with the pulmonary examination and ability to articulate symptoms increase with age. Key symptoms such as localized chest pain can help to direct the examiner to specific areas of potential disease and enhance the examination. Subjective expression of breathlessness or *dyspnea* is easier to elicit at this age.

KEY FINDING

◤ Inspection   Since the chest wall become less compliant with age, the usefulness of *observation* for retractions becomes less important. However, during increased work of breathing, children increasingly will use accessory muscles of respiration, including the scalenes, sternocleidomastoids, intercostal muscles, and abdominal muscles. There is lifting of the shoulders with contraction of the sternocleidomastoids and abdominal muscles during inspiration. Inward motion of the suprasternal notch indicates upper airway obstruction.

Paradoxical breathing (as seen in young infants) may present in children with neuromuscular disease owing to weakness or paralysis of the intercostal muscles. Differential chest excursion may be due to diaphragmatic paralysis or weakness. It also may occur with *spontaneous, acute pneumothorax.*

Chest wall conformation often reflects underlying lung disease. With diffuse obstructive disease such as *chronic asthma* or *CF*, the chest is barrel-shaped with increased anteroposterior and lateral diameters. With restrictive pulmonary disease such as *interstitial fibrosis* or *muscle weakness* (e.g., *muscular dystrophy*), there is contraction of the thoracic diameters often creating a bell-shaped chest. *Pectus excavatum* (funnel chest) and *pectus carinatum* (pigeon chest) become more noticeable in this age group. The pustular lesions of *herpes zoster* will show a typical pattern of distribution along a thoracic dermatome in children as well as adults. Observation of breathing pattern, rate, and rhythm is important. *Tachypnea* occurs chronically in those with persistent airway obstruction (poorly controlled *asthma* or *CF*) and decreased chest wall or pulmonary compliance (*neuromuscular disease, pulmonary fibrosis*, etc.).

Acute tachypnea may indicate *metabolic acidosis,* as seen with hyperpnea in *Kussmaul* type breathing in *diabetic ketoacidosis* or with *salicylate intoxication.* It is, however, the most common finding in acute pneumonitis of infectious origin. *Bradypnea,* or abnormally slow respirations, can be an ominous sign of impending respiratory failure in children with increased work of breathing from any cause. *Apnea* often follows bradypnea in children with fatiguing respiratory musculature but can occur at other times. Cheyne-Stokes breathing consists of periods of increasing hyperpnea alternating with periods of apnea and occurs in children with *congestive heart failure* and *increased intracranial pressure. Obstructive sleep apnea,* as a part of *sleep-disordered breathing,* occurs in this age group. *Obesity* and upper airway obstruction from *tonsillar hypertrophy* contribute to this problem. Caregivers may describe snoring along with respiratory pauses. *Behavioral problems* can result from sleep-disordered breathing in children; daytime sleepiness is less of a feature in this age group than in teens and adults. Children with severe developmental disabilities from cerebral trauma or neonatal asphyxia may have abnormal breathing patterns with periods of hyperpnea alternating with irregular respiratory pauses and snoring.

Acute chest pain may cause splinting (flexion of the trunk toward and decreased respiratory excursion of the affected side) and acute pneumothorax may reveal decreased respiratory excursion with relative hyperinflation of the affected lung.

Inspection of the abdomen, pharynx, and associated structures such as the nose and ears is important to detect coexisting conditions. *Scoliosis* can cause apparent chest asymmetry, and examination of the back and spine is an essential part of the chest and pulmonary examination. Digital clubbing is an associated sign of chronic pulmonary, cardiac, or hepatic disease but does not necessarily correlate with the degree of severity of these conditions, nor is it specific for any one disease. In true clubbing, there is a gradual disappearance of the hyponychial or ungual angle with the dorsal surfaces of like fingers on both hands put together, called Schamroth's sign (FIGURE 8–6). One can distinguish digital clubbing from normal familial nail conformation by examining other family members.

KEY FINDING

▼ **Palpation** Palpation of the trachea for proper (slightly rightward) position is important because deviation can indicate a pulling force owing to atelectasis or tracheal fixation such as with a mediastinal tumor. It also may indicate a pushing force such as *pneumothorax* or a space-occupying *mass.* Additionally, posterior placement may occur with mediastinal tumors. One should palpate the chest wall, especially with the complaint of chest pain or if there is an obvious deformity. Chest wall pain may be due to local trauma from localized *contusion* and may show an overlying area of ecchymosis. *Costochondritis* will reveal pain along the sternal costochondral junction, and the xyphoid may be tender in the case of *xyphoiditis.* In *Tietze syndrome,* a tender, localized, fusiform swelling occurs along the sternal border.

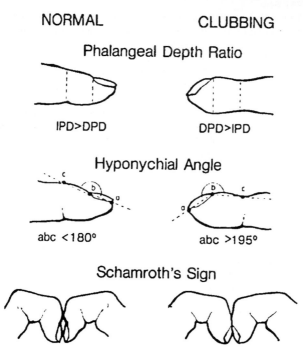

NORMAL   **CLUBBING**

Phalangeal Depth Ratio

IPD>DPD   DPD>IPD

Hyponychial Angle

abc <180°   abc >195°

Schamroth's Sign

FIGURE 8–6   Clubbing and Schamroth's Sign. *Clubbing can be measured by comparing the distal phalangeal diameter (DPD) to the interphalangeal Diameter (IPD), which is less than one in normal subjects. The hyponychial angle is increased in clubbing, as seen in the drawing, and the normal "diamond-shaped" opening produced by opposing the hyponychial angles of opposite finger fisappears with clubbing (Schamroth's sign). (Adapted with permission from Chernick V, Boat TF, Wilmott RW, Bush A (eds):* Kendig's Disorders of the Respiratory Tract in Children, *7th ed. Philadelphia: Saunders-Elsevier, 2006.)*

▼ KEY FINDING

◣ Auscultation   The more cooperative older child (with the "toddler exception") allows the examiner to appreciate subtleties of the pulmonary examination during auscultation. A warm stethoscope is a positive way to begin. Choose an appropriate head size for the size of the child. Auscultate symmetrically all lung segments during a deep inspiration. Wheezing is usually continuous and found during expiration or, with more severe diseases, throughout the respiratory cycle. It results from obstruction of airways with subsequent turbulent airflow. A forced expiration may be useful to bring out wheezing when the examination is not obvious but the history suggests airflow obstruction. Unilateral wheeze suggests ipsilateral obstruction from a foreign body or other endogenous or exogenous airway lesion. Wheezing over the sternum suggests large airway obstruction. Crackles are associated with opening of small airways or fluid in airways. They correlate with a local decrease in breath sounds indicating an area of consolidation. Pleural rubs, sounding like dry, fine crackles, occur with stretching of inflamed pleura and may be present only during inspiration or throughout the respiratory cycle. Stridor is usually acute and indicates an infectious (*epiglottis, pharyngeal abscess*) or *allergic (spasmodic croup)* etiology. Children with previous *subglottic stenosis* or those who are *post-tracheostomy placement* often persist with stridor during childhood. *Egophony,* or change in transmission of spoken sound, becomes a more useful tool in older children. Change from the spoken *e* to an *a* sound heard on auscultation is classic for lung consolidation.

KEY FINDING

■ Percussion As with auscultation, *percussion* becomes a more useful part of the pulmonary examination as children become more cooperative. FIGURE 8–7 demonstrates the technique of percussion. Perform the examination symmetrically, and listen for dullness or hyperresonance. Symmetric hyperresonance occurs in obstructive lung disease such as *asthma* and *CF*. Unilateral hyperresonance occurs with *pneumothorax* or unilateral airway obstruction. Symmetric dullness often occurs in the lung bases with widespread pneumonitis such as in *CF* or *viral illness.* Asymmetric dullness occurs with atelectasis, lung consolidation, or fluid accumulations in the pleural space.

Adolescents

The pulmonary examination in adolescents is similar to that in older children, although conditions occurring primarily during puberty (e.g.,

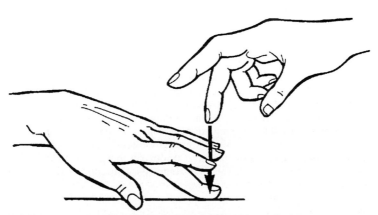

FIGURE 8–7 Technique of Chest Wall Percussion. *(Adapted with permission from Chernick V, Boat TF, Wilmott RW, Bush A (eds):* **Kendig's Disorders of the Respiratory Tract in Children,** *7th ed. Philadelphia: Saunders-Elsevier, 2006.)*

painful breast nodule) or those of a primarily cosmetic nature (e.g., *pectus* deformities) are often areas of focus. Most adolescents are cooperative, especially when there is thoughtful attention to privacy.

▼ KEY FINDING
■ Inspection Asymmetric chest wall conformation occurs with rib abnormalities but more commonly with increasing scoliosis at this age. Therefore, *examination* of the back and spine is essential as in the younger child. This is especially true in adolescents with developmental disabilities or with muscle weakness as in *muscular dystrophies.* Obesity in neuromuscular disease may preclude recognition of decreased anteroposterior and lateral diameter of the thoracic cage, but hyperinflation with airway obstruction will be evident in poorly controlled asthma and advancing CF pulmonary disease. *Pectus* deformities may become particular foci of cosmetic concern for adolescents and their families, and they may seek surgical correction for this reason alone. Breast asymmetry is common in developing adolescents and is noted during the chest wall inspection. Respiratory rate, rhythm, and pattern are essential parts of this examination. With decreasing compliance of the chest wall and increasing muscle mass, increased work of breathing manifests in use of accessory muscles of respiration and tachypnea. Adolescents can readily relate feelings of dyspnea, and the examiner needs to search for correlates in tachypnea and increased depth of respirations. This is especially important in assessing adolescents for psychosomatic respiratory symptoms, such as anxiety-driven hyperventilation. Observation of sighing or a disruptive, loud, honking cough during the examination may lead the examiner to a diagnosis of anxiety-driven symptoms (*sighing dyspnea* and *psychogenic cough*).

▼ KEY FINDING
■ Palpation *Palpation* of the chest wall in adolescents includes the breasts in both males and females. Painful nodules (benign *gynecomastia*) are a common complaint, particularly in early adolescence, and the examiner can allay patient fears surrounding this issue through a careful examination. With athletics, injury to chest wall musculature and *rib contusion* (and even *fracture*) become increasingly common in this age group, and localized pain on palpation can lead to further evaluation. *Costochondritis* and *Tietze syndrome* occur commonly in this age group and probably are the result of stress owing to use of thoracic musculature during activities. *Slipping rib syndrome* with pain over the lower costal margin occurs in adolescence. A "hooking" maneuver whereby the examiner hooks his or her hand under rib margin and gently lifts with subsequent pain suggests this diagnosis. Palpation of the trachea for position and the neck for masses is important.

▼ KEY FINDING
■ Auscultation The technique of *auscultation* (with an adult-size stethoscope) is similar to that in older children. Increasing chest wall muscle mass and breast tissue can make auscultation somewhat more challenging than over the thinner thoracic cage of the younger child.

It is important to record the intensity and location of lung sounds (as defined in TABLE 8–2).

▼ KEY FINDING

◤ Percussion This technique is also similar to that in older children, but again, chest wall development and the increase in thoracic size increase the effort that goes into performing this maneuver. *Percussion* prior to thoracentesis is an important adjunct to imaging in order to optimize placement of a thoracentesis needle.

Synthesizing a Diagnosis

TABLE 8–1 outlines upper airway diagnoses (nose and sinuses) with their salient historical and physical examination points. Consult the text for synthesizing pulmonary problems and findings into diagnoses.

Confirmatory Testing

Laboratory and Imaging

Testing for diseases of the respiratory tract consists of laboratory testing, pulmonary function testing, and imaging. Invasive testing such as thoracentesis, laryngoscopy, bronchoscopy, and endoscopic surgery are in the purview of subspecialists and not discussed here. Level of cooperation, anatomy, and age-related differential diagnosis clearly dictate the type of testing done. TABLES 8–4 and 8–5 contain a review of testing with comments as to indications.

Pulmonary Function

In infants, pulmonary function testing (PFT) requires specialized equipment and skilled operators. All noninfant PFT studies require patient cooperation and therefore are done on children of at least 5 years of age. A good deal of operator skill is necessary to produce an adequate test in children. Complete PFT consists of the components noted in TABLE 8–6. Traditionally, a measure of gas exchange (arterial blood gas) was commonplace, but this is no longer the case with the advent of oximetry. TABLE 8–7 provides examples of obstructive and restrictive pulmonary diseases in children and adolescents.

When to Refer

Referring to a pulmonary specialist is largely a matter of judgment based on the practitioner's sense of the severity and complexity of the condition.

TABLE 8-4 *Laboratory Testing*

Test	Condition	Age*	Comments
Complete blood count	Infection, anemia, hemoglobinopathies, allergy	I, C, A	Fragmented and sickled cells may be present; eosinophils may confirm allergy
Sweat test	CF	I, C, A	May be performed in infants older than 48 hours of age; may be falsely elevated in hypothyroidism, Addison, HIV, among others
Cystic fibrosis DNA analysis	CF	I, C, A	Detects carriers and confirms CF diagnosis
Capillary blood gas	Hypoxemia, hypercarbia, acidosis	I	Usefulness beyond the newborn period doubtful
Arterial blood gas	Hypoxemia, hypercarbia, acidosis	I, C, A	Best measure of efficiency of gas exchange
IgE	Allergy, allergic bronchopulmonary aspergillosis (ABPA)	I (occasionally), C, A	Elevated in atopy, usually above 1000 IU/ml in ABPA; specific IgE testing available
Erythrocyte sedimentation rate, C-reactive protein	Bacterial infection, autoimmune disease	I, C, A	When combined with elevated white blood cell count is a good indication of bacterial pneumonia
Mycoplasma titer (IgM)	Acute *Mycoplasma* infection	C, A	Elevation suggests acute infection
Cold agglutinins	Acute *Mycoplasma* infection	C, A	May be elevated in acute viral infection

*I = infant; C = child; A = adolescent.

TABLE 8-5 *Imaging of the Respiratory Tract*

Test	Condition	Age*	Comments
Chest x-ray	Hyperinflation and hypoinflation, bilateral and unilateral; opacification (consolidation, atelectasis); hilar and parenchymal masses; abscesses; adenopathy; effusion; pneumothorax	I, C, A	Best screening study for pulmonary disease; relatively insensitive in determining parenchymal disease (fibrosis, interstitial fluid, interstitial pneumonitis); adequate inspiration with right hemidiaphragm at eighth rib level
Decubitus chest x-ray	Unilateral airway obstruction (foreign body, etc.), pleural effusion	I, C, A	A "passive examination" suitable for young children, where inspiratory and expiratory films cannot reliably be obtained
Fluoroscopy	*Chest:* Tracheomalacia, unilateral airway obstruction *Esophagram:* Vascular ring, tracheoesophageal fistula, disorders of swallowing and esophageal motility	I, C, A	Radiation exposure should be minimized; in tracheomalacia, the trachea collapse inward during expiration; lesions and structures indenting the esophagus can be visualized (vascular ring, extrinsic masses, etc.)
Chest CT	Assess both mediastinal and intrapulmonary structures in detail; consolidation, interstitial disease, masses, pulmonary nodules, mediastinal masses, and air; pleural air-fluid and chest wall masses	I (sedated), C, A	Most sensitive visualization of thoracic structures in detail but higher radiation than chest x-ray; spiral CT scan best for pulmonary vascular and mediastinal structures; high-resolution CT best for lung parenchyma, including pulmonary nodules

(Continued)

223

TABLE 8-5 *Imaging of the Respiratory Tract (Continued)*

Test	Condition	Age*	Comments
Magnetic resonance imaging	Assessment of vascular structures especially in the mediastinum	I (sedated), C, A	Limited experience in pediatric patients
Ultrasonography	Assessment of character of pleural fluid, lung opacity, and evaluation of upper mediastinal structures; doppler useful to assess vascular malformations	I, C, A	No ionizing radiation; limited usefulness over air-filled spaces; useful to assess fluid level prior to thoracentesis
Anteroposterior and lateral neck x-ray	Subglottic narrowing	I , C, A	Of questionable clinical use in acute but helpful in chronic stridor
Sinus x-rays	Sinus anatomy, mucosal swelling, air-fluid levels, polyps, and masses	C, A	Requires cooperation and useful for "gross" diagnosis of sinus conditions; CT gives more detail
Sinus CT scan	Anatomy of the osteomeatal complex; defines sinus pathology including polyps better than sinus x-ray Essential for infants	I (sedated), C, A	Defines anatomy and pathological changes better than sinus x-rays. More ionizing radiation and requires cooperation.
Bronchoscopy (with video)	Assessment of endobronchial lesions (foreign body, TB, mucus obstruction, masses, laryngeal and tracheal malformations) bronchoalveolar lavage for cell type identification and infection; transbronchial biopsy for masses and post-lung transplant evaluation	I, C, A	Size of airway and bronchoscope limits use in small children; sedation is necessary in young children and infants and desirable in older children

*I = infant; C = child; A = adolescent.

224

TABLE 8-6 *Pulmonary Function Tests in Children and Adolescents*

Spirometry	Measures airflow limitation; standards based on race, gender, and height; common measures include FVC (forced vital capacity), FEV_1 (forced expiratory volume over 1 second), and FEF_{25-75} (forced expiratory flow at between 25 and 75 percent of the vital capacity); FEV_1 and FEF_{25-75} reduced in obstructive lung disease; all reduced in restrictive lung disease; a 12–15 percent improvement in FEV_1 after administering a beta-adrenergic bronchodilator is found with reversible airway obstruction.
Static lung volumes	Measures lung capacity; common measures include TLC (total lung capacity), FRC (functional residual capacity), RV (residual volume), and SVC (slow vital capacity); reduced in restrictive lung disease.
Diffusing capacity	Measures blood volume in pulmonary vasculature; reduced in restrictive diseases with diminished pulmonary blood flow; normal or elevated in obstructive pulmonary disease.

Referral to a specialist or subspecialist does not mean the loss of a patient to a practice because the best approach is shared care between the primary care practitioner and the specialist. This means that good communication between care providers remains vigorous and continuous. Common reasons to refer include

1. Perceived worsening of the condition despite the best efforts to stabilize and ameliorate it.
2. Unknown definitive diagnosis.

TABLE 8-7 *Common Pediatric Pulmonary Diseases Classified by Type of Pulmonary Function Abnormality*

Obstructive pulmonary disease	Bronchiolitis, bronchopulmonary dysplasia, asthma, CF, croup
Restrictive pulmonary disease	Infant respiratory distress syndrome, adult respiratory distress syndrome, viral and bacterial pneumonia, atelectasis, interstitial pneumonia and fibrosis, thoracic muscle weakness, obesity

3. The time involved in pursuing the diagnosis or treating the condition exceeds the amount of time that the practitioner has to devote to it. In the case of many respiratory diseases, education of the patient and parents is essential as part of the management strategy. Since this takes considerable ongoing time, it is often not well suited to the busy practice environment.

4. The resources available to best serve the patient's needs are only available through the specialist and include
   a. A multidisciplinary approach to the problem using a highly skilled team. This is the Center of Excellence concept, an example of which is the national chain of Cystic Fibrosis Foundation–accredited Cystic Fibrosis Care, Teaching, and Research Centers. These centers concentrate the most up-to-date resources to best care for the specialty patient.
   b. Specialized knowledge of up-to-date diagnostic and therapeutic techniques, including procedures that aid in diagnosis and therapy. An example of this is flexible bronchoscopy with biopsy and bronchoalveolar lavage.
   c. Certain states may require an evaluation by a specialist to determine eligibility for state financial assistance programs.

5. Reinforcement of primary care plan and education to enhance adherence to the therapeutic plan (e.g., an asthma action plan and asthma education).

Chapter

9 The Cardiovascular System

Eugene F. Luckstead

The cardiovascular system is subject to both congenital problems occurring during fetal development and those acquired throughout childhood and into adolescence. This chapter focuses on both with age-related considerations. The goals are to

1. Learn pediatric cardiovascular physiology and functional mechanics in the fetal/premature/newborn infant (I), child (C), and adolescent (A).
2. Develop a comprehensive cardiovascular history that will elicit and document pertinent facts in the infant, child, and adolescent. List the key cardiovascular symptoms and expand each symptom as it relates to the diagnosis of specific pediatric cardiovascular disorders in all age groups.
3. Delineate the four cornerstones of examination: observation, palpation, percussion, and auscultation. Discuss the cardiac examination with emphasis on general considerations for infants, children, and adolescents. List the key cardiovascular signs in the infant, child, and adolescent age groups. This list will serve as a core base for a cardiovascular differential diagnosis in patients of each age group.
4. Be able to discuss briefly the most common acyanotic and cyanotic congenital cardiovascular anomalies and include key symptoms and/or signs for each cardiac abnormality. Provide a table that serves as a summary format by listing the "high points" for diagnosing a specific pediatric cardiac lesion. Also include congenital syndromes with cardiac involvement.
5. Be able to discuss the most common acquired heart disease in infants, children, and adolescents. Provide a table that serves as a summary format listing the high points for diagnosing acquired heart disease.
6. Discuss indications and develop a table outline to order specific confirmatory laboratory and/or imaging studies. Such confirmatory testing will be derived from the respective pertinent pediatric cardiovascular history, key signs, and/or symptom presentation in the infant, child, and adolescent with a suspected cardiac abnormality.
7. Know when and how to refer a patient with a suspected cardiovascular abnormality to a specialist. What additional diagnostic tools are available to the specialist, and what are the indications for using them? How do you work together with complex cardiac patients?

Functional Anatomy, Physiology, and Mechanics

Newborns and Infants

Cardiac function is detectable during fetal development by auscultation at 16 to 20 weeks of gestation. Fetal echocardiography during the first trimester now assesses anatomy and physiology earlier. Fetal electrocardiograms (ECGs) diagnose and monitor dysrhythmias in utero. These prenatal diagnostic studies help to anticipate newborn cardiac care and management needs once the infant is delivered. At birth, the 10-point 1- and 5-minute Apgar scores have significant cardiac and vascular components (see Chapter 5).

The placenta-driven fetal circulation has only a minimal respiratory role when contrasted with the newborn circulation, with the patent foramen ovale (PFO) and patent ductus arteriosus (PDA) enabling pulmonary-to-systemic vascular shunting. The PDA and PFO can shunt blood right to left, bidirectionally, or left to right depending on multiple fetal physiologic major organ system needs (FIGURE 9–1). The pulmonary system is largely inactive in the fetal circulation (~8 percent of blood flow), with the placenta functioning as a lung substitute. The ductus venosus serves as a liver diversion bypass shunt in the fetus. After birth, it closes usually in 4 to 5 days.

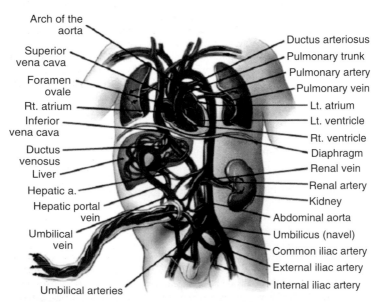

FIGURE 9–1 Fetal Circulation. *(From Van de Graaff KH:* Human Anatomy. *New York: McGraw-Hill, 2002, Fig. 16.42, p. 581.)*

Postnatally, the newborn cardiovascular system changes from a single to a biventricular system. The lungs and heart now assume a codependent, or shared, role. The left ventricle pumps oxygenated blood to the coronary arteries and all major body organ systems except the lungs; the right ventricle provides returning venous unoxygenated blood through the pulmonary arteries to the lungs for oxygenation, which then enters the left atrium and ventricle via the pulmonary veins. After birth, with functioning lungs, markedly higher oxygenated pulmonary venous blood flow enters the left atrium and left ventricle.

The pulmonary and right-sided pressures begin to decrease after birth because of lung expansion, increased lung blood supply, and other metabolic factors. The atrial foramen ovale will close partially or completely from a left to right direction because it no longer has the previously needed fetal right-to-left shunt function. With oxygen stimulation, the ductus arteriosus and ductus venosus will close during the first 12 to 24 hours after birth.

Some newborn infants will still have continued right-to-left and/or bidirectional PFO and PDA shunting from persisting high pulmonary arterial pressures (PPHN): Persistent Pulmonary Hypertension of the Newborn, previously called *persistent fetal circulation*, that can result in varying degrees of central cyanosis in the newborn. Persistent left-to-right shunting at the PDA level may be inaudible, cause a late systolic crescendo murmur, or at a later age develop into a continuous murmur with a peak intensity that occurs over the second heart sound. Peripheral pulses typically are increased in newborns with moderate to large PDA shunts owing to increased venous return to the left side of the heart.

Term newborns tolerate large left-to-right shunts because of their more resistant, less compliant, thickened pulmonary arteriole vascular beds, resulting in a slower decrease from their initial high pulmonary blood pressure at birth; i.e., a slowly maturing pulmonary vascular resistance. However, premature infants have less well-developed pulmonary arterioles depending on their degree of prematurity and gestational age and have more problems adapting to significant left-to-right shunting. Such shunts further compromise their immature pulmonary system, often resulting in congestive heart failure (CHF). This often requires continuing respiratory support measures until either medical or surgical PDA closure resolves the left-to-right shunt respiratory overload. Although it is a cardiac problem, the clinical picture is one of chronic respiratory distress and ventilator dependency.

Childhood and Adolescence

Normal sinus rhythm consists of regular electrical impulses that are generated by the sinus node and travel through the right and left atrial muscles (P wave on the ECG). The electrical impulse then continues to travel through specialized tissue (atrioventricular node, PR interval on the ECG) that conducts electricity to the ventricles at a slower pace. This allows for filling of the ventricles during diastole and then contraction of the ventricles during subsequent systole (the QRS complex on the ECG). The T wave represents the short interval of relaxation prior to the next cardiac cycle. Variance of sinus ryhthm with the respiratory cycle (sinus arrythmia) is a normal phenomenon in children and is not to be confused with pathologic dysrythmias. Disturbances of rate and rhythm are regular features of both intrinsic heart disease and extrinsic metabolic and other conditions that affect cardiac functioning. Many of these are discussed in subsequent sections of this chapter.

Most pediatric patients older than age 10 years will have adult cardiovascular function even though they may be only at the Tanner stage 2/5 maturation levels.

History

A prenatal history is useful to gather information. Family history, especially genetic, is most helpful. Inquire about illnesses and toxic exposures in the mother during gestation. Maternal infections such as rubella cause significant congenital heart disease. How does the newborn appear? Is the infant feeding well, active, and alert? Is the color good?

Infants of diabetic mothers will have a higher risk for congenital heart defects, specifically transient hypertrophic septal cardiac changes from their intrauterine increased insulin stimulation. Such infants are often large for gestational age (LGA) and also may have hypoglycemia and hypocalcemia. These abnormalities are not seen in gestational diabetic pregnancies.

Feeding difficulties and poor growth may occur with easy fatiguabilty, irritability, and/or crying or limited physical activity in infants and children with heart disease. Other notable symptoms are shortness of breath, cyanosis with or without crying, sweating, or alterations in consciousness. Adolescents may report syncopal episodes, palpitations, dizziness, and chest pain. Infants, children, and adolescents with left-to-right shunts often will be taking cardiac or pulmonary medications that also may have side effects. Those who have had palliative or corrective open-heart surgery frequently will be on multiple medications for long periods of time after their initial and/or subsequent surgeries. TABLE 9–1 provides a list of key cardiac history points for all age groups.

TABLE 9–1 *History Checklist*

Infant
- Birth weight and gestational history? Abn/nl ___
- Any cyanosis with crying? Y/n___
- Feeding and activity levels? Abn/nl ___
- Family history of heart problems? Y/n___
- Murmur? Y/n___
- Respiratory problems? Y/n___
- Genetics abnormal in family? Y/n__
- Maternal diabetic history? Y/n___
- Other information from parent about family diseases/syndromes? Y/n_____
- Any other information from family or parent?

(Continued)

TABLE 9-1 *History Checklist (Continued)*

Child

- Birth weight and gestational history? Abn/nl ___
- Any cyanosis with crying? Y/n___
- Feeding and activity levels? Abn/nl ___
- Family history of heart problems? Y/n___
- Murmur? Y/n___
- Respiratory problems? Y/n___
- Genetics abnormal in family? Y/n___
- Diabetic history? Y/n___
- Frequent respiratory illness? Y/n___
- Activity level normal? Y/n___
- Growth parameters okay? Y/n___
- Spells or seizures? Y/n___
- Shortness of breath on exertion (SOBOE)? Y/n___
- Family history of sudden death under 50 years in close relative? Y/n___
- Other information from parent or family? Y/n___

Adolescent

- Birth weight and gestational history? Abn/nl ___
- Any cyanosis with crying? Y/n___
- Feeding and activity levels? Abn/nl ___
- Family history of heart problems? Y/n___
- Murmur? Y/n___
- Respiratory problems? Y/n___
- Genetics abnormal in family? Y/n___
- Diabetic history? Y/n___
- Frequent respiratory illness? Y/n___
- Activity level normal? Y/n___
- Growth parameters okay? Y/n___
- Spells or seizures? Y/n___
- SOBOE? Y/n___
- Family history of sudden death under 50 years in close relative? Y/n___
- Severe chest pain? Y/n___ Describe what makes it better or worse?___
- Severe dizziness with exercise? Y/n___
- Syncope with or after exercise? Y/n___
- Palpitations? Y/n___ Heart racing? Y/n___
- Drug use or abuse? Y/n___
- Migraine, gait unsteadiness, or seizure family history? Y/n___
- Arthritis, joint swelling, rash, and/or pain? Y/n___
- Chest or significant head trauma? Y/n___
- Diet history/sleep history/water intake/meal history? abn/nl___
- Prior tests (ECG/chest x-ray/echo/others)?_____
- Other questions or other symptoms? Y/n___

Abbreviations: Abn = abnormal; nl = normal; Y = Yes; n = no; SOBOE = shortness of breath on exertion.

Physical Examination

KEY FINDING

▼ **Inspection** General *inspection* is critical to the examination in all age groups. Alertness of the infant, cry characteristics, skin color and turgor, finger clubbing, respiratory breathing patterns, and hydration all may relate to cardiovascular status. Capillary "flush" timing can be helpful for circulatory assessment.

Cyanotic newborn infants are often a cardiac emergency when they present with central cyanosis, particularly if they have PDA-dependent lesions. Similarly, associated weak cry or lethargy may suggest significant heart disease. Central cyanosis should be assessed by an oxygen saturation monitor or arterial blood gas determination in both room air and an increased oxygen (preferably 100%, if possible) environment (hyperoxia test).

Acrocyanosis (cyanosis of the extremities) is often present during the first few hours after birth and is assessed by the Apgar scoring system at 1- and 5-minute intervals and, if persistent, for longer intervals. It is usually due to autonomic instability and is rarely of cardiac significance. Localized peripheral cyanosis owing to autonomic nervous system effects is termed the *harlequin effect*. It may be noted for several weeks after birth. These areas of color change corresponding to body segments are caused by infant position change and resolve with maturation of the autonomic nervous system.

Determine infant size as large, small, or appropriate for gestational age by standard growth charts (see Chapter 5). Pedal edema and abdominal *ascites* may reflect cardiac or noncardiac newborn abnormalities and also must be considered in cardiac evaluation. *Dysmorphic* infants or those who have a known syndrome should raise suspicion for frequently associated cardiac anomalies (TABLE 9–2).

Height, weight changes, and sexual maturation are evident between the ages of 8 and 12 years. Growth is different between girls and boys, with female development and sexual maturation occurring 1 to 2 years earlier. Cardiac examination must consider these Tanner stages (1–5) of maturation or pubertal development when examining patients in this age range.

TABLE 9–2 *Cardiac Syndrome: Pediatric Cardiac Anomaly Correlates*

Down syndrome: A-V canal > VSD > tetralogy of Fallot >
 Eisenmenger syndrome
Turner syndrome: C/A > AS > aortic dilatation
Noonan syndrome: PS > pulmonary dysplasia > A-V canal, HCM
Marfan syndrome: aortic dilatation > MVP > aortic aneurysm
Ehlers-Danlos syndrome: aortic dilatation, aneurysm
LEOPARD syndrome: pulmonic stenosis, VSD
Rubella syndrome: PDA, peripheral pulmonic stenosis
DiGeorge syndrome: Tetralogy of Fallot > truncus arteriosus > aortic
 arch anomalies

Abbreviations: A-V = atrioventricular; VSD = ventriculolseptal defect; PS = pulmonary stenosis; HCM = hypertrophic cardiomyopathy; MVP = mitral value prolapse; PDA = patent ductus arteriosus.

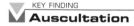

KEY FINDING

Palpation *Palpation* of the precordium is useful to detect location and intensity of the heartbeat. If turbulence of flow is significant (murmur > 3/6, see "auscultation" section below) the examiner will feel a vibration or "thrill" over that area. In addition, extracardiac palpation of the liver and extremities for swelling also identifies fluid accumulation in heart disease.

Peripheral pulse palpation and upper and lower extremity blood pressure measurements are very important, especially during the first 24 to 48 hours after birth. Increased or diminished pulse amplitude and blood pressure measurements may suggest a cardiovascular abnormality. Cardiac heart rate monitoring will show a wide range of normal newborn heart rates during the first 2 to 3 days after birth. Infant heart rates normally can increase to 200 beats/min during this time but also can decrease to 50 to 60 beats/min, especially with an increased vagal effect during the first 1 to 3 days following birth. See TABLE 9–3 for the normal ranges of heart rates in infants, children, and adolescents.

KEY FINDING

Percussion Cardiac *percussion* is important to delineate heart borders and size. Because of the differential density between heart tissue and lung, a dull sound will become more resonant as the border is crossed from heart to lung. In addition to cardiac percussion, percussion of both the lung and the liver is important to assess for dullness in the event of fluid accumulation.

KEY FINDING

Auscultation

General Considerations

Cardiac murmurs are audible sounds in the range between 20 and 2000 Hz that are produced by the heart and blood vessels. Murmurs are by far the most common cause for cardiac consultation in the pediatric age group. Although the large majority of murmurs are innocent or functional, they still must be separated from those that are caused by cardiac anomalies (pathologic murmurs). About 50 percent of school-age children will have innocent murmurs sometime during childhood.

TABLE 9–3 *Normal Pulse Rates for Age*

Age	Pulse Rate
Infant	100–200
Toddler	90–150
Preschooler	80–140
School age	70–120
Adolescent	60–100

Source: APLS: Pediatric Emergency Medicine Course, ACEP/AAP, 3rd edition, 2004, Table 4-3, p. 43.

Auscultation remains an important cardiac physical diagnostic skill for murmur identification. Unfortunately, these skills have eroded, are not taught as well, or have been ignored with increased reliance on newer cardiac imaging such echocardiography, computed tomography (CT) scan, and magnetic resonance imaging (MRI). This deterioration of clinical heart auscultation skills has occurred not only at the medical student level but also at the resident, fellow, and staff levels.

It is important to perform the pediatric cardiac examination in a quiet area with auscultation of the heart sounds at each respective cardiac valve site (FIGURE 9–2). One should routinely examine patients with the stethoscope bell and diaphragm in both the supine and upright positions in newborns, infants, and children. Examine preadolescents and adolescents in the standing and/or left lateral decubitus position to allow an optimal evaluation of the mitral valve. The bell will detect best low-frequency sounds, and the diaphragm will detect best the higher frequencies; medium-frequency sounds are heard equally well with both. The use of selected maneuvers such as position change, held expiration and inspiration, Valsalva maneuver, and exercise often can provide additional findings to differentiate between innocent and pathologic murmurs. Most expert examiners will use a pattern sequence that starts with the first and second heart sounds (S_1 and S_2) at each of the four valve sites. Document other heart sounds and the timing, location, quality, and pitch of a murmur.

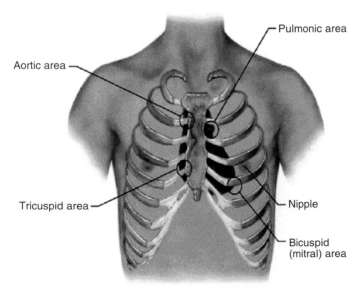

FIGURE 9–2 *Cardiac Valve Areas for Precordial Auscultation.* (*From Van de Graaff KH:* Human Anatomy. *New York: McGraw-Hill, 2002, Fig. 16.13, p. 554.*)

Note changes in sounds and murmurs and splitting of a heart sound, particularly S_2. The first heart sound results from the mitral valve–tricuspid valve closure that occurs early in ventricular contraction. This is best heard with slower heart rates and at the respective mitral and tricuspid valve sites. Mitral and tricuspid valve closure is usually a single S_1 in younger patients. Anything that delays right tricuspid valve closure likely will cause an S_1 split. After the onset of ventricular contraction, the semilunar valves (aortic and pulmonic) open silently to allow ventricular ejection while the atrioventricular (A-V) valves remain closed (FIGURE 9–3).

After ventricular ejection, the semilunar valves close rapidly, producing the second heart sound (S_2). The second heart sound is heard best at the base at the aortic and pulmonic valve sites. Aortic valve closure occurs earlier, and its sound typically is louder than that of pulmonic valve closure.

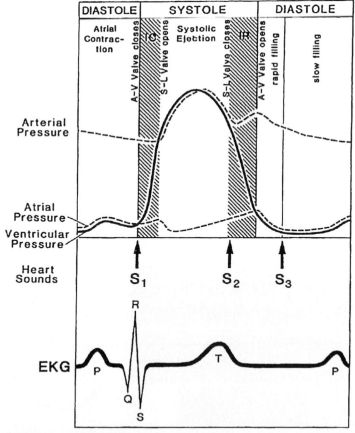

FIGURE 9–3 *The Cardiac Cycle.* (*After CJ Wiggers:* Nelson Textbook of Pediatrics, 17th ed. 2004, Fig. 413–3, p. 1488.)

The normal splitting of the second heart sound is largely influenced by the inspiratory filling effects on the right side of the heart. During expiration, both the aortic and pulmonic valve close nearly at the same time, resulting in a single or narrowly split S_2. It is important to characterize S_2 accurately as to normal splitting and movement with respiration or if there is "fixed" splitting, which is due to persistently increased return to the right side of the heart during diastole. Other sounds, such as an S_3 sound, may be normal unless it is a continuous S_3 gallop in patients with heart failure. On rare occasions, an S_4 sound may be heard and is always abnormal.

Properly obtained blood pressures and pulses in the upper and lower extremities are important, particularly in younger infants and children suspected of having hypertension. The blood pressure cuff should be appropriately sized for age and encircle at least two-thirds of the distance between the elbow and the shoulder (FIGURE 9–4). Machine (Dinamap) pressures are 10 mm Hg higher in systole and 5 mm Hg higher in diastole than auscultation pressures. Palpation of the pulse amplitude in the radial and femoral pulse areas and determination of pulse delay or pulse differences between upper and lower extremities are important to detect cardiac anomalies.

Pathologic Heart Sounds

Systolic murmurs are usually described as holosystolic, systolic ejection, early systolic, midsystolic, or late systolic (FIGURE 9–5). Holosystolic murmurs may result from A-V regurgitation but are more common with *ventriculoseptal defects* (VSDs) in pediatrics.

Systolic ejection murmurs are crescendo-decrescendo (rising and falling) and occur more often from either ventricular outflow tract abnormalities or stenosis of semilunar valves. Diastolic murmurs are less common than systolic murmurs but, when present, are due to semilunar valve regurgitation, stenosis of an A-V valve, or a "functional" stenosis from increased flow across an A-V valve (FIGURE 9–6).

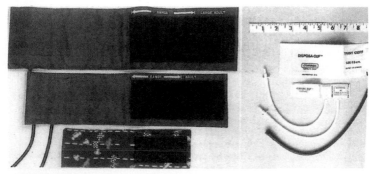

FIGURE 9–4 *Sphygmomanometer Sizes: Large Adult, Adult, and Child Sizes on Left and Infant and Newborn Sizes on Right.*

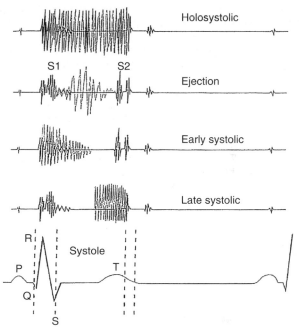

FIGURE 9-5 *Systolic Murmur Classification.*

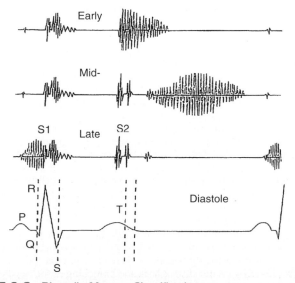

FIGURE 9-6 *Diastolic Murmur Classification.*

Diastolic murmurs are noted in early or protodiastole, middiastole, or late diastole (presystolic). Protodiastolic murmurs are usually from A-V valve insufficiency; middiastolic murmurs are flow-related or stenotic A-V valves with a blowing ejection type of sound, and presystolic murmurs are caused by stenotic or A-V valve obstructions. Continuous murmurs usually are extracardiac in locations distal to the semilunar valves; except for venous hums, most continuous murmurs are pathologic.

Systolic ejection clicks typically are associated with semilunar (aortic/pulmonic) valve stenosis or vessels that are dilated distal to the valve. Midsystolic clicks are associated with A-V (mitral or tricuspid) valve prolapse. Any murmur will need accurate description and documentation regarding timing, grade, intensity, location, duration, pitch, and quality. It is important to locate a murmur in the cardiac cycle. This will be either in systole, diastole, or continuous with reference to the first and second heart sounds. Most examiners should use the Levine grading scale for murmur intensity from grades 1 to 6 in systole and diastole; some will grade diastolic murmurs from 1 to 4 because grade 5/6 and 6/6 diastolic murmurs are very rare.

Innocent Murmurs

Innocent murmurs are usually systolic ejection, are virtually never holosystolic, and usually change intensity with position. Such murmurs usually are grade 1/6 or 2/6 but rarely over grade 3/6; thus palpable thrills are virtually nonexistent. After the newborn age, the vast majority of murmurs are innocent, the most common of which is the Still's murmur, an early and midsystolic vibratory, buzzing, twanging-string, or a harmonic-musical murmur. It is heard best with the stethoscope bell at the left lower upper sternal border and apex areas of the chest in the supine position. Its intensity changes with position, and it originates from left ventricle (LV) outflow or LV papillary muscle sites. The murmur is not holosystolic but occurs in early and midsystole and is usually of low intensity and does not transmit well or radiate to other parts of the precordium. Exercise, anxiety, anemia, fever, and held expiration will increase the intensity. It can be heard in the newborn but more often occurs between 6 months and 8 years of age and less frequently in the adolescent.

The pulmonary outflow systolic ejection murmur is the second most common innocent murmur, becoming increasingly prevalent in preadolescents and adolescents. It is heard best with the stethoscope diaphragm in both children and adolescents at the second and third left intercostal space in the supine position. An increase in right ventricular heart flow or turbulence usually causes the murmur. Exercise, anxiety, anemia, fever, and the maneuver of voluntarily held inspiration will increase the murmur's intensity.

In neonates and premature infants, the murmur of peripheral pulmonary stenosis is quite common but typically will resolve by 3 to 6 months of age. This is a low-intensity systolic ejection murmur over the chest, axilla, and back caused by relative hypoplasia and branching of the newborn pulmonary artery system. With pulmonary vascular system maturation and the resulting decrease in pulmonary resistance, physiologic pulmonary vessel enlargement, and normalizing pulmonary artery pressures, most such murmurs will abate with time.

Venous hums are common in infants and children. They are innocent murmurs that occur in early systole and early diastole and sound like a "to-and-fro hum" continuously throughout the cardiac cycle. Such murmurs are best heard in the sitting position and on the right side either at the base or the third right interspace. This murmur is most commonly noted in the 3- to 8-year age group. The murmur originates from the jugular venous and innominate–superior vena caval system. Most venous hums will either decrease or disappear when the patient is placed in the supine position or if the neck is turned.

An arterial bruit or murmur noted in the carotid vessels at or above the clavicle is the supraclavicular innocent murmur. It is noted more often in adolescents and heard best in the sitting patient with the bell of the stethoscope on the right side, has low intensity, and is heard best in early systole. Origin of the murmur is from increased active blood flow in the brachiocephalic vessels.

A complete and systematic cardiac and peripheral vascular system examination will help to differentiate innocent from abnormal or pathologic murmurs. Obviously, murmurs associated with congestive heart failure, cyanosis, and dysrhythmias are not innocent. TABLE 9–4 summarizes key findings.

TABLE 9–4 *Key Pediatric Cardiovascular Findings*

Cyanosis
Tachypnea
Tachycardia
Murmur
Pulse amplitude/delay abnormality
Hepatomegaly
Apnea
Clubbing
Bradycardia
Irregular cardiac rhythm
Edema/ascites/anasarca
Fatigue on feeding
Pallor
Systolic ejection clicks
Midsystolic clicks
Opening snap
Gallop (S_3/S_4)
Friction rub
Rash
Fever
Chorea
Abnormal heart sounds
Abnormal heart sound location
Arthritis
Cardiac surgical incision

Cardiac Examination of the Newborn: General Considerations

The cardiac physical examination in the neonate, premature or full term, will focus mostly on inspection, palpation, and auscultation. Inspect the infant skin and mucous membrane areas for central cyanosis and the toes and fingers for early clubbing. Palpate infant pulses for amplitude in the upper and lower extremities, the liver for enlargement, the feet for pedal edema, and the abdomen for ascites. Oximetry and/or blood gas determination can confirm any observation of cyanosis.

Murmurs are commonly heard during the first 3 to 12 hours after birth. Most murmurs are functional and relate to newborn transition cardiac changes. Other murmurs are caused by left-to-right ductus arteriosus shunting. Murmurs that persist 24 to 48 hours after birth are more likely to have a pathologic cause.

A newborn with no heart murmur still may have congenital heart disease. Because of the shifts in systemic and pulmonary pressures discussed earlier, there may be little to no differential pressure over a significant cardiac lesion during the transition phase or up to as long as 3 months of age.

Infant Pediatric Cardiovascular Examination: General Considerations

Your initial interaction with a patient and parent often will vary depending on the age of the patient. Avoid speaking too loudly to an infant or child. Involve the parent in the examination, and get the parent's historical input during the cardiovascular system examination. Sitting down rather than towering over infants and children is helpful. Often the infant or toddler will be more comfortable in the parent's arms rather than on the examination table. Newborn or young infants prefer a quiet environment and can be examined while sleeping or quietly alert in the mother's arms. Warm hands after washing and a warm stethoscope are always a good trouble-saving policy when doing the infant cardiac examination.

Children (Ages 1 to 8 Years) Cardiac Examination: General Considerations

Cardiovascular examination of children ages 1 to 3 years may be quite challenging owing to lack of cooperation. A calm, reassuring approach will work best. Let the child slowly accept you as no threat as you talk with the parents; observe the patient as you talk with the parent. Often the child is more comfortable when examined on a parent's lap. Diagnosis of most congenital heart problems occurs during the first 3 to 6 months of life, with some diagnosed later at between 6 and 12 months of age. The clinical presentation will be that of murmurs, cyanosis, and congestive heart failure; some may later present as cardiac *dysrhythmias, hypertension, recurrent pulmonary infections,* and *growth failure.* Certain dysmorphic or genetic-related syndromes will have commonly associated cardiac abnormalities (see TABLE 9–3). Surgical interventional palliative and corrective treatment of many cardiac anomalies will be completed during the first 6 to 12 months of life.

Acquired heart problems can appear at any age but occur most likely after 6 months and are more frequent in the older child, preadolescent, and adolescent. Frequent infections, growth failure, and cardiac *dysrhythmias* may occur at any age.

Assess systemic hypertension in all age groups by use of the recent norms linking age with height at the 50/90/95th percentile levels in both boys and girls. Systolic or diastolic pressures greater than the 95th percentile are significant and merit renal, cardiac, and/or endocrine consultation (TABLE 9–5).

Older infants and children will have their cardiovascular system evaluated by their physician during their regular health care checkup. Measure vital signs, height, weight, and head circumference percentiles until 2 years of age; height percent and weight percent measurements are done only after 2 years of age. Blood pressure measurement should be done routinely on office visits from 1 year on. Dinamap blood pressures are reasonably accurate for the newborn and during the first year of life. Although they run higher than the standard cuff, they can be useful for trending purposes. Abnormalities of blood pressure will need renal, cardiac, and endocrine evaluation in any age group.

In addition to a full cardiac evaluation, the lung examination by percussion, palpation, and auscultation is also part of the cardiovascular examination because of the close heart-lung physiologic relationships in both congenital and acquired cardiac disease.

Preadolescent-Adolescent Diagnostic Cardiovascular Examination: General Considerations

Adolescent examination takes into consideration all aspects discussed earlier for children. Proper technique requires some level of explanation to the adolescent and parent, but the focus of communication must be with the patient. Because of various concerns regarding cardiovascular chest and pulse examination methods and techniques, another medical or staff person always must be present as a witness. Vital sign measurements, ECG, x-ray examinations, exercise stress testing, and echocardiographic studies will require additional personnel.

Obesity and cardiac-related hypertension present definite challenges for the adolescent. Increased aerobic exercise, prudent dietary caloric intake, and low-weight-intensity weight training have shown the most effective results, particularly when there is whole-family "buy-in." Cardiac examination for preparticipation "sports clearance" is now common.

Adolescent patients may have acquired cardiac valve abnormalities and/or congenital heart anomalies that are often either mild or asymptomatic. Also, patients with known prior cardiac surgical palliation or corrective surgery are being seen in greater numbers. Those with known

TABLE 9-5 Blood Pressure Norms

Blood Pressure Levels for Boys by Age and Height Percentile

Age (Year)	BP Percentile →	Systolic BP (mm Hg)							Diastolic BP (mm Hg)						
		Percentile of Height							Percentile of Height						
		5th	10th	25th	50th	75th	90th	95th	5th	10th	25th	50th	75th	90th	95th
1	50th	80	81	83	85	87	88	89	34	35	36	37	38	39	39
	90th	94	95	97	99	100	102	103	49	50	51	52	53	53	54
	95th	98	99	101	103	104	106	106	54	54	55	56	57	58	58
	99th	105	106	108	110	112	113	114	61	62	63	64	65	66	66
2	50th	84	85	87	88	90	92	92	39	40	41	42	43	44	44
	90th	97	99	100	102	104	105	106	54	55	56	57	58	58	59
	95th	101	102	104	106	108	109	110	59	59	60	61	62	63	63
	99th	109	110	111	113	115	117	117	66	67	68	69	70	71	71
3	50th	86	87	89	91	93	94	95	44	44	45	46	47	48	48
	90th	100	101	103	105	107	108	109	59	59	60	61	62	63	63
	95th	104	105	107	109	110	112	113	63	63	64	65	66	67	67
	99th	111	112	114	116	118	119	120	71	71	72	73	74	75	75
4	50th	88	89	91	93	95	96	97	47	48	49	50	51	51	52
	90th	102	103	105	107	109	110	111	62	63	64	65	66	66	67
	95th	106	107	109	111	112	114	115	66	67	68	69	70	71	71
	99th	113	114	116	118	120	121	122	74	75	76	77	78	78	79
5	50th	90	91	93	95	96	98	98	50	51	52	53	54	55	55
	90th	104	105	106	108	110	111	112	65	66	67	68	69	69	70
	95th	108	109	110	112	114	115	116	69	70	71	72	73	74	74
	99th	115	116	118	120	121	123	123	77	78	79	80	81	81	82

Age	BP percentile	SBP							DBP						
6	50th	91	92	94	96	98	99	100	53	53	53	54	55	56	57
	90th	105	106	108	110	111	113	113	68	68	69	70	70	71	72
	95th	109	110	112	114	115	117	117	72	72	73	74	74	75	76
	99th	116	117	119	121	123	124	125	80	80	81	82	83	84	84
7	50th	92	94	95	97	99	100	101	55	55	56	57	58	59	59
	90th	106	107	109	111	113	114	115	70	70	71	72	73	74	74
	95th	110	111	113	115	117	118	119	74	74	75	76	77	78	78
	99th	117	118	120	122	124	125	126	82	82	83	84	85	86	86
8	50th	94	95	97	99	100	102	102	56	57	57	58	59	60	61
	90th	107	109	110	112	114	115	116	71	72	72	73	74	75	76
	95th	111	112	114	116	118	119	120	75	76	77	78	79	79	80
	99th	119	120	122	123	125	127	127	83	84	85	86	87	87	88
9	50th	95	96	98	100	102	103	104	57	58	58	59	60	61	62
	90th	109	110	112	114	115	117	118	72	73	73	74	75	76	77
	95th	113	114	116	118	119	121	121	76	77	78	79	80	80	81
	99th	120	121	123	125	127	128	129	84	85	86	87	88	88	89
10	50th	97	98	100	102	103	105	106	58	59	60	61	61	62	63
	90th	111	112	114	115	117	119	119	73	73	74	75	76	77	78
	95th	115	116	117	119	121	122	123	77	78	79	80	81	81	82
	99th	122	123	125	127	128	130	130	85	86	86	88	88	89	90
11	50th	99	100	102	104	105	107	107	59	59	60	61	62	63	63
	90th	113	114	115	117	119	120	121	74	74	75	76	77	78	78
	95th	117	118	119	121	123	124	125	78	78	79	80	81	82	82
	99th	124	125	127	129	130	132	132	86	86	87	88	89	90	90
12	50th	101	102	104	106	108	109	110	59	60	61	62	63	63	64
	90th	115	116	118	120	121	123	123	74	75	75	76	77	78	79
	95th	119	120	122	123	125	127	127	78	79	80	81	82	82	83
	99th	126	127	129	131	133	134	135	86	87	88	89	90	90	91

(Continued)

TABLE 9-5 Blood Pressure Norms (Continued)

Age (Year)	BP Percentile ↓	Systolic BP (mm Hg)							Diastolic BP (mm Hg)						
		Percentile of Height							Percentile of Height						
		5th	10th	25th	50th	75th	90th	95th	5th	10th	25th	50th	75th	90th	95th
		Blood Pressure Levels for Boys by Age and Height Percentile													
13	50th	104	105	106	108	110	111	112	60	60	61	62	63	64	64
	90th	117	118	120	122	124	125	126	75	75	76	77	78	79	79
	95th	121	122	124	126	128	129	130	79	79	80	81	82	83	83
	99th	128	130	131	133	135	136	137	87	87	88	89	90	91	91
14	50th	106	107	109	111	113	114	115	60	61	62	63	64	65	65
	90th	120	121	123	125	126	128	128	75	76	77	78	79	79	80
	95th	124	125	127	128	130	132	132	80	80	81	82	83	84	84
	99th	131	132	134	136	138	139	140	87	88	89	90	91	92	92
15	50th	109	110	112	113	115	117	117	61	62	63	64	65	66	66
	90th	122	124	125	127	129	130	131	76	77	78	79	80	80	81
	95th	126	127	129	131	133	134	135	81	81	82	83	84	85	85
	99th	134	135	136	138	140	142	142	88	89	90	91	92	93	93
16	50th	111	112	114	116	118	119	120	63	63	64	65	66	67	67
	90th	125	126	128	130	131	133	134	78	78	79	80	81	82	82
	95th	129	130	132	134	135	137	137	82	83	83	84	85	86	87
	99th	136	137	139	141	143	144	145	90	90	91	92	93	94	94
17	50th	114	115	116	118	120	121	122	65	66	66	67	68	69	70
	90th	127	128	130	132	134	135	136	80	80	81	82	83	84	84
	95th	131	132	134	136	138	139	140	84	85	86	87	87	88	89
	99th	139	140	141	143	145	146	147	92	93	93	94	95	96	97

Blood Pressure Levels for Girls by Age and Height Percentile

Age (Year)	BP Percentile	SBP (mm Hg) Percentile of Height							DBP (mm Hg) Percentile of Height						
		5th	10th	25th	50th	75th	90th	95th	5th	10th	25th	50th	75th	90th	95th
1	50th	83	84	85	86	88	89	90	38	39	39	40	41	41	42
	90th	97	97	98	100	101	102	103	52	53	53	54	55	55	56
	95th	100	101	102	104	105	106	107	56	57	57	58	59	59	60
	99th	108	108	109	111	112	113	114	64	64	65	65	66	67	67
2	50th	85	85	87	88	89	91	91	43	44	44	45	46	46	47
	90th	98	99	100	101	103	104	105	57	58	58	59	60	61	61
	95th	102	103	104	105	107	108	109	61	62	62	63	64	65	65
	99th	109	110	111	112	114	115	116	69	69	70	70	71	72	72
3	50th	86	87	88	89	91	92	93	47	48	48	49	50	50	51
	90th	100	100	102	103	104	106	106	61	62	62	63	64	64	65
	95th	104	104	105	107	108	109	110	65	66	66	67	68	68	69
	99th	111	111	113	114	115	116	117	73	73	74	74	75	76	76
4	50th	88	88	90	91	92	94	94	50	50	51	52	52	53	54
	90th	101	102	103	104	106	107	108	64	64	65	66	67	67	68
	95th	105	106	107	108	110	111	112	68	68	69	70	71	71	72
	99th	112	113	114	115	117	118	119	76	76	76	77	78	79	79
5	50th	89	90	91	93	94	95	96	52	53	53	54	55	55	56
	90th	103	103	105	106	107	109	109	66	67	67	68	69	69	70
	95th	107	107	108	110	111	112	113	70	71	71	72	73	73	74
	99th	114	114	116	117	118	120	120	78	78	79	79	80	81	81

(Continued)

245

TABLE 9-5 Blood Pressure Norms

Age (Year)	BP Percentile →	Systolic BP (mm Hg) Percentile of Height							Diastolic BP (mm Hg) Percentile of Height						
		5th	10th	25th	50th	75th	90th	95th	5th	10th	25th	50th	75th	90th	95th
		Blood Pressure Levels for Girls by Age and Height Percentile													
6	50th	91	92	93	94	96	97	98	54	54	55	56	56	57	58
	90th	104	105	106	108	109	110	111	68	68	69	70	70	71	72
	95th	108	109	110	111	113	114	115	72	72	73	74	74	75	76
	99th	115	116	117	119	120	121	122	80	80	80	81	82	83	83
7	50th	93	93	95	96	97	99	99	55	56	56	57	58	58	59
	90th	106	107	108	109	111	112	113	69	70	70	71	72	72	73
	95th	110	111	112	113	115	116	116	73	74	74	75	76	76	77
	99th	117	118	119	120	122	123	124	81	81	82	82	83	84	84
8	50th	95	95	96	98	99	100	101	57	57	57	58	59	60	60
	90th	108	109	110	111	113	114	114	71	71	71	72	73	74	74
	95th	112	112	114	115	116	118	118	75	75	75	76	77	78	78
	99th	119	120	121	122	123	125	125	82	82	83	83	84	85	86
9	50th	96	97	98	100	101	102	103	58	58	58	59	60	61	61
	90th	110	110	112	113	114	116	116	72	72	72	73	74	75	75
	95th	114	114	115	117	118	119	120	76	76	76	77	78	79	79
	99th	121	121	123	124	125	127	127	83	83	84	84	85	86	87
10	50th	98	99	100	102	103	104	105	59	59	59	60	61	62	62
	90th	112	112	114	115	116	118	118	73	73	73	74	75	76	76
	95th	116	116	117	119	120	121	122	77	77	77	78	79	80	80
	99th	123	123	125	126	127	129	129	84	84	85	86	86	87	88

11	50th	100	101	102	103	105	106	107	60	60	60	61	62	63	63
	90th	114	114	116	117	118	119	120	74	74	74	75	76	77	77
	95th	118	118	119	121	122	123	124	78	78	78	79	80	81	81
	99th	125	125	126	128	129	130	131	85	85	86	87	87	88	89
12	50th	102	103	104	105	107	108	109	61	61	61	62	63	63	64
	90th	116	116	117	119	120	121	122	75	75	75	76	77	78	78
	95th	119	120	121	123	124	125	126	79	79	79	80	81	82	82
	99th	127	127	128	130	131	132	133	86	86	87	88	88	89	90
13	50th	104	105	106	107	109	110	110	62	62	62	63	64	65	65
	90th	117	118	119	121	122	123	124	76	76	76	77	78	79	79
	95th	121	122	123	124	126	127	128	80	80	80	81	82	83	83
	99th	128	129	130	132	133	134	135	87	87	88	89	90	90	91
14	50th	106	106	107	109	110	111	112	63	63	63	64	65	66	66
	90th	119	120	121	122	124	125	125	77	77	77	78	79	80	80
	95th	123	123	125	126	127	129	129	81	81	81	82	83	84	84
	99th	130	131	132	133	135	136	136	88	88	89	90	90	91	92
15	50th	107	108	109	110	111	113	113	64	64	64	65	66	67	67
	90th	120	121	122	123	125	126	127	78	78	78	79	80	81	81
	95th	124	125	126	127	129	130	131	82	82	82	83	84	85	85
	99th	131	132	133	134	136	137	138	89	89	90	91	91	92	93

(Continued)

TABLE 9–5 *Blood Pressure Norms*

Age (Year)	BP Percentile →	Systolic BP (mm Hg) Percentile of Height							Diastolic BP (mm Hg) Percentile of Height						
		5th	10th	25th	50th	75th	90th	95th	5th	10th	25th	50th	75th	90th	95th
		Blood Pressure Levels for Girls by Age and Height Percentile													
16	50th	108	108	110	111	112	114	114	64	64	65	66	66	67	68
	90th	121	122	123	124	126	127	128	78	78	79	80	81	81	82
	95th	125	126	127	128	130	131	132	82	82	83	84	85	85	86
	99th	132	133	134	135	137	138	139	90	90	90	91	92	93	93
17	50th	108	109	110	111	113	114	115	64	65	65	66	67	67	68
	90th	122	122	123	125	126	127	128	78	79	79	80	81	81	82
	95th	125	126	127	129	130	131	132	82	83	83	84	85	85	86
	99th	133	133	134	136	137	138	139	90	90	91	91	92	93	93

BP, blood pressure

* The 90th percentile is 1.28 SD, 95th percentile is 1.645 SD, and the 99th percentile is 2.326 SD over the mean.

For research purposes, the standard deviations in Appendix Table B–1 allow one to compute BP Z-scores and percentiles for girls with height percentiles given in TABLE 4 (i.e., the 5th,10th, 25th, 50th, 75th, 90th, and 95th percentiles). These height percentiles must be converted to height Z-scores given by (5% = –1.645; 10% = –1.28; 25% = –0.68; 50% = 0; 75% = 0.68; 90% = 1.28; 95% = 1.645) and then computed according to the methodology in steps 2–4 described in Appendix B. For children with height percentiles other than these, follow steps 1–4 as described in Appendix B.

cardiovascular abnormalities comprise a large and growing population that requires periodic evaluation of their cardiovascular system to confirm compliance, improvement, and normality or to raise concerns of a new cardiac problem.

The following sections summarize recognition and accurate diagnosis of normal cardiac findings and selected congenital and acquired cardiovascular disorders represented in each pediatric age group.

Synthesizing a Diagnosis

Diagnostic Cardiac Examination: Transition from Infant to Child and Adolescent Ages (1 Month → 2 Years → 8 Years → Preadolescent → Adolescence Age 18 Years)

Infancy is an age of rapid cardiovascular and pulmonary transition. Pulmonary arterial circulation matures with a decrease in pressure owing to pulmonary vessel growth and a decrease in pulmonary arteriolar thickness. This will occur from 3 to 6 months of age in the term infant and to a lesser extent in premature infants. Between the ages of 1 and 3 months, murmurs from left-to-right shunts may be heard initially on routine well-child examinations. Traditionally, well-child visits were scheduled at 1- to 2-month intervals to detect such cardiac problems in the preechocardiography era. Milder forms of congenital heart disease such as *aortic* and *pulmonary stenosis,* mild *coarctation of the aorta, atrial septal defects,* and subtle forms of *cyanotic congenital heart defects* may be diagnosed at this time, but some still may go unrecognized until later childhood and adolescence.

Rapid growth occurs in the infant from the age of 1 month to 1 year of age. Infants may present key signs from their cardiac auscultation, pulse, and blood pressure abnormalities that suggest nonshunt types of obstructive congenital heart disease such as diminished leg pulses in *coarctation of the aorta* and *hypoplastic left heart syndrome.* Murmurs that are associated with systolic ejection clicks suggest *pulmonic* or *aortic valve stenosis. Mitral and tricuspid valve stenoses,* when present, usually are part of the left or right hypoplastic heart groups and rarely exist as isolated congenital A-V heart valve stenoses.

One must consider cyanotic cardiac abnormalities such as *transposition of the great vessels, hypoplastic left and right heart syndromes, total anomalous pulmonary venous return, truncus arteriosus, and pulmonary valve atresia with tetralogy of Fallot,* all of which require emergency diagnostic, medical, and surgical management in the first few days of life. Note that clinical examination and ECG examination are often insufficient to make definitive diagnoses of cyanotic heart lesions. Additional studies after diagnostic echocardiograms such as cardiac MRI, cardiac CT scan, cardiac catheterization, and angiography are necessary before definitive surgical management is contemplated.

It is critical to follow growth parameters, vital signs, murmur evaluation and monitoring, and *dysrhythmias.* Continued clinical assessment of compensated congestive heart failure, cyanotic lesion palliation, and/or treatment response levels is paramount. Children with unrecognized left-to-right shunts such as *VSD, A-V canals, PDA,* and *mild coarctation of the aorta (C/A)* may not be symptomatic until 1 to 3 months of age. *ASDs* are difficult to diagnose at less than 6 months of age. Milder forms of *tetralogy of Fallot (Pink tetralogy)* may not be cyanotic until 6 months after birth.

Syndromes with sudden cardiac death risk such as *Marfan* and *long-QT syndromes,* although more common in the adolescent, can present as sudden death in the child. Look for external manifestations of Marfan syndrome such as arachnodactyly, joint hyperextensibility, and ectopia lentis. Certain prolonged-QT-interval syndromes may be associated with congenital deafness. *Hypertrophic* and *dilated cardiomyopathies* have a significant sudden cardiac death risk potential in both children and adolescents. Cardiac dysrhythmias do occur in all age groups, with isolated *supraventricular tachycardias* (SVTs) common in infants and *Wolff-Parkinson-White* (W-P-W) *syndrome* with SVTs noted in all age groups but more prominent in the child and adolescent. *Long-QT syndrome* with its potentially lethal *torsade de pointes* is more frequent in the child and adolescent. Heart block and the need for pacemaker implantation occur more in the child and adolescent with either primary *third-degree heart block* or in the child or adolescent with surgically acquired heart block. Mitral valve prolapse (female incidence 6 percent; male incidence 4 percent) is uncommon before 9 to 10 years of age, except in patients with *Marfan* or *Ehlers-Danlos syndrome.* It may be associated with dysrhythmia. TABLES 9–6 through 9–10 summarize key problems and findings in infants, children, and adolescents.

TABLE 9–6 *Summary of Key Cardiovascular Findings in the Infant*

Cyanosis: TGV, tetralogy of Fallot, hypoplastic right heart, PS, TAPVR (obstr.), Ebstein, truncus arterious
Murmur: PDA, VSD, C/A, PS, AS; A-V canal, TAPVR (nonobstr.), truncus
Heart sounds: ASD, Ebstein, TAPVR (unobstr.)
Pulse abnormalities: AS, C/A, hypoplastic LV, complete & second-degree heart block
Tachycardia: SVT, atrial flutter
Tachypnea: PDA, VSD, C/A, A-V canal, TAPVR, ASD
Hepatomegaly: VSD, PDA, C/A, A-V canal, TAPVR (unobst.)
Edema/ascites: VSD, PDA, C/A, A-V canal, TAPVR (unobst.)
Clubbing; TGV, tetralogy of Fallo, Ebstein, hypoplastic RV (tricuspid atresia, pulmonary atresia)
Fatigue on feeding: VSD, PDA, C/A, A-V canal, TAPVR (unobst.)
Genetic/dysmorphic: A-V canal, VSD, ASD, PDA, tetralogy of Fallot, PS, AS, C/A, coarctation

---

Abbreviations: TGV = transposition of great vessels; TAPVR = total anomalous pulmonary venous return; AS = aortic stenosis C/A= coarctation of aorta, SVT = supraventricular tachycardia; RV = right ventricle.

T٩ᗺᒪᴇ 9-7 *Summary of Key Cardiovascular Problems in the Child and Adolescent*

Chest pain: AS, C/A, HCM, cardiomyopathy, myocarditis, HCM postpoperative Glenn, Fontan circulation, palliative surgery

Syncope: HCM, AS, dysrhythmias, myocarditis, DCM

Joint pain: ARF, SBE, SLE, C/A

Spells/seizure/dizziness: HCM, tetralogy of Fallot, dysrhythmias, high BP

SOBOE: AS, HCM, tetralogy of Fallot, C/A, cardiomyopathy, myocarditis, HCM, postpoperative Glenn, Fontan circulation, palliative OR

Fatigue/exercise intolerance: Cardiomyopathy, myocarditis, HCM, postpoperative Glenn, Fontan circulation, palliative surgery

Abdominal pain: ARF, SLE, DCM

Abbreviations: DCM = dilated cardiomyopathy; ARF = acute rheumatic fever; SBE = subacute bacterial endocarditis; SLE = systemic lupus erythematosus.

Because infants, children, and adolescents are unique, different diagnoses must be entertained at different ages. Acquired cardiac disorders and dysrhythmias can present during infancy, but most occur later in the childhood or in the preadolescent or adolescent years. *Kawasaki syndrome, dilated congestive myocardiopathy, acute myocarditis, bacterial endocarditis,* and others may occur in the infant and child age groups (TABLE 9–11). Acute rheumatic fever is uncommon in children younger than 5 years of age, but if it is present, it will have severe cardiac involvement between the ages of 3 and 5 years; however, it typically presents between the ages of 5 and 15 years, with a peak incidence at age 11.

TABLE 9–8 *Summary of Key Cardiovascular Findings in the Child and Adolescent*

Murmur: VSD, PD, ASD, A-V canal, AS, PS, C/A, tetralogy of Fallot, truncus

Cyanosis: Tetralogy of Fallot, postpoperative Glenn, Fontan circulation, palliative surgery

Heart sounds: ASD, Ebstein, AS, PS, truncus, tetralogy of Fallot

Pulse abnormalities: AS, C/A

Tachycardia: SVT, WPW, CHF (congenstive heart failure)

Tachypnea: ASD, VSD, A-V canal, C/A, CHF, truncus, TAPVR

Hepatomegaly: ASD, VSD, A-V canal, C/A, CHF, truncus, TAPVR

Genetic/dysmorphic: VSD, A-V canal, tetralogy of Fallot, PDA, ASD, truncus

Growth problems: VSD, A-V canal, tetralogy of Fallot, PDA, ASD, truncus

Hypertension: C/A, PDA

Shock: Cardiomyopathy, myocarditis, HCM, postoperative Glenn, Fontan circulation; palliative surgery

TABLE 9-9 *Summary Chart: Diagnosis of Selected Congenital Cardiac Anomalies*

Diagnosis	Key Symptoms	Key Signs	Confirmatory Labs	Confirmatory Images	Age at Diagnosis
PDA	SOBOE	M, ↑pulses		ECG, echo	I > C/A
ASD	SOBOE	M, fix split S_2		CXR, ECG, echo	I/C/A
VSD	None, SOBOE	M, CHF		CXR, ECG, echo	I > C/A
A-V canal	None→CHF	None → CHF	±Hypoxia	CXR, ECG, echo	I
C/A	Shock, CHF	↑BP, ↓P, CHF		Echo, CT, MRI	I/C
Tetralogy of Fallot	Blue (spells)	Blue (spells)	Hypoxia	CXR, ECG, echo	I > C
TGV	Blue, ↑RR	Blue, ±M, ↓S_2, CHF	Hypoxia	CXR, ECG, echo	I > C
TAPVR	Blue, SOBOE	Blue, like ASD, gallop	Hypoxia	CXR, ECG, echo	I > C
Tricuspid atresia	Blue, SOBOE	Blue, ↓S_2, CHF	Hypoxia	CXR, ECG, echo	I > C
Truncus	Blue	Variable M, CHF	Hypoxia	CXR, ECG, echo	I > C
Ebstein	Blue	±M, gallop	±Hypoxia	CXR, ECG, echo	I/C/A
HLHS	Weak, gray	Shock signs	Hypoxia	CXR, ECG, echo	I
HRHS	Blue	Blue (spells)	Hypoxia	CXR, ECG, echo	I

Abbreviations: SOBOE = short of breath on exertion; CXR = chest x-ray; ECG = electrocardiogram; M = Murmur; CHF = congestive heart failure; HLHS = hypoplastic left heart syndrome; HRHS = hypoplastic right heart syndrome; I = infant, C = child, A = adolescent.

TABLE 9-10 *Congenital Heart Disease Based on Presentation*

Key Presentation	ECG	Echo	Common Diagnoses	Age Group
Cyanosis	RVH	Diagnostic	TGV, tetralogy of Fallot,	I/C
	LVH	Diagnostic	TAVPR, truncus arteriosus	I/C
			tricuspid atresia	
CHF w/o cyanosis	BVH	Diagnostic	VSD, A-V canal, C/A	I/C
CHF w/cyanosis	BVH	Diagnostic	Truncus arteriosus, TAVPR	I/C
CHF in premature	LVH	Diagnostic	PDA, C/A, A-V canal	I
Murmur no cyanosis	LVH, BVH	Diagnostic	VSD, PDA, A-V canal, pink tetralogy	I/C
			of Fallot	
Murmur w/SEC	RVH	Diagnostic	PS, tetralogy of Fallot	I/C
Murmur w/SEC	Nl, LVH	Diagnostic	AS, C/A	I/C
Murmur w/fixed S_2		Diagnostic	ASD, partial PVR	I/C/A
Chest pain	Nl, LVH	Diagnostic	AS, HLHS, noncardiac (musculoskeletal)	C/A
Pulses, weak	Nl, LVH	Diagnostic	C/A, AS, HLHS, shock	I/C
Pulses, slow	Nl, heart block	Not helpful	Heart block	I/C/A
Pulses, fast	Nl, SVT, atrial flutter/fib.	Occ diagn.	SVT, WPW, CHF, palpitations	I/C/A
Syncope	Nl, heart block, VF	Not helpful	Long QT, Stokes-Adams, HCM	I/C/A
Sudden death	3° block, VF (torsades)	Occ. diagn.	AS, HCM, long QT	C/A

Abbreviations: RVH = right ventricular hypertrophy; LVH = left ventricular hypertrophy; BVH = biventricular hypertrophy; SEC = systolic ejection click; VF = ventricular fibrillation.

TABLE 9-11 *Summary of Commonly Acquired Pediatric Heart Disease*

Diagnosis	History	Key Symptom	Key Sign	Confirmatory Labs	Confirmatory Test/Image	Age
HCM	Dizzy, syncope	Chest pain	M, arrhythmia		ECG, echo	C/A
ARF	Strep. inf.	Joint & chest pain	M, chorea, joints, SQ nodules, E. margin	+Strep, ASO	ECG, echo, ?MRI	C/A
Kawasaki	Fever > 5 days	Arthralgia	Mucus memb., nodes, conj., rash, palmar erythema	↑ESR, ↑platelets	ECG, echo	I/C
Fontan heart	CHD, surgery	SOB	CHF signs	↓O₂ sat.	ECG, echo CXR	I/C/A

Abbreviations: ECG = electrocardiogram; SQ = subcutaneous; E = erythema; ASO = antistreptolysin O; CXR = chest x-ray; M = mur mur.

Noncyanotic Congenital Heart Defects

Patent Ductus Arteriosus (PDA)

If the PDA is not large, there may or may not be a murmur. Moderate to large PDAs can cause tachypnea, dyspnea, and fatigue with feeding, diaphoresis, growth failure, and frequent pulmonary infections. Increased peripheral pulses (Corrigan or water-hammer), heart overactivity, apnea, and increased pulse and respiratory rates occur on examination. The murmur often will not be continuous and will be a late grade 2–3/6 crescendo systolic murmur stopping at P_2; diastolic spillover will occur when the systolic and diastolic systemic pressures exceed the systolic/diastolic pulmonary pressures, allowing the clinically continuous murmur seen in children and older patients. If the pressures in the lungs are increased, the large *PDA* is silent if systemic and pulmonary pressures are equal. If pulmonary pressure exceeds systemic pressure, the diastolic murmur will emerge again, this time flowing right to left (*Eisenmenger complex*). At this point the patient may be respirator-dependant with congestive heart failure and/or cyanosis. Chest x-ray will show cardiomegaly and increased pulmonary vascularity. The ECG may be normal or show LV hypertrophy in the premature newborn but can show biventricular (BV) hypertrophy in the full-term newborn or child in whom the condition has progressed. Doppler echocardiography is helpful to evaluate flow through a PDA.

Atrial Septal Defect (ASD)

ASDs are one of the most common pediatric and adult forms of congenital heart disease; 80 percent are *secundum,* 10 percent are *ostium primum,* 9 percent are *sinus venosus,* and 1 percent are *inferior vena caval.* When unrecognized in the pediatric years, many problems can result in the adult. In the pediatric ages (I, C, A) there may be minimal or no symptoms. However, larger defects can cause easy fatigue, shortness of breath, and poor growth. Infants and children may have recurrent pulmonary infections.

Most pediatric atrial septal defects (ASDs) are diagnosed by ECG after a pulmonary "flow" murmur is heard or after an abnormal incidental chest x-ray showing increased low-pressure pulmonary vascularity, right ventricular enlargement, and a prominent pulmonary artery segment. ECGs are only mildly abnormal with mild right ventricular (RV) hypertrophy (RV conduction in V_{4R} and V_1), more pronounced with larger defects. Fixed splitting of the second heart sound and a late "scratchy" diastolic murmur occur after 3 to 6 months of age with moderate to large *secundum* ASDs. *Ostium primum* (ASD I) will present earlier because of a mitral valve murmur or a left or indeterminate QRS axis on ECG. All four ASD location sites can be detected by transthoracic and/or transesophageal echocardiograms.

Most small secundum ASDs will close spontaneously in children. Up to 80 percent of secundum ASDs will close by 18 months of age, but after 3 years, spontaneous complete closure of secundum ASDs is unlikely. There are some moderate-sized defects that get smaller and do not have right atrial (RA) and RV overload and thus do not need closure. Children and adolescents will need periodic follow-up after surgical or interventional closure because of atrial dysrhythmias. Cardiomegaly usually resolves 6 to 12 months after ASD closure.

Ventricular Septal Defect (VSD)

VSDs are the most common form of congenital heart defect, comprising 20 percent. Twenty percent of these are associated with other congenital heart anomalies. A murmur identifies VSD initially, although most are hemodynamically insignificant. Tachycardia, tachypnea, poor growth, cardiac enlargement on chest x-ray, and biventricular hypertrophy on ECG help to predict congestive heart failure in patients with larger defects. Complete echocardiographic imaging studies will further confirm VSD size, left ventricular function, cardiac chamber size, and pulmonary blood pressure. Most small VSDs eventually close spontaneously. Small midmuscular VSDs will close during the first 1 to 2 years, but apical muscle VSDs may take longer. Moderate to large VSDs can cause problems with increasing left-to-right shunting at 2 to 4 weeks or later when the pulmonary vascular resistance decreases.

Some large VSDs will decrease to moderate or smaller size over time and may not need surgical closure. Echocardiographic and clinical monitoring during the first 6 to 12 months by a pediatric cardiologist is mandatory. Early surgical correction is indicated for poor growth and high pulmonary artery pressure. *Eisenmenger syndrome* is now a rarity in recognized congenital heart disease. All infants and children with Down Syndrome should have an echocardiogram to rule out moderate to large VSDs and/or A-V (atrioventricular) canal defects.

Murmur intensity and quality are variable. Small defects are often detected earlier in the newborn infant, infant, and child age groups, with a systolic murmur heard best at the middle to lower left sternal border. Smaller defects will have a crescendo-decrescendo quality, and larger defects may be louder, coarser, and holosystolic. Larger defects may be subtle or masked by the high pulmonary pressure for the first 2 to 3 months of life. Mitral diastolic "flow" rumbles may occur at the cardiac apex when the pulmonary-to-systemic blood flow is over 2:1. This is a *functional mitral stenosis* owing to increased left atrial (LA) blood flow. With clinical CHF, an S_3 gallop is often present; *CHF* and *hepatomegaly* may occur later.

When there are other associated cardiac defects such as C/A or PDA, the ECG will be helpful to diagnose the severity of each anomaly. Monitor patients for the VSD size and possible acquired aortic valve insufficiency (5 percent occurrence rates) with large perimembranous and/or large subpulmonic VSDs.

A-V Canal

Atrioventricular (A-V) canals account for 5 percent of all congenital heart defects. They are most common in Down syndrome (20 percent). Failure of the embryonic endocardial cushion to develop causes the A-V canal spectrum of complete, partial (incomplete), and transitional A-V canals. A complete A-V canal consists of an inferior ostium primum ASD, a cleft anterior mitral valve leaflet, a cleft septal tricuspid valve leaflet, and a posterior VSD. In a transitional A-V canal, the common A-V valve is adherent to the ventricular septum, thereby dividing the valve and functionally closing the VSD. A partial (incomplete) A-V canal consists of some of the above-mentioned defects.

Common associations include *heterotaxy syndromes (situs inversus, polysplenia,* and *asplenia), hypoplastic left heart syndrome, tricuspid atresia, C/A, tetralogy of Fallot,* and *Noonan and Down syndromes.* Symptoms include tachypnea, dyspnea, fatigue on feeding, poor growth, and superimposed infections over the infant's first 1 to 2 months of life. Signs include a loud murmur, increased pulmonary second sound, and occasional cyanosis from high pulmonary pressures at birth and later from the large left-to-right shunting. Congestive heart failure is common. Chest x-ray and ECG will make suggestive diagnosis of an incomplete or complete form of A-V canal.

Complete blood count (CBC) with increased hematocrit ($\uparrow$ Hct) and pulse oximetry confirm central cyanosis. Echocardiography delineates the type and severity of A-V canal defect. Surgery between 3 and 6 months of age is needed to prevent Eisenmenger changes, particularly in Down syndrome. Follow-up of surgical repair largely involves monitoring for mitral valve abnormalities and for dysrhythmias.

Coarctation of the Aorta

Coarctation of the aorta (C/A) is a narrowing in the juxtaductal areas just below the origin of the left subclavian artery; occasionally, there will be aortic arch hypoplasia or complete interruption. C/A can occur frequently with other cardiac anomalies (commonly *PDA* and *aortic stenosis*). *VSD, single ventricle,* and *A-V canal defects* can be associated as the *Shone complex. Turner syndrome* with aortic stenosis has a 30 percent C/A association.

The age of detection often predicts C/A severity, with 50 percent of isolated C/A causing symptoms during the first few days of life. Once the PDA closes, left ventricular hypertension can cause the rapid onset of severe CHF, metabolic acidosis, and possibly death if not diagnosed and treated promptly.

Be suspicious of infant or newborn C/A in a patient with differential upper and lower extremity pulse amplitudes and pulse delay from the upper to lower extremities. Document blood pressure recordings. A grade 2/6 systolic ejection heart murmur may be present at the upper chest and/or back. Associated anomalies such as aortic stenosis also may cause the murmur. A systolic ejection click (SEC) is present at the apex or neck with either anomaly.

Confirmatory testing is by echocardiogram. Occasionally, MRI or cardiac CT scan is necessary. Periodic cardiac follow-up is important to assess for hypertension and recurrent pulse discrepancies in the child and adolescent. Assess continually for other associated cardiac conditions.

Aortic Stenosis

Aortic stenosis (AS) can occur at the *subvalvar, valvular,* or *supravalvar* levels. AS is caused most commonly by a bicuspid aortic valve (BAV). It is thickened and less compliant, causing LV outflow tract obstruction.

Critical aortic valve stenosis, the most common cause of CHF on the first day of life, occurs more frequently in the newborn infant. The most severe are infants with a unicuspid valve and/or a valve annulus of less than 5 mm, which can act like a milder but complicated variant of the hypoplastic left heart syndrome. These are pediatric cardiac emergencies and require early balloon dilation and/or surgery. Milder and moderate forms of aortic valve stenosis can be completely asymptomatic in the infant, child, and adolescent.

A heart murmur is the most common finding and consists of a harsh systolic murmur heard best at the aortic area radiating to the neck. There is an associated and referred systolic ejection click (SEC) at the apex, upper chest, or carotid–arterial vessel sites. Some patients with AS or bicuspid aortic valve will have an associated protodiastolic decrescendo murmur at the aortic valve site, obviating the SEC. Symptoms, when present, include chest pain, lightheadedness, or syncope associated with exercise. Occasionally, sudden death can occur. ECGs and chest x-rays usually are normal unless the AS is severe, and subvalvar and supravalvar AS can have earlier ECG changes of LV hypertrophy and strain.

Confirmatory imaging is by echocardiograph Doppler studies, sometimes MRI and cardiac CT scan. Cardiac catheterization and angiography are used mostly to confirm echocardiographic findings and for balloon angioplasty in moderate to severe cases. Note that AS is subtly progressive with increasing pressure gradients across the defect. All treatment is palliative, and careful postoperative and pediatric or adult cardiology follow-up is mandatory.

Cyanotic Congenital Heart Defects

Tetralogy of Fallot, VSD, PS, RV Hypertrophy, Overriding Aorta

Tetralogy of Fallot presents as the prototypic "blue baby." He or she is not always consistently cyanotic but may present with a murmur and intermittent cyanosis (blue spells). The acyanotic patient may become consistently cyanotic during later infancy or early childhood. Cyanotic infants with *Down syndrome* usually have tetralogy of Fallot, although those with A-V canals also can be hypoxic at birth.

On examination of the heart, S_2 is single, and a systolic ejection murmur is present. A systolic ejection click may be present, but the origin is from the dilated aortic root present in most tetralogy of Fallot patients, not their infundibular pulmonic stenosis. Infants that present early with significant cyanosis may have more severe forms of *pulmonary valve atresia* or *severe pulmonary stenosis*. The ECG may show only upright T waves in the right precordial leads initially. The degree of RV hypertrophy usually progresses during the first year, and cyanosis appears during the transition from a "pink" tetralogy.

The large VSD does not cause a murmur because the shunt is right to left; the murmur originates from the infundibular pulmonic stenosis. The chest x-ray in tetralogy of Fallot shows mild right-sided heart enlargement (boot shaped or sheep's nose), and 20 to 25 percent will have a right aortic arch. Pulmonary vascularity is variably decreased. Hypercyanotic or blue spells will have a decreased murmur during the spell with an increase in cyanosis and irritability. Long hypoxic spells can result in death; thus recognition and prompt treatment are necessary. Affected children who are unrecognized or uncorrected have classic "squatting" spells during physical activity. Transthoracic echocardiography with Doppler studies will demonstrate all four components of tetralogy of Fallot. Monitor postoperatively for degree of residual pulmonary stenosis, pulmonary insufficiency, and arrhythmias.

Transposition of the Great Vessels (TGV)

Transposition of the great vessels (aorta and pulmonary artery) is the most common cyanotic congenital heart anomaly in the first month of life. The aorta and the pulmonary artery are transposed and originate from the "wrong" ventricle. Associated other cardiac anomalies include VSD in 25 percent, pulmonary stenosis, and abnormal coronary arteries. Newborn infants with TGV will present with varying degrees of cyanosis depending on the associated number and size of left-to-right shunts (PDA, ASD, and VSD). Peripheral pulses are usually strong.

Most TGVs are diagnosed in the first days of life unless they have large VSDs. Severe cyanosis and metabolic acidosis occur rapidly when there is only a PDA that closes. Tachypnea without dyspnea is common, but a heart murmur is not. The ECG shows moderate RV hypertrophy. Chest x-ray shows decreased vascularity and often an "egg-on-a-string" pattern: right ventricular enlargement and aortic arch and pulmonary artery segments not seen owing to straight anteroposterior alignment of a typical transposition and absent thymus. Transthoracic echocardiography with Doppler will confirm the diagnosis.

Total Anomalous Pulmonary Venous Return (TAPVR)

TAPVR is the abnormal return of the pulmonary venous system to the right atrium, vena cava, or coronary sinus. It may involve all four pulmonary veins (total) or be partial. Vena cava drainage may be *supracardiac* or *infracardiac*. Clinical presentation is severe if venous return is obstructed (more with right superior vena cava and inferior vena cava drainage). A murmur is often not present, and the heart is small and may demonstrate a figure-of-eight ("snowman") appearance if the obstruction is in the superior vena cava. The pulmonary vascularity is decreased, pulmonary edema is present, and there is severe hypoxia and acidosis. This is a surgical emergency.

The milder partial types present as an ASD. Although anatomically different, the physiology and mechanics are similar, with increased return to the right side of the heart during ventricular diastole. Less emergent surgical referral is necessary.

Tricuspid Atresia (TA)

Tricuspid valve atresia is part of the hypoplastic right heart syndrome and can be associated with pulmonary valve atresia. Clinical presentation can be with mild, moderate, or severe cyanosis depending on associated cardiac anomalies (TGV, VSD, PDA, and PS). Congestive heart failure (CHF) with tachypnea, tachycardia, and hepatomegaly also may occur. Heart murmur may be present. ECG findings of left atrial dilatation and LV hypertrophy are an important clue to the diagnosis because most neonatal ECGs should demonstrate right ventricular predominance. Chest x-ray will reflect the amount of pulmonary blood flow, with larger shunts causing CHF and smaller shunts resulting in a smaller heart, decreased pulmonary flow, and more cyanosis. Echocardiography with Doppler will diagnose TA and associated cardiac lesions and will help to guide treatment. Patients without an ASD or VSD will not survive without surgery once the PDA closes.

Truncus Arteriosus

Persistent *truncus arteriosus* is a primitive, rare congenital heart defect owing to lack of embryonic differentiation of the conus arteriosus into a separate aorta and main pulmonary artery. Infants with truncus arteriosus are cyanotic and often demonstrate early findings of CHF. The heart is moderately to severely enlarged on chest x-ray, with 30 percent having a right aortic arch and prominently increased vascularity. Hepatomegaly and peripheral edema with poor feeding and noisy breathing are due to CHF. Heart murmurs may be loud but can be absent in patients with CHF. ECG will show BV and LA hypertrophy. Oxygen saturation levels are 75 to 80 percent in room air. Echocardiography will confirm the large subaortic VSD and large primitive common semilunar valve root with two to eight valve leaflets present. Different pulmonary artery distributions are possible. Early surgery in the first 2 weeks is needed to prevent rapid pulmonary vascular arteriolar damage and to ameliorate CHF. Di George syndrome is often associated with both truncus arteriosus and tetralogy of Fallot.

Ebstein's Anomaly of the Tricuspid Valve (Upward Traction)

With *Ebstein's* anomaly, there is a very large heart and variable cyanosis. There are multiple heart sounds (gallop rhythm). *Tricuspid regurgitation* can be mild to moderate. Always ask about maternal history of lithium use. Also look for *Wolff-Parkinson-White abnormality* on ECG. Definitive diagnosis is by echocardiogram.

Hypoplastic Left Heart Syndrome Spectrum

Aortic atresia and *mitral atresia* are the most common forms. There may be variable LV outflow obstruction. The less severe forms may present similar to coarctation of the aorta (C/A). The more severe forms present in the newborn with shock and poor pulses and a gray color. It is a PDA-dependent lesion, so severe decompensation develops after closure, often resulting in death. Definitive diagnosis is by echocardiography so that early surgical intervention may occur.

Hypoplastic Right Heart Syndrome Spectrum

Pulmonary atresia with intact septum and *tricuspid valve atresia* comprise this group. It is also PDA-dependent and presents similarly to hypoplastic left heart syndrome with cyanosis, metabolic acidosis, and shock.

Complex Congenital Heart Single-Ventricle Defects (Fontan Circulation)

These defects are many and varied but rare. They may appear as a single (double-inlet) ventricle or a double-outlet right ventricle with or without associated cardiac anomalies. They may be acquired as a result of a Fontan surgical procedure. They present with differing degrees of shunting, murmurs, and CHF. They are not able to be diagnosed clinically, so cardiac consultation with imaging is necessary. TABLES 9–8 and 9–9 summarize the diagnosis of pediatric heart disease.

Acquired Cardiac Disease in the Pediatric Patient

Acute Rheumatic Fever and Rheumatic Heart Disease

Diagnosis of *acute rheumatic fever* requires two or more of the *Jones major criteria: migratory arthritis, carditis, chorea, subcutaneous nodules,* and *erythema marginatum.* Also, laboratory evidence of a recent streptococcal infection is required, except for when chorea is present. The common presenting age is 5 to 15 years, with a peak at 11 years. A second peak occurs in adolescents and young adults between 18 and 21 years of age. Although uncommon, rheumatic fever, when present between the ages 3 and 5 years, often causes severe cardiac disease.

The subcutaneous nodule and erythema marginatum are not valid single major criteria, are seen in only 10 percent of patients, and usually accompany carditis. Arthritis is most common and usually is migratory between large joints. Carditis is the second most common form, followed by Sydenham's chorea. Arthritis and carditis often occur together, but chorea and arthritis do not. Chorea is associated with cardiac involvement in 30 to 40 percent of patients.

There is *pancarditis,* but *endocarditis* with *mitral* and *aortic valve insufficiency* also is common. Moderate to severe *mitral regurgitation* presents as a *Carey-Coombs* type of murmur (an apical middiastolic murmur occurring in the acute stage of rheumatic *mitral valvulitis* and disappearing as the valvulitis subsides). Myocardial and perimyocardial disease can present as CHF, pericarditis, or both. *Cardiac tamponade* is a serious complication of acute rheumatic fever.

Mitral insufficiency occurs commonly with *aortic insufficiency. Tricuspid insufficiency* also can occur; pulmonary valve involvement does not. Mitral insufficiency causes a holosystolic murmur grades 1–3/6 and aortic insufficiency, a 1–2/6 protodiastolic murmur. A pericardial friction rub is present in mild to moderate *pericarditis.*

Kawasaki Disease/Syndrome

Kawasaki disease is now the most common form of acquired pediatric heart disease in America. Rheumatic fever is still the most common worldwide. Criteria for diagnosis include *prolonged high fever for over*

5 days, nonspecific rash, enlarged cervical lymph nodes, nonprurulent conjunctivitis, mucous membranous stomatitis and pharyngitis, and *joint redness and swelling.* Delayed or later desquamation occurs at the joint and perianal-diaper skin areas; *Beau's lines* (deep grooved lines that run from side to side on the fingernail) may appear on the fingers and toenails, with some sloughing of skin on the hand and fingers occurring 2 to 3 weeks after onset. Risk for *coronary artery aneurysms* is high, and cardiac failure with S$_3$ gallops and mitral insufficiency heart murmurs can occur. Age of presentation is usually at 1 to 5 years, but male children under 1 year of age will have a more severe disease presentation and higher risk for coronary aneurysm. Four of six criteria are needed to diagnose Kawasaki disease unless there is confirmatory evidence of coronary artery involvement by echocardiogram. Older patents have more atypical presentations and usually are less ill.

Bacterial Endocarditis

Bacterial endocarditis usually occurs in patients who have congenital or acquired heart disease (except for isolated ASDs) or who are immune compromised. Persistent fever, changing murmurs, fatigue, and weight loss are present. Any suspicion of endocarditis warrants confirmatory blood cultures and imaging.

Myocarditis/Myocardiomyopathy

Myocarditis occurs at all ages, often a complication of bacterial, viral, or rickettsial infection. In severe cases the patient presents with *CHF, sudden cardiac death,* or *cardiogenic shock.* Clinical findings consist of depressed heart sounds, friction rubs, CHF, and shock. Infants and children more frequently will have this type of clinical presentation.

Dilated myocardiopathy can have a similar picture. *Hypertrophic cardiomyopathy,* involving the LV outflow tract in the child and adolescent is a known risk factor for sudden cardiac death. Unfortunately, this can be the first cardiac event. Patients may present with a positive family history, chest pain, or syncope and no warning prodrome. Physical examination, if helpful, will demonstrate a systolic ejection murmur that amplifies during a Valsalva maneuver. This is due to diminished right-sided return, moving the ventricular septum to the right and thus opening up a previously tight aortic valve. TABLE 9–10 summarizes the diagnosis of acquired heart disease.

Confirmatory Laboratory and Imaging

A good history and physical examination, unfortunately, are often of little help in infants with cyanotic heart disease, nor are they helpful to detect arrhythmias, prolonged QT syndrome, hypertrophic cardiomyopathy, or coronary artery anomalies. ECGs are necessary to evaluate arrhythmias and prolonged QT syndrome. Consult tables for corrected QT interval norms for age. Infants with *supraventricular tachycardia* (SVT) and *atrial flutter* have heart rates of up to 300 beats/min and will have typical ECG characteristics—lack of beat-to-beat variability and absent P wave. An infant with a slow pulse should have an ECG to document *sinus bradycardia* and identify complete *third-degree* or *Mobitz-type second-degree block,* which may require treatment if the patient is unstable hemodynamically. Echocardiography will diagnose most cardiomyopathies and is helpful to an extent in assessing coronary blood flow. It is also necessary to confirm clinically suspected congenital heart disease.

Holter monitor or longer time-duration event monitors are often helpful in children and adolescents. One can differentiate benign palpitations such as premature atrial and ventricular contractions from *supraventricular tachycardia, atrial flutter/fibrillation,* and *ventricular tachycardia.* Fortunately, most children and adolescents will have benign arrhythmias when monitored. Electrophysiologic studies (EPs) and cardiac cryo- or radioablation for recurrent arrhythmias, particularly for active adolescents, are now a common occurrence.

Modern technology is most helpful to diagnose cardiac disease earlier, but there still is no substitute for frequent physical assessments and basic laboratory work such as glucose, electrolytes, and calcium level determinations to monitor the physiologic consequences of heart disease. TABLE 9–12 lists diagnostic tools cardiologists employ most frequently.

TABLE 9–12 *Commonly Used Confirmatory Tests and Imaging*

Oxygen measurement
Oxygen saturation monitor
Capillary blood gases
Arterial blood gases
Blood pressure measurement
Dinamap
Auscultation
Arterial flush
ECG
Chest x-ray
Holter monitor
Stress treadmill exercise testing
Echocardiography
   M-mode
   Two-dimensional
Doppler: Pulse, continuous Doppler; color-flow Doppler mapping
Stress echo
Cardiac catheterization and angiography
MRI/CT scan

When to Refer

During the neonatal period, infants suspected of congenital heart abnormalities require frequent murmur, blood pressure, pulse amplitude, rate discrepancy, cyanosis, and heart failure assessment. Infants with *aortic* or *pulmonic valve stenosis* and *obstructive anomalies such as coarctation of the aorta* should be diagnosed within the first month. Most cyanotic cardiac lesions will be diagnosed and many will be treated surgically during the neonatal and early infancy periods. All neonates with diagnosed congenital heart disease, as well as postoperative patients, require frequent follow-up in the pediatrician's and cardiologist's office.

Other infants suspected later to have congenital or acquired heart problems should be referred for cardiac consultation and management. Although left-to-right shunts can occur in the newborn, many do not present until 1 to 3 months after birth, when the pulmonary vascular resistance has lessened. Children with *Down syndrome* and moderate to large left-to-right shunts will need the earliest possible diagnosis of cardiac lesions because they develop rapid pulmonary arteriolar changes (*Eisenmenger syndrome*). They all should have echocardiography performed in the newborn nursery *regardless* of physical examination findings, and they should be referred to a cardiologist if any abnormalities are present.

Innocent cardiac murmurs are estimated by pediatric cardiologists to occur in up to 90 percent of children between the ages of 1 and 8 years. A typical pediatrician likely will only see three to five abnormal murmurs that will need specialty referral per each office practice year but will hear many innocent heart murmurs. Any patient infant, child, or adolescent suspected of a cardiovascular abnormality should be referred to a pediatric cardiologist.

Children and adolescents who have congenital and acquired heart disease or may have had prior cardiac palliative or corrective surgery, like infants, need periodic follow-up. Other frequent cardiac symptoms and signs in children and adolescents, such as *chest pain, dizziness* or *presyncope, syncope, palpitations, dysrhythmias, cyanotic spells,* or *seizure-like episodes and hypertension,* merit close observation and possible referral.

Shock (lack of oxygen supply to tissues) in any of the pediatric age groups may result from sepsis, hypovolemia, anaphylaxis, or disturbances of acid-base balance. When related to severe cyanotic or congestive heart failure, it merits emergency cardiology consultation. *Multiorgan system failure* results in all age groups from cardiac, pulmonary, renal, neurologic, and hematologic interdependence.

With the increasing success of palliative and/or "functional" cardiac surgical correction of most congenital heart anomalies, there are a rapidly increasing number of these pediatric patients. This includes approximately 4 to 7 percent of the pediatric congenital heart patient population. This also includes the significant and growing number of complex cardiac single-ventricle (*Fontan circulation*) patients and those

TABLE 9-13 *Indications for Referral to a Pediatric Cardiologist*

All infants under 1 month of age with suspected heart disease
All patients with diastolic murmurs
Murmur sounds pathologic
Hypertension documented by three serial recordings
Concern for possible rheumatic fever
Innocent murmur getting louder
Systolic click sound; S_2 split and ?"fixed"
Exercise-related syncope/dizziness
Severe chest pain (esp. if exercise-related)
Enlarged heart on chest x-ray
Abnormal ECG
Palpitation; fast heart rate concerns
Prior history of congenital or acquired heart problem
Spells or seizure-like activity
Cyanotic clubbing of extremities
Syndromes with known congenital or acquired cardiac abnormalities

children and adolescents with artificial heart valves and homografts, demand pacemakers, and automatic internal defibrillators. These patients will require regular periodic cardiovascular evaluation and monitoring by pediatric and, eventually, adult cardiologists.

Examination of this special group of cardiac patients will require knowledge of what is not only normal but also what is abnormal on *their* cardiovascular physical examination. Do the patient's examination findings constitute a need for medical or surgical cardiac specialty referral for consultation and possible treatment? Is the patient doing well when compared with his or her child and adolescent peer groups? Can the patient participate safely in selected sports and physical activities? TABLE 9–13 is a summary of indications for referral to a pediatric cardiologist.

10 The Gastrointestinal Tract, Liver, Gall Bladder, and Pancreas

Arthur N. Feinberg and Lisa A. Feinberg

The goals of this chapter are

1. To outline physiology, mechanics, and the perturbations that produce symptoms and signs referable to the gastrointestinal (GI) tract
2. To outline functional anatomy in a similar manner
3. To catalogue the key problems in infants, children, and adolescents and discuss how to clarify and prioritize them
4. To learn to perform a complete physical examination referable to GI symptoms and develop a list of key findings
5. To develop a table narrowing GI diagnoses by anatomy, epidemiology, and etiology
6. To outline confirmatory laboratory, imaging, procedures, and referrals to specialists with their indications

Physiology and Mechanics

The GI tract manifests its pathology as pain, vomiting, diarrhea, constipation, or poor feeding. Pain results from infection (or inflammation) or from distension of a hollow viscus. Sensory receptors (e.g., heat and stretch) communicate with the autonomic as well as the central nervous system (CNS). Vomiting may be due to direct mucosal reaction by pathogens, toxins, corrosives, autonomic dysfunction, or obstruction. Diarrhea may be secretory, osmotic, inflammatory, or due to increased or decreased intestinal motility. Constipation may be a function of decreased intestinal motility, obstruction, or functional stool withholding. Poor feeding may be due to aversion or due to pain during a process that causes mucosal pathology of the upper GI tract.

Simply, the GI tract processes all ingested food and breaks down larger molecules of protein, fat, and carbohydrate into smaller molecules. The intestinal mucosa absorbs them and breaks them down into simpler molecules. The mucosa then releases the molecules to the circulation, which then delivers them to all cells of the body to meet growth and energy requirements.

At the level of the upper GI tract, the esophagus propels boluses of ingested food previously chewed into the stomach. The autonomic nervous system mediates coordination of peristalsis and opening/closing of the lower esophageal sphincter. Salivary amylase acts on complex carbohydrates and breaks them down into smaller molecules. At the level of the stomach, the parietal cells' hydrogen ion pump produces hydrochloric acid, mediated through several pathways, neural (autonomic), endocrine (gastrin and pepsin), and paracrine (histamine). Stomach acid and pepsin further break down protein and carbohydrates into simpler, more absorbable molecules (disaccharides, monosaccharides, smaller peptides, and amino acids).

As the food bolus proceeds into the duodenum, multiple enzymes produced by the pancreas (amylases, lipases, and proteases including chymotrypsin, trypsin, and carboxypeptidase) break down proteins and fats further. The liver produces bile, instrumental in fat emulsification, which is stored in the gall bladder. The gall bladder sends bile through the biliary tree (hepatic and cystic ducts), where it meets at the ampulla of Vater with the pancreatic ducts. The duodenum then receives bile and pancreatic enzymes through the sphincter of Oddi. Bilirubin, the major component of bile, comes from broken-down red blood cell hemoglobin conjugated in the liver to a water-soluble form. It is then secreted into the duodenum. The intestine excretes unconjugated bilirubin (fat-soluble), and the kidneys excrete conjugated bilirubin (water-soluble).

The bolus of food now passes down the small intestine, the jejunum and ileum, whose involuted mucosal lining contains the large surface area over which the now-simplified carbohydrate molecules undergo action by brush-border enzymes and are absorbed. Fat molecules, including fatty acids and monoglycerides, are transported into the enterocyte and ultimately are reesterified into triglycerides. Medium-chain triglycerides are absorbed directly into the lymphatic system with no enzymatic action. The intestine hydrolyzes and absorbs amino acids, dipeptides, and tripeptides, breakdown products of proteins. In addition, vitamins A, D, E, and K are the fat-soluble vitamins whose absorption depends on the proper functioning of the GI tract. Also, intrinsic factor from the stomach is necessary for the absorption of vitamin B_{12} in the distal ileum.

The remaining undigested material passes through the cecum into the large intestine. The purpose of the large intestine is to deliver solid waste for excretion. This material contains mainly sloughed intestinal cells, undigested food, bile pigments, and water. As the fecal stream proceeds through the large intestine rhythmically and nonpropulsively, from the ascending colon to the transverse colon to the descending colon, it reabsorbs water, producing more solid fecal matter. The rectum expels stools through a coordinated defecation reflex stimulated by colon distension and mediated through ganglion cells, ultimately causing voluntary relaxation of the external sphincter to pass stool.

The term *jaundice* (*icterus*) derives from the French *jaune* (or Greek *ikteros*), meaning yellow owing to deposition of the bile pigment bilirubin in the skin. The pigment bilirubin is released in an unconjugated state (fat-soluble) and delivered through the circulation to the liver hepatocyte, where the enzyme uridine 5′-diphosphate (UDP) glucuronosyltransferase acts to convert the bilirubin to a water-soluble polar diglucuronide. The biliary tract receives bile-containing bilirubin via bile canaliculi that is stored in the gall bladder and ultimately delivered to the duodenum via the common bile duct, the ampulla of Vater, and sphincter of Oddi. The enzyme bilirubin oxidase deconjugates conjugated bilirubin in the bowel. The gut reabsorbs bilirubin back into the circulation (enterohepatic recirculation). Bile pigments may be increased and deposited into the skin as either conjugated or unconjugated bilirubin.

All symptoms and signs discussed below explain perturbations of any of the structures or functions discussed in the preceding very simplified scheme. After reviewing them, the reader should begin to formulate differential diagnoses. This chapter does not include every diagnosis but rather provides the reader a format for pursuit thereof. Discussion of the appropriate use of laboratory, imaging, and specialist consultation in order to crystallize a diagnosis follows.

Functional Anatomy

FIGURE 10–1 shows the normal gross anatomic structures of the abdomen. The preceding section on physiology addresses function at the microanatomic level.

History

Infants

A full general history is necessary for making a proper diagnosis. This is covered in Chapter 1 and will not be repeated here. Symptoms and signs below refer in particular to the GI tract.

KEY PROBLEM

Vomiting *Vomiting* is a very common symptom in infants and children and may or may not be specific for GI disorders. It is best to address this symptom as to its frequency and timing, as well as its nature, specifically projectile versus nonprojectile, and content (blood, bile, or food particles). Always think of *congenital* causes in infants.

Vomiting that occurs immediately after food ingestion points to high upper GI obstruction such as *achalasia* or esophageal, gastric (*antral web* or *foreign body*), or duodenal obstruction of any kind (*atresia* or *web*). If vomiting occurs within an hour of feeding, consider *pyloric stenosis, overfeeding, gastroesophageal reflux* (GERD), *milk intolerance or allergy,* and most commonly, *gastroenteritis.* Consider the foods recently consumed. Might they be a cause? *Medications* such as erythromycin and prostaglandins may cause pyloric stenosis. Vomiting days after feeding suggests lower intestinal obstruction such as *volvulus, incarcerated hernia, atresia, stenosis, imperforate anus,* or *Hirschsprung disease.* If vomiting is episodic and

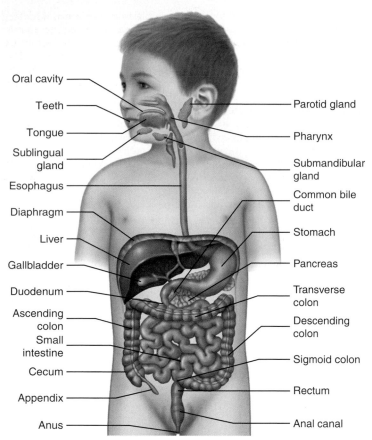

FIGURE 10–1 *Normal Gross Anatomy of the Abdomen.* (*From Van De Graaff KH:* Human Anatomy. *New York: McGraw-Hill, 2002, Fig. 18.1, p. 635.*)

associated with pain (see below), think *intussusception.* As to its nature, projectile vomiting is a warning for pyloric stenosis, whereas dribbling indicates rumination or *achalasia.*

The content of the vomitus is also helpful in developing a differential diagnosis. Gross blood indicates the possibility of *ulcer, esophageal varix of liver disease (portal obstruction),* and *ingestion of a corrosive substance.* Bile in the vomitus bespeaks duodenal obstruction below the sphincter of Oddi, seen in newborns with *annular pancreas* or *duodenal stenosis, duodenal atresia,* or *lower webs. Malrotation/volvulus, intestinal duplications,* and *meconium ileus* originate in the small intestine. Feculent vomitus presents in lower GI obstructions. Intact food particles in vomitus indicate that the food has been in the upper GI tract for too short a period for acid and enzymatic breakdown.

Vomiting may have many non-GI causes such as from the CNS owing to increased intracranial pressure from infection, tumor, or obstruction to cerebrospinal fluid (CSF) flow. Also include *metabolic* derangements, as seen in *organic acidemias* (see Chapter 12 for more detail), *diabetic ketoacidosis, renal failure,* or *renal tubular acidosis.* There are other causes of electrolyte imbalance, including but not limited to *adrenal failure or hyperplasia* and *cystic fibrosis.* GI bleeding owing to non-GI causes should raise the thought of *bleeding diatheses.*

KEY PROBLEM

■ **Diarrhea** *Diarrhea* is an increase in frequency or decrease in consistency of the stools. In infants, the quantity is more than 10 g/kg per day. As with vomiting, diagnostic possibilities for diarrhea depend on its timing, nature, and content. It may be acute or chronic, with a 3-week period considered the cutoff point between the two. If acute, it is most commonly due to *infection* but also may result from acute *toxic* ingestion. If chronic, consider *malabsorption* with multiple causes, such as fat or carbohydrate malabsorption owing to lack of surface area (*short-gut syndrome*) or malfunction of processing at the mucosal level (brush-border enzymes or esterification of fatty acids). Carbohydrate malabsorption owing to *disaccharidase deficiency* produces profuse, watery, explosive diarrhea. Stools that contain excess fat are greasy, float in the toilet, and are most foul smelling. Causes for this are *celiac disease, cystic fibrosis, autoimmune disorders,* and failure of bile salt emulsification of fats owing to hepatobiliary malfunction. Rarer causes include *intrahepatic cholestasis, biliary atresia, lymphangiectasia, abetalipoproteinemia, acrodermatitis enteropathica, eosinophilic gastroenteritis, metabolic diseases* such as *alpha$_1$-antitrypsin deficiency, tyrosinemia,* and *milk allergy.* Consider functional or other disorders of intestinal motility, including *Hirschsprung disease.* "Toddler's diarrhea" occurs commonly in healthy, thriving children between the ages of 1 and 2 years and is due to functionally rapid transit time. The stool contains undigested food particles. *Bacterial overgrowth* owing to sludging of bowel contents also may produce chronic diarrhea.

The content of diarrhea is important in the formulation of a differential diagnosis. Watery diarrhea, often explosive, most commonly bespeaks viral *infections* such as *rotavirus, coronavirus,* and *norovirus.* Also consider *Vibrio cholera* as a bacterial etiology (copious rice-water diarrhea). Gross blood in the stool is a result of *infection,* particularly bacterial, such as *Salmonella, Shigella, Campylobacter, and Yersinia.* History of exposures (animals, travels) helps to determine a pathogen that is causing symptoms. *Anal fissures* are a common cause of bright red blood, often streaky in this age group. Other important causes of bloody diarrhea include *intussusception* (currant jelly stools), *Meckel's diverticulum* (mahogany-colored stools), *malrotation* and *volvulus* causing necrotic bowel, and ischemia. Blood passing through the stomach produces black stools because of the reaction between hydrochloric acid and blood. *Milk-induced colitis* may cause significant blood loss in diarrhea, both gross and microscopic. *Toxic megacolon* is a serious condition associated mostly with *Hirschsprung disease,* causing gross blood loss from the lower GI tract. Stools may vary greatly in color, from brown to green to yellow, all of which are normal owing to bile pigments. Stools with no pigment (white, acholic) raise a concern for biliary obstruction.

Diarrhea may have non-GI etiologies. In this age group one must consider *immune* disorders, *hyperthyroidism* (nocturnal diarrhea), *metabolic* conditions involving excess catecholamines (*neuroblastoma*), and possibly ingestion of laxatives. One always must consider *psychosocial* situations such as *Munchausen by proxy*.

It is important to note that *ingestion* of pigmented foods or drugs, including candies, fruit punch, beets, rifampin, and phenolphthalein laxatives (red in color) and bismuth, activated charcoal, iron, spinach, and licorice (black in color) may mimic hematochezia (red blood in stools) or melena (black blood in stools). Do not misconstrue uric acid crystals in an infant's diaper, often pink or orange, for blood.

● KEY PROBLEM
■ **Constipation** *Constipation* is defined as infrequent passage of stools (<3 per week) or a history of painful passage of hard stools with or without soiling. Salient questions regarding constipation are as follows: Are the stools infrequent but hard and large when they occur? Are the stools infrequent but associated with diarrhea at times? How do the stools look (thin, small, or round)? What is the child's diet? Is there any medication exposure? Is there fecal soiling?

Most commonly, fecal retention during the toilet training process is the cause of constipation in infants. Children may associate bowel training with either pain or fear of loss of stool and will retain it. Anal fissures and irritation can cause secondary constipation. The stools are large, hard, and may even cause bleeding owing to secondary anal fissures. Overflow incontinence occurs because a large, hard stool in the colon will be located in the area of maximal water resorption, thus allowing the proximal water fecal stream to leak through. Often infants will hide and stool in their diapers when they do have a bowel movement, or if they are able to sit on a toilet seat, they often will not plant their feet on the floor in order to the prevent maximal intraabdominal pressure necessary to evacuate the colon.

Organic causes of constipation include *Hirschsprung disease*, which presents with no overflow incontinence and is often associated with poor weight gain. Also consider *anal stenosis, anteriorly displaced anus*, and *anal bands*. *Intestinal pseudo-obstruction* and other motility disorders also cause constipation. Non-GI causes are common in this age group, including *urinary tract infection, metabolic* disorders (*hypothyroidism* and *electrolyte disturbances* such as *hypokalemia* and *hypocalcemia*), *cystic fibrosis* (distal intestinal obstruction syndrome), *renal tubular acidosis*, and CNS problems, specifically those of the lower spinal cord (*spina bifida, tethered cord, syrinx*, etc.). *Congenital* defects in abdominal wall musculature such as *omphalocele, gastroschisis*, and *Eagle-Barrett* (*prune-belly*) syndrome may cause constipation. Consider exogenous causes such as dietary (excess milk intake or low-fiber diet), *medication* such as narcotics and chemotherapeutic agents, and *lead intoxication*.

● KEY PROBLEM
◾ **Pain** *Pain* can be difficult to assess in infants because of lack of verbal communication. It presents mainly as fussiness and crying. Thus localization and nature are virtually difficult to detect. Astute clinical observation of an infant may be most helpful to arrive at a diagnosis. Specifically, timing of the pain may be revealing. If fussiness or crying occurs immediately after feeding, this could be a sign of *gastroesophageal reflux.* If the crying is intermittent and regular, this could be due to spasms associated with intussusception. Pain in the *recumbent position is often associated with* gastroesophageal reflux. Other causes include *malrotation/volvulus, incarcerated hernia, peritonitis, Hirschsprung disease,* and *gastroenteritis.* In addition, consider non-GI causes of abdominal pain such as *genitourinary obstruction, urinary tract infection* (UTI), and *pneumonia.*

● KEY PROBLEM
◾ **Poor Feeding** *Poor appetite* in infants is more often not of GI origin. It may occur in *gastroesophageal reflux* with *esophagitis* if the infant is able to make the association of pain owing to acid reflux immediately after feeding. Most cases of food refusal and subsequent poor weight gain (see below) are nonorganic in nature and require a *psychosocial* approach. However, many non-GI causes of poor intake include poor suck/swallow coordination owing to *CNS abnormality, sepsis, congestive heart failure,* and *renal failure.*

● KEY PROBLEM
◾ **Jaundice** *Jaundice,* as discussed earlier, has an extensive differential diagnosis, especially in the newborn period. See Chapter 5 for a systematic approach to diagnosis. In the 1-month to 2-year age group it may be the result of either unconjugated (prehepatic) or conjugated (posthepatic) bilirubin. Unconjugated bilirubin presents clinically as jaundice of a yellow or orange hue, and conjugated bilirubin appears mainly with a greenish hue. In addition, jaundice associated with hemolytic anemia often will present as a more sallow or waxy hue. Scleral and sublingual areas are typical sites. Technically, unconjugated hyperbilirubinemia is not GI in origin and is a result of hemolysis owing to *infection* [*sepsis, hemolytic uremic syndrome* (HUS)], *immune reactions* and *immunologic* causes, *thalassemia, hemoglobinopathies,* and *red blood cell* (RBC) *enzyme and membrane defects.* It occurs without hemolysis if there is pathology prior to enzymatic conjugation. A severe form is associated with absence of enzyme glucuronyl transferase (*Crigler-Najjar syndrom*e). Intermittent jaundice is characteristic of the more common and benign *Gilbert* syndrome, often as a result of stress, illness, or alcoholic binges. In *Rotor* or *Dubin Johnson syndromes,* the hepatocyte does not release conjugated bilirubin, thus causing jaundice. For other causes of conjugated hyperbilirubinemia, consider *metabolic* disorders such as *cystic fibrosis, alpha$_1$- antitrypsin deficiency, galactosemia, storage and peroxisomal storage mitochondrial diseases,* and *tyrosinemia. Acute hepatitis A, B, C. D, or E, Epstein-Barr or cytomegalovirus,* and *bacterial sepsis* are more common causes. Biliary tract obstructions owing to intrahepatic cholestasis, *stones, choledochal cyst,* or *congenital* malformation of bile ducts (*Alagille syndrome,*

Byler syndrome, and *Caroli disease*) are also other causes of conjugated hyperbilirubinemia. *Alagille syndrome* is associated with other anomalies: vertebral (butterfly), eye (posterior embryotoxon), and cardiac (pulmonary stenosis). Consider drug and *toxic* ingestion.

Carotenemia is often mistaken for jaundice. It peaks at age 9 months, is more orange-yellow in color, and occurs more in acral areas (nose, chin, hands, and feet). It does not affect sclerae and is benign and self-limiting.

Children

KEY PROBLEM

■ **Vomiting** *Vomiting* in childhood has several causes in common with that of infancy. To avoid repetition, we will eliminate certain causes from infancy that do not apply to childhood, such as pyloric stenosis. On the other hand, vomiting owing to *congenital* anomalies, e.g., *annular pancreas, tracheoesophageal fistula* (TEF), *webs, malrotation,* and *volvulus,* may have some residual symptoms that persist during ages 2 to 12 years. *Infectious* causes, usually *gastroenteritis,* are most common.

There are aspects of vomiting in childhood that do not apply to infancy. It may be the earliest presentation of *appendicitis.* Although primary intussusception is not likely in this age group, it may present as a consequence of *Henoch-Schonlein purpura* (HSP) or *Meckel's diverticulum* as a lead point. Ulcer disease as a cause of vomiting becomes more common in childhood, and *inflammatory bowel disease* (IBD) appears. *Neoplasia* begins to play a more significant role in childhood, specifically *lymphoma.* The clinician now must develop a high index of suspicion for *gall bladder disease* and *pancreatitis,* especially in NICU graduates who have received total parenteral nutrition (TPN) and patients with chronic illness. As children after age 2 become more independent and active, they are more subject to abdominal trauma, which could cause obstruction and vomiting secondary to hematoma of the bowel wall, especially the duodenum. One also must consider nonaccidental injury (*abuse*).

Upper GI bleeding has similar causes to those in infancy. Gastric and duodenal *ulcers* and *Mallory Weiss tears* from forceful emesis become more prevalent, as do stress ulcers in trauma and burns. Also, children are more likely to take nonsteroidal anti-inflammatory *medications* and thus are more susceptible to GI bleeding. Non-GI causes of vomiting and bleeding are similar to those outlined during infancy.

KEY PROBLEM

■ **Diarrhea** Causes of *diarrhea* in children are similar to those in infancy. *Infectious* causes, *viral* and *bacterial,* remain the most common. Children are now more likely to venture out of a home setting and encounter pathogens in other areas, such as day-care centers, restaurants, zoos, farms, etc. More exposure to antibiotics increases the risk of *antibiotic-associated colitis.* Thus it is important to elicit a careful history of these exposures. *IBD* and *malignancy* also become more likely to cause diarrhea in childhood. *Toxic megacolon* is now more likely to be a complication of IBD, specifically *ulcerative colitis*.

Lower GI bleeding may result from juvenile polyps. They are benign, usually low in the rectum, and may cause significant gross blood in the stool in the absence of pain. Other rarer causes of *juvenile polyposis* may appear in childhood. *Intussusception* secondary to HSP may produce currant jelly stools, and *Meckel's diverticulum* is associated with painless rectal bleeding (mahogany). Consider anorectal causes of lower GI bleeding such as *rectal prolapse*, often idiopathic, but frequently associated with *cystic fibrosis.* Also, persistent anorectal pathology such as intractable *fissures* may be an early sign of IBD, especially *Crohn disease.* Trauma, both accidental and nonaccidental, is a frequent cause of intestinal bleeding.

KEY PROBLEM
Constipation *Constipation* has similar causes in childhood as in infancy. Constipation that is congenital in origin (*Hirschsprung disease* and *anal stenosis* or *displacement*) may produce residual symptoms, even after treatment. Conditions such as *cystic fibrosis* and *intestinal pseudo-obstruction*, although usually apparent in infancy, will persist throughout life. Psychogenic fecal retention secondary to toilet training plays more of a role in the 2- to 6-year age range but may persist through childhood. *Crohn disease* is now a more prevalent cause of constipation. This is due to periodic areas of narrowing throughout the GI tract called *skip lesions.*

KEY PROBLEM
Pain *Pain* in children becomes a far more significant factor in childhood than in infancy, and a careful history is paramount to accurate diagnosis. There is a wide range of severity of diagnoses, from benign and functional to malignant and/or immediately life-threatening. Subsequently, we will take several aspects of pain and analyze them for their role in assessment.

Intensity of the pain, though subjective, is helpful. There are many standard pain scales, understandable to children. As a general rule, functional pain is relatively mild. The child will mention it frequently but does not appear too distressed and generally does well in between episodes. It is incumbent on the clinician to obtain a careful history to determine if there may be secondary gain involved from school absence. Pain of peptic ulcer disease (PUD), early *appendicitis,* and *gastroenteritis* is more of a moderate to severe nature. The pain associated with *intestinal obstruction, gall bladder disease,* or intraabdominal *malignancy* becomes quite severe. Pain owing to *nephrolithiasis, pancreatitis,* or *peritonitis* from a ruptured viscus can be excruciating. During the evolution of *appendicitis,* the patient may begin with moderate pain. As it progresses to rupture, this may produce immediate relief owing to the relief of pressure, but as peritonitis ensues, the pain quickly worsens.

Location of pain is important in its assessment. Since abdominal viscera begin embryologically as midline structures, pain originating from them generally is midline, with its level of location consistent with the spinal segment to which the afferent nerve fibers travel. Thus foregut pain (distal esophagus, stomach, duodenum, liver, biliary system, and pancreas) produces midline pain from the xiphoid to the umbilicus. Midgut structures (ileum, jejunum, cecum, ascending colon, and proximal two-thirds of the transverse colon) yield periumbilical pain. The hindgut (distal third of the transverse colon and the rest of the large intestine) produces midline pain from the umbilicus to the symphysis pubis. Thus abdominal pain usually will remain midline. The notable exception is that of appendicitis, which classically begins midline and eventually migrates to the right lower quadrant. This is not due to stretching of the appendix but rather to peritoneal irritation by the inflamed viscus. Lateralized pain often is not GI and may be a result of genitourinary pathology (kidney, bladder, ovary, or fallopian tubes).

The timing and quality of the pain are important. Sharp pain indicates a more superficial origin, such as peritoneum, abdominal wall, or skin. Pain originating from the gut is generally dull. Does the pain occur at night as well as during the day? How is it associated with food intake, bowel evacuation, external movement (as in an automobile), posture, or activity? Always ask previously healthy children who develop abdominal pain, "Is this unlike any pain you have had before?" It is important to ascertain whether the pain is associated with other symptoms, such as vomiting, diarrhea, poor weight gain, etc. Cramping or colicky pain should bring to mind *gall bladder disease, nephrolithiasis, gastroenteritis,* or *intussusception,* whereas the initial pain of *appendicitis* is typically steady.

One of the most common complaints in day-to-day pediatric practice is abdominal pain. Several important historical points are most helpful to the clinician to separate functional from organic causes. "Red flags" for organic causes of abdominal pain are age younger than 5 years, fever, weight loss or poor weight gain, joint pain, rashes, vomiting (especially if there is any blood or bile in the vomitus), nocturnal pain that awakens the patient, nonmidline pain, pain that is referred, genitourinary symptoms (dysuria, hematuria, or flank pain), perianal disease (fissures or tags), family history of IBD or ulcers, and blood in the stool. Nonorganic pain, on the other hand, is midline, does not radiate, is usually episodic with symptom-free intervals, and is recurrent but generally does not worsen over time.

Infectious causes, such as *gastroenteritis,* are still the most common. Also consider non-GI causes such as *sickle cell anemia, HSP, HUS, pneumonia, streptococcal infection, rheumatic fever, mesenteric adenitis, hernia, testicular torsion,* and *diabetic ketoacidosis.* Always consider trauma.

KEY PROBLEM

◼ **Jaundice** The approach to *jaundice* in childhood is similar to that of infancy. Many of the diseases that are congenital in origin should have been detected but nonetheless persist throughout. Of interest is *Wilson disease,* a *metabolic* disorder that does not present in infancy but appears in childhood with progressive jaundice, hepatic failure, and neurologic degeneration. The copper-colored Kayser-Fleischer ring of the iris is most helpful in making the diagnosis.

Children are more likely to develop *gallstones* than infants because of their association with a longer-standing hemolytic anemia or previous history of intensive-care treatment with parenteral nutrition. *Infectious* causes such as *hepatitis* becomes more common in this age group, and chronic hepatitis associated with autoimmune disease emerges. There is more likely to be exposure to drugs and *toxins.* Take a careful history for *ingestion* of acetaminophen, valproate, and phenothiazines. *Sclerosing cholangitis from IBD, veno-occlusive disease of the liver, congestive heart failure,* and *cirrhosis of the liver* occur more frequently at this age.

Adolescents (Ages 13 to 21 Years)

Interviewing an adolescent is more difficult than interviewing any other age group. There are issues centering around privacy, modesty, and control. Adolescents are well known for their noncommunication, and the interviewer must make all efforts to elicit a full and truthful history. Adolescents are certain to answer questions differently with and without parents present. It is most desirable to talk to the adolescent alone with assurance of confidentiality. It may be difficult to obtain parental buy-in, but make all efforts to do so. In the interest of honesty and full disclosure, indicate that all information obtained will never leave the room, with the exception of any patient threat of harm to self or others.

The physician must have insight into his or her own feelings and opinions of behavior vis-à-vis drugs, sexuality, etc. This does not preclude pointing out consequences of high-risk behavior, but a nonjudgmental manner will be more credible to the adolescent.

It is difficult to establish rapport with an adolescent at the first visit. Adolescents put great value on peers, and discussing sensitive issues in that context (e.g., "Do your friends take drugs?") is often a way of opening the door to further conversation.

● KEY PROBLEM
◼ **Vomiting** *Vomiting* in the adolescent has similar causes as in children. Infectious *gastroenteritis,* of all causes, *bacterial, viral,* and *parasitic,* remains a common cause of vomiting, as in all age groups. *Appendicitis* and *celiac disease* also are similar to childhood in their incidence. *Achalasia, IBD, ulcers, GERD, gall bladder disease,* and *malignancy* are more prevalent in this age group than in childhood. Posttraumatic *surgical adhesions* are a common cause. Other entities often associated with adolescent behavior now appear. These include *alcoholic gastritis, pancreatitis,* and *gastroparesis* owing to poorly controlled *diabetes mellitus, eating disorders,* and *psychogenic vomiting.* Superior mesenteric artery syndrome (*Wilkie disease*) appears in adolescents, usually female, who are tall and thin, often with weight loss. Loss of fat surrounding the superior mesenteric artery causes subsequent obstruction of the duodenum by the artery that now presses on it.

GI pathology may not always cause vomiting in adolescents. As in children, vomiting in adolescents may be a nonspecific symptom of other infectious diseases, such as *otitis media* and *pneumonia.* *Metabolic* diseases usually have presented by childhood, but *acute intermittent porphyria* is one that is more common in adolescence. Endocrine derangements such as *Addison disease* and other conditions such as *UTI, kidney stones, uremia, hydrometrocolpos,* and *pregnancy* all may cause vomiting. Neurologic disorders such as *infection, head trauma* (*concussion* or *epidural or subdural hematoma*), *Arnold-Chiari malformation, pseudotumor cerebri, migraine, epilepsy,* and *cyclic vomiting* are also important causes of vomiting.

KEY PROBLEM

Diarrhea *Diarrhea* in the adolescent is associated with most of the same conditions outlined in the section on children. Anatomic causes are *short-gut syndrome, protein-losing enteropathy, chronic cholestasis,* and *fecal impaction* with overflow diarrhea. *Infectious* agents are as common as in other age groups. Consider *infectious* etiologies. Bacterial causes include *Salmonella, Shigella, Escherichia coli, Campylobacter, Yersinia, Vibrio cholerae, Clostridium perfringens,* and *C. difficile* (antibiotic-associated colitis). Viral etiologies include *rotavirus, norovirus, adenovirus, cytomegalovirus, astrovirus,* and *calicivirus.* Parasitic agents include *Giardia, Entamoeba, Isospora, Cryptosporidium,* and *Trichuris.* Postgastroenteritis *malabsorption* is due to temporary *lactase deficiency,* and *bacterial overgrowth* is secondary to stasis. *Inflammatory/immune/allergic* causes include *IBD, pancreatitis, celiac disease, collagen-vascular disease, immunodeficiency, HSP, HUS, milk protein allergy,* and *eosinophilic gastroenteritis.* *Toxic/metabolic* causes include pancreatic insufficiency owing to *cystic fibrosis, pancreatitis* (acute and chronic), *Schwachman-Diamond syndrome, Johanson-Blizzard syndrome,* and *Pearson syndrome.* *Liver disease* causing bile acid problems become more common in adolescence. *Poisoning* owing to drug abuse, especially antibiotics, laxatives, and heavy metal ingestions, frequently cause diarrhea. *Neoplasia* such as *lymphoma,* tumors that secrete vasoactive intestinal peptide, and *carcinoid* start in adolescence.

KEY PROBLEM

Constipation *Constipation* in adolescents often occurs as a consequence of poor diet with high fat and low fiber content. *Eating disorders, sedentary lifestyle,* and *depression* are also common causes. Stool withholding and *encopresis* carried over from childhood may occur as well. *Congenital* and *traumatic* causes include *spinal cord anomalies* and *injuries, previous anorectal surgery,* and obstructing extraintestinal pelvic tumors. Primary *malignancy* of the intestine is extremely rare. *Use and abuse of drugs* contribute frequently as a *toxic* cause. Specifically, antacids, anticholinergics, antidepressants, opiates, barbiturates, sympathomimetics, and sucralfate are causes. Consider *IBD, celiac disease, cystic fibrosis, metabolic* causes such as *diabetes mellitus, hypercalcemia, hypokalemia, hypothyroidism,* and *multiple endocrine neoplasias. Irritable bowel syndrome* (IBS) takes on a more significant role in adolescence. *Collagen-vascular disease* becomes more prevalent in this age group and often causes vomiting, constipation, and dysphagia.

KEY PROBLEM

Pain A thorough history including family, occupational, travels, dietary, social, and sexual history is of paramount importance. Is the onset of pain acute or gradual? Where is the pain located? What is the quality? Does it radiate? How intense is it? Are there associated symptoms such as vomiting, diarrhea, or anorexia? Some clinical hints: Most pain in adolescents is of acute onset, although gradual onset and worsening may be due to intestinal obstruction. Colicky pain suggests *cholelithiasis, nephrolithiasis,* or *intussusception.* Pain in the left upper quadrant may indicate constipation or, if dull, boring, and very severe, *pancreatitis.* Sharp shooting pain may be from *pleuritis* or *peritonitis.* Right upper quadrant pain points to hepatitis or *gall bladder disease,* which radiates to the subscapular area. Steady pain in the right lower quadrant raises the suspicion of *pancreatitis, intestinal obstruction,* and *appendicitis.* Back pain associated with abdominal pain may indicate *retrocecal appendicitis.*

Differential diagnosis for acute abdominal pain in adolescence includes *infectious* and *inflammatory* causes, including *gastroenteritis* of all etiologies, *pancreatitis, hepatitis, cholecystitis, diverticulitis, peritonitis, gastritis* (viral, *Helicobacter pylori, peptic ulcer disease,* and *gastroesophageal reflux), vasculitis (HSP, HUS,* and *Kawasaki disease), IBD, appendicitis,* and *mesenteric adenitis.* Consider *obstruction* as an etiology of constipation, including *trauma (hematoma* or *foreign body), intussusception, volvulus, incarcerated hernia, postoperative adhesions,* and biliary causes (*stone, cyst,* and *hydrops*).

Acute abdominal pain may present as a symptom of a non-GI condition. It is often a nonspecific symptom of almost any *infection.* Pain radiating to the back or flank suggests *nephrolithiasis* or *diskitis.* Ureteral colic radiates to the groin, and diskitis radiates to the back. Anatomic diagnoses, *congenital* or acquired, involving the female reproductive tract (*imperforate hymen with hydrometrocolpos, pelvic inflammatory disease, tuboovarian abscess, FitzHugh-Curtis perihepatitis, endometriosis, mittelschmerz, ectopic pregnancy,* or *ovarian cyst* or *torsion*) are common causes. Male reproductive tract disorders such as *testicular torsion, orchitis,* and *prostatitis* are causes of abdominal pain. Consider renal causes such as *UTI, hydronephrosis, abscess,* and *uremia,* as well as cardiopulmonary causes such as *pneumonia, pericarditis, pleuritis,* and *pneumothorax* involving visceral peritoneum, as well as *rheumatic fever.* Musculoskeletal disorders such as *abdominal wall strain, hematoma, abscess,* and *diskitis* are common in adolescence. *Metabolic* diagnoses include *diabetic ketoacidosis, hypercalcemia, multiple endocrine adenomatosis, acute intermittent porphyria, familial Mediterranean fever, hyperlipidemia, hereditary angioneurotic edema, heavy metal poisoning,* and *narcotic withdrawal.*

Chronic or recurrent abdominal pain may be organic in nature and occurs particularly in *IBD, gastroesophageal reflux, chronic hepatitis, chronic pancreatitis, chronic constipation* of all etiologies, *cystic fibrosis,* and *diabetes mellitus.* However, most chronic or recurrent abdominal pain in adolescents relates to functional GI disorders *(FGIDs)* such as IBS, functional dyspepsia (FD), and recurrent abdominal pain (RAP). It is important to separate these diagnoses from organic diagnoses, and the Rome II criteria for *FGIDs* outlined in TABLE 10–1 are helpful.

● KEY PROBLEM
◼ **Jaundice** Differential diagnosis for *jaundice* in the adolescent is similar to that of children but with a higher index of suspicion for *acute*

TABLE 10-1 *Rome II Criteria for Diagnosis of Functional GI Disorders*

	Abd Pain <12 Weeks Out of Year	Bowel Pattern	Organic Pathology	Other
IBS	Upper or lower	<3 stools/wk or >3 stools/d Relief w/stool Change in stool consistency	No	Straining Urgency Feeling of incomplete evacuation Mucus in stool Bloating
FD	Upper	No change	No	
RAP	Upper or lower	Occasional relation to defecation	No	No feigning No evidence of IBS or FD

Abbreviations: IBS = irritable bowel syndrome; FD = functional dyspepsia; RAP = recurrent abdominal pain.

hepatitis, chronic liver disease, and *biliary tract disease,* both infectious and obstructive. Chronic liver disease becomes more prominent in adolescence, and etiologies are *drug abuse, alcoholism, nonalcoholic steatohepatitis* (often associated with obesity), *infection (viral hepatitides A–G, cytomegalovirus, Epstein-Barr, herpes,* and *enterovirus),* bacterial *infections, parasitic infestation, cystic fibrosis, autoimmune liver disease* including *primary sclerosing cholangitis, autoimmune hepatitis, primary biliary cirrhosis,* and *drugs/toxins, Wilson disease, hemochromatosis, alpha$_1$-antitrypsin deficiency (metabolic* causes), *Budd-Chiari syndrome,* and *total parenteral nutrition.* Neoplasms such as *hepatocarcinoma, hemangioendothelioma, leukemia, lymphoma,* and *veno-occlusive disease* also may occur.

Physical Examination

Infants

KEY FINDING

Inspection With any physical examination, it is best first to obtain an overall picture, or *gestalt.* Are there any obvious findings that strike the examiner immediately? Is the child very ill-appearing (toxic or dehydrated)? Are there obvious malformations? Are there any obvious skin findings such as jaundice, bruising, petechiae, or venous distension? What is the nutritional status of the child? What is the shape of the abdomen (distended, flat)? Furthermore, perform a complete physical examination in order to search for non-GI causes of symptoms.

In further detail, obvious external congenital anomalies may well suggest internal GI malformations (e.g., *Down syndrome with a transesophageal fistula, annular pancreas,* etc., or *VATER association with tracheoesophageal fistula* (TEF) or *anal atresia*). Jaundice will bring to mind a list of diagnoses previously discussed. GI causes for bruising or petechiae, although rare in infancy, they may occur with jaundice in *toxoplasmosis, rubella, cytomegalovirus,* and *herpes* (TORCH). Pallor and petechiae also may be present with anemia and thrombocytopenia caused by HUS. Erythematous raw skin located perianally and at the extremities in association with diarrhea in an infant should raise suspicion of *acrodermatitis enteropathica* owing to zinc deficiency. Extensive liver disease can cause venous distension (*varices*), telangiectasia, cyanosis, clubbing, and gynecomastia. A distended abdomen always should lead to further investigation of intestinal obstruction (*intussusception, volvulus,* or *rectal or anal stenosis*). Inguinal or umbilical swelling always should raise the possibility of an *incarcerated hernia.* Poor nutritional state always should suggest the possibility of chronic malabsorptive syndromes. A thin or possibly distended abdomen owing to poor nutrition with visible reverse peristaltic waves indicates an advanced case of *pyloric stenosis* in an infant. Peritoneal fluid accumulation also can cause abdominal distension by *ascites* from *hypoproteinemia of liver disease, renal disease,* or *malabsorption.*

A visual anal examination is most helpful to determine anatomic problems (*fissure, hemorrhoid, stenosis,* and *anterior displaced anus*).

Sometimes signs appearing to be neurologic may be a presentation for GI disease such as *Sandifer syndrome* (sudden hyperextension of the neck and bending of trunk seen in gastroesophageal reflux).

Inspection relating to other systems can be most helpful to explain non-GI causes of typical GI symptoms. Does the enlarged thyroid gland explain diarrhea? Always observe for spinal abnormalities in a neurologic examination. Are there midback tufts of hair, swellings, or dimpling defects? Are there meningeal signs or signs of increased intracranial pressure such as a bulging fontanelle to explain vomiting? Are there obvious genital abnormalities or abdominal wall abnormalities causing intestinal obstruction owing to consequent fecal retention or urinary retention causing UTI, which is often associated with constipation?

Inspection should involve senses other than vision, such as olfaction and even taste. The smell of urine or stool always should initiate further pursuit of incontinence. Fetor hepaticus, a distinctive sweetish smell to the breath, is present in *acute liver failure.* An odor of acetone to the breath indicates caloric deprivation of any cause or *diabetic ketoacidosis.* Many *metabolic* diseases cause distinctive odors, such as cabbage, musky, sweaty socks, and maple syrup urine, which may cause vomiting of a non-GI nature (refer Chapter 12). A salty taste to a patient suggests *cystic fibrosis.*

▼ KEY FINDING
───
◤ Palpation *Palpation* is most helpful in evaluation of the enlarged and/or painful abdomen. Is the abdomen hard or soft? Does it localize? Does palpation of the abdomen elicit any pain or discomfort? Are there any abdominal masses? Are there enlarged organs such as hepatomegaly or splenomegaly? FIGURE 10–2 illustrates the anatomic landmarks by quadrant.

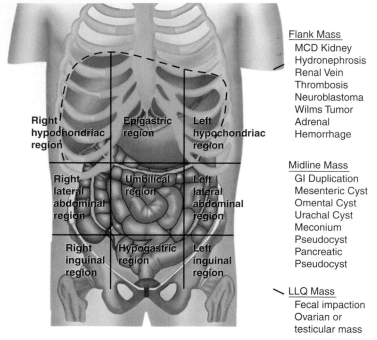

Flank Mass
MCD Kidney
Hydronephrosis
Renal Vein
Thrombosis
Neuroblastoma
Wilms Tumor
Adrenal
Hemorrhage

Midline Mass
GI Duplication
Mesenteric Cyst
Omental Cyst
Urachal Cyst
Meconium
Pseudocyst
Pancreatic
Pseudocyst

LLQ Mass
Fecal impaction
Ovarian or
testicular mass

Right
hypochondriac
region

Epigastric
region

Left
hypochondriac
region

Right
lateral
abdominal
region

Umbilical
region

Left
lateral
abdominal
region

Right
inguinal
region

Hypogastric
region

Left
inguinal
region

FIGURE 10–2 *Normal Anatomic Regions. (From Van De Graaff KH:* Human Anatomy. *New York: McGraw-Hill, 2002, Fig. 2.15, p. 38.)*

Although it is difficult to evaluate pain, abdominal palpation will discern tenderness more easily. It is always a good technique with any palpation examination of an infant, if possible, to put the baby at ease, preferably in the mother's lap, with several distractions to keep his or her mind off the examination. A rock-hard, exquisitely painful abdomen, not voluntary guarding, is indicative of an intestinal *perforation,* spontaneous or traumatic, possibly with *peritonitis,* and is an ominous sign. Since this is almost invariably associated with pain on motion, the baby will prefer to lie still and will cry when moved.

Abdominal masses are generally ominous and require further investigation. Is it unilateral or bilateral? Does it cross the midline? Is it mobile or fixed? Is it painful? Is the mass intestinal or extraintestinal, causing obstruction? Ballottement of masses helps in their evaluation (FIGURE 10–3). Is the examiner palpating excessive stool from a mechanical or functional obstruction? Further investigation in the inguinal or scrotal area may be helpful, with a mass indicating the possibility of an *incarcerated hernia.* A rectal examination is mandatory to determine if there is stool in the rectal vault. The palpation of large, very hard stool in the area indicates fecal retention owing to the toilet training process.

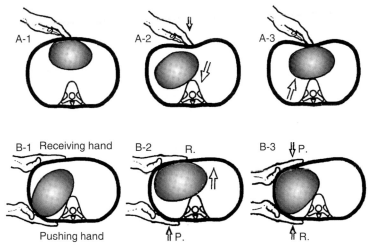

FIGURE 10–3 *Ballottement of Abdominal Masses. The term ballottement is applied to two somewhat different maneuvers. A. One-hand ballottement. The approximated fingers are abruptly plunged into the abdomen and held there; a freely movable mass will rebound upward and be felt with the fingers. This is most commonly employed to feel a large liver obscured by free fluid in the abdominal cavity. B. Bimanual ballottement. (B-1–2). This is used to determine the size of a large mass in the abdomen. One hand (P) pushes the posterior abdominal wall while the receiving hand (R) palpates the anterior abdomen. (B-3) The receiving hand is now in the flank, and the pushing hand compresses the mass to get an estimate of its thickness. (From LeBlond RF, DeGowin RL, Brown DD:* De Gowin's Diagnostic Examination, *8th ed. New York: McGraw-Hill, 2004, Fig. 9.8, p. 519.)*

Hepatosplenomegaly or mass could be due to *liver disease, tumor* (benign or malignant), *choledochal cyst,* portal obstruction, or several *metabolic* disorders. It may be associated with jaundice in infants. It is normal to palpate a 1- to 2-cm liver or spleen tip in an infant, and this should be no cause for concern in an otherwise normal abdominal examination.

Examination of an infant suspected of having *pyloric stenosis* may reveal the classic "olive." Perform the examination with the infant quiet and relaxed, and the "olive" is best felt after vomiting or immediate suctioning of the stomach contents. Feel the mass on the baby's right abdomen as your fingers approach the right subcostal area.

In *intussusception,* the classic abdominal finding of a sausage-shaped mass with an empty right lower quadrant is helpful, if found. If a mass is tender, consider *intraabdominal abscess.* Significant causes of abdominal mass in infants include *neuroblastoma, renal vein thrombosis, Wilms' or other renal tumor, teratoma, ovarian cyst or tumor,* and *adrenal hemorrhage.*

◢ Percussion *Percussion* of the abdomen is most helpful to determine whether distension is mainly gaseous (tympanitic) or fluid (dull sound). In addition, changes in dullness to percussion are helpful in delineating liver and spleen size.

◢ Auscultation Listening to bowel sounds is most helpful in the evaluation of peritonitis and intestinal obstruction. Typically, intestinal sounds are absent with peritonitis and may be increased, with a high-pitch "tinkling" quality to them, in intestinal obstruction. In gastroenteritis, bowel sounds may be hyperactive but also may be hypoactive owing to local ileus. It is an important technique to listen to an abdomen prior to vigorous palpation because this may activate bowel sounds and alter the examination. Localization of bowel sounds can be difficult in a small infant.

Children

◢ Observation As in infants, it is paramount to assess an overall *gestalt*. Is the child of normal height and weight? Does he or she appear ill, toxic, or in distress? Are there other obvious congenital anomalies? Obvious external anomalies may be a hint that there may be other internal GI anomalies, e.g., *Down syndrome with TEF, annular pancreas or VATER association with TEF,* or *anal stenosis.* Although most of these anomalies will have been diagnosed and corrected in infancy, there still may be residual postoperative findings. Initial visualization of the integument can be most helpful to reveal findings that are indicative of conditions that involve the GI tract primarily or secondarily. Purpuric lesions, especially on the buttocks and lower extremities in association with cramping abdominal pain, are part of *HSP.* Petechiae, along with pallor, abdominal pain, and diarrhea, point toward *HUS.* Ecchymoses of the abdomen bespeak *pancreatitis* (flank = Grey-Turner sign; periumbilical = Cullen sign). Chronic *moniliasis* of the skin or nails in the presence of diarrhea should direct one to think of *immunodeficiency. IBD* is frequently associated with skin lesions such as *erythema nodosum, pyoderma gangrenosum,* and *psoriasis.* Cyanosis and clubbing may have a basis in *hepatobiliary disease* owing to formation of microscopic arteriovenous shunts bypassing the pulmonary circulation for oxygenation. Other dermatologic signs of hepatic disease include *spider angiomata* and *caput medusa,* dilated periumbilical varicose veins owing to *portal obstruction.*

Examination of the head and neck may be helpful in diagnosing GI disorders or conditions mimicking them. Ocular examination is most helpful because of the association between *IBD* and *uveitis,* episcleritis, and conjunctivitis. *Papilledema* as a manifestation of increased intracranial pressure may explain the cause of vomiting. Examination of the mouth may reveal *cheilitis, stomatitis,* or *aphthous ulcerations* in patients with *IBD* or *vitamin A deficiency*. One might visualize an enlarged thyroid gland on neck examination, which can be associated with diarrhea.

Examination of the extremities may reveal joint swelling, often associated with *IBD* but also with bacterial enteritis in those susceptible patients who are HLA-B27-positive. Edema may be a result of *hypoproteinemia*, a consequence of either protein *malabsorption* or *primary hepatic disease*.

As in infants, neurologic examination may be most helpful to explain GI symptoms. Always look for spinal abnormalities such as swellings, tufts of hair, or indentations because they can be associated with constipation. Although it is paramount to rule out *meningitis* in a patient with a stiff neck, one may see meningeal signs in bacterial enteritis such as *Shigella*.

Observation of the abdomen is similar to that applied to infants. It is also important to assess the genital region for presence of a *hernia*.

A rectal examination is paramount to arriving at a proper diagnosis. Although the child may be quite anxious over this, it is important to take the time to explain the procedure and calm the child. The parent should be available to help with this. Perform it in all cases of constipation without question. In the most common instance of withholding, there is always excessive stool in the rectal vault. This obviates needless exposure to radiation to confirm this diagnosis. Examine the anus for fissures and skin tags, often associated with constipation. A rectal examination may reveal masses both intraintestinal and extraintestinal or *polyps*. It is also critical in the evaluation of appendicitis because motion of the finger may elicit peritoneal tenderness on the patient's right side.

KEY FINDING

Palpation *Palpation* becomes a more helpful adjunct to diagnosis in a child as compared with an infant. Although children may communicate better than infants, there are still barriers to overcome in performing an accurate palpation of the abdomen. A child may be quite frightened as a physician comes at him or her. Therefore, it is often necessary to calm the child by placing him or her in the mother's lap. Distraction with toys is a useful technique to develop rapport. It should be possible later on, once the child is calm, to use the examination table. An unhurried examination with the patient in the supine flat position is more conducive to an accurate evaluation. Another "trick of the trade" is to examine first with the stethoscope. It may serve to disarm the child, who may not realize that gentle pressure with the stethoscope is a ploy to differentiate voluntary from involuntary guarding.

Good palpation of the abdomen consists of evaluation of all four quadrants. The examiner is always at the patient's right side. Examine the quadrants individually and also directionally, i.e., starting in a midabdominal location and aiming toward each quadrant. Palpate the left upper quadrant by placing the right hand toward the patient's left costal margin while the left hand is placed at the patient's left flank, pushing the spleen anteriorly (FIGURE 10–4). Proper palpation of the right upper quadrant consists of placing the right hand at the right costal margin and the left hand under the patient's right flank, lifting it toward the examiner (FIGURE 10–5). On palpation of either upper quadrant, it is advisable to have the patient take a deep breath. Palpate the lower quadrants

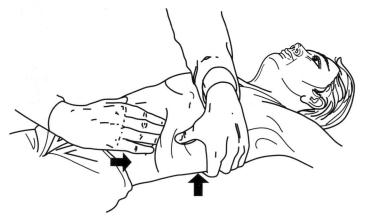

FIGURE 10–4 *Bimanual Palpation of the Left Upper Quadrant. (From LeBlond RF, DeGowin RL, Brown DD:* DeGowin's Diagnostic Examination, *8th ed. New York: McGraw-Hill, 2004, Fig. 9.10, p. 521.)*

with similar technique to evaluate the kidneys for enlargement. Palpation of the right lower quadrant is a critical part of the evaluation for *appendicitis*, with the classic finding of tenderness over McBurney's point. Also, psoas and obturator signs (FIGURE 10–6) are most helpful. FIGURE 10–7 demonstrates the location of pain with regard to specific diagnoses. Elicit peritoneal findings to evaluate a perforated viscus. Localized guarding and rebound tenderness and pain associated with sudden release of the palpating fingers points to peritoneal irritation.

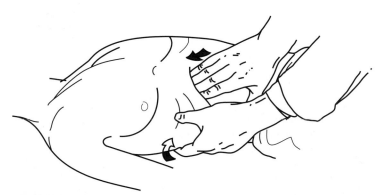

FIGURE 10–5 *Bimanual Palpation of the Right Upper Quadrant. (From LeBlond RF, DeGowin RL, Brown DD:* DeGowin's Diagnostic Examination, *8th ed. New York: McGraw-Hill, 2004, Fig. 9.12, p. 522.)*

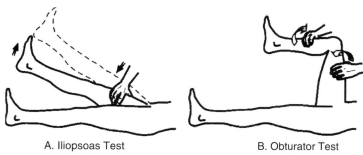

A. Iliopsoas Test   B. Obturator Test

FIGURE 10–6   Tests for Irritation of the Iliopsoas and Obturator Muscles.
Abscesses in the pelvis may be localized by demonstrating irritation of the more lateral iliopsoas or the medial obturator internus muscle. A. Iliopsoas test. The supine patient keeps his or her knee extended and is asked to flex the thigh against the resistance of the examiner's hand. Pain in the pelvis indicates irritation of the iliopsoas. B. Obturator test. The supine patient flexes the right thigh to 90 degrees. The examiner moves the hip in internal and external rotation. Pelvic pain indicates an inflamed muscle. Examine from the side of the limb being tested. (From LeBlond RF, DeGowin RL, Brown DD: DeGowin's Diagnostic Examination, *8th ed. New York: McGraw-Hill, 2004, Fig. 9.13, p. 523.)*

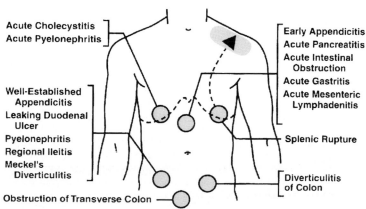

Acute Cholecystitis
Acute Pyelonephritis

Early Appendicitis
Acute Pancreatitis
Acute Intestinal
    Obstruction
Acute Gastritis
Acute Mesenteric
    Lymphadenitis

Well-Established
    Appendicitis
Leaking Duodenal
    Ulcer
Pyelonephritis
Regional Ileitis
Meckel's
    Diverticulitis

Splenic Rupture

Diverticulitis
of Colon

Obstruction of Transverse Colon

FIGURE 10–7   Common Locations of Acute Abdominal Pain. In general, the painful spot is also tender but not always. Note especially that the pain of acute appendicitis is in the epigastrium early and later in the right lower quadrant. Pain in the spleen commonly radiates to the top of the left shoulder. These pains are ordinarily constant, in contrast to the intermittent pain of colic. (From LeBlond RF, DeGowin RL, Brown DD: DeGowin's Diagnostic Examination, *8th ed. New York: McGraw-Hill, 2004. Fig. 9-19, p. 530.)*

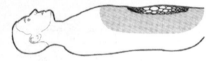

A. Distribution of Tympany   B. Bulging of Flanks

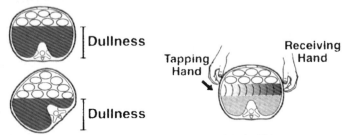

Dullness

Dullness

C. Shifting Dullness

Tapping Hand

Receiving Hand

D. Fluid Wave

FIGURE 10–8 Signs of Ascites. A. Distribution of tympany. In the supine position, free fluid causes the gas-filled gut to float, so an area of tympany forms at the top of the bulging wall. B. Bulging flanks. The weight of free fluid pushes the flanks outward, so they bulge toward the table or the bed; fat in the mesentery also will cause this when the abdominal muscles are weak. C. Shifting dullness. The dependent fluid causes an area of dullness in the lowest part; this shifts to remain lowest with changes in position of the body. D. Fluid wave. A wave in the fluid, elicited by tapping one side of the abdomen, is transmitted to the receiving hand laid on the opposite side; the wave takes perceptible time to cross the abdomen. (From LeBlond RF, DeGowin RL, Brown DD: De Gowin's Diagnostic Examination, 8th ed. New York: McGraw-Hill, 2004, Fig. 9.21, p. 543.)

The classic finding for peritoneal fluid of ascites, the *fluid wave,* is elicited by having an assistant place the outer edge of his or her hand perpendicularly at the midline. The examiner places one hand on one flank and taps on the other. This will elicit the wave (FIGURE 10–8). Is the mass due to hepatosplenomegaly? Is it intraabdominal? The differential diagnosis consists of those mentioned in the infant section but also includes fecal impaction, *appendiceal abscess, hepatitis* and *liver disease,* either primary or secondary to other causes as *infiltrative metabolic disease* or *lymphoma,* and *choledochal cyst.*

KEY FINDING
Percussion *Percussion* of the abdomen is similar in children and infants (see above).

KEY FINDING
Auscultation *Auscultation* of children is similar to that in infants, as discussed earlier.

Adolescents

There are several barriers in this age group regarding privacy and modesty. However, make all efforts to have the patient placed in a gown, albeit awkward and uncomfortable. It is recommended that all examinations be performed in the presence of a nurse or medical assistant of the same gender as the patient not only for legal purposes but also for putting the patient more at ease.

▼ KEY FINDING

Inspection Techniques for *inspection* and findings in adolescents are similar to those in children, as discussed earlier. The examiner should put more emphasis on delayed physical and sexual maturation in IBD.

▼ KEY FINDING

Palpation, Percussion, and Auscultation Adolescent examination is similar to that in children. Right upper quadrant tenderness to *palpation* on deep inspiration, with possible radiation to the right shoulder (Murphy's sign), is due to an *inflamed* or *calculous gall bladder* falling over the examiner's hand and is associated with quick cessation of inhalation. Right upper quadrant tenderness of *Fitz-Hugh–Curtis syndrome* (gonococcal perihepatitis) is more common in this age group. An abdominal mass also should bring to mind complications of IBD, *pregnancy* and its complications, *uterine obstruction, ovarian pathology,* or *any intraabdominal malignancy.*

Summary of Key Findings Derived from the Examination

Based on the careful physical examination of all age groups, we list key findings referable to the GI tract. Also note the importance of non-GI findings that are often associated with primary GI disorders.

- Abdominal distension
- Scaphoid abdomen
- Hepatosplenomegaly
- Abdominal varices
- Abdominal ecchymosis (Cullen and Grey Turner signs)
- Abdominal mass
- Guarding
- Rebound
- Fluid wave
- Hypoactive bowel sounds
- Hyperactive bowel sounds
- Murphy sign
- Inguinal mass
- Anal skin tags and fissures
- Rectal tenderness
- Rectal mass

Synthesizing a Diagnosis

Children are not small adults, and it also must be clear that infants, children, and adolescents are also mutually exclusive groups. TABLE 10–2 lists several diagnoses based on anatomic involvement, etiology, and their relative occurrence vis-à-vis age group. We list age of diagnosis by order of incidence (highest first).

Confirmatory Laboratory and Imaging

This section is presented as two tables. TABLE 10–3 consists of several laboratory diagnostic tests that the primary care physician should consider in the process of arriving at a correct diagnosis or gathering information for further referral. TABLE 10–4 consists of imaging studies for the same purposes. All studies should be viewed as confirmatory for clinical impressions.

When to Refer

The decision to refer to a subspecialist is not always an easy one to make. There are certain conditions that should always warrant referral and that require long-term follow-up by a pediatric gastroenterologist. Other situations may require an initial assessment, with follow-up and treatment done by the primary care physician. Pediatric surgeons are also vital resources in the care of patients with abdominal complaints. Often there may be diagnostic dilemmas with which the subspecialist may be helpful. Both the primary care physician and the specialist should rule out non-GI etiologies, which appear above.

Abdominal pain is a very common complaint, and the etiology is often difficult to determine. Children can be vague when localizing the pain. They often cannot characterize the pain. Many times they are unable to recognize exacerbating or alleviating factors. Dietary history may not be accurate, and a stool history is difficult to obtain in children presumed to be toilet trained. While taking a history is more challenging, it is still the most vital part of the evaluation.

The gastroenterologist can offer additional testing depending on what the history suggests. Esophageal pH or impedance testing can demonstrate correlation between pain and events of either acid or nonacid esophageal reflux. Hydrogen breath testing will evaluate for disaccharidase deficiency, dietary fructose intolerance, or small intestinal bacterial overgrowth. If luminal disease is suspected, esophago-gastro-duodenoscopy (EGD) or colonoscopy may be necessary. Wireless capsule endoscopy now can visualize the small bowel. In children unable to swallow the

TABLE 10-2 Relative Indices of Suspicion for Diagnoses Cited in the Text Based on History and Physical Examination

Anatomic Involvement	Problems and Findings	Diagnosis [Etiology]	Age at Diagnosis [Order of Incidence]
Esophagus	V (instantaneous)	T-E fistula (Cg)	I
	V (instantaneous)	Stenosis/web (Cg)	I, C
	P, V, fussy esp. when recumbent	GERD & esophagitis (Cg)	I, A, C
	V	Achalasia (Cg)	I, C, A
	V (blood), forceful retching	Mallory-Weiss (Tr)	C, A
	V (blood), liver dysfunction	Varices (Cg, Mt, Inf)	A, C
Stomach	V (projectile)	Pyloric stenosis (Cg)	I
	V (dribbling)	Rumination (Ps)	I, C
	V, dist.	Volvulus (Cg)	I, C, rarely A
	P, V, hematemesis	Gastritis, H. pylori (Inf)	A, C, I
	P, V, hematemesis	Gastritis, alcoholic (Tx)	A
	P, V, hematemesis	Peptic ulcer disease (Inf)	A, C, rarely I
Duodenum	V	Atresia, web, annular pancreas (Cg)	I
	P, V, hematemesis	Ulcer (Inf)	A, C, I
	V, dist, recent wt loss	Willkie syndrome (Mt)	A, rarely C
Small intestine	V, D, P	Malabsorption	I, C
		Enzyme deficiency (Cg)	I, C
	D, wt loss	Short-gut syndrome (Cg, Tri)	I, C
	D (greasy), wt loss, dist.	Celiac disease (Cg, Mt)	C, I, A
	P (episodic), V, currant jelly stools	Intussusception (Cg, Inf)	I, C, rarely A
	Painless bleeding (mahogany)	Meckel's diverticulum (Cg)	C, A, I
	V, dist, inguinal or scrotal mass	Incarcerated hernia (Cg)	I, C, A (equal)

(Continued)

TABLE 10–2 *Relative Indices of Suspicion for Diagnoses Cited in the Text Based on History and Physical Examination (Continued)*

Anatomic Involvement	Problems and Findings	Diagnosis (Etiology)	Age at Diagnosis (Order of Incidence)
Large intestine and anus	C, V, D, FTT, dist, abd. mass	Hirschsprung disease (Cg)	I, C
	RLQ pain, rebound, guarding, V, low fever, C, rectal tenderness,	Appendicitis (Inf)	A, C, rarely I
	C, dist, V, abd. mass		
	C, dist, abd. mass	Atresia, stenosis, displaced anus (Cg)	I
	Hematochezia, painless	Stool retention.(F, Ps)	C, A,
	Hematochezia, painful	Juvenile polyps, cong. polyposis (Cg)	C, I, A
	Blood (red streaky), anal tenderness	Tox. megacolon, IBD, polyposis	A (IBD), C (Hirs)
	Blood, anal tenderness)	Hirschsprung disease (Inf, Cg)	I, A, C
		Anal fissure (Tr)	A, C, I (rarely)
		Hemorrhoids (Tr, Mt)	I
Liver	J, ↑ liver, resp. prob.	Alpha₁-antitrypsin deficiency (Mt)	I
	J,↑ liver, malabsorption, liver failure, edema, cabbage odor	Tyrosinemia (Mt)	I
	J	Diglucuronide deficiency (Mt)	I
	J, P, RLQ tender, ↑ liver	Viral hepatitis A–E (Inf)	A, C, poss NB
	J, ↑liver & spleen, petechiae, CNS	TORCH & EBV (Inf)	NB, A, C.
	J, hepatic failure,	Autoimmune hepatitis (Inf)	A, C
	J, mass, wt. loss	Neoplasm	A, C
	Ascites, varices, bleeding, ↑ spleen	Budd-Chiari (Cg)	A, C, I
	Ascites, varices, bleeding, ↑ spleen	Portal hypertension (Cg, Inf, Mt)	A, C, I
	V, HA, liver failure, CNS sx	Reye syndrome (Tx)	C, A, I

Pancreas	J, D (greasy), malabsorption, resp. sx,	Cystic fibrosis (Cg)	I, C
	P (severe), V, abd. ecchymosis	Pancreatitis (Inf, Tr, Mt)	A, C, I
	Malabsorption, D (greasy)	Pancreatic insuff. (Schwachman) (Cg)	C, I, A
Biliary system	J, ↑ liver, malabs., acholic stools	Biliary atresia (Cg)	I
	J, pruritus, malabs., acholic stools	Byler, Caroli, Alagille syndromes (Cg)	I
	J, V, acholic stools	Cholestasis (Cg, Tx, Mt)	I, A, C
	P, V, J, acholic stools, +Murphy	Cholelithiasis (Mt, Tx)	A, C, I
	P, V, J, acholic stools, +Murphy	Cholecystitis (Inf)	A, C, I
	V, J, fever	Ascending. cholangitis (Cg, Inf)	I, C, A
	J, IBD sx,	Sclerosing cholangitis (Cg, Mt, Inf)	A, C
Multi organ	J, P, V, mass	Choledocal cyst (Cg)	I, C, A
	V, D, blood in stool	Food allergy, poisoning (Tx)	All ages equally
	P, V, D (watery = viral; blood = bact)	GI infections (Inf)	A, C
	P, V, D, poor growth, arthritis, erythema nodosum, anal pathol.	IBD (Inf)	A, C
	C, dysphagia, rash, multisystem	Collagen-vascular (Inf)	A, C

(Continued)

TABLE 10-2 Relative Indices of Suspicion for Diagnoses Cited in the Text Based on History and Physical Examination *(Continued)*

Anatomic Involvement	Problems and Findings	Diagnosis (Etiology)	Age at Diagnosis (Order of Incidence)
	P, V, dist.	Volvulus (Cg)	I, C, rarely A
	D, rash	Acrodermatitis enteropathica (Mt)	I, C
	P, D, bloating	Functional GI disease (F, Ps)	A, C
	J, V, D, pallor, petechiae	Hemolytic-uremic syndrome (Inf)	C, I
	P, V, arthritis,	Henoch-Schonlein purpura (Inf)	C, I, rarely A
	J, liver failure, CNS sx, Kayser Fleischer ring	Wilson disease (Mt)	A, rarely C
	P, V, C, dist.	Obstruction due to trauma, adhesion, abd. wall defect (Cg, Tr)	A, C, I
Non-GI origin	V (blood)	Nosebleed, bleeding diathesis (Tr, Mt)	All ages
	V, bulging fontanelle	Hydrocephalus (Cg, Inf, Tr)	I, C
	V, headache, vit. D, tetracycline	Pseudotumor cerebri (Tx)	A, rarely C
	V, dist, poor feeding	Sepsis, CHF, CNS or renal disease	All ages
	V, headache, stiff neck, fever	Meningoencephalitis (Inf)	All ages
	D/C	Hyper/hypothyroidism, meds (Tx, Mt)	All ages
	D, abd. mass	Neuroblastoma (Neo)	C, I
	C + urinary retention	Spinal dysraphism (Cg)	I
	C + urinary retention	Opiates (Tx)	All ages

Symptoms	Condition	Age
C, GU symptoms, fever	Urinary tract infection (Inf, Cg)	All ages
P, fever, V	Mesenteric adenitis (Inf)	A, C
P, fever, V + rash, nodes, red eyes, raw lips	Kawasaki disease (Inf)	C, I
P, V	Uremia, GU obstruction, pneumonia	All ages
V, C	Renal tubular acidosis (Mt)	I
C, ↓ abd. muscle, hypogonadism	Eagle-Barrett syndrome, gastroschisis (Cg)	I
P, C, fussy, hx of pica	Pb intoxication (Tx)	I, C
P (lower quadrant), V	Ovarian cyst/torsion (Cg, Tr)	A, C
P, cervical tenderness, fever	Pelvic inflammatory disease (Inf)	A
P (RUQ), fever	Perihepatitis (Fitz-Hugh–Curtis) (Inf)	A
P (lower quadrant, mid menses)	Mittelschmerz (F)	A
P	Endometriosis (F)	A
P, msss, no menses, bulging hymen	Imperforate hymen (Cg)	A, C
HA, V	Migraine (F)	A, C
V (cyclic)	Cyclic vomiting (F)	A, C
V, C, D, amenorrhea, abraded knuckles, bradycardia, hypothermia	Eating disorders (Ps)	A, C

Abbreviations: P = pain; V = vomiting; D = diarrhea; dist. = distension; C = constipation; J = jaundice; IBD = inflammatory bowel disease; FTT = failure to thrive; HA = headache; RLQ = right lower quadrant; RUQ = right upper quadrant; GU = genitourinary; I = infants; C = children; A = adolescents; NB = newborn; Cg = congenital/genetic; Mt = nutritional/metabolic; Tx = toxic; Tr = traumatic; Neo = neoplastic; Inf = infectious/inflammatory; F = functional; Ps = psychological; CHF = congestive heart failure, CNS = central nervous system.

TABLE 10-3 Basic Confirmatory Laboratory Studies

Test	Comments	When to Order (Suspicion)
Urine		
Urinalysis	Basic urine screen	Abd. pain, (UTI w/WBC, nitrates, biliary obstruction, urolithiasis w ↓urobilinogen)
Urine culture	Identify pathogens	P, fever, dysuria, hematuria
Blood		
Hemoglobin/hematocrit	Determine cause of anemia	Blood loss (Pb intox., polyp., GERD, ulcer, chronic disease, HSP, HUS)
WBC count	Assess infection, inflammation	Fever, abd. pain, (GE, IBD, immune prob.UTI)
Differential WBC count	Distinguish bacterial from viral	GE
Platelet count	Evaluate bleeding	Bleeding, hepatosplenomegaly (↓ in HUS, bleeding diathesis, chronic liver disease, TORCH, immune prob.)
Basic metabolic panel	Na^+, K^+, Cl^-, HCO_3^- BUN, Cr, Glu, Ca^{2+}	Assess hydration, metabolic state (pyloric stenosis w/metabolic alkalosis, acidemia, GE, GI obstruction, DKA, renal BUN, Cr↑, adrenal disorder w/Na↓, K↑)
H. pylori antigen	Identify *H. pylori* (not specific)	Vomiting, hematemesis, pain (peptic ulcer disease)
ESR or CRP	Nonspecific for inflammation	Chronic GI sx, poor growth (IBD, immune disorder)

Test		
Liver function studies	GGT, ALT, bilirubin, alk phos., albumin, globulin, cholesterol, NH_3	Jaundice, hepatomegaly (hepatitis w/↑AST, ALT, biliary obstruction w/↑ alk. phos., hepatic venous occlusion, TORCH, metabolic disease w/↑NH_3)
TORCH, EBV titers	Toxoplasmosis, rubella, CMV, herpes, mononucleosis	Jaundice, petechiae, poor growth, ↑liver, spleen
Hepatitis panel	Test for hepatitis A–C	Jaundice, abd. pain, ↑ liver
Amylase, lipase	Pancreatic function	Severe abd. pain, vomiting, trauma (pancreatitis)
Celiac disease panel	TTG, antiendomyseal Ab	Vomiting, chronic diarrhea, poor growth, occ. constipation
Cu, ceruloplasmin	Wilson disease.	Jaundice, liver failure, encephalopathy
Catecholamines	Dx. neuroblastoma, carcinoid	Diarrhea
Sweat		
Sweat chloride	Diagnostic for cystic fibrosis	Chronic diarrhea, poor growth (CF, pancreatic failure, chronic liver disease)
Stool		
Leukocytes	>5/HPF, bacterial	Vomiting, diarrhea (blood/mucus), fever
Stool culture	Identify bacteria	Vomiting, diarrhea (blood/mucus), fever
Stool for *C. difficile*	Antibiotic assoc. colitis	Diarrhea (bloody), prolonged antibiotic use
Stool for *Giardia* antigen	Identify giardiasis	Persistent diarrhea, vomiting, no fever, wt loss
Stool ova and parasites	Identify other parasites	Persistent diarrhea, vomiting, no fever, wt loss
72-hour fecal fat	Test for fat malabsorption	Poor growth, jaundice, diarrhea

Abbreviations: UTI = urinary tract infection; WBC = white blood cell count; DKA = diabetic ketoacidosis; BUN = blood urea nitrogen; ESR = erythrocyte sedimentation rate; CRP = C-reactive protein; GGT = gamma glutamyl transpeptidase; ALT = alanine amino transferase; TTG = tissue transglutaminase.

TABLE 10-4 Basic Confirmatory Imaging Evaluation

Test	Comments	When to Order [Suspicion]
Imaging		
Plain x-ray studies:		
Flat-plate	Noncontrast (not specific)	P, V, distension, mass (obstruction, perforation, volvulus, tumor, calcification)
Upper GI series	Contrast study	P, V, bleeding (TEF, pyloric stenosis, GERD, esoph. stenosis, achalasia, PUD, IBD, Willkie syndrome)
UGI small bowel follow-through	Contrast study	P, V, D, C, bleeding dist., (IBD, ileus, motility disorder)
Barium enema	Contrast study	P, V, D, C, bleeding (atresia, stenosis, Hirschsprung, polyps, malrotation/volvulus, intussusception)
Abd. CT scanning	W/w/o contrast	P, V, C, dist., mass (trauma, bleeding, intussusception, volvulus, choledocal cyst, tumor, pancreatic pseudocyst multiple non-GI causes of GI symptoms such as ovarian, renal, GYN, CNS)
		P, V, C, mass (pyloric stenosis, duplication cyst, tumor, choledocal cyst, gallstones, non-GI causes of GI symptoms such as ovarian, renal, GYN)
Abd. ultrasound (pylorus, gall bladder, pelvic)	Noninvasive, economical	
Radionuclide scan	Technetium	Meckel's diverticulum

Abbreviations: P = pain; V = vomiting; D = diarrhea; C = constipation; UGI = upper gastrointestinal; GYN = gynecologic; CT = computed tomography; CNS = central nervous system.

298

pill-camera, it can be deployed intraoperatively using endoscopic technique. If these studies detect mucosal abnormalities and there is evidence of IBD, the gastroenterologist typically will follow these patients long term. If screening for celiac disease is positive or equivocal, the pediatric gastroenterologist can perform EGD with biopsy to confirm or rule out the diagnosis. A pediatric gastroenterologist often will follow other, less common mucosal abnormalities.

Vomiting in infants is a very common problem for the general pediatrician. Empirical treatment with H_2 blockers or in some cases proton pump inhibitors is the standard of care. In delayed gastric emptying, a trial of prokinetic medication may be of benefit. Most of the multiple formula changes are unnecessary and costly to the family, but if milk protein or soy intolerance is a concern, a 2-week trial of hydrolysate formula could improve symptoms. Reassurance to the family that this is a common problem and is typically outgrown is often all that is necessary. Vomiting with irritability, even on maximal medical therapy, should prompt a referral to a subspecialist. Other worrisome symptoms include feed aversion, respiratory compromise, leveling of the growth curve, and weight loss. Blood in the emesis always warrants referral to a pediatric gastroenterologist because endoscopy often will localize and potentially treat the source of the bleeding.

In the infant with vomiting who is refractory to medical management, the gastroenterologist may elect to perform endoscopy. Direct examination and biopsy of the mucosa will evaluate for eosinophilic esophagitis or eosinophilic gastroenteritis. In cases were there is delayed gastric emptying but no evidence of pyloric stenosis, pyloric balloon dilation may be helpful.

Referral to a pediatric surgeon may be necessary for patients with reflux refractory to medical management, and fundoplication with or without pyloroplasty may be therapeutic. Bilious emesis in the newborn is a surgical emergency because malrotation with volvulus may present, and without prompt surgical intervention, the gut may rapidly become necrotic. Referral to a surgeon is also necessary is cases of pyloric stenosis because pyloroplasty is the definitive treatment for this disorder.

In older children or adolescents with vomiting, referral is appropriate, again, if they are refractory to medical management with acid blockade and prokinetics. Dysphagia also should prompt a referral to a gastroenterologist because the patient may have esophageal stricture, eosinophilic esophagitis, or achalasia. The gastroenterologist is also able to perform esophageal motility testing, upper endoscopy with biopsy, and pyloric dilation. Antroduodenal motility testing may evaluate for gastroparesis.

Pediatric gastroenterologists may be helpful with failure to thrive refractory to treatment by a generalist. Most often calorie counts and dietary interventions are all that are required, but in patients with the inability to take adequate calories orally, a gastroenterologist may place or assist in placement of a feeding tube. If the patient is receiving adequate calories but is still failing to gain weight appropriately, further investigation to rule out malabsorption or metabolic disease may be necessary, including stool studies, blood work, and possibly endoscopy.

The general pediatrician should manage functional constipation successfully. Strategies include stool softeners and scheduled sitting with rewards. However, it is important to recognize that not all constipation is functional in nature. In cases of Hirschsprung disease, a pediatric gastroenterologist can perform anorectal motility testing, looking for presence of the rectoanal inhibitory reflex. Full-thickness rectal biopsy also may assess for aganglionosis in the outpatient setting. Slow colonic transit also may cause constipation. Evaluation for this may range from noninvasive testing such as ingesting radiopaque markers with serial abdominal flat plates to colonoscopy with motility catheter placement and full colonic motility testing. Often prokinetic agents will treat this condition, or if these are not successful, surgical treatments are available. Often a gastroenterologist will follow patients with chronic constipation owing to organic etiologies. In severe refractory cases, a pediatric surgeon may place an appendocecostomy or perform a partial colectomy. In Hirschsprung disease, surgical treatment is necessary with a Soave pull-through.

Diarrhea in the acute setting is a very common, typically self-limiting problem. The gastroenterologist may see patients with chronic diarrhea more often, typically if it lasts for more than 3 weeks. They will send stool for reducing substances, fecal fat, and alpha$_1$-antitrypsin determinations to look for malabsorptive processes. Other findings in conjunction with diarrhea that should prompt referral include weight loss/poor weight gain, greasy or oily stools, or bloody stools that do not resolve. Laboratory abnormalities that raise the index of suspicion for IBD include low albumin, microcytic anemia, and persistently elevated sedimentation rate. Refer patients with malabsorption. If the gastroenterologist suspects benign diarrhea of toddlerhood, limiting fluid intake to an appropriate level and increasing fiber in the diet typically will correct the problem. The pediatric gastroenterologist may perform a colonoscopy or upper endoscopy depending on the clinical picture and the patient's laboratory evaluation.

Patients with liver disease should have a consult from a pediatric gastroenterologist or pediatric hepatologist. Conditions that warrant referral include direct hyperbilirubinemia, persistently elevated transaminases, neonatal jaundice associated with acholic stools, or dark-colored urine. Acute hepatitis does not usually require referral, although if there is evidence of impaired hepatic function (either laboratory or physical findings), the specialist immediately should refer the patient to a facility with transplant capabilities. Hepatitis B and C should be under the care of a subspecialist, as should other conditions such as chronic hepatitis. Often the pediatric surgeons will manage gallstones, especially if there is bile duct obstruction.

Other subspecialists to keep in mind when evaluating the patient with abdominal complaints include pediatric nephrologists, urologists, and oncologists. In female patients, the obstetrician/gynecologist may be an invaluable consult. Pediatric surgeons treat patients with congenital malformations of the digestive tract, including webs, duplications, and atresia and should treat major congenital malformations such as gastroschisis and omphalocele shortly after birth. Surgeons may consult on patients with abdominal pain. In complex patients, a team approach is often necessary, and multiple subspecialists may partake in the care.

Chapter

11 The Musculoskeletal System

Dilip R. Patel

In addition to the primary conditions affecting the various structures of the musculoskeletal system, numerous systemic conditions also affect the musculoskeletal system, and therefore, any diagnostic assessment of musculoskeletal symptoms and signs must take into consideration relevant assessment of other systems. Neurologic and neurovascular assessment should be an integral part of the evaluation of musculo-skeletal symptoms and signs, especially in traumatic injuries. Because a comprehensive description of the clinical diagnostic methods of the entire musculoskeletal system obviously would be quite extensive, this chapter essentially will serve to introduce the reader to the basic approach to the musculoskeletal diagnosis.

The goals of this chapter are

1. To provide a brief overview of the selected aspects of physiology and anatomy of the musculoskeletal system
2. To review the most relevant symptoms and key aspects of examination of the musculoskeletal system

Physiology and Mechanics

The bony skeleton provides the framework or the structure for the body's various organ systems, as well as the mechanisms for movement and locomotion. Additionally, bone is also the site for mineral metabolism and homeostasis, as well as a site for hematopoiesis. Development of the skeleton, or morphogenesis, begins in the fourth week of life in utero. Bone forms by either the process of endochondral ossification (long bones) or intramembranous ossification (flat bones and clavicles). Chondroblasts, which derive from the mesenchyme, lay down the cartilage framework of the bone, which later consists of osteoblasts. Osteoblasts synthesize and secrete osteoid, which becomes calcified to form the mature bone. The cal-cified cartilage forms the primary ossification center in the middle of long bones, and the secondary ossification centers form at the ends of the long bones. The growth plate, or the physis, forms at the growing ends of the long bones. The anatomic regions of the growing long bones consist of the articular cartilage, the epiphysis, the growth plate, the metaphysis, and the diaphysis. New bone formation continues to occur at the junction between the growth plate, or physis, and the metaphysis in the region of the physis called the *zone of provisional calcification*.

The continued development and remodeling of the bone are a function of osteoblasts (bone-forming cells), osteocytes (mature bone cells), and osteoclasts (bone-breakdown cells). Structurally, bone consists of outer cortical and inner trabecular bone. Bone is involved in the mineral homeostasis of calcium, phosphorous, parathyroid hormone, vitamin D, and calcitonin.

The articular cartilage provides cushioning and functions to reduce friction between two opposing bony surfaces in the synovial joints. The articular cartilage in children and adolescents is relatively more cellular than that of adults. Articular cartilage injuries do not heal well. Injury that involves the articular cartilage and extends to the underlying subchondral bone constitutes an osteochondral fracture. In the knee joint, meniscal cartilages play an important role in reducing friction, stabilizing the joint, and dissipating the load (shock absorption), whereas the intervertebral disks in the spine do the same. Like the articular cartilage, the menisci and intervertebral disks are more resilient in children and adolescents than in adults. In children and adolescents, the intervertebral disk has the annulus fibrosus surrounding it circumferentially, and the disk is sandwiched between the inferior ring apophysis of the vertebra above and the superior ring apophysis of the vertebra below.

Synovial tissue forms the synovial membrane of the joint and bursa, as well as the tendon sheaths. It reduces friction and facilitates smooth motion. The synovium lines the joint capsule of the synovial joint. Ligaments connect two adjacent bones of the joint and are strong fibrous bands that provide mechanical stability to the joint. Skeletal muscles span across joints and bones and attach to the bone either directly or by its tendon. Appropriate neuromuscular functioning and contractions provide for the movements at various joints. Muscle fibers are of two types: type 1, or slow twitch, with high aerobic capacity and type 2, or fast twitch, with high anaerobic capacity. During the growth period, the predominant increase in muscle length occurs at the myotendinous junction. Pathology, both inflammatory and noninflammatory, can affect all the main structures of the musculoskeletal system, as well as the connective and vascular tissues, leading to various conditions or clinical syndromes (such as stress fracture of the bone, arthritis of the joint, osteochondritis dissecans affecting the articular cartilage, and inflammatory conditions that cause tendonitis).

Functional Anatomy

FIGURES 11–1, 11–2, and 11–3 show the movements at the shoulder joint, the thumb, and the ankle, respectively. Anatomy of the shoulder is shown in FIGURE 11–4, and the skeleton of the hand is illustrated in FIGURE 11–5. FIGURES 11–6 illustrates the anatomy of the knee, and FIGURE 11–7 shows that of the ankle. FIGURE 11–8 shows the skeleton of the foot.

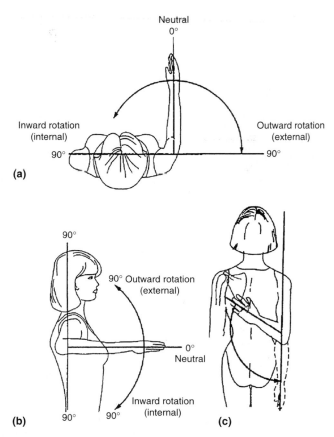

FIGURE 11-1 *Movements of the Shoulder.* *(From Dutton M:* Orthopedic Examination, Evaluation, and Intervention. *McGraw-Hill Medical, New York, 2005, Fig 14-23, p. 439.)*

History

Infants

KEY PROBLEM
She Does Not Move Her Arm Causes of paralysis of one upper extremity detected within the first few days or weeks of life include *trauma* to the brachial plexus, *fracture* of the clavicle or proximal humerus, septic arthritis of the shoulder joint, and *osteomyelitis* of the humerus. Typically, infants with traumatic *brachial plexus neuropathy* or *fracture* of the clavicle or humerus will not be able to move the arm at birth, whereas in case of *septic arthritis* or *osteomyelitis*, the infant will

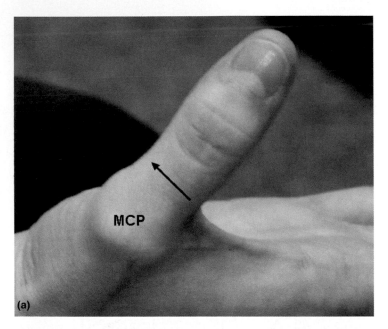

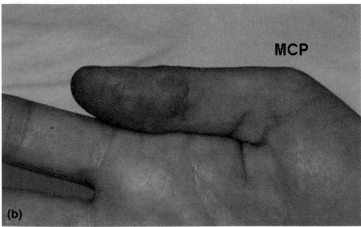

FIGURE 11-2 *A. Movements of the thumb: abduction. B. Movements of the thumb: adduction. C. Movements of the thumb: flexion and extension. D. Movements of the thumb: opposition.*

have normal arm movement preceding the paralysis (pseudoparalysis). Injury to the C_5 and C_6 roots results in *Erb*-type paralysis, whereas injury to C_8–T_1 results in *Klumpke*-type paralysis. There may be a history of a large baby, shoulder dystocia, application of traction during delivery, primigravida, or breech delivery.

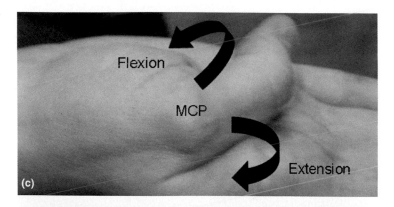

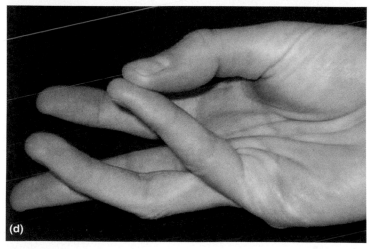

FIGURE 11-2 (Continued)

⬤ KEY PROBLEM

He Is Not Yet Walking Delayed walking is one of the most common and early symptoms of *cerebral palsy* that should prompt further neurologic (see Chapter 12) and developmental evaluation (see Chapter 18). A detailed history of the course and complications of pregnancy, birth, and the early neonatal course is helpful (see Chapters 1 and 5).

⬤ KEY PROBLEM

His Neck Does Not Look Straight In *torticollis* (or wryneck), the head tips to one side, and the chin rotates to the opposite side. The most common cause of torticollis in infants is *congenital* muscular torticollis because of injury and subsequent contracture of the sternocleidomastoid muscle. Causes of torticollis that are present soon

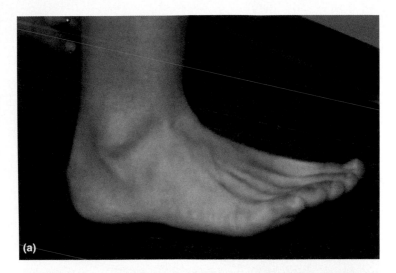

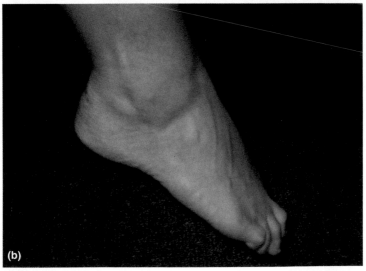

FIGURE 11–3 *A. Movements of the ankle (non-weight bearing): dorsiflexion. B. Movements of the ankle (non-weight bearing): plantar flexion. C. Movements of the ankle (non-weight bearing): inversion. D. Movements of the ankle (non-weight bearing): eversion.*

after or within the first few weeks of life include in utero positional torticollis, traumatic lesions of the sternocleidomastoid muscle, and congenital anomalies of the cervical spine. *Klippel-Feil syndrome* refers to a triad of low hairline, restriction of cervical spine motion, and multiple-level coalitions of the cervical vertebrae.

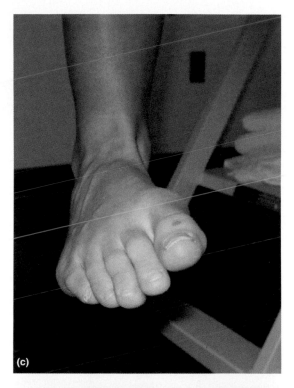

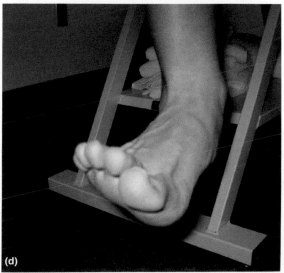

FIGURE 11–3 *(Continued)*

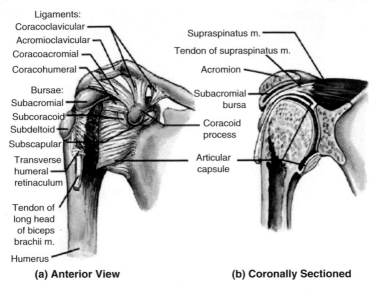

(a) Anterior View   **(b) Coronally Sectioned**

FIGURE 11–4   Anatomy of the Shoulder. *(From Van De Graaff KH:* Human Anatomy. *New York: McGraw-Hill, 2002, Fig. 8.25, p. 216.)*

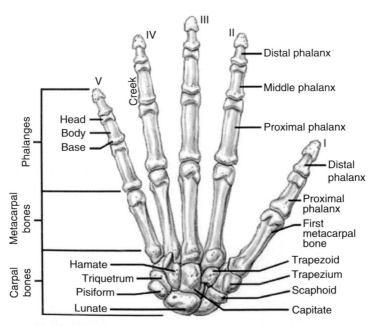

FIGURE 11–5   Bones of the Hand. *(From Van De Graaff KH:* Human Anatomy. *New York: McGraw-Hill, 2002, Fig. 7-9, p. 180.)*

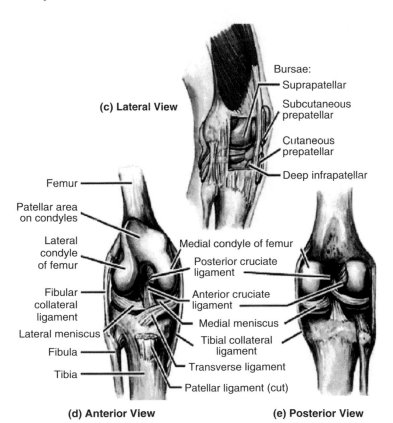

FIGURE 11-6 *Anatomy of the Knee. (From Van De Graaff KH:* Human Anatomy. *New York: McGraw-Hill, 2002, Fig. 8.31, p. 221.)*

The flexion-extension movement occurs at the occiput–C_1 articulation, whereas lateral flexion and rotation occur at the C_1–C_2 articulation. *Developmental, traumatic, inflammatory,* or *metabolic* conditions can affect the stability of these articulations and can lead to progressive *myelopathy* or acute spinal cord *compression*. A higher prevalence of *atlantoaxial instability* occurs in children with *Down syndrome*.

Causes of torticollis that first appears later in childhood include soft-tissue *trauma* to the neck, *inflammatory* conditions affecting the head and neck (including rheumatic diseases), acute *infectious* conditions, and *neurologic* conditions that affect the spinal cord such as a *syrinx* or *a tumor*.

Children

KEY PROBLEM

His Feet Are Turned In Common causes of in-toeing are *internal femoral torsion, internal tibial version, metatarsus adductus,* and

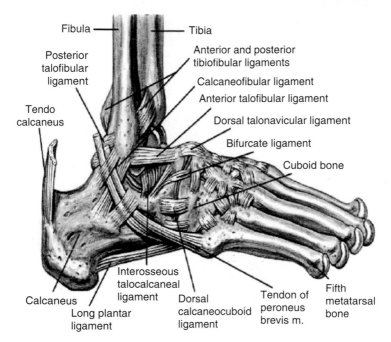

Fibula — Tibia

Posterior talofibular ligament

Anterior and posterior tibiofibular ligaments

Calcaneofibular ligament

Anterior talofibular ligament

Tendo calcaneus

Dorsal talonavicular ligament

Bifurcate ligament

Cuboid bone

Interosseous talocalcaneal ligament

Calcaneus

Long plantar ligament

Dorsal calcaneocuboid ligament

Tendon of peroneus brevis m.

Fifth metatarsal bone

FIGURE 11–7   *Lateral Aspect of the Ankle. (From Van De Graaff KH:* Human Anatomy. *New York: McGraw-Hill, 2002, Fig. 8.33, p. 223.)*

talipes equinovarus. Torsion refers to the position of the foot relative to the body's line of progression during walking and can be external, neutral, or internal. *Version* refers to the angle or inclination within the bone, e.g., the relative angulation between the femoral neck and shaft.

In *internal femoral torsion,* the entire leg rotates internally, and the hips manifest about 80 to 90 degrees of internal rotation with the child in prone position on the examination table, with external rotation limited to 0 to 10 degrees. Internal femoral torsion is the most common cause of in-toeing in children 2 years of age and older. There may be laxity of other joints. Typically, a child with internal femoral torsion sits in a "W" or "television" style. Correction occurs spontaneously by 3 years of age.

A negative value of thigh-foot angle indicates *internal tibial version,* and it is the most common cause of in-toeing in children younger than 2 years of age.

Common causes of out-toeing are *external femoral torsion, external tibial torsion, calcaneovalgus feet,* and *hypermobile pes planus.* External tibial torsion is a common cause of out-toeing. It manifests an abnormally positive thigh-foot angle and is often associated with a *calcaneovalgus foot.* Spontaneous correction typically occurs by age 3 years. External femoral torsion demonstrates excessive hip external rotation and limited internal rotation. Idiopathic *external femoral rotation* is typically bilateral. Unilateral

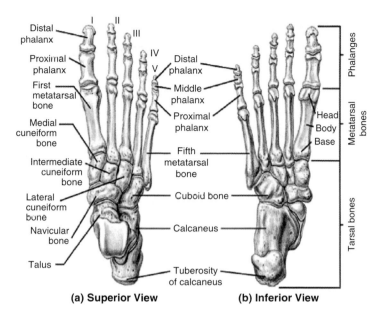

(a) Superior View **(b) Inferior View**

FIGURE 11–8 Bones of the Foot. *(From Van De Graaff KH:* Human Anatomy. *New York: McGraw-Hill, 2002, Fig. 7-19, p. 187.)*

external femoral rotation requires further investigation to rule out hip pathology, such as slipped capital femoral epiphysis.

KEY PROBLEM
She Is Bowlegged

The most common cause of bowlegs, or *genu varum*, is physiologic bowlegs that resolve spontaneously by 2 years of age (FIGURE 11–9). Genu varum is also a characteristic of idiopathic *tibia vara* or *Blount disease* owing to abnormal growth of the medial aspect of the proximal tibial metaphysis. Blount disease can be early onset or late onset, and management requires referral to a pediatric orthopedic surgeon. Other causes of bowlegs are *skeletal dysplasias, rickets,* complication of injury to the growth plate, and local infection or tumor. Bowing of the tibia can be either anterolateral or posteromedial, with predominant direction of the apex of the deformity. Posteromedial bowing of the tibia generally has a good prognosis for correction over time, whereas anterolateral bowing has a worse prognosis and needs evaluation and follow-up by an orthopedic surgeon.

KEY PROBLEM
His Knees Looked Crooked (Knock-Knees)

Physiologic *genu valgum*, or knock-knees (FIGURE 11–10), most commonly occurs between 3 and 5 years of age and typically resolves by 8 years of age. Other causes of genu valgum are skeletal dysplasia, neuromuscular disease, complication of injury to the growth plate, and local infection or tumor.

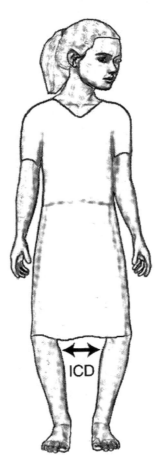

FIGURE 11–9 *Bowlegs or genu varum can be followed by measuring the distance between the child's knees (intercondylar distance) with the ankles held together. (From Rudolph CD, et al (eds):* Rudolph's Pediatrics, *21st ed. New York: McGraw-Hill 2003, Fig. 27-30, p. 2431.)*

KEY PROBLEM

She Has Flat Feet The most common cause of flat feet is *normal-variant flexible pronated flat feet* with loss of the medial longitudinal arch of the foot on weight bearing that requires no treatment. *Tarsal coalitions, neuromuscular disease,* and *Achilles tendon contracture* are the less common causes of rigid flat feet. *Tarsal coalition* or *peroneal spastic flatfoot* manifests rigid and often painful flatfoot associated with peroneal muscle spasms. Tarsal coalition is a result of failure of segmentation or *congenital* fusion of one or more tarsal bones.

KEY PROBLEM

His Back Does Not Look Right See "Adolescent" section below for scoliosis and kyphosis.

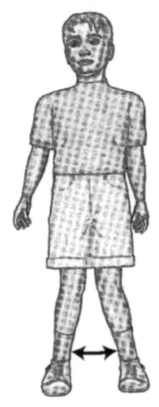

FIGURE 11-10 *Knock-Knees. Genu valgum can be followed by measuring the distance between the ankles, the intermalleolar distance, with the knees just touching. (From Rudolph CD, et al (eds):* Rudolph's Pediatrics, *21st ed. New York: McGraw-Hill 2003, Fig. 27-18, p. 2430.)*

KEY PROBLEM
Back Pain Back pain in children younger than 10 years of age is more likely due to *infectious diskitis, vertebral osteomyelitis,* and *vertebral* or *spinal cord tumors.* In this age group, *tumors* that are more common include *eosinophilic granuloma, acute leukemia, neuroblastoma,* and *astrocytoma.* Younger age, nighttime pain, pain at rest, and severe pain are indicators of significant underlying pathology. Back pain in older children and adolescents is more likely due to acute trauma or *overuse syndromes* (see "Adolescent" section below).

KEY PROBLEM
Limp Pain on weight bearing results in antalgic gait (i.e., less time on affected limb in order to avoid pain) typically caused by *infections, trauma, neoplasms,* or *rheumatic diseases,* whereas neuromuscular conditions that do not cause pain on weight bearing result in a Trendelenburg (circumducting) gait. Painful causes of limp include *transient synovitis* of

the hip, early *Legg-Calve-Perthes disease, septic arthritis, osteomyelitis, fracture, diskitis, slipped capital femoral epiphysis,* and *inflammatory rheumatic joint disease.* Causes of painless limp include *developmental dysplasia of the hip, spastic hemiplegic cerebral palsy* with *hip dislocation, Legg-Calve-Perthes disease, proximal femoral focal dysplasia, congenital coxa vara,* and *congenital bowing of the tibia.*

KEY PROBLEM
Toe Walking Toe walking (*equinus gait*) can be normal before 3 years of age. Common causes of unilateral toe walking are *neuromuscular disease, hemiplegic cerebral palsy, relatively short leg,* and *hip dislocation.* Common causes of bilateral toe walking are *idiopathic* or *habitual* and include *cerebral palsy, neuromuscular conditions, Duchenne muscular dystrophy, myelomeningocele with tethered cord,* and *congenital contracture of the Achilles tendon.*

KEY PROBLEM
My Legs Hurt Acute and localized pain in the leg may be due to *trauma, fracture,* or *infectious* process. More diffuse aching pain should be differentiated from exertional-related undue fatigue indicative of *metabolic* or muscle disease. *Juvenile myalgia* ("growing pains") is highly prevalent in children. Although the etiology and pathophysiology of this condition are not entirely clear, it is nonetheless a common cause of limb pain in children. Pain occurs typically at the end of the day, sometimes at night, and is deep and aching, affecting one or both lower limbs. It is most prevalent between the ages of 2 and 10 years, with a peak at about 5 years of age, and runs an intermittent course over a period of about 2 years. Massage, heat, and analgesics relieve the pain of juvenile myalgia.

KEY PROBLEM
One Leg Is Short Leg-length inequality may be *congenital* or *acquired* and includes *proximal femoral focal deficiency, coxa vara, hemiatrophy-hemihypertrophy, Legg-Calve-Perthes disease, hemiplegic cerebral palsy, infectious osteomyelitis* affecting the growth plate, *trauma to the growth plate,* and *growth arrest* or *overgrowth* owing to *malunion.* Apparent leg-length inequality may occur in neuromuscular disorders affecting lower back, spine, hip, and lower extremities.

KEY PROBLEM
Does Not Move Her Arm Acute *subluxation of the radial head* can occur from a sudden pull of the arm, as in a child pulled by an adult or a child trying to reach for something high and catching himself or herself from falling. There is localized pain laterally over the elbow, mainly on attempt to move the elbow. The child typically will hold the arm close to the chest, with the elbow flexed at about 90 degrees and the arm partially pronated. There is no swelling or local deformity. Closed reduction, gentle supination of the arm, and extension of the elbow followed by flexion are the treatment of choice. In many cases of trauma at this age, the history may not be clear, and there always should be a high index of suspicion for a fracture.

● KEY PROBLEM

Joint Pain Causes of pain around the knee in children include injury to the distal femur and proximal tibia growth plate, *lateral discoid meniscus, chronic juvenile arthritis, septic arthritis, juvenile osteochondritis dissecans affecting the femoral condyles or the patella, acute lymphoblastic leukemia,* and benign and malignant bone *tumors.*

Many young children participate in gymnastics with great intensity, spending up to 30 to 40 hours per week in practice and competition in some cases. Wrist pain is a common symptom seen in young gymnasts and can be due to varied underlying pathology owing to overuse of the soft-tissue structures. *Stress injury* of the distal radial physis presents with activity-related chronic or recurrent pain (bilateral in about 30 percent) of the dorsal aspect of the wrist aggravated during floor exercises, vaulting, and loading the dorsiflexed wrist with localized distal radius and dorsal wrist tenderness. Early recognition of this condition is essential to prevent the complication of premature fusion of the physis and growth arrest. In a child with a history of a fall on an outstretched arm, one should have a high index of suspicion for *fractures of the distal radius* and *scaphoid.*

Early recognition of elbow injuries in children involved in throwing sports is important to prevent long-term complications. Throwing motion in a baseball pitcher imparts tremendous forces around the elbow that can lead to significant soft-tissue and bony injuries. If unrecognized and not treated early, these injuries can lead to long-term complications of elbow flexion contractures, intraarticular loose bodies, early arthritis, and functional limitations.

Stress injury to the proximal physis of the humerus is an important consideration in a child presenting with shoulder pain who is involved in throwing sports. Acute pain also can occur in septic arthritis of the shoulder. Shoulder and upper back pain is also common in children carrying heavy school bags and in children with bad posture.

● KEY PROBLEM

My Heel Hurts *Sever disease* refers to an overuse injury affecting the posterior calcaneal apophysis that presents with activity-related heel pain typically between 9 and 13 years of age. There is a high prevalence in gymnasts, basketball players, and soccer players. Squeezing the heel medially and laterally elicits tenderness. It is a benign, self-limited condition, and its recognition will help to avoid unnecessary investigations, overzealous treatment, or restriction of activities.

Adolescents

● KEY PROBLEM

Limp *Septic arthritis* or *osteomyelitis* can affect joints or bones of the lower limbs, sacroiliac joint, symphysis pubis, or lumbosacral spine, causing a limp. *Slipped capital femoral epiphysis* can present as acute hip pain or insidious, intermittent pain on weight bearing and movement. The hip is typically in external rotation and abduction. Patients with a slipped capital femoral epiphysis should have a referral to an orthopedic surgeon on an emergent basis. Pain from the hip often refers to the knee. Pain in the groin and limp also can be due to a stress fracture of the femoral neck that requires an emergent referral for definitive treatment. Numerous conditions affecting the lower limb joints and bones can cause the adolescent to limp and appear in respective sections of this text.

KEY PROBLEM

Bowlegs *Juvenile Blount disease* is an important consideration in adolescents who present with bowlegs. The juvenile form initially presents with progressively worsening genu varum, typically unilateral, and often seen in obese adolescents. Knee pain is not a consistent feature. The diagnosis is apparent on examination, and radiographic features are characteristic. All patients with Blount disease should have a referral to a pediatric orthopedic surgeon for further evaluation and definitive management.

KEY PROBLEM

Leg Pain Causes of pain in the leg include *acute* or *stress fracture of the tibia* or *fibula, acute* or *chronic exertional compartment syndrome, medial tibial stress syndrome (shin splints), neoplasia* or *infectious osteomyelitis of the tibia or fibula, acute musculotendinous strain,* and *deep vein thrombosis* or *superficial thrombophlebitis.*

The most common site for stress fracture is the tibia and is directly a result of excessive, repetitive stress to the bone, typically from sport participation and running. The pain is constant, dull aching, typically localizes at the junction of the middle and lower thirds of the tibia, with localized tenderness, and worsens with weight bearing.

In chronic exertional compartment syndrome, the symptoms relate to the specific leg compartment affected. The pain typically is concurrent with the same activity, tends to recur at a specific time during the activity, and abates with a variable period of rest. Passive stretching of muscles in the compartment will reproduce the pain.

Pain associated with *fracture, neoplasia* or *infectious osteomyelitis* is a constant and dull aching, occurs at rest, and often at nighttime. Other causes of lower limb pain include *restless leg syndrome* and *peripheral neuropathy.* Pain from nerve is typically sharp, shooting or like pins and needles; vascular pain is throbbing; and articular or bone pain is dull aching pain.

KEY PROBLEM

Neck Pain Pain and stiffness in the neck also occurs in *congenital, inflammatory,* and *infectious* conditions affecting the head and neck region. It can be acute owing to soft-tissue *strain* or *fracture* of the vertebrae or insidious, as seen in *diskitis, cervical spondylolysis,* or lesions of the spinal cord such as *syringomyelia.* Disk *herniation* may present either acutely or insidiously. *Syringomyelia* may be associated with bilateral upper extremity paresthesia.

KEY PROBLEM

Low Back Pain Low back pain is a common complaint in adolescents. Soft-tissue *injuries* (musculotendinous sprains and ligamentous sprains) are the most common cause, followed by postural or mechanical back pain and psychosomatic back pain. The most common identifiable cause of low back pain in adolescents is lumbar *spondylolysis*. Spondylolysis is a stress fracture of the pars interarticularis most commonly affecting L$_5$ and resulting from repetitive hyperextension, such as gymnastics. The pain is insidious in onset, intermittent, and activity-associated. With bilateral spondylolytic lesions at the same level, there may be anterior slippage of the vertebra over the one below, resulting in *spondylolisthesis*.

The most common identifiable cause of thoracic back pain in adolescents is *Scheuermann disease*. *Tumors* such as osteoblastoma, osteosarcoma, and lymphoma and *infection* (*osteomyelitis*) are relatively more likely causes of significant back pain in adolescents that occurs at rest or during nighttime or is persistent.

Disk *rupture* and *herniation* can cause acute or chronic intermittent low back pain. In adolescents, neurologic findings are uncommon. *Slipped vertebral ring apophysis* and *apophyseal ring fracture* can cause acute low back pain. Back pain due to *infectious diskitis, vertebral osteomyelitis,* or *sacroiliitis* may be either acute or insidious and may or may not be associated with systemic symptoms.

Developmental conditions of the spine—*adolescent idiopathic scoliosis, spina bifida occulta,* and *lumbarization* or *sacralization*—are uncommon causes of back pain. Neuromuscular *scoliosis, syringomyelia,* spinal cord *tumors,* and *tethered cord* cause chronic back pain and may be associated with abnormal neurologic findings. Insidious onset, chronic, gradually worsening back pain is often the initial and only symptom of *ankylosing spondylitis, spondyloarthropathy,* or *juvenile chronic arthritis.* Lower back pain may be referred pain from inflammatory bowel disease, renal disease, urinary tract infection, gynecologic conditions, or intraabdominal *neoplasms*.

KEY PROBLEM

Foot and Ankle Pain Stress fracture of the metatarsal or tarsal bones can present with localized pain that is worse with weight bearing during running or jumping. In *tarsal coalition,* there is a fusion or failure of segmentation of two or more tarsal bones. *Talocalcaneal* and *calcaneonavicular coalitions* are the most common types and present with foot pain initially during adolescence that increases with activity and prolonged walking, especially on uneven ground. Pain in *plantar fasciitis,* occurring typically in runners, localizes to the ball of the foot, more prominent in the morning and on weight bearing.

Other causes of foot pain in adolescents are *metatarsalgia, osteomyelitis, puncture wound, sesamoiditis, Morton's neuroma, Freiberg disease, Kohler disease,* and *tarsal tunnel syndrome. Ingrown toenails* are a common cause of toe pain in adolescents.

A bunion, or *hallux valgus,* is a common cause of pain in the great toe, especially in adolescent females who wear shoes with a narrow toe box and high heels. Bunion also may accompany *metatarsus primum varus,* short first metatarsal, and flatfeet.

Pain predominantly in the heel area is characteristic of *Achilles tendonitis, tibialis posterior tendonitis, peroneal tendonitis and subluxation, calcaneal stress fracture, posterior calcaneal bursitis,* and *plantar fasciitis. Sprain* is a common cause of ankle pain in adolescents. Most ankle sprains are inversion type and present with lateral pain. Pain in the medial side associated with eversion injury is indicative of a more significant injury; associated injuries including fractures are possible. Chronic ankle pain can result from inadequately rehabilitated ankle sprain or other associated injuries. The differential diagnosis of delayed recovery or persistent disability following ankle injury includes *inadequate rehabilitation, anterior talar impingement, impingement spurs, peroneal tendon subluxation or dislocation,* osteochondral fracture of the talus, tibiofibular syndesmosis sprain, instability, nerve traction *injury* (superficial peroneal, sural, or tibial), *sinus tarsi syndrome, occult fracture,* and *reflex sympathetic dystrophy.*

◖ KEY PROBLEM
Joint Pain Ascertain evolution of joint pain in terms of the nature of onset, duration, temporal sequence, and progression. Characterize pain based on location, acuity, severity, aggravating and relieving factors, diurnal variation, and progression. Note the circumstances of how the pain started. In case of an acute injury, inquire about the mechanism of injury. In chronic overuse injuries, a detailed history of the volume and intensity of physical activity, as well as the time frame of progression of the activity prior to the onset of pain, is important.

Typically, joint pain owing to septic arthritis is of acute onset, whereas that owing to rheumatic disease or overuse syndrome is insidious. Localized pain may be due to conditions affecting the joint itself or those affecting the periarticular connective tissue, bursae, or tendons. Joint pain may be migratory, affecting multiple joints sequentially, as seen, for example, in disseminated *gonococcal arthritis* or *acute rheumatic fever.* It may be additive, affecting new joints while the joints affected previously are still symptomatic, as seen in *juvenile chronic arthritis* and *spondyloarthropathies.* It may be episodic, affecting one or more joints at a given time, as in *inflammatory bowel disease* or *Lyme disease.*

◖ KEY PROBLEM
Shoulder Pain *Acute septic arthritis,* shoulder dislocation, and fractures present with acute shoulder pain, swelling, and loss of motion. *Acute traumatic biceps tendon strain* or *subluxation* or *supraspinatus musculotendinous* tear also can present with acute pain. The causes of chronic or recurrent shoulder pain in the adolescent include *glenohumeral instability, tears of the glenoid labrum, tendonitis of the long head of the biceps, subacromial bursitis,* and *rotator cuff impingement and tendonitis. Acromioclavicular joint sprain* and *atraumatic osteolysis* of the distal clavicle present with pain in the acromioclavicular joint area. *Scapular dyskinesis, stress fracture* of the scapula, and *suprascapular neuropathy* present with pain that is more widespread and discomfort in the shoulder region and the scapulothoracic area. Shoulder pain occurs in rheumatic diseases and myopathy. Shoulder pain may be referred pain from the neck in spine conditions, including

cervical spinal cord impingement or tumor, syringomyelia, cervical disk herniation, cervical nerve root impingement, brachial plexus neuropathy, and thoracic outlet syndrome. In *Paget-Schrotter syndrome,* the patient develops *thrombosis of the axillary veins* resulting from repetitive physical stress of the shoulder and arm and presents with effort-related shoulder and arm pain that may progress to further signs of vascular compromise.

KEY PROBLEM

Elbow Pain Predominant location is important in evaluating intrinsic causes of elbow pain in adolescents. Lateral elbow pain is characteristic in *lateral epicondylitis (tennis elbow), osteochondritis dissecans of the capitellum,* and *posterior interosseous nerve entrapment.* Medial elbow pain occurs in *flexor-pronator syndrome, medial collateral ligament sprain, ulnar neuritis or compressive neuropathy,* and *medial epicondylitis (golfer's elbow).* Posterior elbow pain is characteristic of *olecranon bursitis, stress fracture of the olecranon, triceps insertional tendonitis,* and *intraarticular loose bodies.* Anterior elbow pain results from biceps strain or tendonitis, flexor-pronator exertional compartment syndrome, and anterior *capsulitis. Juvenile chronic arthritis, infectious arthritis,* and *fracture/dislocations* are also significant causes of elbow pain in this age group.

KEY PROBLEM

Wrist Pain Relatively more common intrinsic causes of chronic or recurrent wrist pain in adolescents include *de Quervain tenosynovitis, distal radial physis stress injury, dorsal soft-tissue impingement syndrome,* and *triangular fibrocartilage complex injury.* Less common intrinsic causes of chronic or recurrent wrist pain are many and include *carpal instability, carpal bone chondromalacia, distal radioulnar joint instability, ganglion cyst, intersection syndrome, Kienbock disease, median nerve entrapment neuropathy, ulnar nerve entrapment neuropathy, stress fracture of the scaphoid, wrist flexor or extensor tendonitis, wrist joint capsulitis,* and *wrist splints.*

KEY PROBLEM

Hip, Groin Pain Causes of the hip and groin area pain include *slipped capital femoral epiphysis, late-onset Legg-Calve-Perthes disease, stress fracture of the femoral neck, stress fracture of the pubic rami, hip flexor adductor tendonitis, iliopectineal bursitis, trochanteric bursitis, iliac crest apophysitis, apophyseal avulsions* (greater trochanter, lesser trochanter, ischial tuberosity), *osteitis pubis, meralgia paresthetica, snapping hip syndrome, iliopsoas abscess, acetabulum injury, malignancy, osteoid osteoma, rheumatic disease,* and *septic arthritis.* Pain in the hip and groin may be referred pain from intraabdominal, pelvic, and renal pathology.

KEY PROBLEM

Knee Pain The most common cause of knee pain in older children and adolescents is idiopathic adolescent knee pain (*patellofemoral syndrome*) that can affect one or both knees. The patient presents with insidious onset poorly localized anterior knee pain that is mild to moderate in severity and aggravated with going up or down stairs and after prolonged sitting. It also can worsen with excessive activity that involves repetitive bending of the knees. Examination of the knee is normal in most cases. This is a benign, self-limited condition, and overzealous treatment or restriction of activities is unnecessary. The differential diagnosis of anterior knee pain includes *patellar or quadriceps tendonitis, prepatellar or infrapatellar bursitis, patellar stress fracture, multipartite patella, juvenile osteochondritis dissecans of the patella, patellar subluxation, Sinding-Larsen-Johansson syndrome, patellar tendonitis, Hoffa's fat pad syndrome,* and *Osgood-Schlatter disease.*

Causes of posterior knee pain are *Baker's cyst* associated with a *meniscal tear, fabella syndrome, gastrocnemius tendonitis,* and *hamstring tendonitis.* Causes of medial knee pain include *medial meniscal tear, pathologic medial synovial plica, pes anserine bursitis, semimembranosus bursitis/tendonitis,* and *juvenile osteochondritis dissecans of the medial femoral condyle.* Predominantly lateral pain is prominent in iliotibial band friction syndrome, popliteus tendonitis, discoid lateral meniscal injury, and disruption of the proximal tibiofibular articulation.

Pain in the knee occurs in systemic *inflammatory* diseases such as *rheumatic diseases, hemophilia,* and *sickle cell arthropathy; infectious* or reactive *arthritis;* benign and malignant bone *tumors;* and *acute lymphoblastic leukemia.* Pathologic conditions of the hip, such as slipped capital femoral epiphysis, Legg-Calve-Perthes disease, and stress fracture of the femoral neck, all may present with pain referred to the knee.

KEY PROBLEM
Stiffness
Stiffness is a feeling of discomfort or tightness associated with movement of a joint following a period of rest typically felt after an hour or so of inactivity. Stiffness usually resolves with activity. Morning stiffness is characteristic of *inflammatory* or *rheumatic* diseases. Patients with *fibromyalgia* complain of generalized stiffness. Stiffness is not true locking of the joint, which is due to a mechanical block.

KEY PROBLEM
Joint Swelling
Characterize joint swelling based on the acuity of onset and progression; precipitating or relieving factors; its location, size, and consistency; and whether it is well defined or diffuse. Internal *trauma* to a joint such as the ligament, cartilage, or intraarticular fracture, *septic arthritis,* and bleeding in a joint from a *bleeding diathesis* such as *hemophilia* all cause acute swelling, whereas *chronic juvenile arthritis* causes insidious onset and progressive swelling. Intermittent swelling is more characteristic of *osteochondritis dissecans* or *intraarticular cartilage injuries.*

KEY PROBLEM
Weakness
Weakness is a true loss of muscle power. It may result from neurologic disease, primary muscle disease, or systemic disease. Acute *cerebrovascular insults* can present with sudden onset of focal weakness or paralysis, whereas insidious onset of weakness is more characteristic of primary muscle disease. *Myopathy* tends to affect

the proximal muscle more, whereas neuropathy tends to affect the distal muscles. Myopathy can be associated with muscle pseudohypertrophy, whereas neuropathy may be associated with paresthesia.

● KEY PROBLEM

◢ **Deterioration of Function** The adolescent may first present with deterioration or inability to perform certain tasks, especially in sports, as a result of joint pain, limitation of motion, stiffness, or weakness.

● KEY PROBLEM

◢ **Constitutional Symptoms** In addition to musculoskeletal features, TABLE 11–1 lists systemic or constitutional signs and symptoms that are common in rheumatic diseases.

TABLE 11–1 *Systemic or Constitutional Symptoms and Signs*

Signs or Symptoms	Condition
Abdominal pain	Inflammatory bowel disease, dermatomyositis, systemic lupus erythematosus, irritable bowel syndrome, Henoch-Schonlein purpura
Alopecia	Dermatomyositis, systemic lupus erythematosus (SLE)
Chest pain	SLE, acute rheumatic fever
Conjunctivitis	Kawasaki disease, systemic vasculitis, Reiter syndrome
Dysphagia	Dermatomyositis, systemic scleroderma
Dyspnea	SLE, systemic vasculitis
Fatigue	Juvenile chronic arthritis, dermatomyositis, fibromyalgia, SLE
Fever	Acute rheumatic fever, infectious arthritis, SLE, systemic vasculitis
Headaches	SLE, fibromyalgia, systemic vasculitis
Hemoptysis	SLE, systemic vasculitis
Iritis	Behçet disease, juvenile chronic arthritis, inflammatory bowel disease
Mucosal ulcers	Behçet disease, Reiter syndrome, disseminated gonococcal disease, inflammatory bowel disease
Raynaud phenomenon and vasomotor instability	SLE, systemic scleroderma, reflex sympathetic dystrophy
Skin rashes	SLE, dermatomyositis, psoriatic arthritis, systemic vasculitis, Henoch-Schönlein purpura, acute rheumatic fever, Lyme disease
Weight loss	Inflammatory bowel disease, malignancy

Physical Examination

Neurologic examination for muscle tone, bulk, strength, and sensation is an integral part of musculoskeletal diagnosis. Chapters 5 and 12 contain components of the neurologic examination. Meticulous examination of the infant must identify and describe any congenital musculoskeletal anomalies. We discuss additional key aspects of the examination below.

Infants

▼ KEY FINDING

Head Note the shape of the head. Measure the head circumference. Note any midfacial deficiencies, retrognathia, mandibular or maxillary hypoplasia, and/or frontal bossing. Head and face anomalies are frequent in a number of genetic syndromes. Feel the anterior fontanel, and palpate skull for swelling or defects.

▼ KEY FINDING

Neck Note swelling, deformity, range of motion, position, or attitude of the head and neck in relation to the chest (*torticollis*). Palpate for any soft-tissue mass in the neck and the cervical spine for deformity. In case of muscular torticollis, a firm, nontender swelling may be palpable in the belly of the sternocleidomastoid muscle. There is restriction of range of motion and the typical position of the head and neck. Avoid hyperextension or flexion movements in Down syndrome when cervical spine anomalies or instability is present. *Hypotonia* and *ligamentous laxity* can predispose to cervical subluxation.

Any degree of loss of the normal cervical *lordosis* or the presence of cervical *kyphosis* is pathologic and should prompt further investigation and pediatric orthopedic consultation. Congenital or developmental cervical kyphosis may be associated with *Larsen syndrome, Conradi syndrome, cervical dysplasia,* or *neurofibromatosis.*

▼ KEY FINDING

Shoulders, Clavicles Note range of motion and symmetry at shoulders and spontaneous movements of the shoulders and arms. In *osteomyelitis* of the humerus, septic arthritis of shoulder, or *fracture* of the humerus, the infant does not move the arm. In fracture of the clavicle, there may be localized swelling, crepitus, and tenderness. The Moro reflex is absent on the side of a brachial plexus traumatic injury, fracture or osteomyelitis of humerus, septic arthritis of the shoulder joint, or fracture of the clavicle. Also palpate the sternoclavicular joint for swelling or crepitus.

▼ KEY FINDING

Chest Wall Observe for *pectus carinatum* or *excavatum* (see Chapter 8). Palpate the ribs, and note any chest wall deficiency. Pectus excavatum (or funnel chest) is usually present from birth, manifested as a depression of the sternum. There is no specific cause in most cases. In some instances it may be associated with connective tissue disorders such as *Marfan syndrome.* Pectus excavatum may be associated with *mitral valve prolapse, Wolff-Parkinson-White syndrome, bronchial atresia,* and *bronchomalacia.* Examination also may reveal narrow anteroposterior diameter of the chest, rounded shoulders, and thoracic *kyphoscoliosis.* Pectus carinatum (or pigeon breast) manifests as a protrusion of the sternum with lateral depression of the ribs. In some cases it is associated with *mitral valve prolapse, coarctation of the aorta,* and *scoliosis.*

KEY FINDING

▼ Upper Limbs

Observe apparent limb asymmetry; muscle atrophy; joint swelling at the elbow, wrist, or small joints of the hand; attitude of the upper extremity; and spontaneous movements. Count fingers, and note any finger or thumb anomalies. In *Erb palsy,* the shoulder is in adduction and internal rotation, the elbow in extension, the forearm in pronation, and the wrist and fingers in flexion (waiter's tip position). In *Klumpke palsy,* the elbow is in flexion, there is supination of the arm, the wrist and fingers are in extension, and the palmar grasp is absent on the side.

Look for congenital anomalies such as *radial club hand, polydactyly, syndactyly,* and *congenital trigger thumb or finger.* Some of the *genetic* syndromes associated with polydactyly are *Carpenter syndrome, Ellis–van Creveld syndrome, Meckel-Gruber syndrome, orofacialdigital syndrome,* and *Rubinstein-Taybi syndrome.* Some of the genetic syndromes associated with syndactyly include *Apert syndrome, Carpenter syndrome, de Lange syndrome, Holt-Oram syndrome,* and *Laurence-Moon-Biedl syndrome.* Multiple joint contractures occur in arthrogryposis multiplex congenita.

KEY FINDING

▼ Spine and Back

Observe for *scoliosis* or *kyphosis.* Note any asymmetry of upper back or scapular region. Observe sitting posture. *Congenital* scoliosis and *kyphosis* result from partial or complete failure of formation, segmentation, or both of the vertebrae. Presence of congenital scoliosis is an indication to look for other congenital anomalies that also may affect the bladder, kidneys, heart, and hearing. *Infantile idiopathic scoliosis* is noticeable during the first 3 years of life; most infants have a left thoracic curve, and it is more common in males, may be progressive, and in some cases may be associated with mental retardation. *Congenital kyphosis* also may be progressive, leading to paraplegia. Presence of a tuft of hair or sinus over the lumbosacral spine should prompt a search for underlying *spina bifida occulta.*

KEY FINDING

▼ Lower Limbs

Observe for asymmetry, posture or attitude, and spontaneous movements of the limbs. Note any limb deficiency.

KEY FINDING

▼ Hips and Groin

Observe posture, asymmetry, spontaneous movements, and swelling. Assess passive hip flexion, extension, internal rotation, and external rotation. Perform the Barlow test and the Ortolani maneuver (see Chapter 5) to assess for *developmental dysplasia* of the hip. The hip is typically in external rotation and abduction in *septic arthritis.* There may be localized findings of *infectious* "red hot" swelling and pain on palpation or movement.

KEY FINDING
Knee Observe the joint for swelling and deformity, and assess range of motion.

KEY FINDING
Foot and Ankle Note congenital anomalies of the foot. In congenital *metatarsus adductus* (FIGURE 11–11), the forefoot is in adduction relative to the midfoot and hindfoot, which are normal; the lateral border of the foot is convex; and the base of the fifth metatarsal is prominent. *Calcaneovalgus foot* is a hyperdorsiflexed foot with forefoot abduction and increased valgus of the heel. *Talipes equinovarus* (clubfoot) is hindfoot equinus, hindfoot and midfoot varus, and forefoot adduction (FIGURE 11–12). *Congenital vertical talus* is the typical rocker-bottom foot, as shown in FIGURE 11–13 (hindfoot equinovalgus, convex plantar surface, and forefoot abduction and dorsiflexion). *Cavus foot* has an exaggerated medial longitudinal arch. It may accompany foot pain and, in older children, a predisposition to ankle sprains. Causes of rigid cavus foot include *cerebral palsy, myelomenigocele,* and *hereditary sensorimotor neuropathies.* Note any congenital anomalies affecting the toes, such as curly toes, overlapping fifth toe, polydactyly, syndactyly, hammertoe, and *mallet toe.*

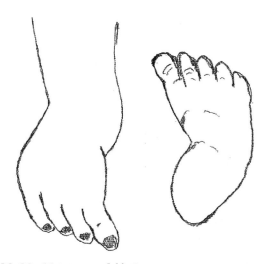

FIGURE 11–11 *Metatarsus Adductus.*

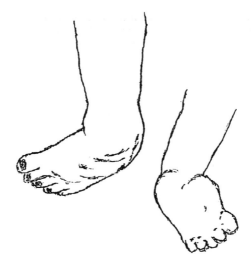

FIGURE 11-12 *Club Foot.*

Children

Gait Normal gait depends on the maturation of the nervous system. A 1-year-old child typically has a wide-based gait, takes short steps, keeps the elbows flexed, and does not have reciprocal movements of the upper extremities. By age 3 years, a normally developing child has acquired most of the characteristics of an adult gait, and by age 7 years, a child's gait is similar to that of an adult.

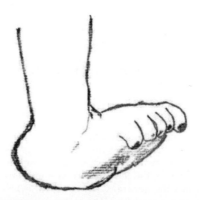

FIGURE 11-13 *Rockerbottom Foot.*

Gait cycle consists of a stance phase and a swing phase. During the stance phase, the limb is in contact with the ground, whereas during the swing phase, the limb is off the ground and advancing forward. Typically, stance phase occupies 60 percent of the gait cycle, whereas the swing phase occupies the remaining 40 percent. *Step length* is the distance between two feet during stance phase when both feet are in contact with the ground (double-limb support). The distance that a limb travels during the stance phase and swing phase is the *stride length,* and the time necessary to complete it is the *step time. Cadence* refers to the number of steps per minute, whereas *walking velocity* refers to the distance traveled per time (meters per second).

Antalgic gait is a result of pain in the lower extremity or back during walking. Because of the pain, there is reduction in the time spent by the affected extremity in stance phase. In Trendelenburg gait there is no pain; it is due to neuromuscular or functional disturbance, and time spent by the affected limb in stance phase is the same as that by the unaffected limb. Gait in a child with proximal muscle weakness demonstrates lurching associated with exaggerated lumbar lordosis. Scissors gait is characteristic of *diplegic* or *quadriplegic cerebral palsy.*

KEY FINDING
Posture Observe sitting and standing posture. Look for asymmetry of the shoulder or pelvis. With the child standing, observe from the front. Note if the patellae are tuned in, neutral, or pointing outward.

KEY FINDING
Torsional Profile *Torsional profile* refers to assessment of the foot progression angle, hip rotation, thigh-foot angle, and shape of the foot.

Foot Progression Angle

Foot progression angle is the angle between the long axis of the foot and the line of progression in which the child is walking. The *long axis of the foot* denotes a line that bisects the heel and extends to second toe, bisecting it. When the long axis of the foot directs inward, the angle is negative, indicating in-toeing, and when it directs outward, the angle is positive and indicates the degree of out-toeing. The normal range of foot progression angle is from –3 to 20 degrees.

Hip Rotation

Assess hip rotation with the child lying prone on the examination table with the hips extended and knees flexed at 90 degrees (FIGURE 11–14). Rotation of the legs outward is a measure of internal rotation of the hips, whereas rotation of the legs inward is a measure of external rotation of the hips. Note the normal values in TABLE 11–2. Note the range and symmetry of hip rotation. Hip rotation is a measure of femoral torsion.

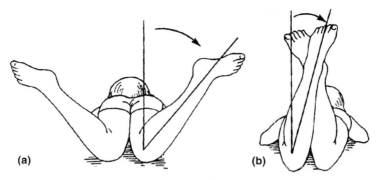

FIGURE 11-14 *Measurement of the hip rotation with the child lying prone. Rotation of the leg outward in the prone position is a measure of hip internal rotation (A), and inward is a measure of hip external rotation (B). (From* Behrman RE, et al. (eds): Nelson Textbook of Pediatrics, *17th ed. Philadelphia: Elsevier-Saunders, 2005, Fig. 665-04, p. 2264, with permission.)*

Thigh-Foot Angle

Measure thigh-foot angle with the child lying prone on the examination table with the hips extended and knees flexed at 90 degrees (FIGURE 11–15). It is the angle between the long axis of the foot and the long axis of the thigh (a line bisecting the posterior thigh). Normal values of the thigh-foot angle are listed in TABLE 11–3. Inward rotation of the foot is a measure of *internal tibial torsion* and has a negative value by convention, whereas outward rotation of the foot is a measure of external tibial torsion and has a positive value.

Foot Shape

With the child prone on the examination table with the knees flexed at 90 degrees, note the shape of the foot.

TABLE 11-2 *Normal Values of Hip Rotation*

Internal Rotation			External Rotation		
Age	Average	Range	Age	Average	Range
1	40 degrees	15–60 degrees	1	65 degrees	40–90 degrees
3	40	15–60	3	55	35–75
5	45	20–65	5	50	30–70
10	45	20–65	10	40	25–55

Range = ±2 standard deviations.
Source: From Rudolph CD, et al (eds): *Rudolph's Pediatrics,* 21st ed. New York: McGraw-Hill, 2003, p. 2424, with permission.

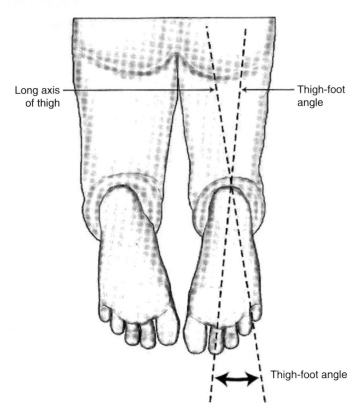

Long axis of thigh — Thigh-foot angle

Thigh-foot angle

FIGURE 11–15 *Measurement of the thigh-foot angle with the child lying prone with the knees flexed at 90 degrees. (From Rudolph CD, et al (eds):* Rudolph's Pediatrics, *21st ed. New York: McGraw-Hill, 2003, Fig. 27-3, p. 2423.)*

KEY FINDING

Neck Observe deformity, normal cervical *lordosis,* and active and passive ranges of motion. Loss of cervical lordosis or *kyphosis* indicates underlying spine or cord anomalies and needs further investigation. *Torticollis* demonstrates the typical attitude of the neck and restricted motion.

TABLE 11–3 *Normal Value of Thigh-Foot Angle*

Age	Average	Range
1	–5 degrees	–30 to +20 degrees
3	+5	–20 to +25
5	+10	–10 to +25
10	+15	+5 to +25

Range = ±2 standard deviations.
Source: From: From Rudolph CD, et al (eds): *Rudolph's Pediatrics. 21st ed.* New York: McGraw-Hill, 2003, p. 2423, with permission.

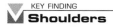 **Lower Limbs** To assess the degree of *genu varum,* have the patient stand with the legs (knees) together, and then measure the distance between the medial malleoli. Similarly, to assess the degree of *genu valgum,* measure the distance between the medial epicondyles of the femur. Assess true leg length with the child supine on the examination table, and measure the distance from the anterosuperior iliac spine to the medial malleolus. Apparent leg length is the distance between the umbilicus and the medial malleolus.

Other Key Areas of Examination

The general approach to examination of other regions and joints is similar in children and adolescents, with some differential age-appropriate emphasis depending on the likelihood of predominant pathology at a particular age. Details of the examination are similar to those described in the section "Adolescents" below.

Adolescents

■ **Gait and Posture** Observe gait for antalgia, Trendelenburg, hemiplegia, or scissoring. Adolescent round back will correct itself by having the patient lie prone on the examining table and hyperextending the back, whereas fixed kyphotic deformity will not. Forward neck and stooping shoulders may be a cause of neck and upper back pain in adolescents.

Observe the normal lordosis of the cervical spine. In spear tackler's spine in football players, the spine becomes a straight column vulnerable to facture-dislocations with flexion injuries. These athletes should not participate further in contact and collision sports.

■ **Shoulders**

Inspection

Note any localized swelling or redness around the shoulder region. Looking from the front, normally the head and neck are in the midline in relation to the shoulders. There may be a step deformity in the acromioclavicular (AC) joint area in case of AC separation. A localized depression laterally over the shoulder occurs in cases of inferior instability with the arm pulled straight down (called the *sulcus sign*). There is flattening of the shoulder contour in anterior dislocation of the shoulder. Note any swelling over the clavicles. In most individuals, the dominant shoulder is relatively low compared with that of the nondominant arm.

From the back with the patient's arms by the side, note any asymmetry of the scapulae. Look for winging of the scapula at rest and with a wall push. Winging at rest occurs in structural abnormalities of the scapula, clavicle, spine, or ribs; winging on wall push suggests long thoracic nerve palsy and spinal accessory nerve palsy. In *Sprengel deformity,* the scapula is poorly developed and high (failure to descend—developmental, congenital).

Palpation

Palpation should localize areas of soft-tissue and bony tenderness around the shoulder joint, AC joints, clavicles, and scapulae. A circumferential tenderness over the proximal humerus is characteristic of *chronic stress injury* of the proximal humeral physis.

Range of Motion and Strength

Active movements at the shoulder joint appear in FIGURE 11–1. Look for asymmetry between the right and left sides, limitation of motion, and pain on motion. From the back, observe the patient's scapula during abduction. Movement at the glenohumeral joint, elevation of the clavicle, and rotation of the scapula—called the *scapulohumeral rhythm*—achieves abduction. During abduction, typically there is a 2:1 ratio of movement at the glenohumeral-to-scapular movement—initial 30 degrees at the glenohumeral joint followed by rest of the 100 to 120 degrees accompanied by 50 to 60 degrees of scapular rotation. Lesions of the glenohumeral joint cause a painful arc during abduction in the range of 45 to 60 to 120 degrees. Assess the strength of shoulder girdle muscles.

Special Tests

Neer test. Forced forward flexion of the arm elicits pain in impingement of the rotator cuff (FIGURE 11–16).

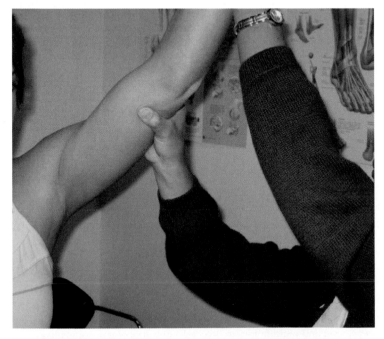

FIGURE 11–16   *Neer Test.*

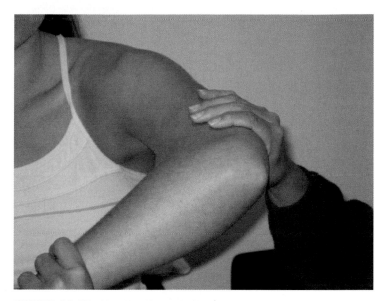

FIGURE 11-17 *Hawkins-Kennedy Test.*

Hawkins-Kennedy test. Internal rotation of arm in abduction and forward flexion also elicits pain in rotator cuff impingement (FIGURE 11–17).

Jobe relocation test. With the patient supine on the examination table, abduct and externally rotate the shoulder fully. The patient feels pain and discomfort in case of anterior instability that will then decrease by applying a posteriorly directed force to move the head of the humerus posteriorly (FIGURE 11–18).

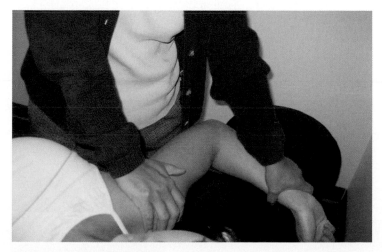

FIGURE 11-18 *Jobe Test.*

Load and shift test. With the patient seated on the table with both arms
by the side, elbows resting in flexion, the examiner stabilizes the
shoulder with one hand and with the other hand grasps the head
of the humerus and attempts to move it anteriorly, posteriorly, and
inferiorly to assess movement (FIGURE 11–19). There is excessive
translation in the direction of shoulder instability.

Supraspinatus test. Test the supraspinatus for weakness or pain on movement against manual resistance. With the patient seated on the table,
apply manual resistance to the arm abducted at 90 degrees, forward
flexed at 30 degrees, and internally rotated (thumbs down or empty-
can sign) (FIGURE 11–20).

Cross adduction. Adduction of the arm across the chest at 90 degrees
of horizontal flexion will elicit pain in lesions of the AC joint
(FIGURE 11–21).

Speed test. To elicit pain in lesions of the long head of biceps, apply manual resistance with the arm held at 90 degrees of abduction, forward
flexed, and externally rotated (palms up) (FIGURE 11–22).

KEY FINDING
Elbow The elbow joint consists of ulnohumeral and radiohumeral
articulations and relates closely to the superior or proximal radioulnar
joint with a continuous joint cavity and capsule.

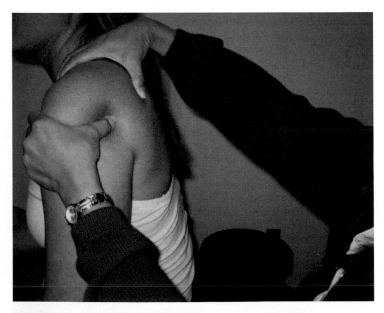

FIGURE 11–19 *Load and Shift Test.*

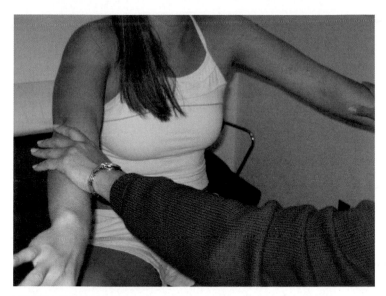

FIGURE 11–20 Supraspinatus Test.

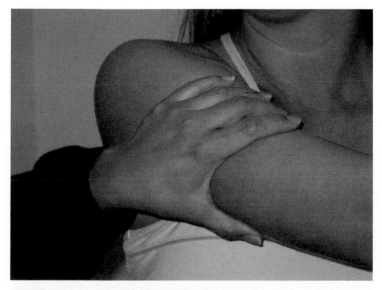

FIGURE 11–21 Cross-Adduction Test.

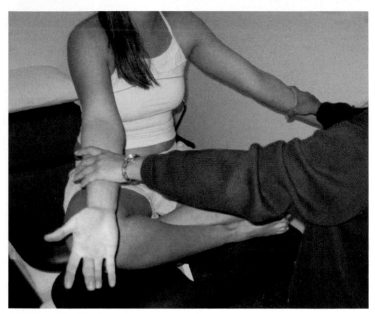

FIGURE 11-22 Speed Test.

Inspection

Observe for swelling, deformity, and asymmetry compared with the un-affected side. Olecranon bursitis causes a well-defined swelling posteri-orly. With the patient standing, arms by the side and extended, note the carrying angle between the axis of the arm and the forearm. Excessive valgus carrying angle increases the stress to the medial structures.

Palpation

Localize any anatomic structure that is tender. There is localized ten-derness over the medical epicondyle in cases of tennis elbow or *medial epicondylitis.* With the arm extended and wrist flexed, have the patient extend the wrist against manual resistance to elicit medial epicondylar pain in tennis elbow. Palpate and note the normal anatomic configura-tion of the medial and lateral epicondyles with the olecranon.

Range of Motion and Strength

Flexion and extension occur at the elbow joint, whereas supination and pronation occur at the proximal radioulnar joint. Note limitation of active and passive range of motion. Note hyperextensibility.

Other Tests

Assess for pain or increased laxity owing to injury of the medial collateral ligament by applying valgus stress with the elbow extended at 20 degrees of flexion. Similarly, assess the lateral collateral ligament by applying a varus stress.

KEY FINDING
Hand and Wrist

Hand

Note the normal attitude of the hand at rest. Inspect the small joints of the hand. Note asymmetry, deformity, contractures, swelling, erythema, and/or skin and fingernail lesions. Have the patient make a fist, and look for symmetry of the knuckles and fingers. Note thenar or hypothenar muscle atrophy. Assess active and passive range of motion of each joint of the fingers and the thumb. See FIGURE 11–2 for movements of the thumb. Test grip strength and strength against manual resistance for each finger and thumb. Localize soft-tissue or bony tenderness.

Mallet finger is an avulsion of the extensor tendon from its insertion on the distal phalanx that results in mallet finger deformity in which the distal interphalangeal (DIP) joint is in flexion and there is loss of ability to extend the finger at the DIP joint.

Boutonniere deformity is an avulsion of extensor tendon central slip insertion at the base of the proximal phalanx that results in a boutonniere deformity in which the proximal interphalangeal (PIP) joint is in flexion and the DIP joint is in hyperextention.

Skier's thumb or *gamekeeper's thumb* is a disruption of the ulnar collateral ligament of the thumb (metacarpophalangeal joint). With the thumb held in extension, stabilize the metacarpal, and apply valgus stress to assess for pain or increased laxity compared with the uninjured hand.

Wrist Joint

Note any swelling, deformity, or redness. Assess active and passive range of motion.

Nondisplaced fractures of the distal radius may present with subtle deformity, localized tenderness, and painful movements at the wrist. Tenderness on the ulnar side may be present in injury of the triangular fibrocartilage complex. The distal radius growth plate is also subject to chronic stress injury, resulting in bony prominence and localized tenderness. Tenderness in the anatomic snuff box is characteristic of a *scaphoid fracture.*

KEY FINDING
Spine and Back

Standing

Observe gait and posture; spine curvature for scoliosis, kyphosis, or lordosis; and alignment of the iliac crests. Look for scoliosis from behind the patient with the patient bending forward trying to touch his or her toes. With the patient standing, assess active range of motion of the lumbosacral spine (flexion, extension, lateral flexion, and rotation). Have the patient stand on one leg at a time and hyperextend the back. This will elicit pain in a case of spondylolysis (one-legged hyperextension test; FIGURE 11–23). In the Trendelenburg test, the side with the weak gluteus

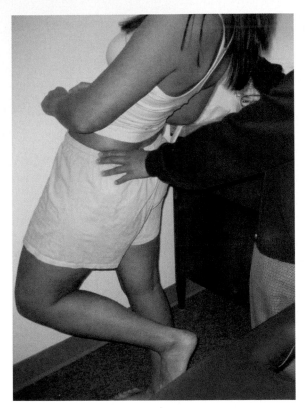

FIGURE 11–23   *The Hyperextension Test for Spondylolysis.*

medius (S_1) will sag, which represents a positive test. Normally, there is no sagging. Test muscle strength. Test the strength of the calf muscles by repeated unilateral heel raises (S_1) and the strength of anterior tibialis by heel walking (L_5). Palpate and localize soft-tissue or bony tenderness.

Supine Back Examination

Note the level of the anterosuperior iliac spines. Measure the leg length from the anterosuperior iliac spine to the medial malleolus. Note thigh or leg muscle atrophy. Test the strength of the following muscles: abdominals (T_6–L_1), hip flexors (L_2), quadriceps (knee extension, L_3), anterior tibialis (foot/ankle dorsiflexion, L_4), extensor hallucis longus (toe extension, L_5), and hamstrings (knee flexion, S_2).

Test sensation to touch and deep tendon reflexes of the lower extremities. With the patient supine on the table, have him or her raise an extended leg one at a time, and note if radiating pain occurs, owing to stretch on the sciatic nerves indicating sciatica.

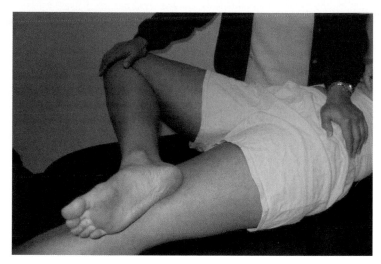

FIGURE 11–24 *Patrick Test.*

To elicit pain owing to sacroiliac joint pathology, have the patient supine on the table, flex, abduct, and externally rotate the leg (FIGURE 11–24); then gently put pressure over the pelvis with one hand and the opposite knee with the other to elicit pain in the sacroiliac region (Faber or Patrick test).

Prone

Differentiate between postural round back and kyphosis by hyperextending the back.

▼ KEY FINDING
◢ **Hips and Pelvis** Hip pathology may cause the patient to limp. Note localized groin swelling or redness. With intraarticular swelling, the hip is in a position of external rotation, abduction, and slight flexion. Note any fixed-flexion contracture at the hip. Note pelvic symmetry with the patient standing. Note any swelling of the thigh.

▼ KEY FINDING
◢ **Knees** Assess active range of motion with the patient standing or lying on the examination table. Test internal and external rotation at the hip with the patient lying prone on the examination table with the hip extended and knee flexed at 90 degrees. Internal rotation will elicit pain and resistance in a patient with an irritable hip because this position places maximum stretch on the joint capsule.

Palpate to localize tenderness in the groin (hip pathology), over the greater trochanter area (trochanteric bursitis), the symphysis pubis (osteitis pubis), and the iliac crest (iliac apophysitis). Note soft-tissue or bony swelling in the thigh.

Inspection

Note the location and extent of any swelling. Intraarticular effusion or bleeding results in a predominantly suprapatellar swelling that is uniform. Note the position of the patella with the patient standing, whether pointing out, straight, or inward. Note if the patella is high riding. A *Baker cyst* causes localized swelling in the popliteal fossa.

Palpation

Localize bony or soft-tissue tenderness. Tenderness over the patella is present in patellar fracture. Circumferential tenderness over the distal femur or proximal tibia may occur in injuries of the growth plate. Note joint-line tenderness in meniscal injuries. In large intraarticular effusion, the patella is ballottable. Assess active and passive range of motion and strength.

Special Tests

Patellar apprehension test. With the patient supine on the examination table with knees extended, apply laterally directed force to the patella. Pain or apprehension indicates patellar *subluxation.*

Lachman test. With the patient supine on the table with the knee at about 30 degrees of flexion, stabilize the femur with one hand just above the knee, and with the other hand just below the knee over the proximal tibia attempt to move the tibia forward (FIGURE 11–25). Loss of a definite endpoint to the motion indicates *tear of the anterior cruciate ligament.*

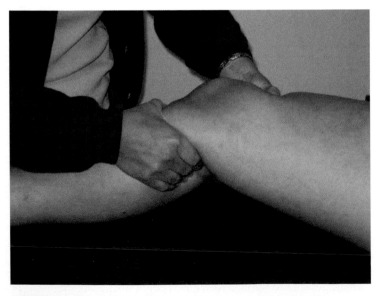

FIGURE 11–25 *Lachman Test.*

McMurray test. With the patient supine on the table with the hip and knee
flexed, with one hand over the knee with thumb on the lateral joint
line, and the fingers on the medial joint line, passively extend and
rotate the knee with the other hand just distal to the knee holding the
leg (FIGURE 11–26). Pain or click will occur with external rotation in

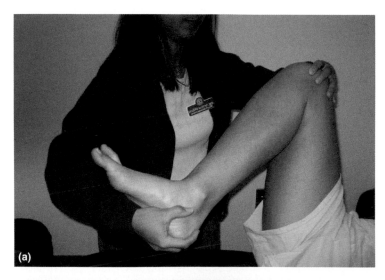

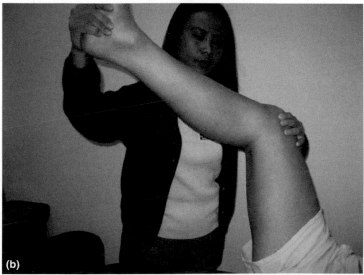

FIGURE 11–26 *A. McMurray Test Starting Position. B. McMurray Test
End Position.*

case of a *medial meniscal tear* and with internal rotation in case of a
tear of the lateral meniscus.

Varus and valgus stress test. With the patient supine on the table with the
knee at 20 degrees of flexion, with one hand just above the knee stabilizing the thigh, apply a varus or valgus stress with the other hand
just distal to the knee. Note pain or increased laxity medially in the
case of medial collateral ligament sprain with valgus stress and laterally in the case of a lateral collateral ligament sprain with a varus
stress.

KEY FINDING

Legs A localized swelling and tenderness over the tibial tuberosity is characteristic of *Osgood-Schlatter disease.* There is tenderness along
the tibia in medial tibial stress syndrome, and localized tenderness is
indicative of a *stress fracture.* Look for any bony swelling. Passive stretch
of the leg muscles will elicit pain in compartment syndromes. Calf tenderness should raise suspicion for *deep vein thrombosis.*

KEY FINDING

Inspection

Significant pain on weight bearing should raise suspicion for severe soft-
tissue disruption or fracture. Examine the ankle ideally with the patient
seated on the examination table with the knee flexed at 90 degrees and
the leg relaxed. Diffuse soft-tissue swelling is characteristic of ankle
sprain. Ecchymosis may develop around the ankle and may extend into
the foot. Intraarticular swelling obliterates the joint and Achilles definition. Note any deformity.

Palpation

Localize tenderness. Palpate the malleoli, anterior tibiofibular ligament,
calcaneofibular ligament, tibiofibular syndesmosis, talus, calcaneus,
tarsal navicular, base of the fifth metatarsal, Achilles tendon, and peroneal tendons. In injury to the distal fibular physis, tenderness localizes
about 2 to 3 cm proximal to the tip of the lateral malleolus. Assess passive and active range of motion.

Special Tests

Anterior drawer test. With the ankle in neutral position, grasp the heel
with one hand and attempt to move the foot forward with the other
hand (FIGURE 11–27). Look for increased anterior motion relative
to the uninjured ankle or a soft endpoint or increased pain, indicative of *sprain of the anterior talofibular ligament.*

Talar tilt. Note increased inversion or pain or soft endpoint with inversion motion indicative of *sprain of the calcaneofibular ligament.*

Squeeze test. With the patient seated on the table with the knee at 90 degrees
and the ankle in a neutral position, squeeze the distal calf. Pain in
the ankle is indicative of *injury to the tibiofibular syndesmosis.*

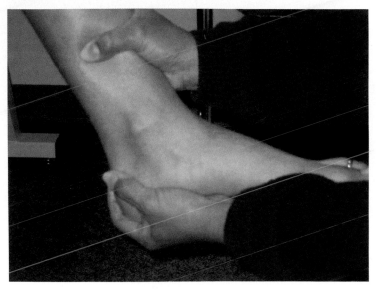

FIGURE 11–27 *Anterior Drawer Test for Ankle.*

External rotation test. Similarly, gently externally rotate the foot. Pain in the ankle is indicative of *injury to the tibiofibular syndesmosis.*

▼ KEY FINDING

▼ **Foot** Observe the patient from behind bearing weight fully. Note excessive pronation and loss of medial longitudinal arches of the feet. Note *pes planus* or *pes cavus* deformities, *bunion, ingrown toenail,* curly toes, or other toe deformities. Localize soft-tissue or bony tenderness. Assess active and passive range of motion of the toes. Elicit localized pain in the foot by squeezing the foot in case of a *Morton neuroma* or a *stress fracture.*

Synthesizing Diagnosis and Further Evaluation

In addition to the history of key symptoms and general history (see Chapter 1), certain aspects specific to musculoskeletal system will aid further in musculoskeletal diagnosis. It is important to gather a past history of similar symptoms and their course. A past history of joint injury is a risk factor for later osteoarthritis. A history of joint or ligamentous injury that has not had adequate rehabilitation is a risk factor for subsequent similar injury (e.g., repeated ankle sprains). A history of multiple fractures may suggest osteoporosis. Spondyloarthropathies evolve over several months to years with intermittent exacerbation and remission of symptoms. Family history may be positive in cases of spondyloarthropathy, psoriasis, gout, and hypermobility syndrome. Psychosocial history is essential in adolescents. Musculoskeletal symptoms are a common presentation in psychosomatic disorders in adolescents. A history of intravenous drug use or sexual activity may aid in the diagnosis of infectious arthritis.

In addition to symptoms and signs limited to the musculoskeletal system, one must consider carefully systemic or constitutional symptoms and signs (see TABLE 11–1) in formulating a differential diagnosis. Some systemic or neurologic conditions can present with numerous musculoskeletal complications, as in patients with cerebral palsy (TABLE 11–4). In infants and young children, certain types of skeletal injuries (TABLE 11–5) in the context of presenting history should raise suspicion of nonaccidental trauma and child abuse. Broad categories of conditions that present with predominant musculoskeletal symptoms and signs are listed in TABLE 11–6.

TABLE 11–4 *Musculoskeletal Abnormalities in Cerebral Palsy*

Gait	Scissoring, hemiplegia, crouch, toe-walking
Upper extremities	Flexion contractures at wrist, elbow, and shoulder
	Thumb-in-palm deformity
Spine	Scoliosis, kyphosis, exaggerated lumbar lordosis
	Sacral sitting posture
Pelvis	Wind-swept deformity
Hips	Flexion contracture and restricted range of motion
	Adductor contracture
	Subluxation and dislocation
	Rectus femoris tightness
Knees	Flexion contracture
	Genu valgus, varum, or recurvatum
	High-riding patella
Ankle and foot	Equinus deformity
	Achilles tightness, gastrocnemius, and soleus tightness
	Calcaneus deformity, calcaneoequinovarus, calcaneoequinovalgus
	Pes valgus, pes cavus, ankle valgus, hallux valgus
	Dorsal bunion
	In-toeing, out-toeing, metatarsus adductus
Rotational deformity	External femoral torsion, internal femoral torsion
	Tibial torsion

TABLE 11-5 *Skeletal Findings Suggestive of Nonaccidental Trauma*

Fractures
    Skull fractures
    Clavicle
    Scapula
    Sternum
    Spinous process
    Vertebral body
    Digits
    Shaft of the long bone
    Ribs

Other findings
    Characteristic metaphyseal fractures (corner or bucket handle)
    Multiple fractures at different ages
    Subperiosteal reaction or elevation
    Lower extremity fractures in nonambulatory children
    Bilateral acute fractures

When to Refer

A consultation with a rheumatologist is necessary in all rheumatic disease patients for further diagnostic workup and long-term management. The appropriate selection and interpretation of specific laboratory tests for rheumatic diseases can be challenging, and a rheumatology consultation can be most helpful.

Orthopedic and neurology consultation may be useful in neuromuscular diseases with orthopedic complications (e.g., cerebral palsy), myopathies, muscular dystrophies, and neuropathies. Findings suggestive of nonaccidental trauma or child abuse should prompt further evaluation by child abuse experts and other consultants.

A consultation with an orthopedic surgeon with special expertise in pediatric conditions is important for the following diagnoses based on initial evaluation:

- Bone tumors
- Congenital skeletal malformations and deformities
- Developmental dysplasia of hip
- Blount disease
- Bone and joint infection
- Legg-Calve-Perthes disease
- Slipped capital femoral epiphysis
- Severe scoliosis or kyphosis
- Significant leg-length inequality
- Complex fractures and dislocations
- Severe ligament injuries associated with joint instability
- Cartilage injuries
- All acute and chronic or stress injuries of the growth plate

TABLE 11-6 *Broad Categories Conditions with Musculoskeletal Symptoms and Signs*

Category	Selected Conditions	Labs and Imaging and Consultation
Developmental variations Seen in early childhood, these are physiologic conditions that correct with normal growth	External femoral or tibial torsion (out-toeing); internal femoral torsion or internal tibial version (in-toeing); physiologic genu varum or valgum	A careful observation is needed. If the condition is unilateral or associated with other signs or symptoms or developmental delay, further evaluation is needed.
Congenital and developmental conditions Characteristic abnormalities noted on examination at birth or soon thereafter during infancy.	Developmental dysplasia of the hip; congenital club foot; Klippel-Feil syndrome	Pediatric orthopedic consultation
Rheumatic diseases Typically present as inflammatory arthritis affecting one or more joints or other articular structures and systemic symptoms such as fever, fatigue, or weight loss. Disease may evolve over months to years. Family history may be positive (e.g., spondyloarthropathy, psoriasis, and gout). Predominant age at onset may vary depending on particular type of the disease.	Chronic juvenile arthritis; systemic arthritis; juvenile ankylosing spondylitis; psoriatic arthritis; juvenile dermatomyositis; scleroderma	CBC, ESR, and CRP are nonspecific indicators of inflammation. Specific rheumatologic tests should be considered in consultation with a pediatric rheumatologist. Plain films may show characteristic findings late in the disease and may not be useful in the initial diagnosis in most cases.

Chronic pain syndromes
Characterized by a chronic, intermittent course of variable intensity of widespread or regional noncharacteristic pain. Most likely to be seen in older children and adolescent age group. Family history may be positive in hypermobility syndrome.

Fibromyalgia; hypermobility syndrome; complex regional pain syndrome

No specific laboratory or imaging studies are characteristic of a specific disease. Depending on the personal experience of the pediatrician, further consultations may be needed to comanage these patients.

Vasculitis
Characteristic symptoms and signs of particular syndrome. Fever, abdominal pain, petechiae, and palpable purpura and mucus membrane inflammation are some of the features.

Henoch-Schönlein purpura; Kawasaki disease

CBC, ESR
Specific tests such as echocardiogram indicated in Kawasaki disease and pediatric cardiology consultation indicated.

Infections
Characterized by a history of exposure followed by joint pain, systemic symptoms, typically of acute onset. Can affect any age group except any age group except sexually transmitted diseases that affect adolescents. A history of unprotected sex in adolescents or intravenous drug users should be ascertained.

Disseminated gonococcal infection and arthritis; Lyme arthritis; postinfectious reactive arthritis; viral synovitis/arthritis; bacterial osteomyelitis

CBC, ESR, and CRP are nonspecific. Culture of appropriate body fluid or tissue for specific etiologic diagnosis. Serology for specific diagnosis in conjunction with typical syndrome.

(Continued)

345

TABLE 11-6 Broad Categories Conditions with Musculoskeletal Symptoms and Signs (Continued)

Category	Selected Conditions	Labs and Imaging and Consultation
Overuse syndromes Most common in the adolescent age group involved in sports and other physical activities. Can affect any soft tissue, bone, joint, cartilage, or growth plate. Characterized by activity-related pain of gradual onset, deteriorating sport performance, and localizing signs such as swelling and tenderness.	Stress injury of the distal physis of the radius; stress injury of proximal physis of the humerus; juvenile osteochondritis dissecans; Osgood-Schlatter disease; stress fractures; tendonitis affecting various tendons; bursitis affecting various bursae; lateral epicondylitis; idiopathic anterior knee pain	Plain radiographs are indicated in growth plate injury, juvenile OCD, stress fractures, joint pain, and swelling. A bone scan may be indicated to make early diagnosis of stress fracture. An MRI or CT scan may be indicated in some cases of juvenile OCD in consultation with an orthopedic surgeon.
Orthopedic conditions Each of the various orthopedic conditions presents with characteristic localizing symptoms and signs.	Legg-Calve-Perthes disease; slipped capital femoral epiphysis; Scheuermann disease	Plain radiography is indicated. Orthopedic consultation for further evaluation and definitive treatment.
Systemic disease Systemic diseases affecting bone and joint (arthropathy) present with other typical characteristics of the systemic syndrome.	Sickle cell disease; hemophilia; diabetes mellitus; sphingolipidoses	Specific laboratory tests are indicated, and management may need specialist consultation.
Metabolic bone disease A metabolic bone disease should be suspected with poor growth, poor nutritional status, recurrent fractures, and progressive joint deformities.	Rickets; idiopathic juvenile osteoporosis; osteogenesis imperfecta; hypophosphatasia; hypothyroidism	Metabolic and endocrinology workup in consultation with a pediatric endocrinologist

Benign neoplasms of the bone Most are asymptomatic and incidental findings on plain radiographs, e.g., aneurysmal bone cysts, fibrous dysplasias, nonossifying fibromas. There may be localized pain. In osteoid osteoma, the pain is characteristically relieved by aspirin.	Osteoid osteoma; osteoblastoma; nonossifying fibromas; aneurysmal bone cysts; fibrous dysplasia	Plain radiographs or CT scan may be indicated. Orthopedic consultation. Most do not need further evaluation or intervention.
Malignant neoplasms of the bone Nighttime pain, dull aching bone pain; adolescents most affected.	Osteogenic sarcoma; Ewing sarcoma	Plain radiographs are characteristic. Orthopedic and oncology consultation
Psychosomatic Important considerations in all adolescents.	Various somatic complaints	Further evaluation may require mental health consultation.
Peripheral neuropathy Characterized by neuropathic pain, paresthesia, and sensory and motor dysfunction in the distribution of the affected nerve. Uncommon in pediatric age group.	Median nerve (carpal tunnel syndrome); ulnar neuropathy; meralgia paraesthetica; tarsal tunnel syndrome	Electromyography, physiatrist consultation

(Continued)

TABLE 11-6 Broad Categories Conditions with Musculoskeletal Symptoms and Signs (Continued)

Category	Selected Conditions	Labs and Imaging and Consultation
Muscle disease Characterized by true insidious and progressive muscle weakness; stretch reflexes affected; sensation remains intact except in sensorimotor diseases; can be seen at any age; however, the particular type may be more prevalent or first recognized in different age groups.	Muscular dystrophies; myopathies	Creatine kinase; genetics consult and testing; metabolic workup
Acute trauma Characteristic history and mechanism of injury with specific localized findings on examination	Soft-tissue injuries; bone fractures; ligament sprains; intraarticular cartilage injuries	Plain radiography is indicated in severe injuries or when fracture is suspected. MRI is indicated in severe musculotendinous and ligament and cartilage injuries in consultation with an orthopedic surgeon.

Abbreviations: CBC = complete blood count; ESR = erythrocyte sedimentation rate; CRP = C-reactive protein; OCD = osteochondritis dissecans.

12 The Neurology System

Arthur N. Feinberg

The goals of this chapter are

1. To outline anatomic and physiologic structure and function of the neurology system
2. To analyze problems that are associated with perturbations in anatomy and physiology and develop a list of diagnostic possibilities
3. To outline common neurologic problems for infants, children, and adolescents and to expand and clarify the history to develop diagnostic hypotheses
4. To localize pathology by eliciting physical findings with a complete and appropriate-for-age neurologic examination
5. To develop a table narrowing neurologic diagnoses by etiology, clinical pattern, and epidemiology (incidence by age group)
6. To develop a plan for appropriate laboratory and imaging usage to substantiate diagnostic hypotheses
7. To discuss appropriate and timely referrals for subspecialty consultation

Physiology and Mechanics

Unlike adults, infants, children, and adolescents are ongoing works in progress; hence all neurologic evaluation must be in the context of an evolving background. Brain development begins prenatally, and rapid development continues during the first 2 years of life. *Neurulation*, the formation and closure of the neural tube, occurs during the first 3 weeks after conception. The ectodemal layer of the embryo forms a plate that converts into a closed neural tube during the third and fourth weeks of gestation. Incomplete or defective formation of the neural tube, *neural tube defects*, is a common malformation of the human central nervous system (CNS). All portions of the CNS and certain endocrine glands evolve from the neural tube. The most rostral portion of the canal, the *anterior neuropore*, closes at about 24 days and then undergoes marked differentiation and cleavage (prosencephalization) to form the forebrain. *Neurogenesis* refers to the development of neurons and their supportive cells (glia) from the inner cells of the neural tube and mainly ends during the third trimester.

The events of neural maturation after the induction and formation of the neural tube include (1) mitotic proliferation of neuroblasts, (2) programmed death of excess neuroblasts, (3) neuroblast migration, and (4) growth of axons and dendrites. At 10 to 15 weeks, the first hemispheric fissures appear, and the smooth exterior of the forebrain converts the pattern of gyri and sulci that will bury 75 percent of the cortical surface.

Cellular proliferation and migration to the hemispheres occur up until the second trimester, during which time the neuroblasts migrate along glial cell fibers with the innermost structures of the cerebrum. The cerebellum and neural crest cells migrate in a different pattern. Once migration has occurred, cell differentiation allows for the development of axons, dendrites, and their connections. Synaptogenesis begins at birth and occurs most rapidly during the first 3 to 4 months of age. Myelination occurs most rapidly from birth until about 2 years of age but continues throughout childhood and is responsible for insulation of axons and increasing conduction velocity.

The neurons, their myelin sheaths, and their connections (synapses) conduct electrical impulses. Simply, individual neurons maintain a difference in electrical potential or polarity (70 μV) across their membranes by energy-dependent (ATP) pumps that force sodium (Na^+) ions outside the cell membrane and potassium (K^+) ions inside the cell. The neurons maintain this resting potential. Depolarization initiates cellular impulses, during which time Na^+ effluxes from outside to inside the neuron and K^+ flows in the opposite direction. After the ionic flux, the cell returns to its original state of potential difference (repolarization). The impulses travel down the original axons toward the cell bodies and then on to the dendrites and synaptic clefts, releasing neurotransmitters presynaptically. These neurotransmitters—epinephrine, norepinephrine, dopamine, and gamma-aminobutyric acid (GABA)—are responsible for cell-to-cell communication. They determine postsynaptically whether impulses are excitatory (depolarization) or inhibitory (hyperpolarization).

The CNS is a complex arrangement of billions of neurons organized into bundles and pathways that serve the several functions discussed in the following section. One can detect the summation of electrical impulses traveling through these pathways by placing electrodes in areas outside the CNS (e.g., electroencephalography or auditory evoked potentials). Although the underlying physics goes well beyond the scope of this chapter, perturbations of electrical potentials and their transmission through multiple cells correlate with changes in these patterns and with neurologic symptoms.

Functional Anatomy

The human neurologic system consists of three main parts: the central (CNS), peripheral (PNS), and autonomic (ANS). The CNS, encased in bone, consists of the cerebrum, cerebellum, brain stem, and spinal cord. FIGURES 12–1 through 12–4 outline the gross anatomy of the CNS. The PNS consists of fibers that coalesce into ganglia and plexuses and then

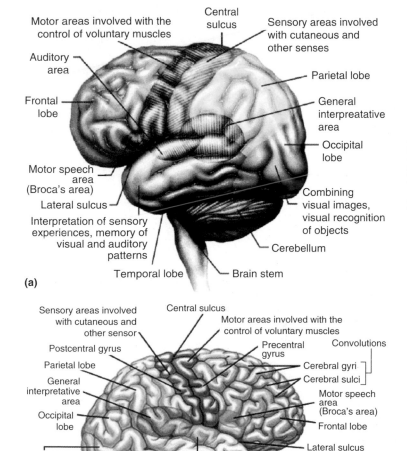

FIGURE 12-1 *A. Surface Anatomy of the Brain. B. Surface anatomy of the brain. (From: Van de Graaff KM:* Human Anatomy. *New York: McGraw-Hill, 2002, Fig. 11.21, p. 366, Fig. 11.19, p. 364.)*

redistribute into peripheral nerves that have either motor or sensory function. The neuromuscular junction and skeletal muscles are also part of this system.

The ANS consists of parasympathetic and sympathetic fibers that innervate smooth muscle of many internal structures, including the heart

Cerebrum and Diencephalon-Cross Section

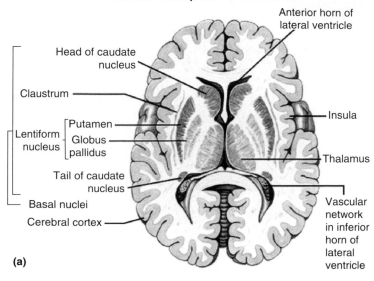

(a)

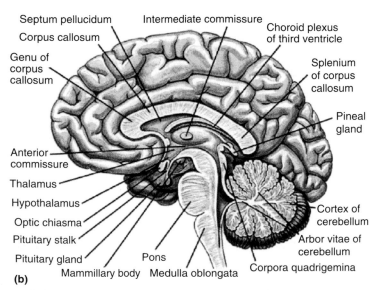

(b)

FIGURE 12-2 *A. Cross Section of the Brain. B. Cross section of the brain. (From Van de Graaff KM:* Human Anatomy. *New York: McGraw-Hill, 2002, Fig. 11.20, p 365, Fig. 11.24, p. 370.)*

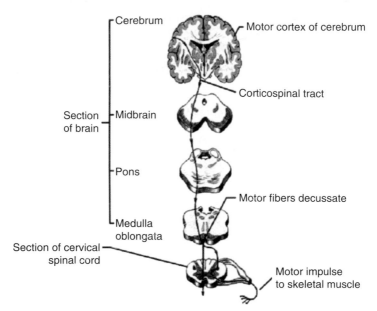

FIGURE 12–3 *Motor Pathways.* (From Van de Graaff KM: Human Anatomy. New York: McGraw-Hill, 2002, Fig. 11.41, p. 387.)

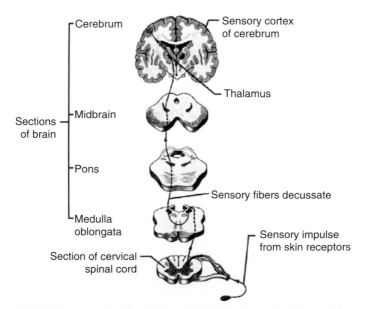

FIGURE 12–4 *Sensory Pathways.* (From: Van de Graaff KM: Human Anatomy. New York: McGraw-Hill, 2002, Fig. 11.42, p. 387.)

and blood vessels and the respiratory, gastrointestinal, and genitourinary systems, which play a significant role in their function. The adrenal medulla and other paraffin cells are also part of the ANS. Autonomic fibers innervate skin glands and hairs.

The PNS, with input from the CNS, originates from cranial, cervical, and sacral roots. Their fibers travel to and aggregate in ganglia, close to the organs which they supply. The sympathetic nervous system, part of the ANS, also with input from the CNS, originates from the thoracic and lumbar roots and aggregates into ganglia that form a chain near the spine. In general, the sympathetic nervous system, mediated by adrenergic fibers, is stimulatory to the cardiovascular and respiratory systems and inhibitory to the gastrointestinal and genitourinary systems. The parasympathetic nervous system, also part of the ANS, mediated by cholinergic fibers, is stimulatory to the gastrointestinal and genitourinary systems and inhibitory to the cardiovascular and respiratory systems.

The functional organization of the CNS is important to understand. In brief, the cerebrum serves all aspects of cognition (intellect, memory, language, attention, and orientation), sensation discrimination (pain, touch, temperature and vibration, proprioception, and spatial discrimination), motor function (pyramidal and extrapyramidal), and mood and affect (fear and anxiety via the limbic system). Complex cognitive function localizes to the dominant hemisphere (usually the left hemisphere in a right-handed person). Sensory input from peripheral receptors with specific segmental representation travels toward the spinal cord (see FIGURE 12–1) and then ultimately to specific point-by-point regions in the parietal lobe posterior to the central sulcus (postcentral gyrus) (see FIGURE 12–2). Voluntary motor function originates from the precentral gyrus, with sensory input, and travels through the pyramidal and extrapyramidal pathways and through the spinal cord and peripheral neurons, and on to the neuromuscular junctions. The medial dominant temporal lobe via the uncus olfactory and limbic system is the pathway for mood and affect. The occipital lobe is the waystation for visual stimuli. The frontal lobe, loosely organized, is involved in behavior and affect.

The cerebellum integrates sensory and motor input for posture, balance, and coordination. Sensory and motor impulses stimulate muscle groups to contract and relax, but the cerebellum coordinates this input into fluid movement.

The brain stem contains the midbrain, the pons, and the medulla. It supplies fibers to the ANS and is therefore involved in unconscious vital functions such as pulse and respiratory rate and reflexive gastrointestinal and genitourinary functions. It also contains nuclei to cranial nerves III to XII. Cranial nerve function is summarized as follows:

Cranial nerve I (olfactory). Sensory nerve receiving input from the nasal passages that pierces the cribriform plate and consolidates into the olfactory bulbs at the bases of the frontal lobes and then on to the olfactory nerves.

Cranial nerve II (optic). Input from the retina with sensory fibers coalescing into the optic nerve, leading to the optic chiasm, and ultimately crossing and looping through the cerebral cortex to the occipital lobe.

Cranial nerve III (oculomotor). The motor nerve that innervates all extrinsic eye muscles except the lateral rectus and superior oblique. Its nucleus lies in the posterior midbrain, and then it branches into separate nuclei for each muscle.

Cranial nerve IV (trochlear). This motor nerve provides innervation for the superior oblique extrinsic eye muscle.

Cranial nerve V (trigeminal). This is the largest cranial nerve, with both sensory and motor components. The sensory division divides into the ophthalmic, maxillary, and mandibular branches. The ophthalmic branch receives input from the cornea, conjunctivae, ciliary body, nasal cavity, sinuses, eyes (not the lids), eyebrows, forehead, and nose. The side of the nose, eyelids, palate, and maxillary gingivae leads to the maxillary branch. The mandibular branch derives from the temporal region, mandibular gingivae, anterior two-thirds of the tongue, lower lip, mandible, and teeth. The motor component of the trigeminal nerve innervates the deep muscles of mastication (temporalis and masseter).

Cranial nerve VI (abducens). This nerve provides motor innervation for the extraocular lateral rectus muscle.

Cranial nerve VII (facial). This complex nerve has sensory, motor, and antonomic functions. Sensory input comes from organs of taste from the anterior two-thirds of the tongue, the ear canal, and the skin behind the ear. Motor fibers innervate facial muscles of expression, as well as the stapedius, stylohyoideus, and posterior belly of the digastricus. Autonomic motor fibers run to the chorda tympani nerve, ultimately leading to secretion in the submaxillary and sublingual salivary glands.

Cranial nerve VIII (acoustic). This is a purely sensory nerve, with the cochlear branch supplying the organ of Corti, serving auditory function, and the vestibular branch leading to the semicircular canals, involved in balance.

Cranial nerve IX (glossopharyngeal). Sensory fibers for pain, touch, and temperature arise from the posterior pharynx and tonsils, and fibers for taste derive from the posterior two-thirds of the tongue. Motor branches innervate pharyngeal muscles.

Cranial nerve X (vagus). This is the most extensive of the cranial nerves—hence the term *vagus* ("wandering"). It consists of sensory, motor, and autonomic branches from the pharynx, neck, thorax, and abdomen. Its cervical branches are the pharyngeal and superior and recurrent laryngeal and superior cardiac nerves. Its thoracic branches are the inferior cardiac, anterior and posterior bronchial, and esophageal nerves. Its abdominal branches are the gastric and hepatic nerves, as well as the celiac and mesenteric ganglia.

Cranial nerve XI (spinal accessory). This is a pure motor nerve that innervates the trapezius and sternocleidomastoid muscles.

Cranial nerve XII (hypoglossal). This nerve serves motor function of the tongue.

The spinal cord contains ascending sensory tracts receiving impulses for touch, pain (lateral spinothalamic tracts), pain and temperature (anterior spinothalamic tracts), and position and vibration sense (posterior columns). It also contains descending centrolateral motor fibers (upper motor neurons and anterior horn cells), which are inhibitory. The dorsal spinal roots contain sensory fibers, and the ventral spinal roots contain motor fibers.

The peripheral nerves are sensory, motor, and autonomic. As mentioned earlier, the sensory nerves receive impulses from the periphery in segmental fashion, as demonstrated in FIGURE 12–1. Peripheral motor nerves contain only lower motor neurons, which conduct impulses to muscle groups via the neuromuscular junction (NMJ) mediated by acetylcholine. The unit of force (strength) is the motor unit, each one consisting of an anterior horn cell, its axon, the lower motor neuron, the NMJ, and all the muscle fibers innervated. The number of muscle fibers per anterior horn cell reflects the fineness of muscle motion. The motor units in the gluteus muscle may have 200 fibers per anterior horn cell, whereas the extraocular muscles are 1:1. It is indeed remarkable to imagine the delicate interplay between sensory and motor fibers, with cerebral and cerebellar input stimulating, inhibiting, and coordinating multiple muscle groups simultaneously, resulting in fluid and purposeful movements.

Problems

A good pediatric neurologic history *always* considers the timeline of development. Infants, children, and adolescents are works in progress, and the nervous system is constantly changing throughout that time. Since presentations to a physician may be based on parental observations, we prefer the term *problem* to *history*. Variations from normal patterns of growth and development throughout the first decades may indicate neurologic disorders. A basic timeline for growth and development appears in Chapter 1. Moreover, neurologic disorders follow a timeline of their own (see FIGURE 12–5). Always consider the following in any neurologic history: "Does the timeline indicate a static, worsening, or

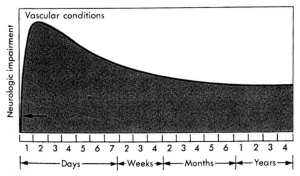

FIGURE 12–5 *Patterns of Onset and Course of Neurologic Conditions. Arrow signifies point of clinical recognition. (From Swaiman KF, Ashwal S (eds): Pediatric* Neurology: Principles and Practice, *3d ed. St. Louis: Mosby, 1999, Fig. 1.1, p. 2, with permission.)*

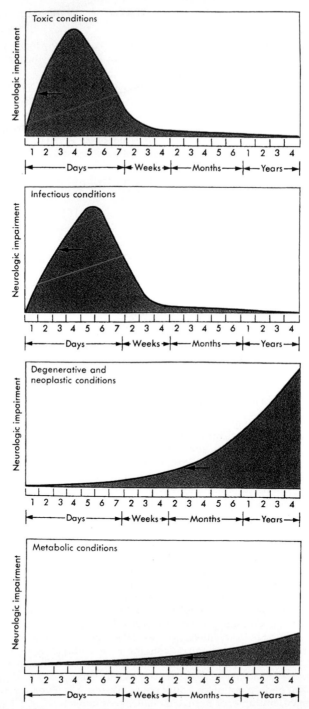

FIGURE 12-5 *(Continued)*

improving condition?" "At what rate is the condition progressing?" "Can we correlate the onset of illness with any event in the history, e.g., febrile illness, injury, or toxin ingestion?"

The next section will present common neurologic symptoms: seizures, headache, altered consciousness, developmental delay, focal weakness, diffuse weakness (hypotonia), clumsiness (ataxia), and movement disorders. Then the standard framework for pediatric diagnosis will be used to place possibilities into the categories "congenital," "infectious," "metabolic/toxic," "traumatic," "neoplastic," and "vascular."

History

Infants

KEY PROBLEM

Seizures A *seizure* is a transitory disturbance in brain function associated with an abnormal electrical discharge of the brain. Since infants are unable to provide a history, clinicians are dependent on caretakers' perceptions. How long do the episodes last? Is consciousness altered or lost? Is there apnea or color change? Do the seizures appear generalized, or are they limited to one part of the body? Does the abnormal movement vary from one part of the body to another? Has the patient been ill or febrile? Has the child's neurodevelopment been normal? Is there a family history of seizures or other neurologic disorders? Has there been any exposure to toxins or drugs?

At this point one can categorize by the standard pediatric framework:

Congenital. Symptoms usually occur earlier in life. If development is delayed, think of chromosomal abnormalities or other syndromes, e.g., neurocutaneous, embryologic malformations (errors in neurulation such as gyral malformations, e.g., *micropachygyria, schizencephaly, lissencephaly,* etc.). Neurocutaneous syndromes such as *incontinentia pigmenti, tuberous sclerosis,* and *neurofibromatosis* are causes of seizures in infancy. Sudden jerking movement of the torso or limbs suggests *myoclonic seizures*. The most violent myoclonic seizure is a sudden flexion at the waist, termed *infantile spasms* (*West syndrome*). With normal development, myoclonic seizures may be a transitory benign movement disorder (essential myoclonic), but myoclinic seizures with delayed or declining development are associated more often with severe brain disorders.

Genetic. Genetically determined *epilepsies* are the most common cause of a first seizure in an otherwise normal child. *Simple febrile seizures* are the most common genetic epilepsy of infancy. If the seizure was short-lived (<15 minutes), not associated with a postictal state, and occurred after the age of 6 months, this is more likely a benign febrile seizure. Such seizures last until age 5 but reach a peak in infancy at around 18 months of age. They are usually single, brief, and generalized and do not predict later nonfebrile seizures. Even when prolonged, multiple, or focal, later epilepsy is unlikely.

Infectious/inflammatory/immune. Consider lumbar puncture for any infant with a fever and a seizure. CNS infections may be *bacterial, viral, fungal,* or *parasitic.* Infants who have seizures secondary to *bacterial meningitis* or *viral encephalitis* are comatose afterwards. Most infections produce generalized seizures. *Herpes simplex encephalitis* may present with focal seizures, but not in infants. *Herpes simplex* types VI and VII are associated with febrile seizures.

Metabolic/toxic. Perturbations in glucose and electrolyte metabolism (Na^+, K^+, Ca^{2+}, and Mg^{2+}) are the usual cause. Inborn errors of metabolism usually cause systemic symptoms (vomiting, failure to thrive, and developmental deterioration). Consider *organic acidemias, aminoacidurias,* and *urea cycle defects.* Always determine if the child ingested any drugs or toxins that may have caused the seizure.

Traumatic (perinatal and postnatal). Always ask for the birth history. *Hypoxic-ischemic encephalopathy* is a common cause of seizures and cerebral palsy. If developmental delay is present, it is often not progressive, and not deteriorating. Always consider postnatal trauma, both intentional and unintentional, including *shaken-baby syndrome.*

Neoplastic. Tumors are very rare in infancy and generally do not present with seizures.

Vascular. Infants may have cerebrovascular accidents owing to both thrombosis and hemorrhage. Consider *arteriovenous malformations* (AVMs), *midline malformations of the vein of Galen, arterial aneurysms, bleeding,* and *clotting disorders.*

Other conditions mimicking seizures include *breath-holding spells,* a genetic disorder of infancy. The patient may turn pale or blue. The child does not hold the breath but stops breathing in expiration. The two forms are *cyanotic,* usually initiated by anger and frustration, and *pallid,* initiated by surprise. The change in facial color differentiates breath-holding spells from seizures. Movement disorders such as *essential myoclonus* may be confused with seizures. Consciousness is maintained.

KEY PROBLEM

■ **Altered Consciousness** This may manifest as agitation and/or confusion. Important areas to question include recent illness, fever, possible ingestion, and past medical and family history of conditions causing alteration of consciousness.

Congenital. Severe *syndromic CNS malformations, hydrocephalus,* and other causes of *increased intracranial pressure* may present with altered states of consciousness.

Infectious. Consider all bacterial, viral, fungal, and rickettsial infections.

Genetic/metabolic/toxic. Always think of *glucose* and *electrolyte imbalances, acidosis,* and their etiologies (endocrine, hepatic, renal, and *inborn errors of metabolism*). It is important to assess the home environment for medications and toxins because infants are always subject to *poisoning,* either accidental or intentional. *Inborn errors of metabolism,* particularly disorders of ammonia utilization, are causes, as are endocrinopathies such as *hypothyroidism* and *hypoadrenalism.* Hepatic, renal, and pulmonary failure alters consciousness through *ammonia toxicity, uremia,* or *severe hypercarbia.*

Traumatic. Head trauma, from concussion to severe intracranial bleeding, may cause alteration of consciousness. This may be intentional or unintentional and may result from shaking as well as direct contact. Prenatal *hypoxic-ischemic encephalopathy* may cause significant damage. Symptoms may be a result of increased intracranial pressure owing to *cerebral edema.*

Neoplastic. Tumors are very rare in infants. If they are located in the posterior fossa, they are usually close to the midline and may cause altered consciousness by blocking the flow of cerebrospinal fluid (CSF).

Vascular. These conditions are also rare and may present as a thrombotic or hemorrhagic *stroke.*

KEY PROBLEM
◢ Developmental Delay/Regression

The first 2 years of life is the period in which health professionals scrutinize neurodevelopment more closely than during any other age interval. Determining the onset of developmental failure is critical. Was the onset precipitous, or was it associated with a life event? Is development progressing slowly or regressing? Are all aspects of development (gross and fine motor, adaptive, language, and personal-social) affected? Consider developmental delay and regression separately.

Developmental Delay

Congenital/metabolic/genetic. Many of these conditions appear in the first 2 years. Consider *neurocutaneous syndromes* in children with consistent skin manifestations. Suspect genetic syndromes such as trisomies if the patient is dysmorphic. They may not cause deterioration but nonetheless are devastating owing to profound delay. *Fragile-X syndrome* is common. Consult sources on congenital malformations for a fuller differential diagnosis. *Hypothyroidism* is a common cause that newborn screening reveals.

Infections/inflammatory/immune. Think of *HIV encephalopathy* or recent bacterial or viral infection. Intrauterine infections (*TORCH*) are frequent causes. Congenital *cytomegalovirus* infection is the most common infectious cause of developmental delay in childhood. In some populations, *HIV* infection is a more common cause.

Traumatic. Mental retardation may well be a consequence of perinatal hypoxia or head injury. *Cerebral palsy* will become apparent in late infancy. Developmental delay is usually static and nonprogressive.

Neoplastic. These conditions are rare in infancy.

Developmental Regression

Congenital/genetic/metabolic. Consider inborn errors of metabolism (*lysosomal storage diseases, mucopolysaccharidoses*) and other genetic disorders that cause gray and/or white matter degeneration. As a rule, the characteristic features of gray matter disorders are early seizures and intellectual deterioration, whereas white matter disorders are macrocephaly and *blindness. Rett syndrome* presents with hand-wringing movements, seizures, and mental deterioration in girls. *Lesch-Nyhan syndrome* presents with self-destructive behavior and mental deterioration. *Mitochondrial disorders* affect organs with high-energy requirements (brain, eye, kidney, heart, and skeletal muscle), and *inborn errors of metabolism* cause seizures and multiorgan failure.

Infectious/inflammatory/immune. Consider progressive *HIV encephalopathy*. Also, slow viral infections (*subacute sclerosing panencephalitis* secondary to *measles*) will cause developmental regression, although it no longer occurs in the United States.

Traumatic/neoplastic/vascular. These conditions usually occur acutely in infancy but do not cause progressive symptoms unless there is a secondary complication such as increasing hydrocephalus.

KEY PROBLEM

Focal Weakness *Focal weakness,* hemiplegia (weakness or paralysis on one side), paraplegia (weakness or paralysis of both legs), and quadriplegia (weakness or paralysis of all four extremities) may be cerebral, spinal, or plexus in origin. *Any hand preference on the part of an infant under 2 years of age is distinctly pathologic.* Facial weakness and dysphagia originate from the lower brain stem and cranial nerves VII, IX, and X. It is always important to determine whether the findings are static or progressive.

Congenital. Consider migration defects as a cerebral cause. Facial asymmetry may arise from cranial nerves owing to aplasia of nuclei of the facial nerve or muscles (*Mobius syndrome*) or as an isolated aplasia of the depressor anguli oris muscle (*asymmetric crying facies*). Congenital malformation of the spinal cord such as *arteriovenous malformation* (AVM), *spina bifida, tethered cord, arachnoid cysts,* and *Chiari malformation* may be responsible for hemiplegia, paraplegia, or quadriplegia, as is external pressure on the spinal cord or nerve roots in such conditions as *osteopetrosis* and *atlantoaxial dislocation* (*Klippel-Feil, Morquio, and Down syndromes*). Caudal regression syndrome (*sacral agenesis*) occurs in infants of diabetic mothers and involves both lower extremities.

Infectious/inflammatory/immune. Meningoencephalitis of *bacterial, viral,* or *fungal* origin rarely causes focal weakness, but brain abscess or *subdural effusion* as a complication of bacterial meningitis will. Cranial or peripheral nerve involvement is usually postinfectious following a viral infection (*Bell palsy, herpes zoster*). Depending on the degree of involvement, *abscess, diskitis, viral myelitis, osteomyelitis* (*bacterial, tuberculous*), and *sarcoidosis* will cause hemiplegia, diplegia, or paraplegia. *Poliomyelitis* was an all-too-common but now oft-forgotten cause of focal weakness.

Genetic/metabolic/toxic. Consider *familial lipoprotein disorders* and *mitochondrial disorders.* Gray and white matter disorders and *demyelinating diseases* are very rare in infancy and will cause paraplegia and quadriplegia.

Traumatic. Any significant brain or spinal cord injury may result in focal weakness and may produce monoplegia or diplegia or quadriplegia depending on which areas are involved. Neonatal or postnatal trauma or hypoxia may produce focal lesions secondary to focal bleeding (*subdural or epidural bleed*) or hypoxia. Birth injury owing to pressure against the uterine wall or difficult forceps delivery may cause peripheral facial nerve palsy. During birth or later in life, the spinal cord may suffer external compression from *vertebral fractures* or *dislocations* resulting in *hematomas* of the cord or its coverings or frank *transection*. Pressure and trauma to the brachial or lumbar plexuses are common causes of focal weakness and may be postnatal as in *Erb palsy* (proximal brachial, inability to externally rotate the humerus, or Porter's tip syndrome) or *Klumpke palsy* (lower proximal and distal brachial, clawed fingers).

Neoplastic. Primary *tumors* causing acute or progressive hemiplegia are very rare in infancy, but metastatic *neuroblastoma* or *Ewing sarcoma* may occur in this age group.

Vascular. Vascular disorders cause hemiplegia, which may be static or progressive. Infants and newborns may have cerebrovascular accidents in utero or soon after birth. This is often associated with a hypercoagulable state such as *protein C and S deficiency* or *factor V Leiden mutation*. Infants may have *AVMs* causing hemorrhagic strokes. Consider neurocutaneous syndromes such as *Sturge-Weber syndrome*, which may cause progressive symptoms. *Bleeding diatheses* such as thrombocytopenia and clotting factor deficiency may cause intracranial hemorrhage. It is important to consider a primary cardiac condition (*cyanotic heart disease, valvular defects*) that may cause thrombi to dislodge and embolize to the brain.

Condition Mimicking Spasticity

Hyperesplexia (now known as *stiff baby syndrome*) is a rare condition in the newborn period presenting as total stiffness in an otherwise alert baby. True spasticity is very unlikely in a newborn. This condition is hereditary and resolves slowly over 3 to 5 years.

● KEY PROBLEM
◐ Hypotonia *Hypotonia may originate from the brain, spinal cord, anterior horn cells, peripheral nerves, neuromuscular junction, or muscle.*

Congenital/metabolic/toxic. Most congenital hypotonia in infants results from malformation (migration and neurulation defects). *All autosomal chromosomal abnormalities produce hypotonia at birth.* Other causes include *oculocerebrorenal (Lowe) syndrome,* consisting of cataracts, mental retardation, and renal tubular acidosis, and *familial dysautonomia (Riley-Day syndrome),* with typical autonomic instability. Include *peroxisomal disorders* and other storage diseases owing to peripheral neuropathy. Most of these disorders are severe and/or progressive and carry a poor prognosis. *Metabolic myopathies, storage diseases, carnitine deficiency,* and *respiratory chain enzyme deficiencies* (*mitochondrial disorders*) cause hypotonia. Heavy metals may cause a *peripheral neuropathy* and subsequent weakness. Neurotoxins such as *botulinum* and that from a tick are a significant etiology of weakness, affecting the neuromuscular junction. Congenital and hereditary disorders involving the anterior horn cell include *spinal muscular atrophies,* which are progressive and bode badly. Congenital mypoathies and congenital muscular dystrophy are rare but are included in the differential diagnosis. Consider *benign congenital hypotonia* if the weakness slowly recovers during infancy, but many patients still have residual language and learning disabilities.

Infectious/immune. Weakness is often an immunologic consequence of a *viral* infection or sometimes *mycoplasmal infection,* as illustrated by *Guillain-Barré syndrome* or other *polyneuropathies. Myasthenia gravis* may occur in infancy and presents as *ptosis* and gradually increasing weakness. Maternal antibodies for *myasthenia gravis* may cause neuromuscular junction (NMJ) blockade in newborns, gradually improving through infancy. Infants may ingest *botulinum* toxin from unprocessed honey and develop neuromuscular junction blockade.

Neoplastic. These processes play little role in infantile weakness.

Vascular. Vascular accidents anywhere in the CNS rarely may cause infantile hypotonia.

Traumatic. Hypotonia owing to cerebral hypoxia may be persistent or occur as an early manifestation of *cerebral palsy,* with the typical hypertonia and spasticity supervening. Trauma and hypoxia to the spinal cord often owing to difficult delivery also play a significant early role in hypotonia.

Conditions Mimicking Hypotonia

Frequently, in a child under age 2, one may misconstrue weakness for ataxia. Nonuse may be secondary to pain because the infant does not want to move the involved extremity. This presents in *osteomyelitis, myositis, septic arthritis, metastatic bone pain,* and *fractures.* Also consider vitamin deficiencies such as *rickets* (pathologic fractures) and *scurvy* (Parrot paralysis). *Hypervitaminosis A* may cause painful bony exostoses.

KEY PROBLEM
■ Clumsiness (Ataxia) *Ataxia* is a broad term for loss of fine control of posture and movement. This occurs primarily in the cerebellum, which coordinates sensory and motor input and output. However, ataxia also may originate from cerebral disorders or sensory deficits. Cerebral deficits manifest as spastic or hemiplegic gaits. Posterior column deficits cause loss of proprioception, resulting in the patient lifting his or her feet high off the ground and slapping them down. *Peripheral neuropathies* may produce a similar gait. Visual compensation occurs in sensory but not cerebellar ataxias.

Congenital. Malformations such as *cerebellar aplasias* and *Chiari* and *Dandy-Walker malformations* are common causes of ataxia in infants. Recurrent ataxias may be hereditary—hence the importance of a family history.

Infectious/inflammatory/immune. Viral and rarely *rickettsial* infections are more likely to cause acute cerebellar ataxia in this age group. This may be progressive and devastating. *Postinfectious ataxia* may occur weeks after an initial infection and is most likely an immune response. This is alarming at first, but patients recover, usually uneventfully, during the ensuing months.

Genetic/metabolic/toxic. Acute toxic ingestions of any kind will cause abnormalities anywhere in the CNS, including the cerebellum. *Heavy metal poisoning* will involve peripheral nerves. Ataxias owing to metabolic conditions may be progressive and carry a poor prognosis. These include spinocerebellar degenerative disorders, progressive ataxias, and various storage diseases. *Inborn errors of metabolism* and *mitochondrial disorders* are also causes of ataxia.

Traumatic. This may occur with localized bleeds or hematomas of the cerebellum. A serious complication of trauma is a *vertebrobasilar occlusion.*

Neoplastic. Most brain tumors in children are subtentorial and present with ataxia. Since they occur more commonly in children than in infants, we will discuss them below.

Vascular. As with cerebral disorders, consider *AVM* and *hypercoagulable states.* Vasculitis is not common in infancy.

■ **Movement Disorders** These are rare in infancy. Please refer to subsequent section on children for further detail. Some genetic progressively degenerative conditions may appear at this time. In particular, in an infant girl, repetitive hand-wringing movements may be an early manifestation of *Rett syndrome.* Seizures and mental deterioration will ensue.

Congenital/metabolic/genetic. Think of embryologic brain malformations, as well as metabolic and neurodegenerative disorders mentioned in the sections on developmental delay and altered consciousness.

Infectious/inflammatory/immune. Movement disorders may be a residual of *meningoencephalitis* of any etiology, notably following the 1918 influenza epidemic.

Traumatic. Think of cerebral anoxia, either perinatal or postnatal, and kernicterus secondary to *bilirubin encephalopathy.*

Neoplastic. Tumors rarely cause movement disorders in infancy.

Vascular. Movement disorders may occur following cerebrovascular accidents in utero or in infancy.

Children

■ **Seizures** Children's *seizures* may be generalized (*grand-mal, petit-mal, tonic, clonic, tonic-clonic, myoclonic*) or *partial* (simple, without altered consciousness, or *complex* with altered consciousness). *Partial* seizures may generalize, secondarily. Seizures will be outlined according to this scheme. Generalized seizures that are not extensions of partial seizures are most often idiopathic and fall under the umbrella of *epilepsy.* An aura often precedes, i.e., feeling strange or changes in sensation or perception. The patient loses consciousness as the seizure begins with the tonic phase and then progresses to the clonic phase. There is usually loss of bladder or bowel control. The seizures may be of short or long duration, and often a postictal state may follow with altered consciousness or focal paralysis (*Todd paralysis*). Absence seizures (petit-mal) present as short alterations in consciousness with staring spells or eyelid fluttering. The patient does not lose consciousness and rarely falls. They appear like eye-rolling or daydreaming and sometimes engender needless punishment. *Hyperventilation* may bring on an episode. *Myoclonic epilepsy* presents as muscle jerks and is not to be confused with benign myoclonic jerks, a normal occurrence. *Myoclonic epilepsy* is usually benign but nonetheless may be associated with learning disabilities and behavioral problems. Complex myoclonic epilepsy may be associated with more severe mental retardation. Progressive myoclonic epilepsy is usually a result of *metabolic* or *mitochondrial* disorders, and outcomes are devastating.

Partial seizures may originate from any area of the cerebral cortex. Simple partial seizures are not associated with alteration of consciousness and often manifest symptoms consonant with their location. Specifically, the postcentral gyrus of the parietal lobe may be the center for alterations in sensation, whereas the precentral gyrus houses the motor strip, and seizures originating from there will present with motor changes (see FIGURE 12-1). *Occipital seizures* will present with flashes of light. *Benign rolandic epilepsy* originates from the rolandic fissure and frequently follows the parietal lobe patterns discussed earlier. The prognosis is excellent. *Complex partial seizures* originate in the temporal lobe, which connects with the limbic circuit. These are associated with auras, alterations of consciousness, automatisms, and lip smacking. The movements are nondirective and repetitive, and the child appears frightened. *Rasmussen syndrome* is of undetermined etiology and causes progressive severe seizures. It typically affects only one hemisphere and responds poorly to medication. Patients may benefit from ablative surgery.

Congenital/metabolic/genetic. Congenital brain malformations are static and will continue throughout childhood. Most of the metabolic causes mentioned in the section on infancy are so devastating that many patients do not survive into childhood or continue to deteriorate very badly. Children as well as infants will ingest *toxins* and *poisons* that may be a cause of seizures.

Infectious/inflammatory/immune. The differential diagnosis is similar to that of infancy. *Simple benign febrile seizures* become unlikely after age 5.

Traumatic. Children, as infants, are subject to similar head trauma and hypoxia.

Neoplastic. Children's brain tumors are usually subtentorial but occasionally may present as a seizure if the tumor is present in the cerebral hemispheres (*astrocytoma, ependymoma,* or *oligodendroglioma*).

Vascular. The differential diagnosis is similar to that of infancy.

Conditions Mimicking Seizures in Children

Rare paroxysmal movement disorders, often familial and causing episodic choreoathetosis, are rare but may be confused with seizures. It is important to differentiate other conditions such as *syncope, hyperventilation, sleep disorders, psychogenic epilepsy,* and *cardiac arrhythmias* from true seizures. *Syncope* often follows an upsetting experience or is associated with standing for a long time. The patient definitely recalls feeling "woozy" and will try hard not to fall. *Hyperventilation* is usually a dramatic event associated with psychological stress. The spasmodic component of an episode is carpopedal, or it may affect the temporal mandibular area. Sleep disorders may present as *narcolepsy* (daytime sleep attacks), *cataplexy* (sudden loss of tone induced by excitement), *sleep paralysis,* and *hypnagogic hallucinations. Psychogenic seizures* may be difficult to differentiate from a true seizure, but often the patient is aroused easily. The patient may not be conscious of what he or she is doing; thus these episodes are not always malingering. *Cardiac arrhythmias* may be life-threatening and can be mistaken for seizures or syncope. If the episode occurs with exertion, spontaneously with no excitatory event, or with no advance warning, or there is a family history of sudden cardiac death, it is important to refer these patients to a cardiologist.

KEY PROBLEM
━━━
■ **Headache** *Headache* is a very common symptom in all children and adolescents. A careful history is critical to determine which headaches merit further evaluation. An accurate account may be difficult to obtain from a child. Ascertain the severity of the pain, the location, the duration, and the timing. Is it associated with vomiting or changes in behavior or affect? There are certain red flags as well as "not to worry" points to consider. Points of concern in the history may be sudden onset of "the worst headache in my life" (vascular disease); morning headache and vomiting, sometimes without nausea (tumor); and sudden severe shooting pain (cervical root and cranial nerve such as *tic douloureux*). Always ask about weakness, numbness, visual disturbance, or alteration of consciousness. A reassuring point may be chronicity (a headache going on for many years is unlikely to be a *tumor* or a *stroke*). If the pain is steady, mild, and never remits, it is usually not due to serious intracranial pathology, but one must consider withdrawal from pain medication or caffeine or posttraumatic headache. *Migraine* and *tension headaches* are most common in children. *Classic migraine with aura* (formerly classic migraine) meets four main criteria: aura, headache, vomiting, and family history. Aura presents with amnesia, confusion, hallucinations such as Alice in Wonderland syndrome, or feeling generally "weird" or "funky." The second phase is associated with severe pain. The patient is often nauseated, vomits, and experiences photophobia and hyperacusis. He or she prefers to be alone in a dark room. The attacks may last several hours or all day. The patient will fall asleep and usually feels better on awakening. *Migraine* may be associated with focal neurologic findings such as hemiplegia, ophthalmoplegia, and vertigo and, although benign, sometimes must undergo further evaluation. However, if the patient normalizes quickly, that history alone may be sufficient not to evaluate further with ancillary studies. *Migraine without aura* (formerly common migraine) is similar to classic migraine minus the aura. Tension headaches are most common and present typically with steady headache, usually circumferential (band around the head pattern), and worsen as the day progresses. There is no vomiting or illness. The patient

may pinpoint worsening to stressful occurrences during the day. Eyestrain and sinusitis may cause headache, but their role is often overstated.

Congenital/genetic/metabolic/toxic. These causes are rare in children. Most genetic and metabolic disorders will present in infancy. Congenital malformations such as *spina bifida* will cause headache owing to hydrocephalus. *Chiari malformation* will present as a headache in childhood. *Arachnoid cysts* and *AVM* bear mentioning because they may appear initially in childhood, adolescence, or even adulthood. However, small children often ingest toxins, so one must suspect lead poisoning, other heavy metals, or any acute ingestion. Also consider *carbon monoxide inhalation, hypoxia, hypoglycemia, uremia,* and *electrolyte disturbances.*

Infectious/inflammatory/immune. *Meningoencephalitis* and *abscesses* of *bacterial, viral, fungal,* or *parasitic* origin will cause headaches either by direct CNS invasion or by myalgias in the cranial region. Also, *viral acute disseminated encephalomyelitis* (ADEM) will cause headaches.

Traumatic. Acute head injury may cause *epidural* or *subdural hemorrhage, contusion,* or *cerebral edema.* Posttraumatic headache is quite common, may last several months, and is often associated with mild cognitive deficits. However, if the headache worsens over time, or if the patient's academic performance falters or he or she appears apathetic, it is important to consider a *chronic subdural hematoma.*

Neoplastic. Tumors may cause headache mainly owing to increased intracranial pressure from obstructive hydrocephalus. Most posterior fossa tumors (*medulloblastoma, astrocytoma*) will present in this manner owing to their proximity to the midline. Supratentorial tumors (*astrocytoma, ependymoma, pineal tumor,* and rarely, *medulloblastoma*) will present with headache and perhaps other focal neurologic symptoms or seizures.

Vascular. Consider *AVM* and *aneurysm* if the onset is sudden and severe. *Vasculitis* becomes more prominent in children; one must consider conditions such as *connective tissue disorders,* hypersensitivity vasculitis (*Henoch-Schoenlein purpura*), and *hypertension* with its many etiologies.

● KEY PROBLEM
◤ **Altered Consciousness** Since children are more communicative, we are now able to assess the level of coma in a patient. Refer to the commonly used Glasgow coma scale in TABLE 12–1.

Congenital/genetic/metabolic Most of these etiologies will have been determined in infancy.

Infectious/inflammatory/immune. Consider *bacterial, viral, fungal,* and *parasitic infections* and *abscesses.* Also include encephalopathies that may not be due to direct invasion of organisms such as *toxic-shock syndrome, Reye syndrome, Lyme disease,* and *hemorrhagic shock* and *encephalopathy.* Postviral *ADEM* frequently will affect children.

TABLE 12-1   Glasgow Coma Scale

Eye opening	
Spontaneous	4
To speech	3
To pain	2
None	1
Best motor response	
Obeys commands	6
Localizes	5
Withdraws	4
Abnormal flexion	3
Abnormal extension	2
None	1
Verbal response	
Oriented	5
Confused conversation	4
Inappropriate words	3
Incomprehensible sounds	2
None	1
Total	15

Traumatic. As stated earlier, *concussion, contusion, intracranial hemorrhage,* and *cerebral edema* all may be responsible for altered states of consciousness. Secondary hypoxia and ischemia also may be a contributing factor.

Vascular. As with seizures and headache discussed earlier, consider *embolism, hypertensive encephalopathy,* and the multiple causes of *vasculitis.*

Systemic Conditions

Keep in mind that conditions other than primary neurologic ones may cause alterations of consciousness, usually as a consequence of a metabolic derangement. Always think of *osmotic disorders* that result from *diabetic ketoacidosis, hypoglycemia* with its many etiologies, *sodium imbalance* owing to *renal* or *adrenal* disorders, and the *syndrome of inappropriate ADH* secretion from primary cerebral or pulmonary lesions. Endocrine disorders such as *hypothyroidism, hypoadrenalism,* and *hyper/hypoparathyroidism* are known to cause alterations of consciousness.

KEY PROBLEM
Developmental Delay/Regression Most of the causes for developmental delay or regression are diagnosed in infancy. Many of the metabolic and storage diseases have juvenile forms that present after age 2 years. Neurocutaneous syndromes such as *neurofibromatosis* and *tuberous sclerosis* become more apparent in childhood.

KEY PROBLEM
Hypotonia (Generalized Weakness) Most of the causes for *hypotonia* in infancy were addressed earlier. Children with

proximal weakness usually present with abnormal gaits (toe-walking or waddling), easy fatigue, frequent falling, slow regressing motor development, or specific disabilities such as climbing stairs, getting up from a sitting position (Gower sign), elevating the arm or shoulder, or weak hand grip. There also may be weakness of facial or neck muscles. This section will be divided into proximal and distal weakness.

Proximal

The typical presenting complaint is inability or loss of ability to walk upstairs. The gait may be waddling. The patient may toe-walk as a distal compensation for the proximal weakness. Many of the conditions causing progressive proximal weakness are hereditary—hence the importance of a family history.

Congenital/metabolic/genetic. Juvenile spinal muscular atrophies of varying types occur in different age groups. *Muscular dystrophy* occurs in many forms. Hereditary conditions affecting peripheral nerves and muscles also include juvenile progressive bulbar palsies, which are progressive and severe. *Metabolic myopathy* may be due to enzyme deficiency, storage diseases, or *carnitine deficiency. Thyroid, parathyroid,* and *adrenal* disorders of any type may present with proximal myopathy.

Infectious/inflammatory/immune. Bacterial *myositis* may cause weakness and is usually quite painful. Consider *HIV* and other viruses, as well as collagen-vascular diseases, particularly *polymyositis of lupus* and *dermatomyositis. Guillain-Barré disease* and postviral *ADEM* also cause weakness in childhood.

Traumatic. Localized pain and weakness may be a consequence of trauma with resulting muscle *hematomas.* The hematomas may heal slowly and often leave residuals, such as *calcifications,* causing long-lasting discomfort.

Neoplastic. Primary muscle tumors are rare, but one always must be mindful of *rhabdomyosarcoma.*

Vascular. Muscle disorders owing to vasculitis are a consequence of the inflammatory conditions mentioned earlier.

Distal

Distal weakness presents with the inability to flex the foot and subsequent easy tripping and repeated ankle sprains. The patient will try to compensate for the foot drop by overuse of proximal muscles to raise the foot higher off the ground, thus resulting in the typical steppage gait. This appears in peripheral neuropathies or myopathies.

Congenital/genetic/metabolic. These conditions may be due to motor neuron disease (*juvenile amyotrophic lateral sclerosis* or *spinal muscular atrophies* and *hereditary neuropathies*). Neuropathy can be a result of many *drugs,* particularly anticancer medications, antiretroviral medications, and antibiotics, especially chloroquine, isoniazid, and nitrofurantoin. Consider *heavy metal exposure. Uremia* may cause peripheral neuropathy with a higher incidence in patients on dialysis.

Infectious/inflammatory/immune. These conditions are associated with *ADEM, acute motor axonal polyneuropathy,* and *chronic inflammatory demyelinating polyradiculopathy,* all variants of *Guillain-Barré syndrome.*

KEY PROBLEM
Focal Weakness

Congenital. Most congenital causes appear in infancy and will progress or remain static during childhood.

Metabolic/genetic/toxic. These conditions occur in infancy and often progress to major disability or death in childhood.

Infectious/inflammatory/immune. Refer to the corresponding section under "Infants" above. Postviral *ADEM* attacks the entire CNS, so these symptoms may involve both brain and spinal cord.

Traumatic. These conditions become more prevalent in children because of their newly found ability to wander off, compounded by inordinate curiosity and lack of judgment. Accidents may account for subdural and epidural hematomas of the brain and spinal cord and external cord compression owing to vertebral fractures and dislocations. The location and severity of the lesion determine the degree of hemiplegia, diplegia, or quadriplegia.

Neoplastic. Malignancies increase in incidence during the childhood years. Primary brain tumors are discussed in other sections of this chapter. Supratentorial tumors, less common than subtentorial tumors, will cause hemiplegia. Metastatic tumors, especially *neuroblastoma* and *Ewing sarcoma,* will cause spinal compression with ensuing hemiplegia, diplegia, or quadriplegia.

Vascular. Vasculopathies take on a major role in childhood hemiplegia. Also, patients with severe *sickle cell disease* may experience *stroke. Vascular malformations* and *coagulopathies* occur in childhood as well as infancy. *Homocystinuria* will cause a vasculopathy predisposing to hypercoagulability. *Heart disease,* although often congenital, may be more likely to cause symptoms in children. For example, as right-to-left shunts and cyanosis proceed, *hyperviscosity* and *embolism* are more likely to occur in childhood. *Atrial myxomas* and rhabdomyomas also may release emboli to the brain. Consider *rheumatic heart disease* as well as *mitral valve prolapse. Vasculitis* becomes more prominent in childhood, specifically hypersensitivity [*Henoch-Schonlein purpura* (HSP)], *hemolytic-uremic syndrome* (HUS), *Kawasaki disease,* and *collagen-vascular disorders* of all types. *Moyamoya* disease is a rare chronic progressive vasculopathy often presenting with unilateral weakness.

KEY PROBLEM
Clumsiness (Ataxia)
The conditions affecting infants discussed earlier are also causes of *ataxia* in childhood. *Vasculitis* is more prominent in childhood. Postinfectious/immune conditions include the *Guillain-Barré disease, Miller-Fisher syndrome* with ataxia, ophthalmoplegia, and areflexia, which are sensory ataxias. *Demyelinating diseases* such as *multiple sclerosis* also cause ataxia from multiple origins. More prominent in childhood are *basilar migraine* and *posterior fossa tumors,* which

may cause progressive symptoms. Consider the *spinocerebellar degenerative disorders*. Although *Friedreich ataxia* is genetic in origin, it usually presents in childhood and is also progressive.

Vertigo as a consequence of *labyrinthitis,* benign paroxysmal vertigo, and *Meniere disease* are not of cerebellar origin but can be misconstrued for ataxia.

● KEY PROBLEM
Movement Disorders
Movement disorders are involuntary, occur without changes of consciousness, often are stereotypic, and improve when sleeping. They are due to disorders of the cerebral basal ganglia. *Chorea* is a random rapid movement that is usually recurrent but not rhythmic. The movements do not affect one part of the body. They often appear during a purposeful movement but have no fixed form to them. *Ballismus* is a violent jerk of a limb originating from the shoulder or pelvis. It is an extreme form of chorea. *Athetosis* is a writhing movement of the limbs occurring alone or in association with chorea (choreoathetosis). *Tardive dyskinesia* presents with abnormal buccal-lingual movements. These movements also may occur with chorea. *Tics* are habit spasms that are more stereotyped and repetitive than chorea. The patient may control tics for a time but often feels a compulsion to make this movement. When tics become vocal and become more severe and affect daily functioning, they fall into the category of *Tourette syndrome.* Tics that involve facial muscles, throat clearing, or sniffing present similarly to allergies and often cause needless medical evaluations.

Congenital/genetic/metabolic/toxic. These conditions include progressive ataxias and spinocerebellar, gray, and white matter degenerative disorders. These are commonly associated with *drugs* such as anticonvulsants, antiemetics, psychotropic agents, stimulants, oral contraceptives, and theophylline. Choreoathetosis was very common years ago when bilirubin encephalopathy from ker*nicterus owing to Rh incompatibility* was prevalent.

Infectious/inflammatory. Sydenham chorea is a major manifestation of acute rheumatic fever. *Collagen-vascular disease*, especially *lupus,* also may cause movement disorders.

Traumatic. Movement disorders may occur after injuries, both perinatal and postnatal.

Neoplastic. Tumors involving the basal ganglia are very rare.

Vascular. Poststroke complications may present as movement disorders.

Adolescents

Much of the differential diagnoses are covered in previous sections, so this section will refer only to problems unique to adolescents.

● KEY PROBLEM
Seizures
Refer to the section on children. A thorough history may uncover exposures that might precipitate a seizure, such as drugs, carbon monoxide, loud noises, or excessive photic stimuli from video

games. *Juvenile myoclonic seizures (of Janz)* appear in early adolescence and consist of jerking movements, usually of the shoulder and arm that are worse in the mornings. The patient is usually most perturbed that a comb or hairbrush flies across the bathroom during use. There is no loss of consciousness. The patients generally do well and respond to treatment.

● KEY PROBLEM

◼ Headache *Headaches* in adolescents are very common, and their causes were listed in the preceding section. *Migraine* and *tension headaches* are most common. Also, *cluster headaches* appear in adolescence, characterized by severe pain in bursts, unilateral, around one eye. The pain increases to almost unbearable levels and eventually subsides, only to repeat itself daily or more frequently. The episodes remit after several months, and the patient may be symptom-free for years after. The patient reports redness and tearing of the ipsilateral eye as well as stuffiness of the ipsilateral nostril. Other causes of headache in adolescents are consequences of their lifestyle and include use of oral contraception, *caffeine withdrawal, drug use (marijuana, cocaine, nicotine)*, and *rebound headaches* from injudicious use of pain medications. Rapid ingestion of ice cream or *monosodium glutamate* also may be problematic. Headaches owing to increased *intracranial pressure* are similar to those outlined previously. Use of vitam*in A* and *steroids* will cause this type of headache. Also include benign *intracranial hypertension (pseudotumor cerebri)* in this group, often affecting overweight females. The patient may experience vomiting and visual difficulty. As in many cases of increased intracranial pressure, there may be bilateral lateral rectus muscle palsies causing esotropia. *Brain tumors* are more likely to originate in the cerebral cortex or meninges, causing more localized pain. Headaches also may originate from non-CNS areas such as teeth, sinuses, and the temporomandibular joint (TMJ*)*.

● KEY PROBLEM

◼ Altered Consciousness Refer to causes of altered consciousness discussed earlier. During adolescence, one must pay particular attention to *ingestions* of substances. *Syncope* is more prominent and may present like a true neurologic disorder. Behavioral problems including *conversion disorders, anxiety,* and *depression* are common causes of alterations in consciousness. *Cardiovascular disorders,* particularly hypertrophic cardiomyopathy and advancing *aortic stenosis,* may cause loss of consciousness and sudden death or leave residual damage owing to cerebral hypoxia. Often an adolescent will complain of "dizziness." It is important to determine whether this is vertigo (perception of motion either of patient or of the room) or dizziness (no perception of motion, more light-headedness). Most causes are benign, such as *presyncope, orthostatic hypotension,* and *hyperventilation.* However, significant neurologic causes may be *acoustic neuroma, posterior fossa tumor, migraine (vertebrobasilar), transient ischemic attack* (TIA), CNS infection, and demyelinating disease. Also consider substance ingestion and metabolic disorders such as *hypoglycemia* and *electrolyte imbalance.* Symptoms may also arise from otic and labyrinthine disorders.

KEY PROBLEM

■ **Developmental Delay, Hypotonia, Focal Weakness, Diffuse Weakness, Ataxia, Movement Disorders** These are not unique to adolescents, but oral contraception and drug ingestion play a more significant role. Refer to their differential diagnoses earlier.

Physical Examination

Infants, Children, and Adolescents

A good neurologic examination is critical to determine the location of a particular problem. It is not a diagnostic tool in and of itself but helps, along with a good history, to arrive at a working diagnosis. This section precents one neurologic exam that is appropriate for all age groups with the understanding an infant is often difficult to evaluate.

The neurologic examination is divided into the following components: cerebral, cerebellar, brain stem (cranial nerves and brain stem reflexes), spinal reflexes, sensory, and motor. This section discusses how to elicit examination findings and how to correlate them with the location of a particular lesion.

It is critical to perform a good general physical examination. Always inspect for dysmorphism in any developmentally delayed patient. This will lead to a diagnosis of chromosomal abnormalities or other metabolic disorders (e.g., coarse facies in mucopolysaccharidoses). Neurologic disease may be associated with cutaneous findings. Observe the patient's posturing and joint mobility as a general indicator of tone. Therefore, careful examination for alterations in skin pigmentation, hemangiomas, nevi, and angiokeratomas with their locations is very important. A Wood's lamp may help to elicit pigmentary lesions. Decreased pigmentation is present in *phenylketonuria* (PKU) and other disorders of tyrosine metabolism. Palpate the fontanels always to assess intracranial pressure. Olfaction is most helpful to elucidate *inborn errors of metabolism.* Maple syrup odor (especially from earwax) points to *branched-chain ketoaciduria.* Patients with *phenylketonuria* (PKU) smell musty. *Organic acidemias* such as *glutaric and isovaleric acidemia* smell like sweaty socks. *Tyrosinemia* and *methioninemia* emit odors reminiscent of boiled cabbage. Transillumination of the skull may show large collections of CSF. Hepatosplenomegaly is often present in *metabolic storage diseases.* Urine and stool retention may be a sign of spinal cord disease. Auscultate cardiac findings such as *congestive failure,* which may occur with *muscular dystrophy.* Test for the Trousseau sign (tetany of hand after arterial occlusion for 3 minutes with a sphygmomanometer) and the Chvostek sign (tap anterior to ear on facial nerve to elicit ipsilateral jaw contraction for *hypocalcemia* in patients with seizures, jitteriness, or altered consciousness).

KEY FINDING

▼ **Cerebral** Simple observation should come first. Are there any malformations of the head? Is it enlarged or small? Do not forget palpation,

TABLE 12-2   Mini Mental Status Exam

Orientation
_____What is the (time) (date) (day) (month) (year)?
_____Where are we (state) (county) (city) (hospital)?

Registration
_____Name three objects and ask patient to repeat them until all are learned. Record the number of trials.

Attention and Calculation
_____Ask the patient to subtract serial 7s five times.

Recall
_____Ask patient to recall the objects mentioned under *Registration* above.

Language
_____Name objects (pencil, watch, etc)
_____Three stage command
_____Reading
_____Writing
_____Copying geometric figures

Source: Adapted from LeBlond RF, DeGowin RL, Brown DD: *De Gowin's Diagnostic Examination.* New York: McGraw-Hill, 2004.

percussion, and auscultation. Are the suture lines pronounced? Is the fontanelle large, small, tense, or depressed? Does the skull sound tympanitic? Is there a cranial bruit? Evaluating cerebral function can be extremely complex. We commonly use the standard Mini Mental Status Examination (TABLE 12–2). However, bear in mind that subtlety and nuance abound when evaluating other functions such as thought, perception, intellect, mood, and behavior. It is helpful to compare a patient's mental status with that prior to the onset of a particular problem. Knowledge of normal and abnormal cognitive and language development is critical when assessing infants, children, and adolescents.

▼ KEY FINDING
M Cerebellar The cerebellum acts as a "waystation" with input from joints, muscles, tendons, and the vestibular system and output to the cerebral cortex, motor strip, and basal ganglia. The cerebellum enables us to react to stimuli in a coordinated fashion. Testing for cerebellar function consists of

Stationary testing (equilibration or Romberg sign). Stand patient upright with both feet together and eyes closed. Watch for ability to maintain balance. The examiner may, after warning the patient, push him or her gently to one side to determine the ability to equilibrate. In general, falling over is usually to the side of the lesion.
Gait examination. Input to gait originates in the cerebral cortex and goes through the entire CNS, ultimately to the muscles. Thus gait is

important to evaluate all CNS function. The term *ataxia* merely means poor coordination, but the pattern can indicate the involved part of the CNS. The ataxic gait of cerebellar dysfunction is wavering or lurching and broad-based. There is no visual compensation. It is important to note that weakness and ataxia may be confused. It is always helpful to perform a "heel to shin" maneuver with the patient rubbing his or her heel along the other shin while lying down. This will test for coordination while taking gravity out of the equation.

Diadochokinesia. This is the ability to substitute quickly a motor impulse with an opposing one. Elicit this by asking the patient to tap his or her finger quickly or slap the thighs with his or her palms alternating rapidly with the dorsum of his or her hands. Also test the rebound sign (Stewart-Holmes) by grabbing the patient's fist with the patient's elbow flexed. Then request the patient to pull the fist toward him or her and release the grasp on the fist. In cerebellar disease, the patient will rebound awkwardly or may strike himself or herself.

Dyssynergia and dysmetria. Dyssynergia refers to impairment of voluntary movements, usually fractionated or jerky. *Dysmetria* refers to the inability to judge distances during voluntary movement. Test this by the finger-to-nose test. Abnormalities will include an action tremor or past-pointing.

Fine motor skills. These are often impaired in cerebellar disease and awkward with intention tremors.

Titubation. Head bobbing is seen in conditions involving the cerebellar vermis.

Labyrinthine tests. Labyrinthine disorders may resemble those of cerebellar origin. The Romberg sign and past-pointing may be similar. The presence of nystagmus will indicate labyrinthine over cerebellar pathology. Nystagmus consists of lateral jerking of the eye with a fast and slow component. The nystagmus is "left" or "right" depending on the fast component. This may be spontaneous, but the examiner may elicit it by placing the patient supine with the neck extended over the edge of the table by 30 degrees and then rotated to one side by 45 degrees. Nystagmus may occur in this position, but it may be necessary to return the patient to the sitting position to observe the abnormal eye movements. The examiner should perform this maneuver with the patient's head rotated to each side. Nausea and vomiting may accompany the nystagmus.

KEY FINDING

Brain Stem Cranial nerve function and brain stem reflexes are the means to evaluate brain stem function. Cranial nerve function was outlined earlier. This section reviews how to elicit findings.

Olfactory I. Use a substance with a familiar odor such as coffee, chocolate, or tobacco. Have the patient identify it with his or her eyes closed. *Anosmia,* or lack of a sense of smell, occurs in *trauma to or tumors of the inferior temporal lobe.*

Ophthalmic II. Careful funduscopic examination is important and often difficult in infants and children. Approach the patient calmly in a relatively darkened room. Ask the patient to look directly ahead at a point designated on the opposite wall, or have the parent stand directly behind you and have the child look at the parent. Then tell the patient that your head will soon be in the way, but try to look through it to the same previously designated spot or person. Then, as you approach the patient's eye with the ophthalmoscope, adjust the lens to the correct focal length to yield the sharpest image. The optic disc should be flat, sharp, and red-orange in color with a more yellow optic cup located centrally. Blood vessels should be of consistent diameter and not engorged. Venous pulsations should be visible. Blurred discs and engorged vessels without venous pulsations raise a concern for increased intracranial pressure owing to hydrocephalus, cerebral edema, or tumor. Pale discs may be a sign of optic atrophy or demyelination. Please consult Chapter 7 for further detail. Also, the macula, which is located temporally, about three disc diameters from the optic nerve, may be cherry red in certain lysosomal storage diseases. Visual-field examination is an important measurement of optic nerve function and is discussed in Chapter 7.

Oculomotor III, trochlear IV, and abducent VI. The abducent nerve innervates the lateral rectus muscles. The trochlear nerve innervates the superior oblique muscle, and the abducent nerve innervates the lateral rectus muscle. The oculomotor nerve innervates all the others. Note in FIGURE 12–4 how each muscle moves the eye. Gaze paralysis is usually due to external compression of extraocular muscles, as seen in trauma, tumor, or infection (orbital cellulitis). Test the nerve function by having the patient gaze in all directions. Lateral rectus paralysis will allow the eyes to deviate nasally at rest. The patient will be unable to gaze laterally when asked to do so. This appears unilaterally with the lesions discussed earlier or bilaterally with increased intracranial pressure causing tension on the cranial nerve, which has the longest pathway outside the brain stem. Superior oblique palsy will force the eyes superiorly and temporally at rest. There will be lack of motion of the eye with downward medial gaze (FIGURE 12–6).

Trigeminal V. The sensory division of this nerve is divided into three branches, ophthalmic, maxillary, and mandibular. Note the distribution in FIGURE 12–7. The motor division innervates the muscles of chewing (temporalis and masseter). Test this by evaluating the muscle mass as the patient bites down hard or by observing malalignment of the teeth with the patient's mouth open. With bilateral involvement, the patient will not be able to close the jaw tightly.

Facial VII. Sensory fibers of the facial nerve originate from taste buds on the anterior two-thirds of the tongue and sensory nerves of the ear canal and behind the pinna. Autonomic fibers allow for secretion from submaxillary and sublingual salivary glands. Motor fibers innervate the muscles of facial expression, the stapedius, the stylohyoid, and the posterior belly of the digastricus. Test seven different poses: (1) rest (look for eye or mouth droop or flattened nasolabial folds), (2) elevation of eyebrows, (3) frowning, (4) tight closing of the eye, (5) showing teeth, (6) whistling and puffing the cheeks, and (7) natural smile. Facial paralyses may be due to upper

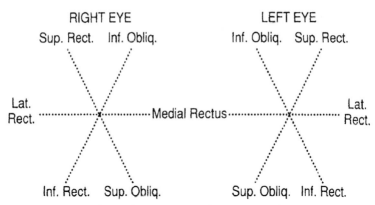

RIGHT EYE
Sup. Rect.   Inf. Obliq.

LEFT EYE
Inf. Obliq.   Sup. Rect.

Lat.
Rect. ················Medial Rectus················ Lat.
Rect.

Inf. Rect.   Sup. Obliq.

Sup. Obliq.   Inf. Rect.

FIGURE 12–6 *The Cardinal Positions of Gaze. Each of the six positions is the result of synergists and antagonists acting with a specific muscle. Paralysis of the specific muscle prevents the eye from attaining the cardinal position for the muscle. (From LeBlond RF, DeGowin RL, Brown DD:* DeGowin's Diagnostic Examination. *New York: McGraw-Hill, 2004, Fig. 14–16, p. 832.)*

or lower motor lesions. As you review neuroanatomy, remember that the upper motor neurons innervate muscles above the palpebral fissure bilaterally. Thus a facial nerve upper motor neuron or brain stem lesion will not affect muscles above the palpebral fissure owing to innervation from the contralateral side as well. A lower motor neuron lesion occurs in the final common pathway between the upper and motor neurons and will affect the ipsilateral side only.

Auditory VIII. Hearing loss may be neural or conductive. A crude measure of hearing could be response to a whisper or ability to hear various pitches using tuning forks with ranges of 256 to 1024 Hz. Tuning forks are helpful to distinguish between air conduction and bone conduction. Normally, air conduction is greater than bone conduction; thus a patient will hear a tuning fork better when placed in front of the ear (air conduction) than when placed against the mastoid

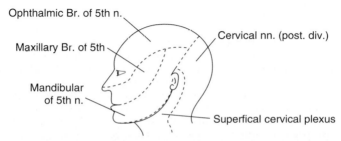

Ophthalmic Br. of 5th n.

Maxillary Br. of 5th

Mandibular
of 5th n.

Cervical nn. (post. div.)

Superfical cervical plexus

FIGURE 12–7 *Distribution of the Sensory Branches of the Trigeminal V Nerve. (From LeBlond RF, DeGowin RL, Brown DD:* DeGowin's Diagnostic Examination. *New York: McGraw-Hill, 2004, Fig. 14–1B, p. 802.)*

process (bone conduction). If a patient has a neural or conductive hearing loss, there will be diminished air conduction. With a pure conductive hearing loss, vibration of the mastoid will overcome the air-conductive defect, and the patient will be able to report a sound because the auditory nerve is still functioning. In the case of a pure neural loss, the patient still will be unable to hear with air or bone conduction or hear equally poorly with both. This is the basis of the Rinne test, which demonstrates that bone conduction is greater than air conduction with a conductive hearing loss. The same principle applies to the Weber test, which is more useful with unilateral hearing loss. With the tuning fork on the top of the patient's head, he or she will hear better on one side if the conductive loss is on that side or if a neural loss is on the opposite side. In addition, audiometry is helpful. Conductive hearing losses are generally low frequency, and neural hearing losses are at the higher frequencies.

Glossopharyngeal IX. Test taste in the posterior third of the tongue. This nerve also provides pain touch and temperature sensation in the pharynx. It intimately relates to the vagus nerve, and the maneuvers for testing are similar.

Vagus X. This nerve supplies the pharynx, as does cranial nerve IX, but also carries sensory and motor fibers to the neck, thorax, and abdomen. Test the pharyngeal mucosa for sensation, as well as the gag reflex. Determine if there is any asymmetry of the palate or uvula. Hoarseness may be a sign of vocal cord dysfunction, and some examiners may be capable of performing indirect laryngoscopy with a mirror. Bulbar palsy with difficulty swallowing may indicate involvement in a pathologic process. Irregularities in cardiac and gastrointestinal function may suggest glossopharyngeal or vagus nerve involvement and may indicate an overall autonomic disorder.

Accessory XI. This is the motor nerve to the trapezius and sternocleidomastoid muscles. Turn the patient's head to one side and attempt to bring his or her chin back to the midline (sternocleidomastoid). Test the trapezius muscle by having the patient shrug his or her shoulders against the resistance of your hands. Look for scapular asymmetry (winging).

Hypoglossal XII. This is the motor nerve for the tongue. Have the patient stick his or her tongue out, and observe for asymmetry. The tongue will deviate toward the weak side. Also check for tremors and fasciculations (writhing movements).

Brain stem reflexes. These reflexes test involvement of the cranial nerves or of their nuclei. The pupillary reflex tests sensory II and ipsilateral oculomotor III. Elicit the consensual papillary reflex by shining light in one eye and looking at the other. This tests sensory II and contralateral III. The ciliospinal reflex (pinching the skin on the back of the neck will elicit papillary dilation) tests sensory cervical nerves, the efferent cervical sympathetic chain, and oculomotor III. The corneal reflex (touching the cornea causes blinking of the eyelids) tests afferent V and motor VII. The jaw reflex (tapping the jaw with subsequent closing) tests sensory and motor V. The gag reflex tests sensory and motor IX and X.

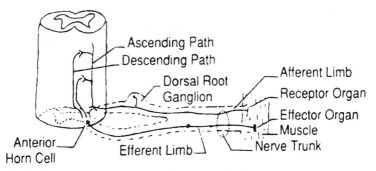

FIGURE 12–8 *The Reflex Aarc. (From LeBlond RF, DeGowin RL, Brown DD: DeGowin's Diagnostic Examination. New York: McGraw-Hill, 2004, Fig. 14–4, p. 807.)*

▼ KEY FINDING

■ Spinal Reflexes The reflex arc in simplest terms is a pathway consisting of afferent and efferent limbs connected by the spinal cord at one level (FIGURE 12–8). A sensory stimulus, usually in the form of a tendon tap on a slightly stretched muscle or skin stroking, will elicit a response along the afferent (sensory) path to the cord and back through the efferent (motor) path to induce a muscle twitch. The grade of the response will evaluate any perturbations of that pathway (TABLE 12–3). The particular muscle tested will help to localize the area(s) of pathology, as indicated in TABLE 12–4. Diminished or absent reflexes indicate disruption of the reflex arc owing to injury, nerve inflammation, demyelination, or infiltration. Hyperreflexia with extra beats of clonus occurs in spasticity. The cause is loss of the normal cortical inhibition of the descending pyramidal tracts, thus creating an amplified reflex response. Pathologic reflexes such as the Babinski sign (fanning of the toes with stroking the lateral aspect of the foot) or the Hoffmann sign (flexion of the thumb as a response to flexing the ipsilateral third finger distal phalanx) or a grasp or palmomental reflex indicate diffuse cortical pathology. Note that many of these abnormal responses in children are normal for newborns that have not developed enough myelin to conduct cerebral inhibitory impulses.

TABLE 12–3 *Measuring Reflex Response*

0
No response
1+
Detectable, but weak
2+
Easily detectable
3+
Brisk with at most a few beats of clonus
4+
Sustained clonus

Source: From LeBlond RF, DeGowin RL, Brown DD:*DeGowin's Diagnostic Examination.* New York: McGraw-Hill, 2004.

TABLE 12–4 *Tendon and Skin Reflexes*

Reflex	Location	Afferent (How to Elicit)	Efferent (Response)
C_5–T_1	Pectoralis	Press pectoralis tendon with thumb. Tap and aim toward pt's axilla	Pectoralis will contract
C_{5-6}	Biceps	Grab around pt's elbow and tap biceps tendon under your thumb	Elbow will flex
C_{5-6}	Brachioradialis	Hold wrist with forearm relaxed in pronation; tap above styloid process	Elbow will flex and arm will supinate
C_{6-7}	Pronator	Suspend wrist vertically; tap distal radius	Forearm will pronate
C_{7-8}	Triceps	Hold elbow at 90 degrees; tap just above elbow	Elbow will extend
T_{5-8}	Upper abd. skin	Run pin from midaxillary line to midline starting at lower thoracic cage	Umbilicus will deviate ipsilaterally
T_{8-9}	Upper abd. muscle	Tap midcostal margin and xiphoid	Abd. muscles will contract ipsilaterally
T_{9-10}	Midabd. muscle	Tap finger at midline between xiphoid and umbilicus	Abd. muscles will contract ipsilaterally
T_{9-11}	Midabd. skin	As in upper abd. skin, but at umbilical level	Umbilical will deviate ipsilat.
T_{11-12}	Lower abd. skin	As in medial abd. skin but at iliac crest	Umbilical will deviate ipsilat.
T_{11-12}	Lower abd. muscle	Tap along symphysis pubis	Lower abd. muscles will contract
L_{1-2}	Cremasteric	Stroke inner thigh	Ipsilateral testis will elevate
L_{2-4}	Quadriceps	Tap patellar tendon	Knee will extend
L_{2-4}	Adductor	Leg in slight adduction; tap adductor magnus tendon on medial femoral condyle	Leg will adduct
L_4–S_2	Hamstring	Grab knee around popliteal fossa; tap fingers over hamstring tendon medially	Knee will flex

(*Continued*)

TABLE 12–4 *Tendon and Skin Reflexes (Continued)*

Reflex	Location	Afferent (How to Elicit)	Efferent (Response)
L_4–S_2	Plantar	Run blunt point over lateral aspect of plantar surface toward ball of foot	Toes and foot will plantar flex
L_5–S_2	Achilles	Tap Achilles tendon with foot dorsiflexed	Foot will plantar flex
$S_{1–2}$	Anal	Stroke perianal area	Anal sphincter will contract

Source: Adapted from LeBlond RF, DeGowin RL, Brown DD: *DeGowin's Diagnostic Examination.* New York: McGraw-Hill, 2004.

Abbreviations: abd = abdomen; ipsilat = ipsilateral; pt = patient.

▼ KEY FINDING

■ Sensory The sensory input from the cutaneous nerves to the spinal cord and then to the cerebrum was discussed earlier. See FIGURE 12–9 for the point-by-point representation to locate the level of the pathology. Furthermore, the sensory modality tested will help to determine the specific locations within the level of cord or cerebral cortex involved.

The anterolateral ascending somatosensory pathways mediate superficial pain (prickling or burning), light touch, temperature, and itching (or tickling). The examiner will poke the patient with a sharp object or a feather over wide areas and locate the level where the sensation is the most or least intense. Test the patient for warm and cold sensations in a similar manner. Pathologic sensory deficits relate to specific dermatomes and appear with spinal cord compression, tumor, or infiltration. Certain patterns such as "stocking" or "glove" anesthesia suggest *conversion reactions.*

Deep pain position (proprioception) and vibratory sense are a function of the posterior columns. Test position sense by asking the patient to close his or her eyes, grasping the patient's finger or toe on the lateral aspects and moving it slightly up and down. The patient, without looking, should be able to report the direction of digital movement. Test vibratory sense with a tuning fork at 128 Hz. Place the fork over prominent bony areas such as the medial and lateral malleoli of the ankles, styloid processes of the wrist, or the tibial plateau. Posterior column problems may manifest with gait problems. Because of proprioception deficits, the gait may be tentative and/or broad-based and misconstrued for cerebellar or labyrinthine ataxia.

Higher sensory function such as stereogenesis, two-point discrimination, and graphesthesia is located in the cerebral cortex, specifically in the parietal area in the precentral gyrus. Refer to FIGURE 12–10 for the point-by-point distribution. Test stereogenesis by placing various familiar objects (e.g., coins) in the patient's hand and having him or her identify them with closed eyes. Test two-point discrimination by using two safety pins, pricking the patient and asking if he or she feels two

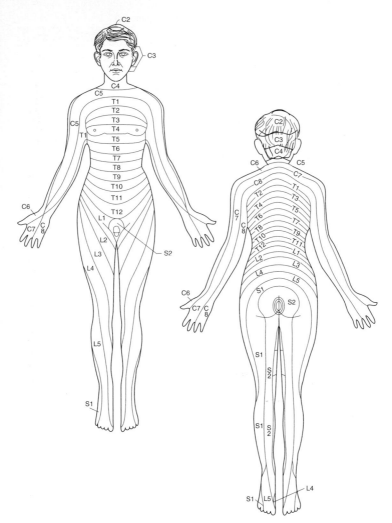

FIGURE 12-9   *Dermatome Representation of Cutaneous Sensation.*

needles. Then bring the needles closer and closer, repeating the process. Determine the distance between the needles when the patient no longer can feel both of them. To test graphesthesia, write numbers with a blunt point on the patient's hand, and ask him or her to identify what they are.

<hr>

KEY FINDING

▼ **Motor** Examine for muscle atrophy or hypertrophy. Distal muscular atrophy bespeaks neuropathy, whereas proximal weakness points to myopathy. Test the patient for tone and strength. Assess tone

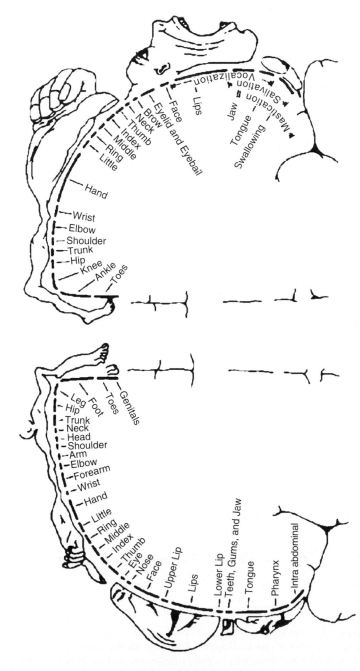

FIGURE 12-10 "Homunculus" Representation of Cortical Sensory (left) and Motor (right) Areas of the Parietal Lobe.

by having the patient relax and then move the limb passively. Some patients are unable to relax and may have to be distracted to keep their minds off the examination. Increased tone may indicate spasticity, and decreased tone may indicate spasticity, neuropathy, or myopathy. Muscle groups involved may help to indicate the level of pathology. Testing gait is helpful to evaluate muscle strength and involvement. A foot drop suggests peripheral weakness, as seen in neuropathy. The patient may attempt to compensate for the foot drop by using a steppage gait (lifting the knees high to keep the feet off the ground). In cases of proximal weakness, as in muscular dystrophy, the patient is unable to get off the floor unless he or she "climbs up" his or her legs using his or her hands (Gower sign). Sometimes the patient will compensate for general weakness by employing a broad-base gait. Ataxia may be similar but is generally more awkward. Hysteria, conversion reaction, and malingering may appear as a bizarre, contorted gait. Patients will claim weakness but somehow never seem to fall, or if they do fall on rare occasion, they generally protect themselves very well. It requires far more strength not to fall when in such a deviated position than the patient claims to have. Another sign for hysteria is the Hoover sign. Have the patient lie supine, and cradle both heels in your palms while resting your hands on the table. Ask the patient to raise one leg at a time. Normally, the other heel will press downward. This does not occur in hysteria.

Synthesizing a Diagnosis

TABLE 12–5 is a summary of diagnoses discussed herein. They are subclassified by etiology, epidemiology (age of occurrence), clinical pattern, and anatomic location. Some of the etiologic diagnoses are classes of diseases (e.g., "white matter degenerative") because further studies and consultations are required to make specific rare diagnoses (e.g., *Canavan disease*).

Drug ingestions and poisoning are difficult to assess by individual neurologic symptoms because they may act on many parts of the CNS. However, combinations of symptoms and physical findings constitute "toxidromes," which the physician may employ to elucidate the possible substance ingested (TABLE 12–6). TABLE 12–7 lists neurologic symptoms with the drugs and toxins that cause them.

Confirmatory Laboratory and Imaging

General Comments

Arriving at neurologic hypotheses occurs after a careful history and physical examination are completed. Ancillary studies are useful to test them. Sometimes a diagnosis is readily apparent, and we know exactly

TABLE 12-5 *Summary of Diagnostic Categories with Their Histories and CNS Locations*

Diagnosis by Etiology	History Age at Dx	History Pattern	History Problems	Localization by Neuro Examination, Other Findings
Congenital malformation				
I. Chromosomal	I	Birth, static	Sz, AC, DD, hyp.	Ce, dysmorphic
II. Brain malform.				
A. Embryologic lissencephaly, agenesis of corpus callosum	I	Birth, severe, static Variable in severity	Sz, AC, DD, hyp S, DD	Ce, poss. dysmorphic Ce, poss. dysmorphic
Brain stem aplasias	I	Static	Focal weakness (FW)	BS, cranial nerves (cr nn)
Cerebellar aplasias	I	Static	Sz, DD, at., nyst, ↑↓reflexes AC, FW	Cb, occ. BS & SC
B. Other				
Spina bifida & cord malform.	I	Acute onset, static	HA, at., FW, (bulbar) DD	Ce, ↑HC
Chiari I	I,C,A	Slow onset, prog	At., DD	Cb, BS, cardioresp
Chiari II (spina bif.)	I	Sudden, prog.	At, bulbar sx, DD	Cb, BS, cardioresp
Dandy-Walker	I	Sudden, static	Hyp., DD	Cb, BS (cr nn IX, X) ↑HC
Hydrocephalus	I	Var. onset, prog.		BS (Cr nn VI) ↑HC,
Arachnoid cysts	I	Slow, progressive	HA, DD, FW, at.	Ce, Cb

(Continued)

TABLE 12-5 Summary of Diagnostic Categories with Their Histories and CNS Locations *(Continued)*

Diagnosis by Etiology	Age at Dx	History		Localization by Neuro Examination, Other Findings
		Pattern	Problems	
Genetic/metabolic				
I. Inborn errors of metabolism	I	Birth, prog.	Sz, AC, DD, hyp.	Ce, SC
II. Mitochondrial disease	I	Childhood, prog.	Sz, at, FW, dementia, sensory	Ce, Cb, Cr nn II, VII, SC, PN
III. Gray matter degeneration	I, C	Prog, severe	Sz, AC, DD, hyp.	Ce
IV. White matter degeneration	I, C	Prog, severe	Sz, AC, DD, hyp., blind, deaf	C, BS, SC, ↑HC
V. Storage diseases	I, C	Prog, severe	Sz, AC, DD, hyp., FW, bulbar sx	Ce, Cb, BS, SC, PN, cherry red macula, coarse facies
VI. Spinal muscle atrophy	I, C	Prog, severe	Hyp., bulbar sx, ↓ref	BS, SC wasting
VII. Muscular dystrophy and myopathy	C, I, A	Prog, variable sev.	Hyp, ↓ reflexes	Occ DD, M, cardiac, wasting or hypertrophy
VIII. Progressive ataxias	A, C, I	Prog, variable sev.	At, ↓ pos. & vibr., ↓reflexes	Cb, BS, SC
Spinocerebellar degeneration	A, C, I	Prog, variable sev. ↓ propriocept.	At, dementia, sensory, hyp, MD At., DD, ↓ reflexes,	Ce, Cb, BS, SC, PN

IX Neurocutaneous				
Tuberous sclerosis	I, C	Birth, variable sev.	Sz, DD	Ce,SC pigm, angiokeratoma
Neurofibromatosis I	I, C	Birth, variable sev.		6 café-au-lait, neurofibroma, Lisch nodules, axillary freckling
Neurofibromatosis II	I, C	Birth, variable severity (sev)	Pain, brain tumors Hearing	Ce, BS, SC, fewer skin signs, acoustic neuroma
Toxic/metabolic				
Hypoglycemia	I, C, A	Acute, may be self-limited if treated, or a small ingestion. May progress if not treated. Some drugs affect specific parts of CNS. Some affect multiple parts of CNS	Jittery, Sz, diaphoresis Jittery	Ce PN, Trousseau/Chvostek Ce, PN
Hypocalcemia	I, C, A		Sz, AC, irritability ($\uparrow$Na$^+$)	Ce, PN
Hypo/hypernatremia	I, C, A		Sz, AC	Ce, PN
Uremia			Sz, AC, hyp., at., MD (See Tables 12–7, 12–8)	Ce Cb, BS, SC, PN, NMJ, M (See Tables 12–7 and 12–8)
Ingestions (medications, poisons, or illicit drugs)	I, C, A			
Infectious/ inflammatory				
Infectious	I, C, A	Acute, may recover or leave static residuals	Sz, HA, AC, FW	Ce, Cb, Cr.nn,
Inflammatory (often postviral)	I, C, A	Chronic	Sz, HA, FW, hyp.	Ce, Cb, BS, SC, PN, NMJ

(Continued)

TABLE 12-5 Summary of Diagnostic Categories with Their Histories and CNS Locations *(Continued)*

Diagnosis by Etiology	Age at Dx	History		Problems	Localization by Neuro Examination, Other Findings
		Pattern			
Guillian-Barré (GB)	Acute inflamm demyel polyneuro-pathy I, C, A	Ascending paralysis, ↓reflexes, Cr nn III palsy, autonomic instability			SC (ant. horn), Cr nn, PN
CIDP (chronic inflammatory demyelinating polyneuropathy)	C, A	Prolonged G-B Similar to G-B. Longer recovery, affects entire CNS			Ce, Cb, BS, SC, PN
ADEM	C, A				
Myasthenia gravis	I, C, A	Weakness, fatigue, ptosis, thymoma			NMJ
Traumatic/hypoxic					
Acute	I, C, A	Variable		Sz, HA, AC, FW	Ce, Cb, BS, SC,
Residuals	I, C, A	Static		Sz, HA, AC, DD, FW, at, MD	Ce, Cb, BS, SC
Neoplastic					
Cortical	C, A, I			HA, FW, MD	Ce

388

Choroid plexus papilloma, glial tumor, PNET, pinealoma, meningioma				
Subtentorial (postfossa) PNET, glial tumor, ependymoma, hemangioblastoma	C, I, A	Slow onset, progressive. PNET may be more rapid onset	HA, AC, DD, at.	Cb
Middle fossa			HA, visual field changes	Cr nn III, delayed puberty
Optic glioma, pituitary tumor	C, A, I			
Brain stem Glioma	C, I, A		FW, AC, at.	BS
Vascular CVA thrombotic Clotting disorder, homocystinuria, dehydration, embolism from CHD or tumor, or endocarditis	All ages	Acute onset, may be calamitous, may leave residuals static residuals	Sz, AC, HA At., AC, HA FW, Cr nn sx. (cranial nerve symptoms)	Ce, Cb, BS Thin body habitus

(Continued)

TABLE 12-5 Summary of Diagnostic Categories with Their Histories and CNS Locations (Continued)

Diagnosis by Etiology	Age at Dx	History Pattern	Problems	Localization by Neuro Examination, Other Findings
CVA hemorrhagic AVM, aneurysm, ataxia telangiectasia, Sturge-Weber Vasculitis/ vasculopathy, HUS, HSP, Kawasaki, collagen-vascular, moyamoya		Acute severe headache Infections, cancer Port-wine hemangioma		

Abbreviations: I = infants; C = children; A = adolescents; Ce = cerebral; Cb = cerebellar; BS = brain stem; Cr nn = cranial nerves; SC = spinal cord; PN = peripheral nerves; NMJ = neuromuscular junction; Sz = seizures; AC = altered consciousness; HA = headache; DD = developmental delay; FW = focal weakness; hyp. = hypotonia; at. = ataxia; MD = movement disorder; sx = symptoms; HC = head circumference; PNET = primitive neuroectodermal tumor; CVA = cerebrovascular accident; CHD = congenital heart disease; AVM = arteriovenous malformation; HUS = hemolytic-uremic syndrome; HSP = Henoch-Schonlein purpura; pigm. = pigmentation; ADEM = acute disseminated encephalomyelitis; chr = chronic; prog = progressive; sev = severity; var = variable; meds = medications; SC = subcutaneous.

TABLE 12-6 *Toxidromes*

Toxidrome	Presentation	Vital Sign Changes	Causative Agents
Anticholinergic	Delirium, flush, ↑ pupils, urinary retention, constipation, seizures, memory loss	Tachycardia, hyperthermia, hypertension	Antihistamines, scopolamine, jimson weed, angel trumpet, atropine, tricyclic antidepressants (TCAs)
Cholinergic	Confusion, weakness, salivation, lacrimation, diarrhea, emesis, diaphoresis, miosis, seizures	Bradycardia, hypothermia, tachypnea.	Organophosphates, carbamates, mushrooms
Hallucinogens	Disorientation, hallucinations, panic, sweating, diarrhea, seizures	Tachycardia, tachypnea, hypertension	Amphetamines, cannabis, cocaine, phencyclidine (PCP)
Opiates	Drowsiness, miosis, shock	↓ Resp, bradycardia, hypothermia, ↓ bp	Opiates, propoxyphene, dextromethorphan
Sympathomimetics	Delusions, paranoia, diaphoresis, piloerection, mydriasis, anxiety, seizures (sz)	Tachycardia, hypertension	Amphetamines, ephedrine, other "cold medicines," albuterol, ma huang
Sedative/hypnotic	Coma, stupor, confusion, sedation,	↓ Respirations, apnea	Barbiturates, benzodiazepines, alcohol, anticonvulsants

Abbreviations: resp = respiration; bp = blood pressure.

TABLE 12-7 *Neurologic Symptoms Caused by Drugs and Toxins*

Symptoms	Toxins
Seizures	Heavy metals, amphetamines, tricyclics, theophylline, heavy metals (Pb, As)
Altered consciousness	Pb, As, barbiturates, opiates, psychotropics, immunosuppressives (cyclosporine, OKT3), amphotericin B
Behavior changes	Barbiturates, corticosteroids, theophyllines, lead poisoning
Ataxia	Psychotropics, anticonvulsants, antihistamines
Movement disorders	
Chorea	Anticonvulsants, antiemetics, oral contraceptives, psychotropics, stimulants, theophylline
Dystonia	Antiemetics, antipsychotics, metoclopramide, Hg
Neuropathy	Anticancer drugs, antimicrobials, antiretrovirals, colchicines, gold, Pb, As, Hg
Deafness	Antimicrobials (aminoglycosides, vancomycin), furosemide, cisplatin, ASA

Abbreviations: ASA = acetylsalicylic acid; As = arsenic; Hg = mercury; Pb = lead.

where to look to confirm a single answer (e.g., unequivocal history of a drug ingestion confirmed by a single drug level determination). More often, history and physical examination may enable us only to clarify whether the condition is congenital, genetic/metabolic, toxic, infectious/inflammatory, traumatic, neoplastic, or vascular. Thus further laboratory and imaging testing becomes necessary to narrow down hypotheses. The goal of this section is to help the generalist select available confirmatory tests relevant to his or her scope of practice.

Key Laboratory Findings

Blood, CSF, and urine studies (TABLE 12–8).

Key Electroencephalographic (EEG) Findings

EEG may be helpful but sometimes is overrated. Clinical history and physical examination should take priority in assessing whether the patient "had a seizure." If the history and physical assessment clearly indicate that a seizure occurred, discount a normal EEG. Similarly, about 10 percent of the population may have occasional spikes on an EEG, but their condition meets no clinical criteria for a seizure. Formerly, EEGs were most useful to locate a cortical lesion, but recent imaging techniques have supplanted them. Some specific EEG patterns are still helpful when imaging is not (TABLE 12–9).

TABLE 12–8 *Laboratory Studies*

Diagnostic Group	Indications	Comments
Congenital		
Chromosomes	Dysmorphism or malformation	See Chapter 6
Genetic/metabolic		
Basic metabolic panel	Sz, HA, AC, hypotonia (hyp.)	Routinely
Ca^{2+}, PO_4^{3-}, Mg^{2+} (Magnesium)	Sz, AC, hypotonia (hyp.)	Routinely
Anticonvulsant levels	Sz, AC, hyp., ataxia (at.)	Any patient on medication
pH, NH_3, lactate/pyruvate	Sz, AC, DD, hyp., at., FTT	High index of suspicion in infants for
Organic acids, blood, and urine	↓ pH, normal or ↑ NH_3 = org.	inborn errors of metabolism
	Acidemia	
Urea cycle aa, blood, and urine	Nl pH, ↑NH_3 = urea cycle	
	Nl or ↓pH, nl NH_3 = aminoaciduria	
Vitamin D levels	Sz, AC, hypocalcemia	Metabolic bone disease
Copper/ceruloplasmin	Suspect Menkes, Wilson disease	Suspicion based on history and physical
		examination (PE).
Endocrine studies:		
Thyroid: T_4, TSH	DD, AC, hyp.	Clinical suspicion based on PE. See
		Chapter 13
Adrenal cortical hormones	Sz, AC, ↓Na^+, ↑K^+ AC, hyp.	See Chapter 13
Creatine phosphokinase (CPK) levels	Weakness	Myopathies, mitochondrial, SMA

(Continued)

TABLE 12-8 *Laboratory Studies (Continued)*

Diagnostic Group	Indications	Comments
Toxic		
Specific drugs (medications or drugs of abuse), blood, and urine	Sz, HA, AC, hyp., ataxia (at.)	Routinely, especially with unclear history; refer to toxidromes
Anticonvulsant levels	Sz, AC, hyp., At	Consider over/under dosing
Vitamin A and D levels	Sz, HA, AC, bone pain, abnormal Ca^{2+} (calcium) and PO_4^{2-} (phosphate)	Overdosing, underdosing
Botulinum toxin	Hyp., cr nn findings	Infants fed unprocessed honey
Infectious/inflammatory		
Meningoencephalitis		May need to obtain imaging first
CBC		↑WBC, left shift for bacterial ↓WBC, right shift for viral
CSF cells	Fever, Sz, AC, hyp., at, FW, stiff neck, +Kernig, Brudzinski signs	↑PMN (polymorphonuclear cells) for bacterial, early viral ↑Mononuclear cells for viral, Tb, fungal, ↑ red blood cells (RBC) in herpes
CSF chemistries		↓Glucose for bacterial, ↑ protein for all types
Bacterial cultures, viral cultures, titers, PCR		Confirmatory studies after history, physical, and preceding labs
Abscess	Fever, Sz, AC, FW	Should obtain imaging first
Complete blood count (CBC)		↑WBC, left shift
Cerebrospinal fluid (CSF)		
Postviral		
Guillain-Barré	Hyp., ↓ reflexes, cr nn III findings Autonomic instability, ascending paralysis	Small ↑white blood cells (WBC), ↑protein Previous viral or *Campylobacter* infection
Cerebrospinal fluid (CSF)		

Demyelinating disorders		
Multiple sclerosis	Sz, AC, FW, cr nn sx, sensory	↑CSF protein
CSF		Relapses and remits ↑IgG, ↑oligoclonal bands
ADEM	Similar to multiple sclerosis in presentation	Similar to multiple sclerosis in presentation
Traumatic		See Imaging Studies; CSF, blood, and protein may be elevated, but this is nct helpful in diagnosis
Neoplastic	HA, Sz, AC, At, FW	See Imaging Studies; CSF, protein may be ↑; lumbar puncture (LP) not indicated
Vascular		
CVA	HA, Sz, AC, FW	Imaging more specific for diagnosis
Tests for hypercoagulability, Protein C, S, factor V Leiden mutation, D-dimer.		
CSF: RBC for subarachnoid blood. Xanthochromic w/ old blood, ↑ protein from blood		
Sickle cell studies, Hgb electrophoresis		
Collagen-Vascular studies ANA, Anti DNA, RF		

Abbreviations: Sz = seizures; HA = headache; AC = altered consciousness; at. = ataxia; FW = focal weakness; cr nn = cranial nerves; ADEM = acute demyelinating encephalomyelitis; SMA = spinal muscular atrophy; aa = amino acids; nl = normal; DD = developmental delay; hyp = hypotonia; Na = sodium; K = potassium; Hgb = hemoglobin; ANA = antinuclear antibody; RF = rheumatoid factor; NH$_3$ = ammonia; w/ = with.

TABLE 12–9   EEG Patterns

Condition	Clinical: EEG Pattern
Petit-mal	See text: 3/s spike and wave, occur with hyperventilation
Infantile spasms	See text: hypsarrhythmia—chaotic high-voltage asynchronous
Encephalopathy	Sz, AC, progressing DD, diffuse slowing
Landau-Kleffner (syndrome)	Acquired aphasia: spike and long waves centropemporally
Lennox-Gastaut (syndrome)	Sz, MR, 1.5-2/s spike and wave
Otahara syndrome	Sz, profound DD, burst suppression
Rolandic epilepsy	Generally benign sz: centrotemporal spikes
Juv. myoclonic epilepsy of Janz	4-6/s spike and wave, occur with photic stimuli
Partial seizures	See text: use EEG if imaging is not helpful and clinical picture is in doubt
Pseudoseizures	Normal EEG pattern in the face of an episode
MR, nonprog	Not indicated
ADD, LD	Not indicated

Abbreviations: Sz = seizures; AC = altered consciousness; DD = developmental delay; nonprog = nonprogressive; MR = mental retardation; ADD = attention deficit disorder; LD = learning disability.

Key Neuroimaging Findings

Recent technology enables us to diagnose several conditions more accurately. However, studies have shown that not all MRI results correlate with findings at autopsy. Therefore, we must continue to test clinical hypotheses and should not order neuroimaging studies as a "fishing expedition." Clinical history and physical findings should continue to play a significant role in formulating a diagnosis.

Ultrasonographic studies are more helpful in patients with fontanels. In newborns, they are useful for detecting CNS hemorrhage, hydrocephalus, and malformation of the vein of Galen. Doppler ultrasounds also detect vascular blockages or overcirculation in *arteriovenous malformations (AVMs)*.

X-ray studies, including CT scans and MRI, are today's most helpful diagnostic adjuncts. Plain skull films are rarely, if ever, indicated. Neuroimaging is necessary for all patients with seizures who demonstrate any focality. CT scans are most helpful to detect blood, as in trauma (*hematoma* or *epidural or subdural collections*) or hemorrhagic stroke. They detect *congenital malformations, calcifications, hydrocephalus, cysts, porencephalic cysts,* and *cortical brain tumors.* They also detect infarction, focal encephalitis (herpes), and demyelination at later stages. When enhanced with contrast material, they are helpful to delineate increased vascularity, as in *AVMs* and *tumors.* MRIs, if available emergently, are helpful to diagnose early focal encephalitis and transient ischemia. They are also the first-choice indication for evaluating *sellar and posterior fossa tumors, demyelinating disease (multiple sclerosis, ADEM), progressive dementia, encephalopathy,* and *movement disorders.* If a finding on CT scan is suspicious for a focal lesion, order an MRI for confirmation. Also, if a CT scan is not helpful to confirm a strong clinical suspicion, MRI is necessary.

When to Refer

The many reasons for consultation include one or more of the following: patient comfort, diagnosis, and management. Consistent with the scope of this book, this section discusses referrals for diagnosis. Case management is a separate consideration, and the neurologist and pediatrician should be partners in care, with one or the other taking the primary role. After taking a careful history and completing a physical examination, the primary care physician should obtain neurologic consultation when questions remain unanswered. Often a conversation between the pediatrician and the neurologist before referral saves time and expense. A single diagnostic test suggested by the neurologist and ordered by the pediatrician may obviate the need for further consultation. *As a rule, only order diagnostic tests if they will influence patient management.* Too often an unnecessary imaging study done at the parent's request identifies an unrelated normal variant that leads to further anguish and expense. A thoughtful consultant orders tests sequentially, and one who orders panels of tests at the onset has no idea what is wrong and is fishing for an answer. The urgency for consultation should be a clinical decision based on rapidity of onset and progression of symptoms. In practice, parental concern and tolerance for delay often dictate urgency.

Congenital. CT scan detects most major malformations. MRI is required to observe many *migrational defects* and to further clarify the extent of many congenital anomalies. *Inborn errors of metabolism* may cause structural abnormalities of the brain, and genetic consultation is helpful even in the absence of dysmorphic features (see Chapter 6).

Genetic/metabolic. Every pediatrician should be aware of the specific diseases that comprise the newborn screen in the state of birth. Most inborn errors of metabolism have characteristic clinical features that lead to specific evaluation. Computer-based resources such as *Online Mendelian Inheritance in Man* (OMIM) and *Geneclinics* provide guidelines for evaluation and diagnosis. See Chapter 5 for state screening.

   After initial screening, separate *organic acidemias* from *urea cycle defects* and *aminoacidopathies.* Acidosis owing to *inborn errors of metabolism* and some *aminoacidopathies* will have an increased anion gap. Some *aminoacidopathies* have normal pH and ammonia levels. Acidosis is characteristic of *organic acidemias,* some *aminoacidopathies,* and *carboxylase deficiencies. Urea cycle disorders* typically have elevated ammonia levels with normal pH. See TABLE 12–10 and consult a neurology text for more details about each of these metabolic disorders, as well as *mitochondrial, gray matter, white matter, myopathic,*

TABLE 12-10 *Rarer Congenital/Metabolic/Genetic Diagnoses*

Diagnosis	Clinical Points
I. Inborn errors of metabolism	
a. Aminoacidopathies	
Phenylketonuria (PKU)	Seizures, vomiting, DD, musty odor, fair skin, ↑ phenylketones
Tyrosinemia (type I)	Boiled cabbage odor, hepatorenal disease, PN, ↑ fumarylacetoacetate
Branched-chain ketoaciduria	Maple syrup urine (skin, cerumen); MR Sz, spasticity ↑Leu, Iso, Val.
b. Urea cycle defects	↑NH₃, normal pH, AC, MR, ↑ornithine, citrulline, argininosuccinate
c. Organic acidemias	Acidosis, nl or ↑NH₃ level, Sz, DD, vomiting
Isovaleric acidemia	"Sweaty sock" odor, AC Sz, coma, occ ↑NH₃, and hypoglycemia
MCAD	Sz, lethargy, coma, "tomcat urine" odor, FTT, eczematoid rash, ↑ infection
Biotin deficiency	Skin rash, Sz, hyp., MR, ↑ infection, biotin or biotinidase deficiency
Methylmalonic acidemia (MMA)	Sz, lethargy vomiting, acidosis, ↑NH₃. May have nl dev.; occurs in attacks
Propionic acidemia	Similar to MMA +MR, and MD
II. Mitochondrial disorders	
a. MELAS syndrome	Myoclonic epilepsy, lactic acidosis, and stroke
b. MERRF syndrome	Myoclonic epilepsy with red ragged fibers
c. Kearns-Sayre syndrome	Retinal degen, ophthalmoplegia, at., heart block, ↑CSF protein
d. Leigh disease	Hyp, spasticity DR, MD, lactic acidosis, cardiomyopathy
e. Alper	Sz, DR, blindness, lactic acidosis, grey matter degen., cirrhosis of liver
III. Gray matter degeneration	
a. Lesch-Nyhan	Hyp., MD, MR, aggressiveness, self-mutilation, ↑uric acid level
b. Rett	Females, hand-wringing, Sz, DR, at., autism, microcephaly
c. Menkes	Kinky hair, lethargy, myoclonic Sz, ↓ serum Cu, and ceruloplasmin
d. Ceroid lipofuscinosis.	Sz, DR, blindness, pigmented CNS and eyes; infantile and juvenile forms.

IV. White matter degeneration

a. Alexander disease (dis) — DR, Sz, ↑ head size, MRI criteria for dx, Rosenthal fibers on biopsy

b. Pelizaeus-Merzbacher dis. — Head nod, at., MD, DR, optic atrophy, demyelination on MRI

c. Canavan disease — DR, hyp. at first, then spastic, ↑ head, optic atrophy

d. Adrenoleukodystrophy — DR, at., behavioral change, blindness/deafness, adrenal insuff., ↑ long chain FA

V. Storage diseases

a. Gaucher type II, infantile — Hyp. → spasticity, head retraction, sucking prob., pursed lips, DR, ↑ spleen, ↓glucocerebroside activity

b. Tay-Sachs GM$_2$ gangliosidosis — ↑ Startle, DR (motor and mental), cherry red macula, ↑ in AJP, hex. A defic.

c. Sandhoff GM$_2$ gangliosidosis — Like Tay-Sachs + hepatosplenomegaly (HSM); hex. A and hex. B deficiency

d. Niemann-Pick (sphingomyelin) — DR, FTT, blindness, opisthotonus, emaciation, HSM, cherry red macula

e. Metachromatic leukodyst — At., DR quadriplegia; infantile and juvenile; arylsulfatase A deficiency

f. Mucopolysaccharidoses — Coarse facies, gibbus deform., corneal clouding, deafness, DR; see individual types for degree of variation

VI. Spinal musc. atrophy

a. Werdnig-Hoffman (SMA I) — Infantile form, hyp. (in ureters), facial weakness, swallowing problem, fasciculations

b. Kugelberg-Welander (SMA III) — Juvenile form, gait instability, proximal weakness, tremor, ↓ reflexes

VII. Neuropathy

a. Charcot-Marie-Tooth disease — Childhood, slow onset, pes cavus, foot drop, distal weakness (peroneal → gastrocnemius), ↓ reflexes and position sense

VIII. Myopathy

A. Musc. dystrophy (limb-griddle)

a. Duchenne (DMD) — Onset < 5 y, ↓ motor dev., prox. weakness, +Gower sign, toe-walking, pseudohypertrophy, prog. weakness, ↓ reflexes, contractures, cardiac, LD

b. Becker (mild form of DMD) — Onset >10 y, shoulder girdle → humerus → facial muscles, occ. blind and deaf

c. Facioscapulohumeral — Emery-Dreifuss (onset age 5, slow progression, contractures, cardiomyopathy),

d. Others — Betlem (onset age 2, slow prog., contractures)

399

(Continued)

TABLE 12-10 *Rarer Congenital/Metabolic/Genetic Diagnoses (Continued)*

Diagnosis	Clinical Points
B. Cong. myopathy	
a. Nemaline myopathy	Variable clinical forms, face, neck proximal weakness, rods on biopsy
b. Central core disease	Mild hypotonia at birth, slow prog, weakness prox. > distal, upper ext. > lower, contractures, scoliosis, hip dislocation, malignant hypothermia, bx diagnosis
c. Others	Myotubular myopathy, multiminicore disease
IX. Neurocutaneous	
a. Incontinentia pigmenti	Sz, MR, bullae → pigment whorls → depigmented whorls; spasticity, Sz, MR, other ectodermal defects (hair, eyes)
b. Linear nevus sebaceous	Unilateral linear nevus, hemihypertrophy, ocular abn., Sz, MR, FW, ↑ head size
	Ataxia, dev regression, ↓ reflexes, ↓ proprioception
c. Hypomelanosis of Ito	Sz, MR, eye abnorm, whorls of hypopigmentation, ↑ head size
X. Progressive ataxias.	
Spinocerebellar degen.	
b. Abetalipoproteinemia	Retinitis pigmentosa, low cholesterol, acanthocytosis
c. Refsum disease	Retinitis pigmentosa, polyneuropathy, ataxia, ↑ phytanic acid
d. Friedreich ataxia	Children and adults, progressive, ataxia, pes cavus, ↓ position and vibration, cardiac failure

Abbreviations: Sz = seizures; DD = developmental delay; PN = peripheral nerves; AC = altered consciousness; MR = mental retardataion; FTT = failue to thrive; hyp. = hypotonia; MD = movement disorder; at. = ataxia; DR = developmental regression; AJP = Ashkenazi Jewish Population; at = ataxia; cong = congenital; degen = degeneration; def = deformity; dev = development; ext = extremity; HSM = hepatosplenomegaly; insuff = insufficiency; nl = normal; occ = occasional; Cu = copper; leu = leucine; iso = isoleucine; val = valine; Hex A = hexosaminidase A; leukodyst = leukodystrophy; MELAS = mitochondrial encephalopathy lactic acidosis, strokelike episodes; MSUD = Maple Syrup Urine Disease; SMA: spinal muscular atrophy.

lysosomal storage, spinocerebellar degenerative diseases, and *spinomuscular atrophies.* Note the recent advances in molecular genetics, and always include a geneticist in consultation with patients with these conditions.

Neurocutaneous syndromes such as *neurofibromatosis I and II* and *tuberous sclerosis* are usually clinical diagnoses with some help from imaging. However, molecular genetics studies are available for tuberous sclerosis and are employed to differentiate genotypes.

Infectious/inflammatory. Specific bacterial, viral, fungal, or rickettsial cultures or other serologic or immunologic evidence of infection, e.g., fluorescent antibodies, obtained by antibody titers is most helpful to determine an etiology of an acute infectious or postinfectious process, e.g., *rubella, measles, EBV,* or *campylobacter in Guillain-Barré disease.* It still may be necessary for the neurologist to order nerve conduction velocities or electromyography to differentiate neuropathy from myopathy. Imaging studies may be helpful, examples of which are localization in the temporal lobe of *herpes encephalitis* and demyelinating lesions in *ADEM.*

Traumatic. Most acute trauma is diagnosed immediately during the acute event. History, physical examination, and imaging studies are usually sufficient to elucidate the diagnosis.

Neoplastic. The primary care physician may identify tumors, but the neurologist and/or neurosurgeon is necessary to delineate the specific histologic type. If neuroimaging studies are normal and there is still clinical suspicion of a space-occupying lesion, a neurologist is helpful to review findings and to consider additional studies.

Vascular. The primary care physician always should be mindful of clotting disorders, vasculitides, and congenital malformations that may cause thrombotic or hemorrhagic strokes. If CT scan and MRI are normal and the clinician still suspects vascular disease, arteriography may be necessary.

13 The Endocrine System

Martin B. Draznin and Manmohan Kamboj

The goals of this chapter are

1. To summarize developmental, anatomic, and functional aspects of the endocrine system(s)
2. To review symptoms that suggest an endocrine disorder as presented by infants, children, and adolescents and to suggest different endocrine diagnoses that may explain these symptoms
3. To present details of physical findings that are due to endocrine disorders and discuss how they support consideration of endocrine diagnoses
4. To provide a systematic approach to laboratory evaluation based on the history and physical examination
5. To assist with the decision about when a consultation with an endocrinologist is helpful

Anatomy and Developmental Physiology

There is truly a plethora of substances that can act as hormones. Hormones are produced in one cell, transmitted to another cell by means other than direct cell-to-cell contact (as in neuronal transmission of signals), interact with specific receptors of the target cell, and have an effect on a specific function or functions of that cell. There is often a *negative-feedback loop* operating between the hormone-secreting cell and the hormone target cell to maintain homeostasis and avoid oscillation of the effects of the hormone. One typically thinks of the hypothalamic-pituitary-endocrine gland axes as being of major importance; however, the gastrointestinal tract can be considered to interact in a pseudoendocrine manner with the pancreas by providing changing concentrations of nutrients as a signal. Gut-derived peptides not only signal satiety but influence release of insulin and growth hormone. The central nervous system (CNS) is also involved in meal-related activation of the pancreas. The immune system and endocrine system have numerous interactions as well. For purposes of diagnosis, we will limit this chapter to the more classically defined endocrine subsystems, their development and function, and disorders that manifest when they malfunction. FIGURE 13–1 shows the anatomic location of the endocrine glands.

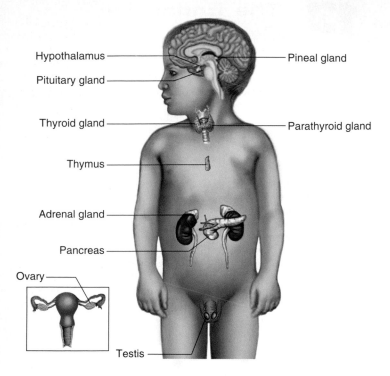

Hypothalamus

Pituitary gland

Thyroid gland

Thymus

Adrenal gland

Pancreas

Ovary

Pineal gland

Parathyroid gland

Testis

FIGURE 13-1 Endocrine Organs. *(From Van de Graaff KM:* Human Anatomy. *New York: McGraw-Hill, 1998.)*

The role of hormones begins in utero. One critical function is sexual differentiation. This process requires chromosomal components to cause the gonad to differentiate either to ovary or testis. The gonad then migrates caudally to a location appropriate for the sex of the embryo under the influence of human chorionic gonadotropin (hCG) and, later, pituitary luteinizing hormone (LH). The testes release testosterone to virilize the external genitalia and mullerian inhibiting hormone to suppress the persistence of the uterus and fallopian tubes to complete male differentiation. Female structures seem to develop without requiring any further stimulus at this stage. There is evidence that male and female brains contain subtle structural differences owing in part to androgen exposure during the gestation, but there also may be genetic differences.

The thyroid gland coalesces from branchial clefts and migrates to the front of the lower neck by 40 days of gestational age. Its secretion of thyroid hormone gradually increases throughout gestation, more during the third trimester, and then with the postdelivery surge of thyroid-stimulating hormone (TSH), it increases dramatically. The peripheral deiodination of T_4 during gestation is preferentially to the inactive reverse

T_3 form. On delivery, the newborn preferentially produces T_3; thus the gland works in concert with the peripheral tissues, as well as the hypothalamus and pituitary, to control thyroid economy. Deficiency of both fetal and maternal thyroid hormone leads to profound hypothyroidism at birth with attendant high risk of severe developmental delay if not rapidly treated. Calcitonin from the thyroid C cells is involved in calcium accretion by bones in utero.

Parathyroid hormone is relatively inactive, but a parathyroid hormone–like peptide is of vital importance in tissue differentiation and development in many organ systems. The vitamin D receptor is very important in embryogenesis.

Adrenal hormones generated in the fetal zone of the adrenal pass through the placenta. They are vital in maintaining the pregnancy to term. The fetal pancreas is capable of secreting insulin to allow nutrients entry to cells. Insulin acts as a growth peptide in utero.

Following delivery, the endocrine systems mediate growth and development, energy metabolism, balance of fluids and electrolytes, control of circulating calcium within a narrow range of concentration, and sexual maturation and function. Symptoms owing to endocrine dysfunction may be very subtle or quite dramatic. Signs also may not be readily apparent early in the course of an endocrine disorder. Numerous other conditions may suggest an endocrine problem when none is present.

History

Infants

Infants have a limited repertoire of symptoms, exhibit a few more signs than symptoms, and do not speak for themselves. Thus the ability to interpret parents' understanding of their problems is the key to progress in making a diagnosis.

There are few symptoms that by themselves declare an endocrine diagnosis. As with any subspecialty area, a thorough general history is the foundation on which to base endocrine-specific questions. Presenting problems that are due to endocrine dysfunction include changes in general well-being, disordered growth, disordered energy metabolism, disordered sexual development or function, alterations of skin and its appendages, and altered gastrointestinal motility, thirst, and urine output. The review of systems from the general history touches on endocrine function at many levels.

We address growth disorders by focusing on the complaint—too little or too much growth—in a comprehensive manner; i.e., when was the problem first noted, how has the growth changed, does it cause difficulties for the patient, and did other family members have problems or concerns with their growth? Other helpful questions include whether the parent replaces clothes and shoes because they are worn out or because they are outgrown, whether the patient can keep up with age peers in all activities, what psychosocial stressors may have occurred, changes in appetite, use of stimulant medications for attention-deficit/ hyperactivity disorder (ADHD), pregnancy, delivery, and neonatal growth characteristics. It is important to understand what and how much the patient actually eats and to elicit symptoms of chronic renal, gastrointestinal, cardiac, pulmonary, or inflammatory disorders because poor growth statistically is more likely to be due to undernutrition or chronic nonendocrine disorders than to deficiency of hormones that promote growth.

Disorders of sexual differentiation usually manifest early in life. Questions that are useful in a family history are whether there are any other affected family members, whether there were any early infant deaths, whether there were any exposures of the mother to androgenic agents during the pregnancy or if she experienced virilization, or for undervirilized males, if there was any exposure to putative endocrine disruptors or estrogenic compounds. Sexual maturation may occur precociously or very late, and a family history again is of primary importance, especially because a history of delayed onset of puberty in healthy parents suggests that the child has a different pattern of growth and development from the norm rather than a disorder. Exposure to exogenous sex steroids should be investigated; these may be present in cosmetics in the case of estrogen and also in substances used by body builders such as skin bronzing treatments that also contained testosterone, to name two sources.

Disorders of energy metabolism suggesting thyroid problems present with changes in activity, in tolerance to heat or cold, in duration of sleep, and in an increase in fidgeting or a decrease in the ability to pay attention; even emotional lability may be due to hyperthyroidism. Hypothyroid patients may have increased gut transit time or frank constipation; hyperthyroid patients may have hyperdefecation or diarrhea. Precocious puberty with a "muscular" appearance owing to pseudohypertrophy of calf muscles may occur in school-age hypothyroid children. Adolescent females may experience menometrorrhagia to the point of becoming anemic with hypothyroidism; conversely, hyperthyroid adolescents may have scanty to absent menses.

Adrenal insufficiency may lead to fatigue, mental status changes, chronic diarrhea, and collapse. It may be insidious, so the diagnosis may be delayed until obvious signs are found.

Skin changes in endocrine disorders include pallor, plethora, striae, early acne, subcutaneous deposits of glycoproteins (myxedema), thickening and darkening of intertriginous areas (pseudoacanthosis nigricans), tanning (the color in Addison disease is unusual), and "bronzing" of the skin, including areas that receive little or no sun exposure. Some of these will be part of the complaint, whereas the examiner may have to elicit others.

Increased thirst and urine output can mark diabetes mellitus or diabetes insipidus. The preferred fluid may be a clue because cold water seems to be most satisfying to persons with diabetes insipidus. Questions should focus on onset, timing, whether the increase in drinking preceded or followed the increased urine output, whether sleep is affected or there is enuresis, and how much liquid intake is needed to satisfy thirst.

Disorders of calcium metabolism affect rapidly growing bone as well as the function of nerves and muscles because calcium flux across cell membranes is a critical signaling mechanism for many vital cellular processes. Excess calcium adversely affects renal function, whereas calcium deficiency may lead to elevated parathyroid hormone, which may induce phosphaturia and even a Fanconi syndrome-like effect with glycosuria and aminoaciduria.

KEY PROBLEM
Constitutional Infants may show little energy, poor feeding, weak cry, poor muscle tone, and other nonspecific variations of activity. The older they are, the more specific the parents can make their characterizations. The endocrine and endocrine-related conditions that may present with these complaints include *hypoglycemia, dehydration, hypothyroidism,* and *electrolyte imbalance.* Jitteriness, tremors, agitation, excessive crying, and inconsolability may be signs of *hyperthyroidism, hypoglycemia,* or *hypocalcemia.* Relation of these symptoms to timing of feedings and relief with food may suggest hypoglycemia. Heat or cold intolerance is not likely to be a complaint related to infants, but mottling of the skin may indicate hypothyroidism. Altered consciousness or frank seizures may be hard to discern at times in infants but become more typical with increased age, and their investigation should include tests for hypoglycemia and hypocalcemia.

KEY PROBLEM
Growth Issues Small stature is a common complaint in older children but may occur even in newborns. *Intrauterine growth retardation* (IUGR), *placental disorders, Turner syndrome, Russell-Silver syndrome,* and *growth hormone resistance* can yield a small neonate or may appear later in infancy. Overgrowth, usually defined as a birth weight above 90th percentile, is associated with *maternal diabetes* and *genetic syndromes,* including *Beckwith-Wiedemann* syndrome in early infancy. Later, excessive size may be secondary to exogenous obesity. Underweight infants who present with failure to gain weight or who lose weight may have *undernutrition, hyperthyroidism,* or *diabetes mellitus,* whereas overweight infants usually are overfed but may occasionally have an *overgrowth syndrome* or *hyperinsulinemia* (see anthropometric measurements under "Physical Examination" below).

KEY PROBLEM
Abnormalities of Skin and Cutaneous Appendages Infants may have hairiness, which may be hypertrichosis owing to *hyperinsulinemia* or some *medications* (e.g., diazoxide), or it may be a familial pattern. Their hair may be coarse, dry, and brittle in hypothyroidism. The skin may appear pale, thickened, and waxy if *hypothyroidism* has persisted for weeks or months without treatment. There may be a history of unusual pigmentation that might include café-au-lait spots with an irregular border, tending to be unilateral in *McCune-Albright*

syndrome. Fingernails and toenails may be unusual, such as the hyper-convex nails in *Turner syndrome.*

KEY PROBLEM

Abnormalities of the Head A "ping pong ball skull" suggests *neonatal rickets.* Persistence of an open posterior fontanel or a very large anterior fontanel suggests *hypothyroidism.*

KEY PROBLEM

Abnormalities of the Eyes Parents may observe nystagmus, especially if it is associated with signs of poor visual fixation, suggesting *septo-optic dysplasia,* often associated with hypothalamic-pituitary deficiency. A defect of the iris also may accompany hypothalamic malformation.

KEY PROBLEM

Abnormalities of the Ears Deafness may be part of hereditary syndromes such as *Pendred syndrome,* which also includes *hypothyroidism,* but deafness is also a consequence of untreated hypothyroidism.

KEY PROBLEM

Abnormalities of the Neck Swelling in the anterior neck may be due to thyroid enlargement as a result of iodine deficiency, enzymatic defects of thyroid hormonogenesis, *maternal antithyroid medication* leading to increased TSH stimulation in utero, or transplacental passage of thyroid-stimulating immunoglobulin from *maternal Graves disease* leading to *neonatal Graves disease.* A cystic midline mass may be a *thyroglossal duct cyst.* An orifice in the midline that drains clear fluid may be a thyroglossal duct sinus.

KEY PROBLEM

Respiratory Symptoms Irregular breathing may indicate CNS effects of *hypoglycemia* or *hypocalcemia.* Hyperventilation or hyperpnea often occurs in new onset of *diabetes mellitus* in infants.

KEY PROBLEM

Cardiovascular Symptoms High heart rate is often apparent in *hyperthyroidism,* whereas low heart rate accompanies *hypothyroidism* but is less likely to be discovered by parents.

KEY PROBLEM

Gastrointestinal Symptoms Abdominal pain may indicate *diabetic ketoacidosis, adrenal failure,* or *hypercalcemia.*

KEY PROBLEM

CNS Symptoms Parents usually will not comment on reflexes but may comment on stiffness (consider *hypocalcemia* as an endocrine cause) or floppiness (consider *hypercalcemia*). Abnormality of gait may be due to *rickets.* The bending of the limbs is due to walking on them when there is an enlarged and abnormal zone of osteoid that cannot calcify. These bones are also painful on weight bearing.

KEY PROBLEM
Breast Changes Early breast development may represent retained neonatal breast buds that enlarge slightly or may be due to a *functioning ovarian follicle, exogenous estrogen exposure,* or *precocious puberty.* Infants may have physiologic galactorrhea.

KEY PROBLEM
Male Genitalia Abnormalities Undescended testes may be physiologic when due to *prematurity,* or they may be due to syndromes. A virilized female infant with *congenital adrenal hyperplasia* may appear to be a male with undescended testes. Enlarged, firm testes may be physiologic or due to *tumor, torsion, hydrocele,* etc. *Microphallus* can accompany *hypopituitarism, androgen insensitivity,* or *premature testicular failure* and loss. Hypospadias can accompany disorders of sexual differentiation and some syndromes.

KEY PROBLEM
Premature Appearance of Pubic Hair When just on the scrotum or labia majora in infants, this may be a benign finding and will not progress. However, when there is progression or spread over the pubes, *congenital adrenal hyperplasia* and *androgen-producing tumors* are more likely.

KEY PROBLEM
Menstrual Disturbances Postdelivery estrogen withdrawal may eventuate in vaginal bleeding in normal female neonates.

KEY PROBLEM
Polyuria and Polydipsia *Diabetes insipidus* may lead to very frequent feeding in infants or increased thirst in toddlers and increased urine output. *Diabetes mellitus* may present in a similar manner.

Children

KEY PROBLEM
Constitutional Children may complain of fatigue or have reduced exercise tolerance, increased sleep, lethargy, etc. from *hypothyroidism, hypoglycemia, dehydration, electrolyte and/or calcium abnormalities, adrenal insufficiency,* or *diabetes mellitus.* They may have irritability, agitation, difficulty concentrating in school, and emotional lability from *hyperthyroidism, hypocalcemia,* or *hypoglycemia.* Heat intolerance may accompany hyperthyroidism, whereas cold intolerance is a frequent complaint with *hypothyroidism.* Fainting may be due to *hypoglycemia, adrenal insufficiency,* or *hypocalcemia.* Seizures may be due to hypoglycemia or hypocalcemia.

KEY PROBLEM
Heat or Cold Intolerance
Children and adolescents are more able to articulate these symptoms, and they will be uncomfortable in a warm or cool office setting. Think *hypothyroidism* for cold intolerance and *hyperthyroidism* for heat intolerance.

KEY PROBLEM
Growth
Children notice that they are shorter than their peers, as do their parents. A change in the rate of growth also may be the complaint, well before the child is actually short. Causes include the physiologic, such as familial short stature and constitutional delay of growth and maturation. Others include *malnutrition, chronic illness, inflammatory bowel disease, congenital syndromes such as Turner syndrome* and others, *hypothyroidism, growth hormone deficiency,* and *Cushing syndrome.* Excessively tall stature may be secondary to *exogenous obesity, precocious puberty, genetic overgrowth syndromes,* and *growth hormone excess owing to tumor.*

KEY PROBLEM
Weight
Underweight children have too little intake or too much expenditure of nutrients. *Hyperthyroidism* and *diabetes mellitus* cause wasting of energy and nutrients, and *diabetes insipidus* substitutes drinking of water for eating and also may suppress appetite if there is electrolyte imbalance. Overweight in children is occasionally due to hormone deficiency, as in *hypothyroidism,* or hormone excess, as in *Cushing syndrome.* These usually are readily distinguishable from exogenous obesity because hormone-induced obesity almost always accompanies diminished linear growth. Overgrowth syndromes may be associated with overweight. *Prader-Willi syndrome* is usually associated with short stature and delayed puberty, even with growth hormone deficiency.

KEY PROBLEM
Skin and Cutaneous Appendages
Stretch marks accompany weight gain and may occur in exogenous obesity or *Cushing syndrome.* Dark skin in creases and around the neck may be a complaint. Generalized hairiness or just increased hair in androgen-sensitive areas may be a concern. Hair that breaks suggests *hypothyroidism,* whereas hair that falls out in a diffuse manner suggests *telogen effluvium,* with synchronization of follicles after an endocrine change, and leads to more profuse loss. More circumscribed hair loss suggests *alopecia areata,* an autoimmune condition that may accompany *autoimmune endocrinopathy.* Thick, waxy skin is characteristic of *hypothyroidism,* whereas thin skin accompanies *Cushing syndrome.* Pigmented patches are seen in infants and may signify *McCune-Albright syndrome,* whereas generalized bronzing, with absent tan lines (i.e., areas not exposed to sun are also hyperpigmented), suggests *Addison disease. Candidiasis* of nails suggests *polyglandular autoimmune endocrinopathy,* hyperconvex nails occur in *Turner syndrome,* and onycholysis occurs in *Graves disease.*

KEY PROBLEM
Head Abnormalities Children complain of headache, which may be due to *increased intracranial pressure* associated with *tumors* in the region of the pituitary, as well as *pseudotumor cerebri* associated with starting/cessation of endocrine hormone therapy, including starting growth hormone. *Hypoglycemia* may trigger migraine headaches.

KEY PROBLEM
Eye Abnormalities Children have less frequent and less severe exophthalmos with *Graves disease* than do adults but may complain of dry, red, or burning eyes. Diplopia on upward or lateral gaze may indicate extraocular muscle involvement. Visual field defects may manifest as tripping over or running into objects that are low and to one side and indicate a search for a *pituitary mass lesion*. Nystagmus is associated with *septo-optic dysplasia*. Blurring of vision may be due to *hyperglycemia* with swelling of the crystalline lens and loss of accommodation.

KEY PROBLEM
Ear Abnormalities Deafness associated with *hypothyroidism* is the same as in infants.

KEY PROBLEM
Neck Abnormalities Thyroid enlargement with or without pressure symptoms can be a complaint in *hypothyroidism* or *hyperthyroidism* or *thyroiditis*, as in infants. Pain is a usual accompaniment of acute or *subacute thyroiditis*; it is not often part of *chronic thyroiditis* or *Graves disease*. Swallowing may be difficult in the presence of a large *goiter*.

KEY PROBLEM
Cardiovascular Symptoms Palpitations, or a high and regular heart rate, indicate increased adrenergic effect that may be due to *hyperthyroidism*, whereas most children will not complain of a slow heart rate.

KEY PROBLEM
Gastrointestinal Symptoms Pain in diabetic ketoacidosis or *Addison disease* may be quite severe and suggests other conditions such as *appendicitis* or *gastroenteritis*. Constipation may be due to *hypothyroidism*, whereas *hyperthyroid* children may have increased numbers of bowel movements in a day or even diarrhea.

KEY PROBLEM
Neurologic Symptoms These are the same as with infants.

KEY PROBLEM
Breast Changes Early development of breasts, younger than 8 years of age, may be *isolated premature thelarche* without true precocious puberty or may signal a more serious condition. Questions to ask include possible exposure to estrogen-containing medications or

cosmetics. Androgen symptoms such as sexual hair, acne, or body odor suggest puberty rather than an isolated growth of breast tissue. Discomfort in the breast bud and asymmetry in size are not usually symptoms suggesting pathology, although chest wall tumors and indolent infections may give rise to masses in the area of the breast. Galactorrhea may be due to medication or increased pituitary release of prolactin. *Gynecomastia,* breast growth in males, may be prepubertal, in which case there may be no identified pathology, or there may have been exposure to exogenous estrogen.

KEY PROBLEM
Male Genitalia Abnormalities
Undescended testes may be idiopathic, part of a syndrome, or due to a *disorder of sexual development.* Enlarged testes may be due to onset of puberty, genetic causes such as *fragile-X syndrome* or autonomous testicular function in the absence of pituitary activation, or *tumors,* including adrenal rest tissue in poorly controlled *congenital adrenal hyperplasia.* Painful testes may be due to *torsion* or *tumor.*

KEY PROBLEM
Polyuria and Polydipsia
These may be due to *diabetes insipidus* or *diabetes mellitus.* A form of *diabetes insipidus* can be due to *hypercalcemia.*

Adolescents

KEY PROBLEM
Constitutional
Since adolescents have a different wake/sleep cycle than adults and children yet are expected to be awake and alert in the early morning for school, it is often difficult to differentiate pathologic fatigue from a mismatch of physiology with schedule. *Hypothyroidism, adrenal insufficiency, diabetes mellitus, hypoglycemia,* and *hypocalcemia* are all possible causes of nonspecific fatigue. As for shakiness and agitation, they can be associated with *hyperthyroidism,* hypoglycemia, or hypocalcemia. Emotional lability from hyperthyroidism also may be harder to differentiate from the typical adolescent experience of strong and shifting emotions. Heat and cold intolerance are still helpful clues to hyper- or hypothyroidism. Poor athletic performance even though training hard may be a sign of reversible *hypopituitarism;* in females it would accompany menstrual irregularity. Fainting spells and seizures may begin with adolescence; hypoglycemia and hypocalcemia are still the most profitable areas to pursue. *Adrenal insufficiency* may manifest with orthostatic hypotension and fainting.

KEY PROBLEM
Heat or Cold Intolerance
This is similar to children and adolescents.

KEY PROBLEM

Growth Short stature in adolescents is often due to delay of on-set of puberty and not to a disorder of growth. Delayed puberty may or may not be a physiologic variant; *hypogonadal hypogonadism* or primary *gonadal failure* may be the cause. All causes of short stature in children apply to adolescents as well. Tall stature is similar in this regard and with delayed puberty may indicate *Klinefelter syndrome.* Complaint of underweight, isolated or associated with undergrowth, can be part of *diabetes mellitus, hyperthyroidism,* or *undernutrition.* Overweight adolescents almost all have exogenous obesity, but rare overgrowth syndromes may include obesity. Adolescents with *Cushing syndrome, hypothyroidism,* and *Prader-Willi* syndrome are usually not tall.

KEY PROBLEM

Skin and Cutaneous Appendages There may be complaints of stretch marks in children; acne may be extreme in hyper-androgenic states such as undertreated *congenital adrenal hyperplasia* or the *metabolic syndrome–polycystic ovarian syndrome* continuum. Hirsutism in females suggests androgen excess; generalized hairiness may just be hypertrichosis. Hair changes such as increased falling hair from a sud-den change in endocrine balance and dryness and breaking in hy-pothyroidism are important symptoms. Patchy hair loss again is more from autoimmune causes. The dry, waxy skin of *hypothyroidism* may be a complaint. A very unusual tan involving areas that are not sun-exposed may indicate *Addison disease.* Nail abnormalities are similar to those in children.

KEY PROBLEM

Head Abnormalities Symptoms are much as in children.

KEY PROBLEM

Eye Abnormalities Adolescents are more likely than chil-dren but less likely than adults to have exophthalmos. Other eye complaints in *Graves disease* are the same as experienced by children. Adolescents are more likely to articulate visual field defects as blind spots, although they too may just trip over or bump into objects that are in the blind spot. Blurring of vision and loss of accommodation can accompany *diabetes mellitus* until the blood sugar levels are controlled.

KEY PROBLEM

Neck Symptoms Adolescents are more likely to notice a pressure sensation and/or mass in the neck from a *goiter;* there may be painful symptoms from *subacute* or *acute thyroiditis.* The causes are similar to those in children.

KEY PROBLEM

Cardiovascular Symptoms Adolescents may notice and be concerned about heart rhythm disturbances or rapid rate more than children. They are more prone to orthostatic hypotension of a physiologic nature.

KEY PROBLEM
Abdominal Symptoms These are much the same as in children owing to *diabetes with ketoacidosis* or *Addisonian crisis*. Diarrhea associated with *Graves disease* and constipation owing to *hypothyroidism* are still useful symptoms to pursue.

KEY PROBLEM
Neurologic Symptoms Adolescents are more aware of loss of function or tightness of muscles as with *hypocalcemia* and shakiness from *hypoglycemia* or *hyperthyroidism* and may complain of these symptoms or answer in the affirmative on the review of symptoms.

KEY PROBLEM
Breast Changes Galactorrhea in males or females is more common and can be due to hyperprolactinemia from a *pituitary adenoma* or to *medication* or chronic nipple stimulation. Mild gynecomastia with small breast buds that regress spontaneously is physiologic in male puberty. Persistent gynecomastia is still usually not due to an endocrine disorder, but it also may indicate *disorders of androgen synthesis, Klinefelter syndrome, feminizing adrenal tumors, aromatase hyperactivation, drugs and medicines* (including spironolactone, cimetidine, phenothiazines, cannabis, and others), and *testicular failure.*

KEY PROBLEM
External Male Genitalia Abnormalities Undescended testes are the same as in infants and children. Testicular masses may be *tumors;* if painful and enlarged, they may be due to *torsion* or *hydrocele.*

KEY PROBLEM
Female External Genitalia Abnormalities Virilization occurs when the androgen levels are high enough to produce clitoral hypertrophy. This may be associated with male-pattern hair loss. Virilization occurring postnatally does not induce labial fusion and ambiguity, except for the increased size of the clitoris.

KEY PROBLEM
Menstrual Disturbances Primary amenorrhea occurs in physiologic delay of puberty, in *Turner syndrome*, in disorders of sexual differentiation, and in gynecologic abnormalities. Oligomenorrhea occurs in *hyperthyroidism*, the female athlete triad, and the first year or so after menarche in some adolescents until they start having mostly ovulatory cycles. Secondary amenorrhea occurs in *pregnancy, polycystic ovarian syndrome, hyperthyroidism,* and the *female athlete triad.* Menorrhagia/ metrorrhagia occurs in *hypothyroidism.*

KEY PROBLEM
Polyuria and Polydipsia These occur in *diabetes insipidus* and *diabetes mellitus.*

KEY PROBLEM

Menstrual Disturbances Premature menses in childhood require evaluation for precocious puberty or pseudopuberty and for exposure to exogenous estrogen. Primary amenorrhea suggests *ovarian dysgenesis* as in *Turner syndrome,* other *disorders of sexual differentiation, hematocolpos,* a thick hymen, or absence of a uterus. Secondary amenorrhea may be due to pregnancy, polycystic ovarian syndrome, androgen excess from uncontrolled *congenital adrenal hyperplasia,* or tumors. Oligoamenorrhea may be part of the female athlete triad; it may be due to hyperthyroidism or significant weight loss from other causes. Menorrhagia and metrorrhagia may be due to *hypothyroidism.*

Physical Examination

Endocrinology is quantitative, and how much of what, when, and where are central themes. Measurements of stature and body proportion are only useful if done consistently and correctly throughout the growth and development of the patient. Proper plotting of values, at the precise age and on the correct chart, will maximize ability to interpret these values. Measure length in infants supine on a flat, firm surface with a fixed surface at right angles to the horizontal backboard at one end, against which an assistant gently holds the vertex of the skull. The examiner gently but fully stretches the legs and places the bottom of the heels on another right-angle surface that slides to adjust to the length of the infant. Measuring in any other fashion introduces significant errors. Measure heights with feet flat on a stationary surface instead of the movable doctor's office scale. The back of the heels, the sacrum, the thoracic spine, and the occiput should all touch this plane with the knees fully locked. Pull the head gently upward with pressure on the mastoid processes while the Frankfort plane (outer canthus of the eye to the top of the auditory canal) is parallel to the floor. Measurement at the vertex of the skull is then possible. While a wall-mounted stadiometer-like device is preferable, a metal tape and right-angle triangle used for mechanical drawing can work as well. The most recent growth norms are listed in Chapter 2.

Growth velocity is critical to assess, especially around the time of adolescence (TABLE. 13–1). This should be part of a generalist's evaluation of growth.

Measure the anterior fontanel from each opposite apex of its diamond shape; record both sagittal and coronal distances.

Proceeding caudally, palpate the thyroid gland. Move the skin overlying the gland without allowing the examiner's fingertips to slide on the skin; the sensation will be like wearing a glove. If the fingertips slide on the skin, that tactile impression may interfere with feeling the gland. Depending on the age of the child and the skill of the examiner, palpation from behind, from the side, or from directly in front of the

TABLE 13–1 *Average Growth Velocity per Year*

Age	Cm/yr
First year	25
Second year	10
3–4 years	7
5–7 years	6
7 years–puberty	5
Puberty	10.3

patient may be more appropriate. Younger patients do *not* trust or tolerate examiners coming at them from behind. A helpful technique to bring the thyroid into relief from behind the strap muscles is to allow the patient's head to hang over the end of the examination table in the supine position. Again, do this in such a way as to avoid frightening the patient. Measure the length of each lobe, measure the distance between the upper poles of the thyroid across the neck, measure the diameter of the neck at the level of the isthmus, and measure the cephalad-to-caudal distance across the isthmus. Feel for, and measure, if possible, a "Delphian" lymph node just above the isthmus or for a pyramidal thyroid lobe arising from the cephalad edge of the isthmus. These measurements make it much easier to compare thyroid size at subsequent visits than guesses of thyroid weight or estimates such as "twice normal size."

Quantify breast buds and early to middle-development breast tissue by measuring the diameter at the base of the tissue in a plane parallel to the floor when standing for ready comparison with later examinations. It may be difficult to differentiate breast gland tissue from adipose tissue unless the patient is of normal body habitus.

Perform genital measurements as follows: Express testicular volume in milliliters, comparing the patient with the Prader orchidometer standards. Stretch the penis and measure the length from the base of the shaft at the pubic symphysis to the tip of the glans. This may require pressing the end of the ruler down into a significant fat pad for an accurate measurement. Likewise, measure clitoral length from the suspensory ligament to the tip of the glans. Do not include the preputial skin. Also measure the diameter of just the erectile tissue. Measurements of a non-endocrine-specific nature such as limb lengths are helpful to assist in endocrine evaluations. Tanner staging has been the "gold standard" for objective evaluation of pubertal status and appears in FIGURES 13–2 through 13–4.

Infants

▼ KEY FINDING
V **Constitutional** Poor tone, poor suck, poor feeding, lethargy, and fussiness are all nonspecific but indicate a need to evaluate for

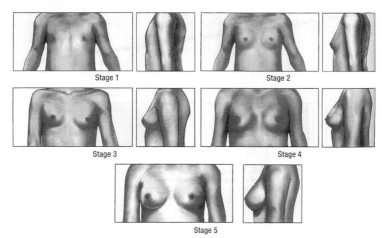

Stage 1

Stage 2

Stage 3

Stage 4

Stage 5

Stage 1   Preadolescent: juvenile breast with elevated papilla and small flat areola.
Stage 2   The breast bud forms under the influence of hormonal stimulation. The papilla and areola elevate as a small mound, and the areolar diameter increases.
Stage 3   Continued enlargement of the breast bud further elevates the papilla. The areola continues to enlarge; no separation of breast contours is noted.
Stage 4   The areola and papilla separate from the contour of the breast to form a secondary mound.
Stage 5   Mature: areolar mound recedes into the general contour of the breast; papilla continues to project.

FIGURE 13–2 Sexual Maturity Rating: Breasts. *(From Greydanus DE, Patel DR, Pratt HD:* Essential Adolescent Medicine. *New York: McGraw-Hill, 2006.)*

hypoglycemia, hypocalcemia, and *hypothyroidism.* Agitation, jitteriness, tremors, or increased tone may suggest hyperthyroidism, hypocalcemia, and hypoglycemia. Increased mottling of skin in older infants suggests hypothyroidism.

KEY FINDING
General Observation of the Infant *Lymphedema* of hands and feet is frequent in *Turner syndrome*, as is neck webbing and low posterior hairline. A shield-shaped chest with widely spaced nipples and narrow shoulders is also a clue to Turner syndrome. A *rachitic* rosary, broadening of the costochondral junctions (in the anterior axillary line not the midclavicular line in newborns), and flared wrists suggest rickets. Bowing of the legs occurs on walking; prewalking infants have flared distal ends of the femora, which are harder to see and feel than the changes in the wrists.

KEY FINDING
Measurements Small-for-dates infants may have IUGR, other syndrome diagnoses, chromosomal disorders such as *Turner syndrome,* or *hypopituitarism.* Large infants may be infants of diabetic mothers, have overgrowth syndromes, or have *Beckwith-Wiedemann syndrome.* Underweight but normal-length infants usually are malnourished. The

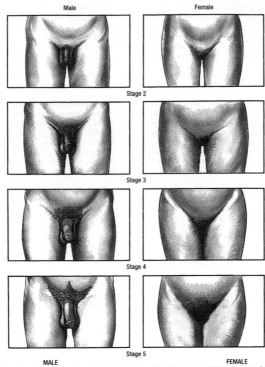

	MALE	FEMALE
Stage 1	Preadolescent: no pubic hair present; a fine vellus hair covers the genital area.	Preadolescent: no pubic hair present; a fine vellus hair covers the genital area.
Stage 2	A sparse distribution of long, slightly pigmented hair appears at the base of the penis.	A sparse distribution of long, slightly pigmented straight hair appears bilaterally along medial border of the labia majora.
Stage 3	The pubic hair pigmentation increases; the hairs begin to curl and to spread laterally in a scanty distribution.	The pubic hair pigmentation increases; the hairs begin to curl and to spread sparsely over the mons pubis.
Stage 4	The pubic hairs continue to curl and become coarse in texture. An adult type of distribution is attained, but the number of hairs remains fewer.	The pubic hairs continue to curl and become coarse in texture. The number of hairs continues to increase.
Stage 5	Mature: the pubic hair attains an adult distribution with spread to the surface of the medial thigh. Pubic hair will grow along linea alba in 80% of males.	Mature: pubic hair attains an adult feminine triangular pattern, with spread to the surface of the medial thigh.

FIGURE 13–3 *Sexual Maturity Rating: Pubic Hair. (From Greydanus DE, Patel DR and Pratt HD:* Essential Adolescent Medicine. *New York: McGraw-Hill, 2006.)*

growth curve will assist in the short and underweight infant because nutritional causes usually manifest first with underweight, then the length "falls off the chart," and finally, the head circumference suffers if there is no correction of prolonged undernutrition. *Diabetes mellitus* or *hyperthyroidism* may lead to underweight in infancy. Overweight infants are almost all over-nourished; rarely, *Cushing syndrome* in infancy leads to overweight with diminishing linear growth. Infants with persistent hyperinsulinemia may be overgrown owing to constant hunger and feeding as protection from hypoglycemia.

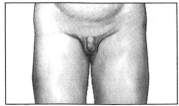

Stage 1

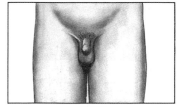

Stage 2

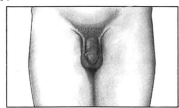

Stage 3

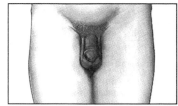

Stage 4

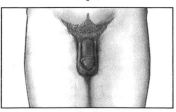

Stage 5

Stage 1 Preadolescent: testes, scrotum, and penis identical to early childhood.
Stage 2 Enlargement of testes as result of canalization of seminiferous tubules. The scrotum enlarges, developing a reddish hue and altering its skin texture. The penis enlarges slightly.
Stage 3 The testes and scrotum continue to grow. The length of the penis increases.
Stage 4 The testes and scrotum continue to grow; the scrotal skin darkens. The penis grows in width, and the glans penis develops.
Stage 5 Mature: adult size and shape of testes, scrotum, and penis.

FIGURE 13–4 Sexual Maturity Rating: Male Genitalia. *(From Greydanus DE, Patel DR, Pratt HD:* Essential Adolescent Medicine. *New York: McGraw-Hill, 2006.)*

▼ KEY FINDING
Skin and Cutaneous Appendages Infants may have hypertrichosis owing to drugs or *hyperinsulinemia*. Prolonged *jaundice* can be a sign of *hypothyroidism*. Nails may be small and hyperconvex and appear to curve up at the tips of the fingers in *Turner syndrome*. Dry skin and myxedematous changes may be a sign of acquired as well as long-standing *congenital hypothyroidism* in infants. Hair that is dry and breaks suggests hypothyroidism but also nonendocrine syndromes (see Chapter 16).

▼ KEY FINDING
Head Abnormalities The "ping pong ball skull" in *neonatal rickets* has very thin bones that feel flexible. The anterior fontanel becomes large in hypothyroidism with growth of the brain and lack of

bony growth, so its absence in the newborn is unreliable. An open pos-terior fontanel after a month or two of age is associated with *congenital hypothyroidism.*

KEY FINDING
Eye Abnormalities Pendular nystagmus may be hard to detect early on, but poor fixation may be a clue to optic nerve involve-ment such as *septo-optic dysplasia* or other midline defects in the CNS associated with the hypothalamus. *Colobomata* of the iris and retina sug-gest midline CNS defects as well. Persistent myelination of the corneal nerves occurs in *multiple endocrine neoplasia (MEN) type 2b.*

KEY FINDING
Ear Abnormalities The helix of the ear is often unusual as in *DiGeorge syndrome.* Deafness is associated with *Pendred syndrome* and can result from late treatment of *congenital hypothyroidism.*

KEY FINDING
Neck Abnormalities The newborn thyroid is hard to feel; thus a *goiter* would suggest a disorder of thyroid hormone synthesis. This may be hereditary or may be due to iodine deficiency in utero or in later infancy, maternal Graves disease with transplacental transfer of thyroid-stimulating immunoglobulins, or transplacental *transfer of an-tithyroid drugs* such as propylthiouracil. A fluctuant mass in the anterior midline of the neck is consistent with a *thyroglossal duct cyst.* A *thy-roglossal duct sinus* is rare.

KEY FINDING
Cardiovascular Tachycardia may be due to *Graves disease,* bradycardia to *hypothyroidism.* Hypotension is associated with *adrenal insufficiency,* as in salt-wasting *congenital adrenal hyperplasia, adrenal hemorrhage,* etc. There is an association of congenital heart disease with *DiGeorge syndrome (conotruncal defects).* Diminished and delayed femoral pulses in *Turner syndrome* are due to *coarctation of the aorta.*

KEY FINDING
Neurologic Hyperreflexia may occur in *hyperthyroidism,* and increased tone and reflexes may be seen in hypocalcemia, especially the Chvostek sign and the Trousseau sign. *Hypothyroidism* causes hypore-flexia with "hung up" deep tendon reflexes. Test anosmia in adolescents with delayed onset of puberty in whom *Kallmann syndrome* is under con-sideration. Coffee grounds and orange peels are good substances to use.

KEY FINDING
Breast Abnormalities While the breast tissue noted in the full-term neonate is usually up to 1 cm in diameter, it may be more. If it enlarges during the first year of life or emerges for the first time later in infancy, an evaluation for etiology is in order. Consider a spon-taneously active *ovarian follicle, precocious puberty* (either *central* or *pe-ripheral*), and *exposure to exogenous estrogen.* Galactorrhea is physiologic

soon after birth. Expression of more than colostrum, persistence out of the neonatal period, or new onset after the neonatal period should trigger a search for an endogenous or exogenous source of stimulus for prolactin release.

⊠ External Female Genitalia Neonatal genital examination should have revealed any ambiguities. Rarely, an infant with virilization will go undetected. The newborn endocrine screen for congenital adrenal hyperplasia is useful to find affected males because they typically do not appear abnormal at birth, but it also has been instrumental in identifying the rare virilized undiagnosed female. The clitoral index is normally less than 16. This is the product of length and the diameter, in millimeters, of the erectile tissue only, ignoring preputial size. The distance from the anus to the posterior edge of the vaginal opening or fourchette should be less than 50 percent of the distance from the anus to the pubis (anogenital ratio normally less than 50 percent). There should not be fusion or rugation of the labia majora in a female newborn.

⊠ External Male Genitalia Testes should be in the scrotum by 32 weeks of gestational age and usually have a volume of 1 to 3 ml. Nondescent may indicate *hypopituitarism,* especially when associated with micropenis. *Androgen insensitivity* syndromes are associated with *maldescent of the testes* as well. The median penis stretched length at birth is 3.5 cm, with a diameter of about 1 cm. Microphallus (<2.5 cm in length at full term) can occur with hypopituitarism, vanishing testes, and androgen insensitivity syndromes. Testicular torsion can occur in infancy. Isolated mild *hypospadias* is not usually due to endocrine disorders, but the more severe forms may be due to androgen receptor mutations or disorders of sexual differentiation, as well as other genetic syndromes. Enlargement of the penis with no enlargement of the testes suggests an adrenal source of excess androgen or an exogenous androgen exposure.

⊠ Premature Pubarche Premature *adrenarche* can be idiopathic or due to *precocious puberty, congenital adrenal hyperplasia* that did not significantly virilize female external genitalia (in males there is no external sign), exposure to *exogenous androgens,* or the rare *androgen-producing tumors* of adrenals or gonads.

Other Key Findings

Diabetes insipidus and *diabetes mellitus* in infants may present with a well-appearing infant or one that is profoundly dehydrated and acidotic depending on circumstances. No particular physical findings are of specific help in making this diagnosis.

Children and Adolescents

Approach to physical findings in adolescents and children is similar to that in infants. Please refer to the preceding section.

▼ KEY FINDING
Constitutional Fatigue and lethargy are nonspecific. Endocrine causes such as *hypoglycemia, hypothyroidism,* and *adrenal insufficiency* may present with a very tired-appearing child.

▼ KEY FINDING
General Puffiness of hands and feet, webbed neck, low posterior hairline, and other findings suggestive of *Turner syndrome* may be obvious to the examiner, also noting the widely spaced nipples and shield-shaped chest. Bowed legs and flaring of the wrists are easy to see, whereas the rachitic rosary again is part of the chest examination. Bony abnormalities such as the *Madelung deformity* or short fourth metacarpals are also readily apparent.

▼ KEY FINDING
Agitation, Tremors The *hyperthyroid* school child or adolescent may seem to have *ADHD*. *Hypoglycemia* leads to epinephrine release with tremors, clammy skin, and a feeling of dread. *Hypocalcemia* can cause muscle irritability as well. These signs can progress to frank syncopal episodes or seizures.

▼ KEY FINDING
Measurements Refer to the "History" section for the conditions associated with short stature, tall stature, underweight, or overweight. Repeated accurate measurements spaced 6 or more months apart yield rate-of-growth information that helps to distinguish between a pattern of growth that is a variant and a disorder of growth. Variant patterns of growth ultimately yield normal adult size. A key feature is that they usually have appropriate growth velocity, whereas growth disorders are most often characterized by abnormal rates and poor outcome.

▼ KEY FINDING
Skin and Cutaneous Appendages The stretch marks of obesity are usually thinner and pink or pale, whereas those from *Cushing syndrome* are wider and purpler; there is a sensation of fullness in stretched skin from obesity, whereas the striae of Cushing syndrome are associated with cutaneous atrophy. *Acanthosis nigricans* is dark and "velvety" and found in intertriginous areas. Attempts to scrub it off may have traumatized the skin. There is thickening of the skin with deep creases in this lesion. Very fair-skinned individuals may have a lighter-colored lesion, with less melanin, but the other characteristics are the same. In children and adolescents this is usually a consequence of insulin resistance. Hirsutism is the growth of hair in a sexually inappropriate manner. Facial and body hair in females growing in a male pattern may be due to androgen excess or can be idiopathic with normal

hormone levels. Hypertrichosis, increased hairiness of the rest of the body, may accompany *hyperinsulinemia* or exposure to *medications* such as minoxidil or be familial. Dry or breaking hair or hair that falls out more than usual can be due to hypothyroidism. Skin that is dry and waxy or sallow in appearance and nonpitting edema (*myxedema*) owing to accumulation of glycoprotein in the subcutaneous layer are features of hypothyroidism. Pretibial myxedema also may be present in *Graves disease*. Café-au-lait spots with irregular border suggest *McCune-Albright syndrome*. A generalized bronzing of the skin with no tan line is more typical of Addison disease or out-of-control congenital adrenal hyperplasia. A more subtle manifestation is hyperpigmentation just of skin creases and the knuckles. Nail changes appear in *Graves disease* with onycholysis, in Turner syndrome with hyperconvexity, and in *Candida infection* associated with *autoimmune polyendocrinopathy*.

▼ KEY FINDING

Eyes Exophthalmos is common in *Graves disease* but also occurs occasionally with *Hashimoto thyroiditis*. The distance from the outer canthus of the orbit to the anterior surface of the cornea is usually less than 15 mm. This is measured with an inexpensive Luedde exophthalmometer or with one of the more costly exophthalmometers employing prisms. Chemosis of the sclera is often apparent even when the patient can fully close the eyes during sleep. There may be stare and lid lag, with or without exophthalmos. Extraocular muscle involvement may lead to partial paralysis of gaze in one or more directions. Visual field defects may be due to optic nerve pressure from lesions in or near the pituitary. Nystagmus occurs in *septo-optic dysplasia*, often associated with *hypothalamic-pituitary deficiency*. Occasionally, iris *coloboma* and/or coloboma of the retina is associated with hypothalamic-pituitary deficiency. Persistent myelination of the corneal nerves occurs in *MEN 2b*. Cataracts may be present in diabetes mellitus, sometimes paradoxically during improvement of glycemic control. Retinal changes of *diabetes* include *exudates, microaneurysms*, occasional *hemorrhage*, and uncommonly in this age group, *neovascularization*.

▼ KEY FINDING

Ears External ear malformations suggest genetic disorders (see Chapter 6). Deafness is associated with the *Pendred syndrome* and with inadequately treated congenital hypothyroidism for some period after birth.

▼ KEY FINDING

Neck *Goiters* from iodine deficiency, hereditary deficiency of enzyme(s) needed in thyroid hormone synthesis, *chronic lymphocytic thyroiditis*, and *Graves disease* are usually painless, whereas those from acute and *subacute thyroiditis* are painful. A bruit over the thyroid gland denotes hypermetabolism with increased blood flow in *Graves disease*. A *Delphian lymph node* may be present in *autoimmune thyroid disease;* it is located just above the isthmus. It differs from a pyramidal lobe, a normal variant of thyroid formation. *Thyroglossal duct cysts* may present in childhood and adolescence as a cystic or fluctuant mass in the anterior neck, and there may be recurrent episodes of infection, pain, and swelling before the diagnosis becomes apparent.

KEY FINDING

Cardiovascular Tachycardia with or without widened pulse pressure (systolic pressure minus diastolic pressure is often more than 50 percent of systolic pressure) and "water-hammer pulses" suggest increased adrenergic sensitivity owing to *Graves disease*. Bradycardia is common in *hypothyroidism*. A systolic flow murmur may be present in Graves disease, whereas diminished heart sounds owing to pericardial effusion suggest hypothyroidism.

KEY FINDING

Abdominal Pain and tenderness of *diabetic ketoacidosis* can mimic appendicitis or ureteral obstruction. The abdominal pain of *Addisonian crisis* also may suggest a "surgical abdomen."

KEY FINDING

Neurologic Increased deep tendon reflexes can occur in *hyperthyroidism* or *hypocalcemia*. The Chvostek sign and the Trousseau sign are detectable in *hypocalcemia*. Fine-intention tremor and fasciculation of the tongue on protrusion are frequent in *Graves disease*. To amplify the hand tremor, place a small, light piece of paper on the dorsum of the outstretched hand. It is possible to demonstrate an intention tremor by asking the patient to firmly grasp and shake both the examiner's hands (the examiner crosses hands to make it easy for the patient). Decreased deep tendon reflexes may occur in *hypothyroidism* or *hypercalcemia*, the "hung up" or late and prolonged reflex is a sign of hypothyroidism.

KEY FINDING

Breasts Onset of thelarche in girls is normal after age 8. Initiate an investigation for precocious puberty or exogenous estrogen exposure for girls manifesting thelarche earlier than 8. The tissue may be tender or painful in early stages because the capsule is under tension. Asymmetry of breast development is sometimes distressing to child or parent; however, it is usually not permanent or pronounced by late adolescence or adulthood and is most often physiologic. There are some non-endocrine-related malformations of breast tissue to consider. Delayed onset of development of breast tissue, i.e., no development by age 13, indicates a need to evaluate the child for causes of delayed puberty, e.g., *ovarian failure, chronic illness, malnutrition, hypogonadism of pituitary origin*, etc. *Galactorrhea* may be due to medication, *prolactinoma,* chronic irritation of the nipple, and in adolescents, during a pregnancy and postpartum; lactation is physiologic. *Gynecomastia*, development of breast tissue in males, is of unclear etiology in preadolescents. Certain drugs may induce it, and rarely, estrogen-producing *tumors* are causes. *Adolescent gynecomastia* is a physiologic process; estradiol is derived from testosterone by adipocytes in the skin of the chest when testosterone levels are at early pubertal levels, and there is spontaneous resolution of breast hypertrophy in most males. Persistence or continued growth of the tissue may not be consistent with endocrine disorder, but *Klinefelter syndrome, anorchia,* other *acquired testicular failure, defects of testosterone synthesis, androgen receptor defects, feminizing adrenal tumors, drugs, aromatase overactivity,* and possibly *hyperprolactinemia* may be causes.

KEY FINDING

Male External Genitalia Testicular enlargement is one of the first signs of puberty; it is normal after 9 years of age, associated with a thinned and pendulous scrotum. Hard and/or irregular enlargement of testes may be a sign of *tumor.* Hydrocele and torsion may be painful. *Hydroceles* will transilluminate; *torsion* and *tumors* will not. Delayed onset of puberty, no changes by age 14, merits an evaluation. It may be due to extreme constitutional delay of growth and maturation, it may be familial, or it may be due to defects anywhere in the hypothalamic-pituitary-testicular axis or to chronic illness. Precocious puberty with early enlargement of testes may be *central* from activation of hypothalamic and pituitary hormone release, it may be *peripheral* as in familial gonadotrophin-independent precocious puberty, and it may be due to *McCune-Albright syndrome.* If the phallus grows and pubic hair appears but the testes remain small, consider *adrenal androgen excess,* as in simple virilizing *congenital adrenal hyperplasia* or *tumor.* Exogenous *exposure to testosterone* also may produce this picture. Microphallus may be due to *androgen insensitivity* or *hypopituitarism. Hypospadias* has similar etiologies as in infants. Premature onset of pubic hair may be physiologic if there is no enlargement of the testes or phallus and bone age is not advanced. Otherwise, it may be the earliest manifestation of precocious puberty or androgen excess of endogenous or exogenous origin.

Synthesizing a Diagnosis

TABLE 13–2 presents a summary of problems and findings related to endocrinologic diagnoses.

TABLE 13–2 *Synthesizing a Diagnosis from Endocrine Signs and Symptoms*

Signs and Symptoms	Age Group	Possible Disorders
IA. Constitutional		
Exhaustion, lethargy, easy fatigability	Infants	Hypoglycemia Dehydration Electrolyte abnormalities. Hypothyroidism
	Children and adolescents	All the above Diabetes mellitus Adrenal insufficiency

(Continued)

TABLE 13-2 *Synthesizing a Diagnosis from Endocrine Signs and Symptoms (Continued)*

Signs and Symptoms	Age Group	Possible Disorders
Palpitations	Children and adolescents	Hyperthyroidism
Agitation, jitteriness, tremors	I, C, A	Hyperthyroidism Hypocalcemia Hypoglycemia
Heat or cold intolerance	I, C, A	Hypothyroidism Hyperthyroidism
Syncope or seizures	I, C, A	Hypoglycemia Hypocalcemia
IB. General physical		
Puffiness of hands and feet	Infants	Turner syndrome
Neck webbing and Low hair line	I, C, A	Turner syndrome
Widely spaced nipples, and Widened chest wall	I, C, A	Turner syndrome
Pectus excavatum, and Rachitic rosary Bowing of legs	I, C, A	Rickets
Short fourth metacarpal, Madelung deformity (dinner fork deformity of wrist and forearm)	I, C, A	Turner syndrome Albright hereditary osteodystrophy
II. Anthropometric measurements		
Short stature	Infants	IUGR Placental insufficiency Turner syndrome (in females) Russell-Silver syndrome
	Children	Genetic short stature Turner syndrome Growth hormone deficiency Hypothyroidism Malnutrition Celiac disease Cushing syndrome Prader-Willi syndrome
	Adolescents	Constitutional delay Delayed puberty Same as above in children

(Continued)

TABLE 13–2 *Synthesizing a Diagnosis from Endocrine Signs and Symptoms (Continued)*

Signs and Symptoms	Age Group	Possible Disorders
Tall stature	Infants	Beckwith-Wiedemann syndrome
		Genetic overgrowth syndromes
	Children	Genetic overgrowth syndromes
		Growth hormone–producing tumors
		Acromegaly
		Obesity
		Precocious puberty
	Adolescents	Same as above
		Klinefelter syndrome
III. Weight		
Underweight, failure to thrive, failure to gain weight, or weight loss	I, C, A	Undernutrition
		Hyperthyroidism
		Diabetes mellitus
Overweight	Infants	Over nutrition
		Overgrowth genetic syndromes
		Hyperinsulinemia
	Children and adolescents	Over nutrition
		Metabolic syndrome
		Overgrowth genetic syndromes
		Prader-Willi syndrome
		Cushing syndrome
IV. Skin and cutaneous appendages		
Stretch marks (pale or purplish)	Children and adolescents	Obesity (pale)
		Cushing syndrome (purplish)
Acanthosis nigricans (dark, velvety pigmentation on the neck, flexors)	Children and adolescents	Insulin resistance
Hirsutism (abnormal hair growth on face in females)	I, C, A,	Ethnic
		Hyperandrogenism
		Polycystic ovarian syndrome
		Virilizing forms of CAH
Hypertrichosis (generalized increased hair growth)	I, C, A	Hyperinsulinemia
		Drugs
		Ethnic

(Continued)

TABLE 13–2 *Synthesizing a Diagnosis from Endocrine Signs and Symptoms (Continued)*

Signs and Symptoms	Age Group	Possible Disorders
Coarse, dry, brittle hair, generalized hair falling/breaking	Children and adolescents	Hypothyroidism Hypothyroidism Post-Partum
Patchy hair loss	Children and adolescents	Autoimmune endocrine disease
V. Skin		
Dry, thickened, waxy skin	I, C, A	Hypothyroidism
Thin plethoric skin with purple striae	I, C, A	Cushing syndrome
Café-au-lait spots (hyperpigmented macules) Irregular margins (coast of Maine) Regular margins (coast of California)	Children and adolescents	McCune-Albright syndrome Neurofibromatosis
Generalized bronze pigmentation of skin	I, C, A	Addison disease
VI. Nails		
Candidiasis	Children and adolescents	Polyglandular autoimmune endocrinopathy
Onycholysis	Children and adolescents	Graves disease
Hyperconvex nails	I, C, A	Turner syndrome
VII. Head		
Ping pong ball skull	Infants	Neonatal rickets
Headaches	I, C, A	Pituitary tumors Treatment with growth hormone Hypoglycemia Hyperglycemia
Open posterior fontanel	Infants	Neonatal hypothyroidism
VIII. Eyes		
Exophthalmos, lid lag, Partial gaze paralysis	Children and adolescents	Graves disease
Visual field defects	Children and adolescents	Pituitary tumors

(Continued)

TABLE 13–2 *Synthesizing a Diagnosis from Endocrine Signs and Symptoms (Continued)*

Signs and Symptoms	Age Group	Possible Disorders
Nystagmus	I, C, A	Septo-optic dysplasia with hypothalamopituitary deficiency
Coloboma of iris	I, C, A	Hypothalamic-pituitary defects
Persistent corneal nerve myelination	I, C, A	MEN 2b
Cataract	Adolescents	Diabetes mellitus
Retinopathy	Children and adolescents	Diabetes mellitus
IX. Ears		
External ear abnormalities	I, C, A	Genetic syndromes, DiGeorge syndrome
Deafness	I, C, A	Pendred syndrome
X. Neck		
Thyroid gland enlargement (goiter)	Infants	Iodine deficiency Enzymatic defects of thyroid hormonogenesis
	Children and adolescents	As in infants above Graves disease Hashimoto thyroiditis Iodine deficiency Subacute hypothyroidism
Painful goiter	Adolescents	Subacute thyroiditis
Bruit over the thyroid gland	Children and adolescents	Graves disease
Delphian node	Children and adolescents	Autoimmune thyroiditis
Cystic neck mass in midline anteriorly	I, C, A	Thyroglossal duct Ectopic thyroid gland
XI. Cardiovascular findings		
Tachycardia	I, C, A	Graves disease
Bradycardia	I, C, A	Hypothyroidism

(Continued)

TABLE 13–2 *Synthesizing a Diagnosis from Endocrine Signs and Symptoms (Continued)*

Signs and Symptoms	Age Group	Possible Disorders
Hypotension	I, C, A	Addison disease Salt-wasting CAH
Hypertension	Children and adolescents	Cushing syndrome Metabolic syndrome Pheochromocytoma Turner syndrome
Widened pulse pressure	I, C, A	Graves disease
Diminished heart sounds	Children and adolescents	Pericardial effusion due to hypothyroidism
Flow murmurs	Children and adolescents	Graves disease
Congenital heart disease	I, C, A	In association with DiGeorge syndrome
Coarctation of aorta	I, C, A	Turner syndrome
XII. Abdominal signs and symptoms		
Abdominal pain and tenderness	I, C, A	Diabetes mellitus in ketoacidosis Addison disease
XIII. Neurologic signs and symptoms		
Hyperreflexia	I, C, A	Hyperthyroidism
Chvostek sign	I, C, A	Hypocalcemia
Trousseau sign	I, C, A	Hypocalcemia
Hyporeflexia "Hung up" deep tend on reflexes	I, C, A	Hypothyroidism
Anosmia	Children and adolescents	Kallmann syndrome
XIV. Breasts		
Early breast development	Infants	Generally normal, physiologic
Premature the larche of infancy (unilateral or bilateral)		May have to rule out causes of precocious puberty if indicated
Premature thelarche in early childhood (2–8 years), unilateral or bilateral in females	Children	Rule out causes of precocious puberty. Benign follicular cyst Exogenous exposure to estrogens or phytoestrogens

(*Continued*)

TABLE 13–2 *Synthesizing a Diagnosis from Endocrine Signs and Symptoms (Continued)*

Signs and Symptoms	Age Group	Possible Disorders
Painful and tender early pubertal breast buds	Children	Normal
Asymmetric breast development	I, C, A	Local exogenous exposure to estrogens or phytoestrogens
		Rule out local infections, inflammations—if indicated
Galactorrhea	Infants	Physiologic in early infancy
	Children	Medicinal/drug intake, e.g., risperidone, prolactinoma
		Local infection
	Adolescents	As above in children
		Pregnancy and postpartum
Gynecomastia—breast tissue development in males	Infants	Normal in early infancy
	Children	Prepubertal gynecomastia—not physiologic
		Estrogen producing tumors
		Drugs/medications (below)
	Adolescents	Physiologic
		Klinefelter syndrome
		Anorchia
		Acquired testicular failure
		Biosynthetic defects of testosterone synthesis
		Androgen receptor defects
		Hyperprolactinemia
		Feminizing adrenal tumors
		Aromatase overactivity
		Drugs: cimetidine, spironolactone, digitalis, phenothiazines, marijuana
		Hormonal treatments: estrogens, hCG, testosterone

(*Continued*)

TABLE 13-2 *Synthesizing a Diagnosis from Endocrine Signs and Symptoms (Continued)*

Signs and Symptoms	Age Group	Possible Disorders
XV. External male genitalia		
Undescended testes (cryptorchidism)	Infants	Prematurity
		Delayed testicular descent
		Genetic—in multiple family members
		Genetic syndromes—25% chance of Intersex problem in cryptorchidism and Hypospadias
		Androgen insensitivity syndrome
	Children and adolescents	Genetic—in multiple family members
		Genetic syndromes—25% chance of intersex problem in cryptorchidism and hypospadias.
		Androgen insensitivity syndrome
Symmetric bilateral testicular enlargement—soft, smooth, and regular on palpation	Children and adolescents	Pubertal onset
Asymmetric bilateral testicular enlargement—hard and irregular on palpation	I, C, A	Testicular tumors
Painful testicular enlargement	I, C, A	Testicular torsion
Transillumination +/−		Hydrocele
		Rule out tumors
Microphallus	I, C, A	Hypopituitarism
		Androgen insensitivity
Hypospadias Tertiary/penoscrotal	Infants	Disorders of sexual differentiation
		Opitz syndrome
		Androgen receptor abnormalities
First-degree/coronal/ glandular	Infants	Generally no endocrine abnormality

(Continued)

TABLE 13-2 *Synthesizing a Diagnosis from Endocrine Signs and Symptoms (Continued)*

Signs and Symptoms	Age Group	Possible Disorders
XVI. Premature pubarche		
Premature appearance of pubic hair	Infants and children	Idiopathic premature adrenarche Simple virilizing CAH Nonclassic CAH Androgen-producing tumors need to be ruled out
XVII. Menstrual disturbances		
Primary amenorrhea	Adolescents	Turner syndrome Rokitansky-Kuster-Hauser syndrome Disorders of sexual differentiation
Secondary amenorrhea	Adolescents	Pregnancy Polycystic ovarian syndrome Anovulatory cycles—few years postmenarche
Oligomenorrhea	Adolescents	Hyperthyroidism
Menorrhagia/ metrorrhagia	Adolescents	Hypothyroidism
XVIII. Others		
Polyuria	I, C, A	Diabetes insipidus
Polydipsia		Diabetes mellitus

Abbreviations: I = infants; C = children; A = adolescents.

Laboratory, Imaging, and Referral for Endocrine Disorders

The endocrine evaluation depends on the signs and symptoms of the patient. Nonendocrine causes are more common for growth disorders, so nonendocrine tests are essential before ordering a complete endocrine evaluation. A stepwise approach actually may save time as well as money compared with a shotgun approach to laboratory testing. Hormones do mediate growth, but most patients with a growth complaint do *not* have an endocrine cause. TABLE 13-3 lists the suggested laboratory tests for short stature. The order in which to obtain these tests relates to the particulars of the case. It is easiest to start with knowledge of the rate of growth and current bone age. If the rate is appropriate and bone age is similar to height age (age at which height is 50th percentile),

TABLE 13-3 *Diagnostic Workup for Endocrine Disorders*

Endocrine Disorder	Laboratory	Imaging	Further Testing
Growth workup			
1. Short stature	CBC, ESR, CMP, FT$_4$, TSH IGF-1, IGFBP3 Karyotype	Bone age	Refer to pediatric endocrinologist Refer Growth hormone stimulation test Genetic workup—if indicated
2. Tall stature	IGF-1	Bone age	Karyotype
3. Obesity—nutritional	Workup depends on BMI 2-hour OGTT Lipid profile Insulin level		
Thyroid workup	FT$_4$, TSH TPO, ATG, TSI	Thyroid ultrasound Thyroid scan	Refer Thyroglobulin levels Serum calcitonin levels
Puberty workup			
1. Precocious puberty	FSH, LH, Estradiol/testosterone, 24-h urine FSH, LH	If Indicated: bone age pelvic ultrasound MRI of pituitary and abdomen	Refer Tumor markers if indicated Refer
2. Delayed puberty	FSH, LH Testosterone (males) Estradiol (females) Karyotype	Bone age Pelvic ultrasound (females)	Kallman gene males

Adrenal workup		
1. Premature adrenarche	17-OHP, DHEAS, androstenedione	Bone age	Refer
			ACTH stimulation test
2. Addison disease	Serum cortisol		Refer
			ACTH level
			Low-dose ACTH stimulation test
			Metyrapone test
3. Congenital adrenal hyperplasia (CAH)	17OHP, DHEAS, androstenedione, 11-deoxycortisol		Refer
	Serum electrolytes		ACTH stimulation test if non-salt-wasting CAH
	Serum aldosterone		
	Plasma renin activity		
Disorders of calcium metabolism			
Hypocalcemia	Serum calcium, phosphorus, alkaline phosphatase	X-ray of wrist and knee for rickets	Refer
Hypercalcemia	PTH		Bone density (only if required)
Rickets	Vitamin D levels (25-hydroxyvitamin D; 1, 25-hydroxyvitamin D)		
Parathyroid gland disorders	Urine calcium: urine creatinine ratio		

(*Continued*)

435

TABLE 13-3 *Diagnostic Workup for Endocrine Disorders (Continued)*

Endocrine Disorder	Laboratory	Imaging	Further Testing
Diabetes insipidus	24-h intake/output Serum electrolytes Urine electrolytes Serum osmolality Urine osmolality		Refer Water deprivation test Serum AVP levels
Diabetes mellitus			
1. Diabetes mellitus 1	Blood sugar Urine glucose and ketones Anti-GAD 65 antibodies Anti-islet antibodies Anti-insulin antibodies hemoglobin A1c (not diagnostic)		Refer
2. Diabetes mellitus 2	Fasting/random/2-h postprandial blood sugars Insulin levels 2-h OGTT with insulin levels C-peptide		Refer

| *Hypoglycemia* | Critical serum sample in spontaneous hypoglycemia for CMP, cortisol level, growth hormone, insulin level, free fatty acids, ketones, ammonia, lactate, total and free carnitine, acyl carnitine profile. Urine—ketones and organic acids | Refer Supervised fast study (includes baseline critical as well as hypoglycemic blood samples) |

Abbreviations: CBC = complete blood count; CMP = comprehensive metabolic panel; FT$_4$ thyroid hormone; TSH = thyroid stimulating hormone; TPO = thyroperoxidase antibodies; ATG = Anti-thyroglobulin antibodies; IGF-1 = insulin-like growth factor 1; IGFBP3 = insulin-like growth factor binding protein 3; 2-h OGTT = 2-hour oral glucose tolerance test; 17-OHP = 17-hydroxyprogesterone; DHEAS = dehydroepiandrostenedione sulfate; FSH = follicle-stimulating hormone; LH = luteinizing hormone; ACTH = adrenocorticotrophic hormone, PTH = parathyroid hormone; AVP = arginine vasopressin; GAD = glutamic acid decarboxylase; CMP = complete metabolic panel.

it may be best to follow the growth for a half year to a year before any testing. Normal rate implies a variant pattern of growth rather than a disorder of growth. If the rate is not appropriate, the next level of tests, screening for chronic illness, is in order. Include thyroid hormone levels, insulin like growth factor 1 (IGF-1), and insulin-like growth factor binding protein 3 (IGFBP3) in this level; *consider a karyotype in short girls or in boys with more than a few minor malformations to find Turner or other syndromes.* One may request specific genetic probes as well. Request stimulation testing by the endocrinology consultant if there is a possibility of growth hormone deficiency. *An important note:* Random growth hormone levels are not useful, and the exercise stimulation test is only a screen. A genetics consultation may be necessary to diagnose the cause of short stature in some children and adolescents. Tall stature is rarely due to an endocrinopathy, and true pituitary giants are very rare. *Exogenous obesity* is frequently a cause of tall stature. *Precocious puberty* also may manifest with early overgrowth before external changes become visible. Elevation of IGF-1 may occur in growth hormone excess. *Klinefelter syndrome* may manifest with tall stature before the pubertal problems appear—thus a karyotype may be in order.

Obesity is rarely a product of endocrine disorders because those which cause obesity are not common, whereas exogenous obesity unfortunately is common. Obesity in some children and adolescents leads to *impaired glucose tolerance* or frank *diabetes.* Evaluation for glucose intolerance requires a 2-hour oral glucose tolerance test with simultaneous glucose and insulin levels. The proper preparation for the test includes 3 days of adequate carbohydrate intake (e.g., 300 g or more in adults and approximately 50 percent of daily calories in children and adolescents).

Thyroid Testing

For hypothyroidism, free T_4 and TSH will identify the biochemical state, antithyroglobulin and anti-thyroid peroxidase antibodies will identify autoimmune thyroid disease (*chronic lymphocytic thyroiditis* a.k.a. *Hashimoto thyroiditis*). In infants, an ultrasound and radionuclide uptake and scan (^{123}I, where available) to locate and evaluate function of the gland are recommended when hypothyroidism is present to find the uncommon hereditary forms in which enzyme deficiency leads to goitrous hypothyroidism. In hyperthyroidism, thyroid-stimulating immunoglobulins identify Graves disease. Thyroglobulin levels, calcitonin levels, pentagastrin stimulation tests, and other studies in cases of thyroid nodules or suspected tumors are best for the consultant to perform.

Disorders of Puberty

In early puberty, normal or precocious, the elevation of LH and folliclestimulating hormone (FSH) may be present only overnight; daytime serum levels may be misleadingly normal. Likewise, estradiol is notoriously difficult to measure in infants and children because normal levels are well below the threshold of the usual commercial kits. Testosterone levels may be more reliable. Bone-age films are very useful to assess the degree of advanced skeletal maturation and are helpful in determining the severity or duration of a growth problem. Pelvic ultrasound is useful to search for activated ovarian follicles. Tumor markers such as β-hCG and alpha-fetoprotein may be helpful to search for steroid-producing tumors. In toilet-trained and cooperative children, 24-hour urine LH and FSH determinations can detect elevation when the serum levels are not elevated during the day. Stimulation testing of gonadotrophin release is best left to the consultant. Reserve brain imaging (with attention to hypothalamic and pituitary regions) for demonstrated cases of central precocious puberty. In males, 50 percent are idiopathic, and in females, 95 percent are idiopathic, the number with CNS pathology being about the same in males and females. One should order ultrasound or CT scan of the abdomen to search for adrenal tumors after discovery of elevated precursor hormones or tumor markers and not as the initial test. In delayed puberty, bone-age films should correlate well with the size and Tanner stage of the patient. Gonadotrophins may be low or high depending on etiology; sex steroid hormone levels may be useful, with the caveat that estrogen is hard to measure. Karyotype for *Turner syndrome* and *Klinefelter syndrome* diagnosis is very useful when clinical signs support those diagnoses (and sometimes when they seem unlikely). Kallmann gene analysis of the X chromosome is only positive in those 25 percent of cases involving the X chromosome and probably should be reserved for the consultant to order. Delayed puberty may be a consequence of *chronic illness* (see short stature evaluation for appropriate evaluation).

Adrenal

Evaluation of premature adrenarche calls for determination of androgen precursors such as serum 17-hydroxyprogesterone. Order adrenal androgens, dehydroepiandrostenedione sulfate (DHEAS), and androstenedione, as well as testosterone, determinations. Bone-age advancement beyond height age does not occur in simple premature adrenarche; thus bone age is an important test to get early in the evaluation. The consultant endocrinologist should perform adrenocorticotropic hormone (ACTH) stimulation testing where appropriate. Testing for Addison disease reveals low serum cortisol and elevated ACTH levels. Also assess for *hypoglycemia, hyponatremia, and hyperkalemia.* There is controversy between adherents of the low-dose ACTH test versus the metyrapone test for Addison disease; the consultant should perform whichever one he or she prefers. *Congenital adrenal hyperplasia* (CAH) is included in the newborn screening test in all but a few states in the United States. 17-Hydroxyprogesterone, DHEAS, androstenedione, 11-deoxycortisol, cortisol, possibly ACTH, serum aldosterone, and plasma renin activity and serum electrolytes are helpful. In case of suspicion of non-salt-wasting or nonclassic congenital adrenal hyperplasia (CAH), ACTH stimulation testing is usually under the supervision of the endocrinologist.

Disorders of Calcium Metabolism

The initial evaluation of hypocalcemia includes determination of serum ionized calcium, phosphorus, alkaline phosphatase, parathyroid hormone, 25-hydroxyvitamin D, and 1,25-dihydroxyvitamin D levels. X-rays of wrists and knees are helpful to diagnose rickets. Urine calcium and phosphorus excretion and ratio of urinary calcium to creatinine are useful. Bone density measurements in infants and children by dual energy x-ray absorptiometry (DEXA) are hard to interpret; use of adult norms and so-called T scores will yield unreliable estimates of low density; age-adjusted Z scores are the appropriate comparison. It is not advisable to go to the expense of this test in the absence of significant bone pain, fractures with minimal trauma, etc. The consultant is best to evaluate the bone density analysis. For *hypercalcemia,* similar lab testing is helpful; there is also a good assay for the parathyroid-related peptide associated with malignancies. Imaging of the parathyroid glands is necessary for preoperative evaluation but adds nothing to the initial diagnosis.

Diabetes Insipidus

The first morning void, along with serum electrolytes, may be diagnostic if there was no overnight drinking of fluids; otherwise, a supervised water deprivation test may be necessary. Again, this should be in the domain of the consultant. Serum osmolality, serum electrolytes, and simultaneous urine osmolality determinations on a spot basis may be diagnostic. Urine electrolytes may reveal the cause of polyuria that is not particularly dilute and is not due to diabetes insipidus.

Type 1 Diabetes Mellitus

Plasma glucose above 200 mg/dl on a random draw or a fasting plasma glucose above 126 mg/dl, either one episode with accompanying symptoms or if found on more than one occasion, would be diagnostic of diabetes. One or more of anti-insulin, anti-islet cell, and anti-GAD 65 antibodies accompany new-onset type 1 diabetes in the majority of cases. Approximately one-third of cases present with *diabetic ketoacidosis;* one-third with symptoms of polydipsia, polyuria, and weight loss with hyperglycemia and glycosuria; and the remainder on routine urine analysis or blood test in patients with no symptoms. It is useful to get consultation on the diagnosis and treatment of type 1 diabetes.

Type 2 Diabetes Mellitus

Random or casual postprandial blood sugar levels may be diagnostic; otherwise, a formal 2-hour oral glucose tolerance test is necessary. This test requires basal and 2-hour determinations of glucose and is more helpful with simultaneous insulin level determinations. At presentation, up to 25 percent of youth with type 2 diabetes patients may have urinary ketosis, even ketoacidosis, so evaluation is critical if there are features of both types. Endocrinologic referral is usually necessary for further evaluation and treatment.

Hypoglycemia

The *critical serum sample* at the time of hypoglycemia should include glucose, electrolytes, cortisol, growth hormone, insulin, alanine, free fatty acids, ammonia, and lactate determinations. Total and free carnitine and acyl carnitine profile urine for ketones and organic acids are also useful to evaluate inborn errors of metabolism. If spontaneous hypoglycemia occurs in an unpredictable pattern and the sample is unobtainable, consultation and a supervised fast to induce hypoglycemia and obtain the critical sample is in order.

14 The Renal System

Alfonso D. Torres and Donald E. Greydanus

The goals of this chapter are

1. To outline the basic anatomy, embryology, and physiology of the renal system
2. To provide renal disease history and physical examination principles
3. To give relevant clinical manifestations of renal disease in fetal life, infancy, childhood, and adolescence
4. To list differential diagnostic considerations for nephrology syndromes
5. To list imaging and laboratory studies in renal disease

Anatomy, Physiology, and Development

Anatomy of the Urinary System

The urinary system consists of paired kidneys with ureters, a urinary bladder, and a urethra. The kidneys are bean-shaped organs located in the retroperitoneal space in the posterior aspect of the abdomen at each side of the spinal column. A fibrous capsule contains each kidney and normally is separable from the surface. In chronic renal disease the capsule adheres to the kidney because of fibrosis. The kidneys lie in perinephric fat; the upper pole of each kidney is at the level of the twelfth thoracic vertebra and the lower pole at the level of the third lumbar vertebra. FIGURES 14–1 and 14–2 show the gross anatomy of the urinary system and the kidney. TABLE 14–1 lists the combined *weight* of kidneys at different ages. The renal *length* correlates with age, body weight, and body length. In the healthy term newborn it is around 5 cm, with a range of 4 to 6 cm; in the adult, the average length of each kidney is 11 cm.

The adrenal glands are located above each kidney, although tumor and hemorrhage of the gland may displace the kidney downward. The contractions of the diaphragm displace the kidneys downward during inspiration. In the anteromedial aspect of each kidney there is a slit called the *hilus*, the site for the entrance of the renal artery and nerves and the

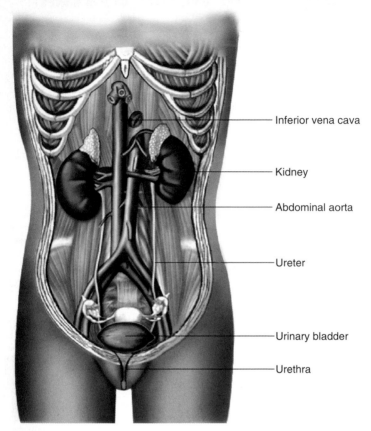

FIGURE 14–1 Urinary System. *(From Van De Graaff KM:* Human Anatomy. *New York: McGraw-Hill, 2002, Fig. 19.1, p. 676.)*

exit of the renal vein, lymphatics, efferent nerves, and renal pelvis. The relatively large size of the kidneys in the newborn period allows for palpation. Fetal lobulations in the kidneys of newborns are of no clinical consequence and disappear during infancy.

On a bisected surface of a kidney, two distinctive areas are identifiable. There is a a pale inner area (the *medulla*) and a darker superficial region (the renal *cortex*) with a thickness of about 1 cm in the adult kidney. The medulla divides into 8 to 12 conic regions, the renal *pyramids*, with cortical tissue separating them called the *columns of Bertin*. The base of the renal pyramid is located in the outer medulla. The tips of the pyramids form the renal papillae, which contain the opening of the collecting ducts; a minor calyx surrounds each papilla.

The minor calyces form the major calyces. The upper collecting system consists of the calyces, the renal pelvis, and the ureter. The walls of

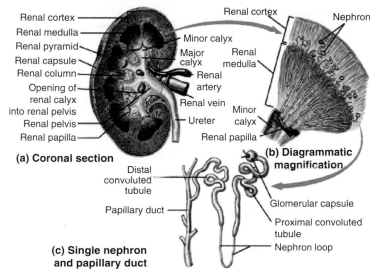

Renal cortex
Renal medulla
Renal pyramid
Renal capsule
Renal column
Opening of renal calyx into renal pelvis
Renal pelvis
Renal papilla

(a) Coronal section

Renal cortex

Nephron

Minor calyx
Major calyx
Renal medulla
Renal artery
Renal vein
Ureter
Minor calyx
Renal papilla

(b) Diagrammatic magnification

Distal convoluted tubule

Papillary duct

Glomerular capsule

Proximal convoluted tubule

Nephron loop

(c) Single nephron and papillary duct

FIGURE 14–2 Structures of the Kidney. *(From Van De Graaff KM:* Human Anatomy. *New York: McGraw-Hill, 2002, Fig. 19.5, p. 679.)*

the upper collecting system contain smooth muscle that contracts to help transport urine to the lower collecting system (bladder). Each ureter originates in the lower part of the renal pelvis at the level of the ureteropelvic junction (UPJ) and extends down to the bladder, entering at the level of the superior angles of the trigone. The lower angle of the trigone is the opening of the bladder neck.

Kidney Components

Light microscopic examination of the kidney reveals components that constitute the substance of the kidney, including *nephrons, blood vessels, interstitial tissue,* and *nerves.* The nephron is the structural and functional

TABLE 14–1 Mean Combined Weight of Both Kidneys at Different Ages

Age	Weight, g	Age, yrs.	Weight, g
0 Birth	24	4	119
3 mos.	41	6	140
6 mos.	53	8	157
1 yrs.	70	10	171
2 yrs.	91	12	183
3 yrs.	107	Adult	300

Source: From Oliver JT, Rubenstein M, Meyer R, Bernstein J. Congenital anomalies of the urinary system—III: growth of the kidney in childhood—determination of normal weight. *Journal of Pediatrics* 61:256–261, 1962.

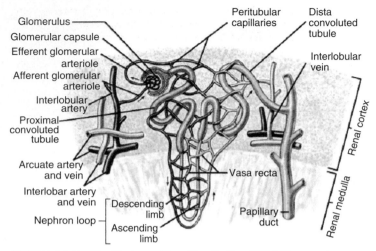

FIGURE 14–3   The Nephron. *(From Van De Graaff KM:* Human Anatomy. *New York: McGraw-Hill, 2002, Fig. 19.7, p. 680.)*

unit of the kidney; its function is urine formation (FIGURE 14–3). The components of a nephron include the glomerular corpuscle, or glomerulus, a tuft of specialized capillaries surrounded by a capsule (Bowman's capsule); the proximal convoluted tubule, originating from the tubular pole of Bowman's capsule; followed by the loop of Henle, the distal convoluted tubule, and the collecting duct. The glomeruli, the proximal convoluted tubule, most of the loop of Henle, the distal convoluted tubule, and the cortical collecting ducts are located in the renal cortex. There are two populations of glomeruli, those with the long loop of Henle extending to the tip of the renal papillae, found deep in the renal cortex adjacent to the outer medulla, and those more superficial in the renal cortex, possessing shorter loops of Henle that also lie mainly in the renal cortex. The difference in the length of the loop of Henle may have functional implications, specifically in the ability of the kidneys to concentrate urine with preservation of volume.

Blood Supply and Lymphatic Drainage

The blood enters the kidneys via the renal arteries that originate from the aorta. Usually there is a single renal artery for each kidney, but variations are frequent. In the adult, 20 to 25 percent of cardiac output goes to the kidneys. The renal artery enters the renal sinus and divides into anterior and posterior branches in the hilar region. Three segmental arteries (superior, middle, and inferior) arise from the anterior branch that supplies blood to the anterior half of the kidney. The posterior branch provides blood to the posterior half of the kidney, except for the upper pole, which receives blood from the anterior branch. There is no anastomosis between the segmental arteries, and if a segmental artery occludes, the renal segment will die.

The veins that drain the kidney are not segmental. The left renal vein is longer than the right and crosses posterior to the superior mesenteric artery and anterior to the aorta, emptying into the inferior vena cava. The right renal vein drains directly into the inferior vena cava. The lymphatic fluid in the kidney drains into lymphatic vessels that pass through the renal sinus and hilum to drain into the lumbar lymph nodes.

Physiology of the Urinary System

Innervation of the Kidney

The kidney receives sympathetic fibers that originate in the spinal cord (segments T_8–L_2) and synapse in the renal ganglia in the renal plexus. Stimulation of these nerves causes vasoconstriction and decreases blood flow to the kidneys. Sensory fibers travel the sympathetic pathway to segments T_{10} and T_{11}. Renal pain refers to the flank regions within these dermatomes. Parasympathetic innervation to the kidneys is unclear.

Innervation to the Ureter

The ureter receives sympathetic fibers from the renal plexus and preaortic plexuses. Visceral afferent fibers travel the sympathetic nerves, and ureteral pain is referred to dermatomes T_{11}–L_2

Innervation of the Bladder

The parasympathetic innervations of the bladder consist of the pelvic splanchnic nerves (S_{2-4}) originating from the inferior hypogastric plexus. These parasympathetic fibers innervate the detrusor muscle involved in reflex bladder contraction during micturition. Sympathetic innervation of the bladder is involved in urinary retention by inhibition of activity of the detrusor muscle and increasing urethral resistance. Relaxation of the external urethral sphincter and pubococcygeus muscle is necessary to initiate micturition. Visceral afferents travel along the pelvic splanchnic nerves.

Renal Microcirculation

The nephron is the basic structural and functional unit of the kidney, with between 800,000 and 1,200,000 nephrons occurring in each human kidney. It consists of the renal corpuscle (glomerulus and Bowman's capsule) and the renal tubule. The renal tubule has several segments, including the proximal convoluted tubule with its straight part, the loop of Henle with its thin descending and ascending parts, the thick ascending segment of the loop of Henle, the distal convoluted tubule, and the collecting duct.

In order to understand the function of the nephrons, it is necessary to understand their relationship to renal microvasculature. Blood enters the kidney via the interlobar arteries that are tertiary branches of the renal arteries. The interlobar arteries travel between the renal pyramids and give off the arcuate arteries that travel along the corticomedullary junction. The arcuate arteries give off small arteries, the interlobular arteries, that ascend to the cortex. The afferent glomerular arterioles branch off the interlobular arteries. The afferent glomerular arterioles enter Bowman's capsule, branching into the glomerular capillaries that then drain into a portal vessel, the efferent glomerular arteriole. The efferent arteriole then takes the blood to a second capillary network called the *peritubular capillaries*.

Glomerular filtration results from intraglomerular capillary pressure under the influence of independent contraction and dilation of the afferent and efferent glomerular arterioles. The peritubular capillaries are specialized vascular structures that facilitate reabsorption of the renal interstitial fluid from the renal cortex and renal medulla. A branch of the efferent arteriole descends straight into the renal medulla. These terminal branches of the efferent arterioles are the *arteriolae rectae*. These vessels enter the peritubular capillary network at various levels; the peritubular capillaries enter venules that ascend the medulla toward the cortex in mirror image of the arterial side, the *venae rectae*. These vessels are collectively called the *vasa recta* (vasae rectae) and act as a countercurrent exchange system that helps to maintain the osmotic gradient in the renal medulla.

Changes in Renal Function at Birth

During intrauterine life, the maternal kidneys maintain fetal fluid volume, electrolyte, and acid-base homeostasis. The placenta functions as a dialyzer. The fetal kidneys contribute to the formation and maintenance of the amniotic fluid volume. Agenesis of fetal kidneys or inability of the kidneys to function during fetal life, for example, because of certain medications, results in oligohydramnios and lung hypoplasia. At birth, the renal response to the new environment and success in maintaining homeostasis correlates with gestational age, as well as events that have taken place during intrauterine life. These include congenital malformations and intrauterine growth retardation of diverse causes that may permanently affect renal function. All newborn infants void during the first 24 hours after birth regardless of their gestational age. After the second day of life, oliguria is urine flow of less than 1 ml/kg per hour. Polyuria exists when the urinary output is more than 2000 ml/ 1.73 m^2 per day and needs further investigation. After delivery, renal blood flow increases significantly owing to several factors, including a decline in renal vascular resistances because of an increase in prostaglandin synthesis and an increase in systemic arterial blood pressure.

Glomerular filtration rate (GFR) doubles at the end of the first week of life in term infants. Infants born before 34 to 35 weeks of gestation have a slower rate of GFR increase owing to incomplete nephrogenesis; however, it increases rapidly after the 35th week of gestation. In full-term infants, the serum these reflects the mother's creatinine level, and these decrease by 50 percent at the end of the first week. In preterm infants, the rate of decline of serum creatinine at birth is slower, reflecting the stage of nephrogenesis. In children, GFR corrected for surface area of 1.73 m^2 reaches adult levels by 2 years of age. At birth, renal tubular function changes with GFR, and the fractional excretion of sodium (FENa) is high. Infants born before 35 weeks of gestation, who have a low sodium intake may develop symptomatic hyponatremia owing to tubular immaturity and sodium wasting. Term neonates can dilute urine very well to levels of 25 to 35 mOsm/liter; however, they have a limited ability to concentrate urine to more than 600 to 700 mOsm/liter. Preterm infants can concentrate urine up to 500 mOsm/liter.

Development of the Kidneys

The most common causes of chronic kidney disease and the need for dialysis and transplantation for infants, children, and adolescents up to 18 years of age are *congenital* abnormalities or *genetically* determined renal and urologic diseases. The general use of prenatal ultrasonographic evaluation of pregnancies has resulted in prenatal findings of renal and urologic abnormalities of clinical consequences. The physician at a minimum must deal with this information and notify the parents of the potential consequences of these findings. Therefore, a basic understanding of the embryologic development of the kidneys and urinary tract is essential.

The kidneys develop from the intermediate mesoderm. In mammalians, kidneys develop in intrauterine life as the *pronephros,* the *mesonephros,* and the *metanephros.* The first evidence of the pronephros in humans occurs at the end of the third gestational week and degenerates by the fifth week. The earliest stage of development of the mesonephros in humans is in the fourth week. It functions as a transient kidney, serving as an excretory organ for the embryo. The mesonephric tubules lack the loop of Henle, the macula densa, and the juxtaglomerular apparatus, and the tubules open laterally into the mesonephric ducts, which connect to the urogenital sinus. The mesonephros obtains its maximal size by 8 weeks and regresses by 16 weeks with only some elements retained as parts of the reproductive organs in the male. The metanephros, or definitive kidney, originates from the interaction of the ureteric bud arising from the lower end of the mesonephric duct at the fifth week as it enters the urogenital sinus. The ureteric bud comes in contact with the metanephric mesenchyme at the twenty-eighth day of gestation and begins dichotomous divisions. The ureteric bud dilates at its growing tip, and this area becomes the ampulla, which interacts with the metanephric mesenchyme, forming a cap and inducing the formation of future nephrons. This process gives the metanephros a lobulated appearance. In humans, nephrogenesis is complete by 34 to 35 weeks (238–245 days).

Reciprocal inductive influences of the ureteric bud and the metanephric mesenchyme activate numerous genes sequentially. The formation of the collecting system results from the initial few divisions of the ureteric bud, given origin to the renal pelvis, major and minor calyces, and collecting ducts. By the 6 to 9 weeks, the kidneys ascend from the pelvis to the lumbar site below the adrenal glands.

Urine production in the human fetal kidney begins between the tenth and twelfth gestational week and increases significantly during the third trimester. Urine volume is around 5 ml/h at 20 weeks of gestation and increases up to 50 ml/h at 40 weeks. The fetal metanephric kidney has a relatively low blood flow and GFR compared with the adult. The normal fetal urine is hypotonic in relation to plasma because the fetal kidney also conserves less sodium than the adult kidney. Fetal urine is hypotonic and has a high sodium content and a large volume compared with that of a term newborn. The evaluation of these parameters and beta$_2$-macroglobulin in fetal life is, on occasion, helpful to assess the health of the kidneys in fetal life.

Prenatal and Perinatal Period

There are few specific manifestations of renal diseases; however, there are many general manifestations, including effects on growth and development. The clinical manifestations of renal diseases evolve with the age of the patient from the prenatal period to adolescence and young adulthood. The impact of the generalized use of prenatal ultrasound has been high, and at a minimum, it imposes on the clinician the responsibility to deal with the available information in order to help make decisions in the best interest of the fetus and the expectant parents. These advances in our ability to evaluate the fetus have, in effect, created a new branch in pediatric urology/nephrology—perinatal urology. The incidence of fetal urologic abnormalities detectable by prenatal ultrasound is between 0.2 and 0.9 percent (TABLE 14–2). Up to 57.2 percent of fetal anomalies of the urinary tract manifest as hydronephrosis by high-resolution ultrasonography.

Hydronephrosis is a finding and not a specific diagnosis obtained prenatally or after delivery by appropriate studies. *Renal ectopia*, most often pelvic, occurs with a frequency of 1 in 1200 live births and is diagnosable by prenatal sonography. *Renal agenesis* may be detectable as early as the twelfth week of gestational age. Unilateral renal agenesis occurs in 1 in 1100 to 1500 live births. There are no specific findings in the mother or in the newborn when the contralateral kidney functions normally; however, by fetal sonography, the absence of a paravertebral reniform mass on transverse and parasagttal planes is sufficient to confirm the diagnosis. Additionally, the use of color Doppler sonography can establish the presence or absence of a renal artery.

Bilateral renal agenesis is a very rare condition. The bilateral absence of a paravertebral reniform masses, the absence of renal arteries, and anhydramnios establish the diagnosis. *Sirenomelia,* a severe complex of congenital malformations, is also associated with bilateral renal agenesis. The fetus with bilateral renal agenesis, as well as any other with

TABLE 14–2 *Renal and Urologic Abnormalities Detectable by Prenatal Ultrasound*

Upper Urinary Tract	Lower Urinary Tract
Hydronephrosis	Urethral disorders
Renal dysplasia	Bladder disorders: exstrophy
Duplex kidney	Bladder enlargement
Polycystic kidneys	
Renal agenesis	
Ureterocele, vesicoureteral reflux	

prolonged anhydramnios, has a peculiar facies, prematurely senile-appearing with a prominent skin fold beginning over the eye that is in a semicircle over the inner canthus that extends over the cheek. There is blunting of the nose, and the ears are low set. Patients with Potter anomaly frequently have pulmonary hypoplasia owing to anhydramnios and insufficient amniotic fluid to expand and allow normal development of the fetal lung. The severity of the lung involvement is the major determinant of the survival of these infants.

Renal diseases in the immediate newborn period are mostly related to congenital abnormalities of the kidneys and the urinary tract (TABLE 14–3). Many of these conditions are detected prenatally by high-resolution ultrasonography and then confirmed after delivery by direct physical examination, repeated ultrasound, or other imaging studies.

TABLE 14–3 *Congenital Renal Disorders*

Anomalies in number
  Unilateral renal agenesis
  Bilateral renal agenesis
  Supernumerary kidneys
Anomalies in volume and structure
  Hypoplasia
  Dysplasia (there are more than 30 syndromes associated with renal dysplasia)
  Renal cystic diseases
  Multicystic dysplastic kidney
  Autosomal recessive polycystic kidney disease (ARPKD)
  Autosomal dominant polycystic kidney disease (ADPKD)
  Medullary cystic kidney disease
  Syndromes associated with renal cysts
Anomalies of ascent
  Simple ectopia
  Pelvic kidney
Anomalies of fusion
  Fused ectopia
Obstructive uropathy or urinary tract dilatation
  Ureteric–pelvic junction obstruction, unilateral or bilateral
  Ureteric-vesical junction obstruction, unilateral or bilateral
  Megaureter, unilateral or bilateral
Urethral level of obstruction
  Posterior urethral valves
Renal masses
  Hydronephrosis
  Multicystic dysplastic kidney
  Renal vein thrombosis
  Congenital nephroblastic nephroma
  Multilocular cystic nephroma
  ARPKD (autosomal recessive polycystic kidney disease)
  ADPKD (autosomal dominant polycystic kidney disease)
  Nephroblastomatosis (Beckwith-Wiedemann syndrome)

TABLE 14–4 *Manifestations of Renal Disease from 0 to 2 Years of Age*

Poor feeding	Poor urinary stream	Jaundice
Vomiting	Bladder distension	Seizures
Failure to gain	Oliguria	Fever
Rapid respiration	Polyuria	Dehydration
Abdominal masses	Hypertension	Jaundice
Enlarged kidneys	Hematuria	Screaming
or bladder	Edema	on urination
Other external abnormalities		Malodorous
or stigmata		urine

A prenatal ultrasound may miss some conditions, such as posterior urethral valves, but the condition will declare itself after birth by the presence of a distended bladder. Findings include oliguria and a suprapubic firm mass owing to a contracted, hypertrophied bladder. Other causes include vascular diseases, acute renal injury as a consequence of infection or shock, complications of therapeutic interventions, including invasive procedures, and the administration of potentially nephrotoxic medications. Other genetically determined conditions that may manifest in the perinatal period include *autosomal recessive polycystic kidney disease* (ARPKD) and, more rarely, *autosomal dominant polycystic kidney disease* (ADPKD). These hereditary conditions manifest as bilaterally enlarged kidneys with oligohydramnios and Potter anomaly.

TABLE 14–4 lists pre- and perinatal manifestations of renal disease in the newborn. Although single malformations of the urinary tract are few, there are consistent patterns of multiple congenital abnormalities. These include malformations, deformations, and disruptions that result in specific syndromes. Currently, more than 500 described syndromes are associated with renal or urinary tract abnormalities. In many cases, nonrenal malformations associated with specific syndromes may alert the clinician to the need to investigate for kidney and urinary tract abnormalities. Some of the extrarenal abnormalities often associated with renal or urinary tract disorders appear in TABLE 14–5.

TABLE 14–5 *Extrarenal Abnormalities Associated with Renal or Urinary Tract Disorders: Newborn, 0 to 28 Days*

Low-set or malformed ears
Stigmata of chromosomal trisomies (18,21)
Anal atresia
Absence of radius
Vertebral anomalies
Tracheoesophageal fistula
Aniridia
Visceromegaly
Anomalies of the spinal cord
Congenital ascites
Hemihypertrophy

S KEY SYNDROME

▼ **Neonatal Hypertension** Systolic and diastolic blood pressures have a linear correlation with gestational age and weight. Hypertension at this age is blood pressure falling above the 95th percentile for infants of similar gestational or postconceptual age. In severely ill infants in the neonatal intensive care unit (NICU), intraarterial catheters are usually in place and provide a means for direct measurement of blood pressure. In less critical situations, the most commonly used method for blood pressure measurements is an oscillometric device, which is much less invasive. The causes of hypertension in the neonate are multiple (TABLE 14–6).

Clinical Presentation

The clinical presentation of hypertension in the newborn may be an incidental finding during routine monitoring of vital signs, congestive heart failure, cardiogenic shock, seizures, and stroke. These conditions are hypertensive emergencies that require immediate treatment. Other manifestations of hypertension include feeding difficulties, tachypnea, apnea, irritability, or lethargy. After discharge from the nursery, manifestations of hypertension may be failure to thrive, irritability, vomiting, and seizures.

Note that renal diseases play a significant role in hypertension, but there are multiple other causes as well. The evaluation of hypertension in the neonate starts with a complete maternal history, including obstetric history, medications, nonprescribed drugs, and drugs of abuse (e.g., alcohol and tobacco). Document events of labor and delivery (such as fetal distress, placental abruption or birth asphyxia). The physical examination of the infant should be complete, with attention to the presence of congestive heart failure and evidence of volume overload (manifested as liver enlargement) or unilateral abdominal mass (as seen in *renal vein thrombosis, renal tumor,* and *adrenal tumor*). Bilateral renal enlargement owing to polycystic kidney diseases may be detectable in the newborn period. Assess the quality of the peripheral pulses, absence of which can indicate *aortic coarctation* or *thrombosis.* Determination of blood pressure in the four extremities is necessary in evaluation of the hypertensive neonate. Ambiguous external genitalia in the newborn may be associated with hypertension and may be an indicator of abnormal adrenal function requiring further evaluation. Systolic hypertension and tachycardia bring up the possibility of *hyperthyroidism.*

S KEY SYNDROME

▼ **Acute Renal Failure in the Neonate** Acute renal failure is a sudden decrease in GFR resulting in accumulation of nitrogen waste products and inability to maintain acid-base-electrolyte homeostasis and preserve water balance. Acute renal failure in neonates is a GFR of less then 50 ml/1.73 m^2 per minute. Because the placenta is an excellent dialyzer, uremia is not present at birth. This is true even in infants with severe hypoplastic kidneys, severe obstructive uropathy, and even absence of the kidneys. In these circumstances, the most telling manifestations of severe renal disease are severe oliguria, lung hypoplasia, and *Potter syndrome.*

TABLE 14-6 *Causes of Hypertension in the Neonate*

Renovascular	**Acquired renal parenchymal disease**	**Medications/intoxications**
Thromboembolism	Acute tubular necrosis	*Infant*
Renal artery stenosis	Cortical necrosis	Dexamethasone
Midaortic coarctation	Interstitial nephritis	Adrenergic agents
Renal venous thrombosis	Obstruction (stones, tumors)	Vitamin intoxication
Compression of the renal artery	**Pulmonary**	Theophylline
Renal parenchymal disease	Bronchopulmonary dysplasia	Caffeine
Congenital	Pneumothorax	Pancuronium
Polycystic kidney disease	**Cardiac**	Phenylephrine
Multicystic dysplastic kidney	Thoracic aortic coarctation	*Maternal*
Tuberous sclerosis	**Endocrine**	Cocaine
Ureteropelvic junction obstruction	Congenital adrenal hyperplasia	Heroin
Renal hypoplasia	Hyperaldosteronism	**Miscellaneous**
Congenital nephrotic syndrome	Hyperthyroidism	Total parenteral nutrition
Neurologic	**Neoplasia**	Closure of abdominal defect
Pain	Wilms tumor	Adrenal hemorrhage
Intracranial hypertension	Neuroblastoma	Hypercalcemia
Seizures	Nephroblastic nephroma	Traction
Subdural hematoma		Extracorporeal membrane oxygenation (ECMO)

Source: From Vozzelli MA, Foreman JW: "Neonatal hypertension." In Spitzer AR (ed): *Intensive Care of the Fetus and Neonate*, 2d ed. Philadelphia, Elsevier-Mosby, 2005, Chap. 78, p. 1238.

Acute renal insufficiency in the newborn (TABLE 14–7) is divisible into three different categories: prerenal, intrinsic renal, and obstructive. As many as 23 percent of newborns in the NICU have evidence of acute renal failure; however, more than 70 percent of these infants have prerenal azotemia that responds rapidly to a fluid challenge. The incidence of intrinsic renal failure is between 6 and 8 percent in newborns, and the most common cause is asphyxia. The development of oliguric acute renal failure in association with severe hypoxia can be a result of prolonged fetal bradycardia, Apgar score of less than 5 at 5 minutes after delivery, and a base deficit of 14 or less at 1 hour after delivery. The presence of these observations is associated with 38 percent of intrinsic renal failure. During the physical examination, pay particular attention to the presence of the *Potter sequence*, kidney size, abdominal masses, palpable bladder, umbilical vessels, external genitalia, abdominal wall musculature abnormalities, imperforate anus, and other external malformations known to be associated with abnormalities of the kidneys and urinary tract.

History

Infants

Serious kidney diseases in infants, similar to newborns (TABLE 14–8), may be entirely asymptomatic, or the findings may point to other organ system involvement.

KEY PROBLEM

Growth Retardation, Poor Feeding, Failure to Thrive Short stature has significant consequences for the quality of life of children, adolescents, and adults. Some of the more dramatic associations occur in children with *cystinosis* and those with early age of onset *end-stage renal disease* (ESRD); however, numerous other renal diseases affect growth even in the presence of well-preserved GFRs. Children with a body mass index (BMI) greater than the 75th percentile or less than the 5th percentile are at increased risk for health problems that are cumulative and additive to the renal disease risk. Obtain head circumference measurements in all children with chronic kidney disease early in life during the period of rapid brain growth rate, from birth to 2 years of age. In general, brain growth is independent of somatic growth, except in severe, symmetric, intrauterine growth retardation, in which the generalized growth disturbance involves all organ systems, resulting in renal hypoplasia and poor brain growth. These infants often advance to ESRD and also will likely have neurologic compromise. Growth failure in infancy and childhood associated with chronic kidney diseases includes tubulointerstitial disorders, glomerular diseases, and obstructive nephropathy. These are also associated with multiple congenital malformations (TABLE 14–9). See TABLE 14–10 for multiple factors associated with growth retardation in chronic kidney diseases in early infancy.

TABLE 14-7 *Causes of Acute Renal Failure in the Neonate*

Prerenal Failure	Obstructive Renal Failure	Intrinsic Renal Failure
Hypovolemia	Posterior urethral valves	Acute tubular necrosis
Fetal hemorrhage	Urethral diverticulum	Renal dysplasia/hypoplasia
Neonatal hemorrhage	Urethral stricture	Polycystic kidney disease
Dehydration	Eagle-Barrett syndrome	Renal tubular dysgenesis
Hypoalbuminemia	Megacystis/megaureter	Congenital infection (CMV, *Toxoplasma*, syphilis)
Systemic hypertension	UPJ obstruction	Pyelonephritis
Renal hypoperfusion	Closure of abdominal wall	Arterial or venous thrombosis
Cardiac surgery	Hematocolpos	Disseminated intravascular coagulation
Congestive heart	Renal calculi	Nephrotoxins, patient and maternal (NSAIDs,
failure	Fungal balls	amphotericin B, aminoglycosides, captopril)
	Neurogenic bladder	Hemoglobinuria/myoglobinuria

TABLE 14–8 *Important Symptoms and Signs Suggesting Renal or Urinary Tract Disease in Neonates and Infants from 1 to 24 Months of Age*

Key Problems		Key Findings	
Poor feeding	Dysuria	Hypertension	Poor urinary
Vomiting	Malodorous	Dehydration	stream
Failure to gain	urine	Pallor	Hematuria
Polydipsia	Fever	Enlarged	Proteinuria
Polyuria	Edema	kidneys	
	Seizures	Distended	
		bladder	

Children

The family history provides clues regarding the possibility of genetically transmitted diseases such as autosomal dominant polycystic kidney disease in the father or mother. One can see autosomal recessive tubular disorders, such as, for example, *nephropathic cystinosis,* or X-linked hereditary nephritis (as in *Alport syndrome*), or the existence of vesicular reflux in a sibling that has been diagnosed as having vesicoureteral reflux after evaluation for a febrile urinary tract infection.

TABLE 14–9 *Chronic Kidney Diseases Associated with Growth Failure*

Fanconi syndrome
Infantile nephropathic cystinosis
Primary infantile hyperoxaluria type 1
Distal type 1 renal tubular acidosis
Proximal type 2 renal tubular acidosis
Nephrogenic diabetes insipidus
Familial X-linked hypophosphatemic rickets
Chronic hypokalemias (Bartter syndrome, Gitelman syndrome)
Idiopathic hypercalciuria
Pseudohypoaldosteronism type 1
Infantile nephronophthisis (NPH2)
Juvenile nephronophthisis (NPH1)
Autosomal recessive polycystic kidney disease (ARPKD)
Glomerular diseases associated growth failure in infancy and early childhood
Congenital nephrotic syndrome [Finnish type *NPHS1* gene mutation (nephrine)]
Diffuse mesangial sclerosis
Denys-Drash syndrome
Focal segmental glomerulosclerosis [*NPHS2* gene mutation (podocin)]

TABLE 14-10 *Factors Associated with Growth Retardation in Renal Diseases*

Disturbances in Water, Electrolyte Metabolism, and pH	Bone Disease	Hormonal Alterations	Uremia
Hyposthenuria Depletion of Potassium Sodium Phosphorus Calcium Magnesium Metabolic acidosis	Osteomalacia Osteofibrosis Osteoporosis Renal osteodystrophy	Reduction of activity of growth hormone Somatomedin Thyroid hormone Testosterone	Uremic toxins accumulation Protein-caloric malnutrition Other nutritional deficiencies

Obstetric and perinatal histories provide information about the existence of prenatal renal and urologic abnormalities detected by prenatal ultrasound. These include *hydronephrosis* and traumatic events complicating birth and the immediate perinatal period, including asphyxia, infection, and *renal vascular thrombosis*. The general medical history is important because of the effects of renal dysfunction on multiple organ systems and because many syndromes with external abnormalities are associated with renal malformations and abnormalities of renal function. For example, there may be progressive hearing loss and glomerulonephritis as in *Alport syndrome*. The presence of congenital cataracts, mental retardation, and proximal tubular dysfunction is part of *Lowe syndrome*. Abdominal pain, blood in stools, palpable purpura, and nephritis occur in *Henoch-Schönlein purpura* with *nephritis*. Hemorrhagic colitis, anemia, thrombocytopenia, and acute renal failure make the diagnosis of *hemolytic-uremic syndrome*.

Documentation of micturition history, including the frequency and quality of the urinary stream, is necessary and essential, particularly in boys. The age at which the child achieved daytime and nighttime bladder control in relation to other members of the family is also important, as is the history of urinary tract infections.

Many children with chronic kidney diseases manifest growth retardation; therefore, it is important to obtain a dietary history to evaluate adequacy of protein and other nutrient intake. In the past, severe malnutrition and intellectual impairment was common among infants with chronic kidney diseases.

● KEY PROBLEM
◤ **Dysuria, Frequency** These are the cardinal manifestations of urinary tract infection and are covered in Chapter 19.

● KEY PROBLEM

Enuresis Enuresis may be primary or secondary. Refer to Chapter 19 for more detailed discussion.

● KEY PROBLEM

Flank Pain This is also related to infection, particularly of the upper urinary tract, although clinical history and findings are neither highly sensitive nor specific to be able to separate upper from lower *urinary tract infections* (UTIs). The presence of flank pain also must bring to mind the possibility of a renal tumor or stone.

● KEY PROBLEM

Discolored Urine See Chapter 19, see hematuria below.

● KEY PROBLEM

Acute Renal Colic *Renal colic* is a complex of acute symptoms involving the collecting system and ureter (TABLE 14–11). Factors contributing to pain are acute urinary obstruction, renal interstitial edema, stretching of the renal capsule, and passage of a stone causing direct irritation to the mucosa of the collecting system and ureter.

In general, nonobstructing stones located in the calyx cause pain only periodically; this pain is usually a deep, dull ache in the flank or in the back with mild to moderate severity. The pain relates to the state of hydration. Acute increase occurs after ingestion of large amount of fluids, causing transient obstruction to the flow of urine. Stones located in the renal pelvis that are large enough to obstruct the ureteropelvic junction (UPJ) (i.e., several millimeters in diameter) cause severe pain in the costovertebral angle below the twelfth rib. This pain radiates to the flank and the ipsilateral upper abdominal quadrant; if located in the right side; the differential diagnosis includes *acute cholecystitis* and *biliary colic.* If the stone is located in the left, the differential diagnosis includes acute pancreatitis and acute gastritis.

Congenital UPJ obstruction may cause similar symptoms after drinking large amount of fluids or when associated with infection. Usually the severity of pain will compel the patient to seek immediate medical attention. Stones located in the upper ureter cause pain radiating to the costovertebral angle, flank, and lumbar area. Stones located in the midureter cause referred pain to the middle and lower abdomen. On the right side, the differential diagnosis will include acute appendicitis

TABLE 14–11 *Causes of Renal Colic*

Urinary obstruction (the most common cause as from a kidney stone)
Clots lodged in narrow ureteral parts (with hematuria and urinary tract obstruction)
Fungal bezoars
Accumulation of tumor cells in the ureteral lumen
Polyp

and ovarian cyst in the female. If the stone is located in the left ureter, the differential diagnosis includes an ovarian inflammatory process and intestinal disease. A stone in the distal ureter causes referred pain to the inguinal area, testicle in the male and labia majora in the female. The differential diagnosis in males includes *testicular torsion* and *epididymitis.* Calculi in the intramural portion of the ureter may cause symptoms of urgency, frequency, and dysuria.

The classic description of renal colic has three phases: *onset, constant,* and *abatement.* The pain starts at night or in the morning hours. The *onset* is abrupt, awakening the patient from sleep, and migrates to the flank and in the testis or vulva; it is persistently severe, although it may worsen with excruciating paroxysms. The pain reaches its peak in half an hour, and the patient is restless. During the *constant phase,* the pain remains with the same intensity for a variable period of time and, without treatment, may last for several hours. During the *abatement phase,* the pain gradually decreases in severity but may occur spontaneously without the administration of analgesics. The patient gradually drifts to sleep, but unfortunately, the abatement phase lasts only minutes.

KEY PROBLEM
Oliguria TABLE 14–12 outlines normal voiding frequencies and urine volume by age. *Oliguria* in pediatric patients is simply the insufficient passage of urine to maintain homeostasis. In this population, the urine volume indicating oliguria is less than 240 ml/m² per day; this urine volume is less than 1 ml/kg per hour and is insufficient to excrete the normal daily osmotic load resulting from normal nutritional intake. The consequences of oliguria are retention of products of protein metabolism and *prerenal azotemia.* Oliguria may result from many causes, as listed in TABLE 14–13. Oliguria by itself does not imply renal injury.

KEY PROBLEM
Polyuria Polyuria is an increase of urine volume (see Table 14–12). It is usually associated with hypotonic urine. The causes of polyuria

TABLE 14–12 *Average of Volume of Urine Excreted Daily and Urine Volume*

Age	Frequency of Voiding/Day	Volume, ml
1–2 days	2–6	30–60
3–10 days	5–30	100–300
10–60 days	5–30	250–450
2–12 months	5–30	400–500
1–3 years	6–8	500–600
2–5 years	6–8	600–700
5–8 years	6–8	650–1000
8–14 years	6–8	800–1400

TABLE 14–13 *Causes of Oliguria*

1. Severe restriction of water intake
2. Increase in water loss from
   a. Sweating
   b. Burns
   c. Diarrhea
3. Edematous states from:
   a. Nephrotic syndrome
   b. Congestive heart failure
4. Intrinsic acute renal failure
5. Chronic renal insufficiency

are multiple (TABLE 14–14). *Nephrophthisis–medullary cystic disease complex* is associated with polyuria, polydipsia, and progressive renal insufficiency. The polyuria results from the inability to concentrate urine owing to interstitial fibrosis and tubular damage. Polyuria with an abnormal osmotic load occurs in untreated diabetes mellitus and during administration of mannitol.

Some children develop psychogenic polydipsia or the habit of excessive water drinking with resulting polyuria. It may be difficult to distinguish between *nephrogenic diabetes insipidus* and compulsive *psychogenic* water drinking. In *psychogenic water drinking,* the child usually sleeps well through the night with no nighttime drinking, and there is no failure to thrive. In *nephrogenic diabetes insipidus,* the infant becomes irritable and has feeding difficulties and failure to thrive. Hypernatremic dehydration is common if the condition is not treated. In psychogenic polydipsia, moderate water restriction and regular diet correct the polyuria. Water restriction in nephrogenic and central diabetes insipidus is dangerous.

TABLE 14–14 *Causes of Polyuria*

Congenital nephrogenic diabetes insipidus
Neonatal Bartter syndrome
Post correction of obstructive uropathy
Nephrophthisis–medullary cystic disease complex
   (associated with polyuria, polydipsia, and progressive renal
   insufficiency)
Complete or partial vasopressin deficiency
Polycystic diseases of the kidneys
Nephrotoxic drugs (such as lithium)
Diabetes mellitus
Genetically-transmitted nephrogenic diabetes insipidus
Psychogenic polydipsia
Mannitol

Physical Examination Including Urinalysis

Infants

A complete physical examination is always necessary. Refer to the section on children below for details.

▼ KEY FINDING
Hypertension Evaluation of *hypertension* in infancy is similar to that in a neonate. Refer to the section above.

▼ KEY FINDING
Hematuria This may be gross *hematuria* (visible blood in the urine) or detected by dipstick or microscopic evaluation of the urinary sediment. In the presence of red or brown discoloration of the urine, a methodic approach is necessary to distinguish the presence of blood from that of other material that may be confused with blood (TABLE 14–15). The first step is the centrifugation of the urine and observation of the urine sediment and supernatant. If the sediment is red, there is blood. If there is no sediment, hemoglobin or myoglobin may be present. In order to distinguish *hemoglobinuria* from *myoglobinuria,* a simultaneous observation of the serum supernatant is useful. A clear supernatant favors myoglobinuria, whereas the presence of a red supernatant indicates hemoglobinuria (TABLE 14–16).

The presence of red blood cell (RBC) casts or a high number of dysmorphic RBCs suggests that the blood is of glomerular origin. As demonstrated by electron microscopy, the dysmorphic cells develop by the mechanical disruption of the RBCs as they travel through small defects in the glomerular basal membrane. In some rare cases, dysmorphic RBCs have been seen in association with bladder malignancies. Normal morphology of the RBCs indicates an extraglomerular origin of the bleeding.

Children

Make a rapid assessment to determine how sick the child looks, assessing the existence of the circulation, perfusion, and shock and the adequacy

TABLE 14–15 *Causes of Discolored Urine Suggesting Hematuria*

Associated with Diseases	Associated with Food or Drug Ingestion
Hemoglobinuria	Aminopyrine, azo dyes
Myoglobinuria	Beets, blackberries
Porphyrinuria	Chloroquine, desferrioxamine
Alkaptonuria	Ibuprofen, methyldopa, nitrofurantoin
Homogentisic acidiuria	Rifampin, sulfasalazine
Melanin, methemoglobinuria, tyrosinemia	Urates, alanine, cascara, resorcinol, thymol

TABLE 14–16 Causes of Hemoglobinuria

Diseases	Drugs and Chemicals	Miscellaneous
Hemolytic anemias	Aspidium	Cardiopulmonary bypass
Hemolytic-uremic syndrome	Carbon monoxide	Freshwater drowning
Paroxysmal nocturnal hemoglobinuria	Fava beans	Mismatched blood transfusion
	Poisonous mushrooms	
	Potassium chloride	
	Sulfonamides	

of ventilation. The mental status and level of consciousness may indicate neurologic involvement. Assess growth and nutrition by plotting the anthropometric measurements in the appropriate growth curves.

Determining the vital signs is important, including temperature, pulse, blood pressure, and respiratory rate and depth. A peripheral to central temperature gap of more than 2°C indicates poor cardiac output. Tachycardia is an early manifestation of intravascular volume depletion, and a rapid threadlike pulse with cold and clammy extremities and prolonged capillary refill time precedes hypotension in infants and children developing hypovolemic shock. The state of hydration is sometimes difficult to assess. In cases of rapid weight gain or weight loss, the change mainly reflects changes in water. Blood pressure in children changes with age, body size, and gender. An exaggerated decline in blood pressure (orthostasis) indicates a decreased intravascular volume. Oliguria, edema, and hypertension, on the other hand, represent an increased intravascular volume. Patients with edema may have intravascular volume depletion in the presence of increased total body water. Also, examination of the oral mucosa for pallor and the skin for birth marks may give clues to the nature and duration of any renal involvement.

There is a well-known association of ophthalmologic abnormalities and renal diseases. Cataracts can occur in *Lowe syndrome* or in *galactosemia* associated with renal tubular dysfunction. Posterior lenticular cataracts result in patients with prolonged steroid use. Deposition of crystals in the corneas is common in infantile *hyperoxaluria type 1* and *cystinosis*, whereas scleral calcifications appear in patients with hypercalcemia and hyperphosphatemia in advanced chronic kidney disease. *Keratoconus*, a conical abnormality of the cornea, occurs in Alport syndrome.

Abnormalities of the retina are observed in many conditions associated with renal diseases. Abnormal pigment is present in *cystinosis* and *Alport* syndrome, whereas retinitis pigmentosa is characteristic of *Laurence-Moon-Biedl syndrome,* a condition that leads to ESRD owing to renal medullar dysplasia. Retinal cystine crystal deposition is common in cystinosis, and retinal calcium oxalate crystals are part of infantile hyperoxaluria type 1. The effects of hypertension manifest in the retina vasculature with narrowing of the arteries and exudative papilledema of hypertensive encephalopathy. Bilateral hemorrhages and severe hypertension are components of malignant hypertension. *Diabetic retinopathy* occurs in older adolescents that acquired type 1 diabetes early in life. The retinopathy correlates with the development of diabetic nephropathy. Aniridia and hemihypertrophy occur in *Wilms tumor* (nephroblastoma). Deformities of the external ear are associated with renal abnormalities in *branchio-otorenal syndrome,* and progressive hearing loss is present in *Alport* syndrome. Nerve deafness is associated with genetically transmitted distal renal tubular acidosis. *Acute tubular necrosis* and ototoxicity may be a consequence of aminoglycoside treatment.

In the newborn, the kidneys are usually palpable. In older children it becomes more difficult but possible with practice. Place the right middle and ring fingers in the patient's left-side angle formed between the last rib and the spine, lift the left kidney, and palpate it with the left hand. In order to palpate the patient's right kidney, place the fingers of the left hand in the patient's right costovertebral angle, lift the right kidney, and palpate it with the right hand. With practice, it becomes easier to palpate the lower pole of both kidneys. In the supine position, percussion of the kidneys is not useful to determine their size because of bowel interference.

Enlargement of the kidneys is detectable by palpation in cases of *autosomal recessive polycystic kidney disease, Beckwith-Wiedemann syndrome* in infants with nephromegaly, and bilateral enlargement of the kidneys with oliguric renal failure owing to massive bilateral renal leukemic infiltration. Localized renal enlargement is apparent in unilateral *hydronephrosis* or renal tumor. Abdominal distension from ascites occurs in the *nephrotic syndrome* and is also part of the *triad syndrome (prune-belly syndrome).* A round, firm mass is sometimes palpable in the suprapubic area in the male newborn with hypertrophic bladder wall owing to *posterior urethral valves.*

Liver enlargement occurs in infants that have hepatic fibrosis and portal hypertension in association with autosomal recessive polycystic kidney disease and in adolescents with severe *glycogen storage disease* complicated by *focal segmental glomerulosclerosis. Infectious and inflammatory diseases* such as *subacute bacterial endocarditis, acute pyelonephritis,* and *shunt nephritis* will cause renal enlargement. *Collagen-vascular diseases,* such as lupus nephritis and juvenile rheumatoid arthritis, also may cause renal enlargement.

In the female with external ambiguous genitalia, consider the possibility of adrenal hyperplasia with salt wasting and hyperkalemia or the *Denys-Drash syndrome* with pseudohermaphroditism, cryptorchidism, and proteinuria. Renal biopsy and genetic analysis will confirm the correct diagnosis. Cryptorchidism is also a component of the *triad syndrome* (prune-belly syndrome). Imperforate anus and displacement of the anus accompany abnormalities of other organ systems, including the kidneys and urinary tract.

Neurologic manifestations are common in association with renal diseases. Seizures may occur in severe hypertension, electrolyte abnormalities (such as hyponatremia, hypernatremia, hypocalcemia, and hypomagnesemia), *systemic lupus erythematosus* (SLE) with renal or CNS involvement, and the *hemolytic-uremic syndrome.* Cerebrovascular events may occur during hemodialysis, resulting in seizures or strokes.

Skeletal manifestations in renal disease include *rickets* of chronic renal tubular disorders or of vitamin D–resistant rickets in the familial hypophosphatemias. Renal *osteodystrophy* may manifest with bone pain and tibial deformities. *Avascular necrosis* may be a consequence of chronic steroid therapy, such as in the treatment of lupus or after renal transplantation. Deformities of the spine occur in patients with meningomyelocele. *Scoliosis* is common in children after renal transplantation. Joint involvement of SLE (*lupus*) and *Henoch-Schönlein purpura* often accompany acute nephritis.

Routine Urinalysis

Routine urinalysis is a very important tool for the clinician. Dipstick technology provides a rapid and practical method for determination of blood, protein, glucose, pH, nitrate, and leukocyte esterase. Microscopic examination of the urinary sediment is usually in the purview of the laboratory technician, although the experienced clinician should be able to perform the urinalysis skillfully. The urinalysis is so essential, convenient, and cost-efficient that we will consider it part of the physical examination.

▼ KEY FINDING
▉**Hematuria** Hematuria may be gross or microscopic. It may originate from the kidney or extrarenal structures. It is incumbent on the clinician to take a thorough history of present illness and family history and to perform a complete physical examination to locate the source of the bleeding. A microscopic examination of the urine sediment is most helpful to arrive at a diagnosis. Association with proteinuria greater than 2+, cuboidal epithelial cells, or RBC or WBC casts suggests renal parenchymal involvement. Also, dysmorphic RBCs in the urine indicate renal involvement, whereas normal RBC morphology is more likely to indicate lower urinary sites of bleeding. TABLE 14–17 indicates renal diagnoses related to history and clinical findings. TABLE 14–18 outlines causes of extraparenchymal urinary bleeding.

▼ KEY FINDING
▉**Proteinuria** The American Academy of Pediatrics recommends that asymptomatic children have a screening urinalysis four times from infancy to adolescence. Many experienced pediatric nephrologists have questioned this recommendation. In several countries urine screening tests are routine at school and may on occasion detect asymptomatic abnormalities with clinical consequences.

The normal glomerular basement membrane (GBM) restricts the filtration of protein from the plasma. The permeaselectivity of the GBM is a result of the actions of the cells at both sides of the GBM, the normal negative electric charge, and the GBM proper. Albumin, for example, with a molecular weight of 69 Da and a negative electric charge, passes the glomerular filter only in small amounts of 10 mg/liter of glomerular filtrate, and normally, the proximal tubule actively reabsorbs whatever gets through. Membrane pore size and electric charge characteristics prevent loss of large-molecular-weight proteins. Low-molecular-weight

TABLE 14–17 *Common Components of the Clinical Evaluation of Hematuria*

History of	*Suggests*
Dysuria	UTI, upper or lower
Fever	Infection, vasculitis [collagen-vascular, Henoch-Schoenlein purpura (HSP)]
Sinusitis, cough, headache, epistaxis	Wegener granulomatosis
Flank pain	Stones, acute obstruction, infection, cysts, tumor
Intermittent gross hematuria	Nephritis, hypercalciuria, tumor
Antecedent viral illness	Post infectious nephritis and others, IgA nephropathy
Cola-color urine, edema, hypertension	Glomerulonephritis
Bloody diarrhea	Hemolytic-uremic syndrome
Family history of	*Suggests*
Microhematuria	Thin basement membrane disease, hereditary nephritis, stones
Hearing loss	Hereditary nephritis (Alport)
Renal failure	Hereditary nephritis, polycystic kidney disease
Anemia	Sickle cell disease
Physical findings of	*Suggests*
Hypertension	Acute or chronic glomerulonephritis
Edema	Glomerulonephritis, membraneous nephropathy, focal sclerosis
Bruising	Coagulopathy, collagen-vascular disease
Heart murmur, fever	Subacute bacterial endocarditis
Purpura	Systemic infection, HSP
Flank mass	Polycystic kidneys, obstruction, tumor, multicystic dysplasia

Source: From Greydanus DE, Patel DR, Pratt HD: *Essential Adolescent Medicine.* New York: McGraw-Hill, 2006.

TABLE 14–18 *Causes of Extraparenchymal Urinary Bleeding*

Urinary infection
Hypercalciuria or nephrolithiasis
Abdominal or flank trauma
Urinary tract malformations
Instrumentation of lower urinary tract (medical and nonmedical)
Hemoglobinopathy
Medications
Tumor
Hemorrhagic diathesis

Source: From Greydanus DE, Patel DR, Pratt HD: *Essential Adolescent Medicine.* Ne~ York: McGraw-Hill, 2006.

proteins pass through the GBM, but they are rapidly reabsorbed in the proximal tubule by endocytosis, an energy-consuming mechanism involving the megalin system. The proximal tubule then metabolizes the reabsorbed proteins. Tamm-Horsfall proteins are also present in the urine, originating in the renal tubules.

Significant glomerular proteinurias can result from functional or structural abnormalities of the GBM. *Proteinuria* may be selective, indicating predominantly albumin, or nonselective, when all the plasma protein may leak through. Overflow glomerular proteinuria is seen when an abnormally large amount of proteins are present in plasma, such as in *myeloma*. Significant tubular proteinuria occurs when large amounts of low-molecular-weight proteins pass in the urine. Usually it is the result of dysfunction of the proximal renal tubule owing to such diseases as *cystinosis, Fanconi syndrome,* or *Dent disease*. Typical markers of tubular proteinuria include beta$_2$-microglobulins, alpha$_1$-microglobulins, and retinol-binding protein.

Orthostatic proteinuria occurs when the individual is standing or active but is not present when the person is supine or resting. This proteinuria is best detectable by a properly collected 24-hour "split" urine collection for measuring total protein and creatinine in each container. The test reveals normal protein excretion during the night-time collection and significant proteinuria during the daytime collection. Orthostatic proteinuria is more common in tall, slender, rapidly growing, and active adolescents. Renal biopsy is not necessary, and there is no need for treatment. In general, the prognosis is excellent.

Transient proteinuria occurs in association with exercise, fever, and dehydration; it is most likely a consequence of hemodynamic changes. It alone does not have renal pathologic implications.

Chronic persistent proteinuria leads to tubulointerstitial disease and renal injury; it needs to be investigated, and long-term follow up is indicated. Refer to the discussion on nephrotic syndrome.

Synthesizing a Diagnosis

Infants

S KEY SYNDROME

▼ **Urinary Tract Infection** Poor feeding, vomiting, fever, and malodorous urine suggest *urinary tract infection,* often *acute pyelonephritis,* in infancy. The physical examination will reveal irritability, or lethargy, abdominal distension, abdominal and back tenderness, jaundice, and/or rapid respiratory rate. Appropriate culture of body fluids will help to establish the correct diagnosis and guide treatment.

S KEY SYNDROME

▼ **Acute Renal Failure** The etiology of acute renal failure in fancy is similar to that of newborns. Refer to the section above.

S KEY SYNDROME

▼ **Renal Tubular Acidosis** *Renal tubular acidosis* (RTA) is a
syndrome characterized by the inability of the kidney to maintain normal bicarbonate concentration in the presence of normal hydrogen
ion production resulting from the normal metabolic processes in the
body. The consequence is titration of bicarbonate and other buffers
resulting in the development of hyperchloremic, normal-ion-gap
metabolic acidosis. RTA reflects renal tubule functional abnormalities.
There are several types of RTA, the classification of which is based on
history and related to the chronologic order of the description of the
abnormalities and to the location of the abnormality on the site of the
nephron. More recently, with better understanding of the molecular
structure, function, and location of the different ions and transporters involved in hydrogen production and secretion in the
nephron, a more precise classification is possible. Currently, three types
of RTA are recognized: *proximal, or type 2, RTA; distal, or type 1, classic
RTA;* and generalized distal nephron dysfunction resulting in *type 4, or
hyperkalemic and hyperchloremic, RTA.*

Proximal RTA Type II

Patients with proximal RTA develop hypokalemia. Bicarbonate wasting
is associated with volume depletion, resulting in stimulation of the
renin-angiotensin-aldosterone system that increases sodium reabsorption and potassium excretion. Hypokalemias may be symptomatic,
resulting in muscular weakness, hyposthenuria, and polyuria. Symptoms of proximal RTA in the infant and child include recurrent vomiting,
polyuria, polydipsia, growth retardation, failure to thrive, and muscle
weakness often related to hypokalemia, which occurs frequently. In general, patients with proximal RTA do not develop nephrolithiasis or
nephrocalcinosis.

Normally, the proximal tubule reabsorbs approximately 90 percent
of the filtered bicarbonate, maintaining serum bicarbonate concentration
within normal limits (24 to 28 mmol/liter). These levels are just below
the threshold for proximal tubule bicarbonate reabsorption. In proximal
RTA, the threshold is decreased, allowing excretion of bicarbonate in
the urine. This results in a limited form of metabolic acidosis. This defect
causes the filtered bicarbonate to escape to the lower segments of the
nephron, increasing the urine pH. When the serum bicarbonate concentration is below the threshold, the distal mechanism of proton excretion results in decreased urinary.

Isolated primary RTA may be sporadic or familial. In some cases it
may be transient, particularly in infancy and childhood, but it is permanent in adult-onset disease. The condition may be autosomal dominant or autosomal recessive, and it may be isolated or associated with
mental retardation or hearing loss. The most common cause is
dysfunction of the Na^+-H^+ exchanger (NHE3 antiporter). It occurs in
mitochondrial myopathies that also affect the kidneys. *Osteopetrosis* associated with carbonic anhydrase 2 deficiency (*Sly syndrome*) involves
both proximal and distal RTA.

TABLE 14–19   *Syndromes with Proximal Renal Tubular Acidosis*

Nephropathic cystinosis
Lowe syndrome
Hereditary fructose intolerance
Tyrosinemia
Galactosemia
Wilson disease
Metachromatic leukodystrophy
Silver-Russell syndrome (dwarfism)
Dent disease

Proximal RTA is a component of several syndromes listed in TABLE 14–19. It is also associated with dysproteinemias, including multiple myeloma and light-chain disease. Other renal diseases associated with proximal RTA are *medullary cystic disease, early rejection of kidney transplant, chronic renal vein thrombosis, drugs,* and *toxins including gentamicin ifosfamide,* and *outdated tetracycline.*

Fanconi syndrome is a condition of multiple etiologies consisting of dysfunction of the proximal tubule resulting in abnormal amounts of amino acid loss in the urine, glucosuria, phosphaturia, hypophosphatemia, abnormalities in vitamin D metabolism, and bicarbonate wasting. These abnormalities manifest clinically as polyuria, dehydration, metabolic acidosis, proteinuria, hypokalemia, hypouricemia, rickets, and failure to grow. Fanconi syndrome may be congenital and associated with multiple abnormalities of metabolism or may develop secondary to toxic agents or as a consequence of autoimmune diseases.

Cystinosis is an inherited disease owing to a defect in the egress of cystine from lysosomes. It results from mutations in the gene *CTNS* that encodes cystinosin, a protein present in the membrane of lysosomes and necessary for the egress of cystine from lysosomes. Malfunction of cystinosin results in accumulation of cystine in lysosomes, causing cellular damage and cell death. There are three recognized forms of cystinosis. *Nephropathic* cystinosis is the most severe, presents in early infancy, and is associated with progressive renal disease. In these patients, the severe mutation is present in both chromosomes. In *ocular* cystinosis, there is one chromosome that carries a severe mutation, but the other chromosome mutation is not severe, and the patient is able to produce some amount of normally functioning cystine. The third form of cystinosis is *adolescent* cystinosis, a slowly progressive disease that affects the kidneys and eyes.

Infants with *nephropathic* cystinosis manifest polyuria, polydipsia, anorexia, dehydration, and failure to thrive. Patients with nephropathic cystinosis have the biochemical abnormalities found in the *Fanconi syndrome,* including glucosuria, aminoaciduria, proteinuria, hypophosphatemia, phosphaturia, loss of bicarbonate in the urine, hyperchloremic metabolic acidosis, hypokalemia, and hypouricemia. Most infants with nephropathic cystinosis are blond and have growth failure and rickets. In addition, they also have ocular manifestations, including progressive photophobia owing to accumulation of cystine crystals in the conjunctiva and cornea (as noted during slit-lamp examination). The ophthalmologic examination also reveals peripheral retinopathy. The condition affects mainly Caucasians but also occurs in African-Americans and other ethnic groups. The definitive diagnosis of nephropathic cystinosis is through laboratory findings of elevated levels of intracellular cystine in leukocytes or fibroblasts containing between 5 and 10 nmol/mg of protein.

Classic Hypokalemic Distal RTA

Distal RTA, also known as *RTA type 1*, results from the inability of this tubular segment of the nephron to excrete H^+ and acidify the urine to a pH of less than 5.5 (TABLE 14–20). The responsible transporters in this segment include the electrogenic H^+-ATPase or proton pump, the electroneutral H^+, K^+-ATPase, and the HCO_3-Cl exchanger. The presentation of classic distal RTA is characterized by a progressive positive acid balance, hyperchloremic metabolic acidosis, volume depletion, and hypokalemia,

---

TABLE 14–20   *Classic Hypokalemic Distal Renal Tubular Acidosis*

Primary
Familial
1. Autosomal dominant
    a. *AE1* gene mutation
2. Autosomal recessive
    a. With deafness
    b. Without deafness
Sporadic
Endemic
    Southeast Asia
Secondary to systemic disorders
Disorders of calcium metabolism with nephrocalcinosis or
    hypercalciuria
Primary hyperparathyroidism
Hyperthyroidism
Vitamin D intoxication
Medullary sponge kidney
X-linked hypophosphatemia
Autoimmune diseases
Hyperglobulinemia purpura
Cryoglobulinemia
Sjögren syndrome
HIV nephropathy
Drugs and toxins
Amphotericin B,   Toluene
Ifosfamide   Mercury below
Lithium   Classic analgesic nephropathy
Associated with genetically transmitted diseases
Hereditary elliptocytosis   Ehlers-Danlos syndrome
Hereditary sensorineural deafness   Jejunal bypass with
                                             hyperoxaluria
Osteopetrosis with carbonic anhydrase deficit Marfan syndrome

---

along with calcium, magnesium, and phosphate wasting that results in bone disease. Nephrocalcinosis and nephrolithiasis result from the elevated urinary pH and hypocitraturia associated with chronic metabolic acidosis. UTIs occur more frequently in the presence of nephrolithiasis.

Chronic kidney disease leading to ESRD may develop in these patients if not treated. In infants and preadolescent children, growth retardation and rickets cause significant morbidity. Tachypnea, polyuria, vomiting, poor feeding, and protein-caloric malnutrition are also common in infants and young children. Severe acidosis may be life-threatening in infants. Chronic hypokalemia causes muscular weakness and, in the more severe cases, death from muscular paralysis and cardiac dysrhythmia. The condition may hereditable as an autosomal dominant or autosomal recessive disorder in some cases associated with deafness.

The condition may be familial or present as an isolated disorder. There is an endemic form in Southeast Asia. Hypokalemic distal RTA may be secondary to many systemic disorders, including *autoimmune diseases, tubulointerstitial nephritis, hypercalciuria, nephrocalcinosis, drugs,* and *toxins.*

Distal RTA Type IV

Distal RTA type 4 is the most common form of RTA and demonstrates hyperkalemia, mild metabolic acidosis, and preservation for acidification of the urine to pH below 5.5. It usually is associated with mineralocorticoid deficiency, as in congenital adrenal hyperplasia, mineralocorticoid resistance (pseudohypoaldosteronism type I), or more generalized distal tubular dysfunction (*interstitial nephritis* and *reflux nephropathy*). It also can be due to medications such as spironolactone, captopril, heparin, prostaglandin inhibitors, and others.

Mineralocorticoids stimulate H^+ secretion by the alpha intercalated cells and sodium reabsorption by the principal cell in the distal convoluted and cortical collecting duct of the nephron, thus enhancing K secretion. The absence of aldosterone and the tubular resistance to the effects of aldosterone and other mineralocorticoids interfere with these mechanisms, resulting in sodium loss along with hydrogen and potassium retention; there is also decreased ability to excrete ammonium. Patients with distal type 4 RTA do not have nephrocalcinosis or urolithiasis most likely because the urinary citrate is normal. Clinical manifestations in the infant and young child include failure to thrive, abnormal external genitalia, dehydration, lethargy, salt wasting, and hyperkalemia.

Other Syndromes: Glomerulonephritis and Nephrotic Syndrome

Acute glomerulonephritis and the nephrotic syndrome are rare occurrences in early infancy. The major problems are often nonspecific as listed earlier. Specific findings are hematuria in nephritis and edema with or without hematuria in *nephrotic syndrome.*

Several forms of the congenital nephrotic syndrome are due to gene mutations resulting in defective synthesis of proteins of the podocyte filtration diaphragm. Consequently, they have the potential to transmit to future generations.

The most severe form of primary congenital nephrotic syndrome is the *Finnish type of congenital nephrotic syndrome*. It is an autosomal recessive disease owing to a defect in the gene *NPHS1,* and the most severe mutation leads to absence of the protein nephrin, an integral protein of the podocyte filtrating apparatus. The clinical presentation starts in utero with the development of *polyhydramnios,* resulting in preterm delivery around 36 weeks of gestation. The physical examination reveals a small infant with the placenta weight 25 percent of the infant's weight. Edema develops soon after birth; abdominal distension is prominent, and an umbilical hernia is usually present. The fontanels are wide open, and hypotonia increases in severity as age advances. Feeding difficulties are always present, whereas diarrhea, vomiting, and malnutrition are common; infections are a constant threat. Laboratory studies show marked proteinuria of more than 20 g/liter of urine when plasma protein is greater than than 15 g/liter.

The *Denys-Drash syndrome* consists of a triad of male *pseudohermaphroditism,* progressive *glomerulopathy,* and development of *Wilms tumor* or *gonadal tumor.* The glomerulopathy is usually consistent with diffuse *mesangial sclerosis* with *nephrotic syndrome* of early or variable onset. The syndrome is due to mutations in the *WT1* gene and multiple mutations of the gene for the *Denys-Drash syndrome* (DDS). TABLE 14–21 lists the causes of *primary* and *secondary* congenital nephrotic syndrome.

Children

Congenital abnormalities of the kidneys and the urinary tract continue to dominate the causes of renal diseases, particularly in patients younger

---

TABLE 14–21   *Causes of Congenital Nephrotic Syndrome*

Primary
Congenital nephrotic syndrome Finnish type
Isolated diffuse mesangial sclerosis
Denys-Drash syndrome
Congenital nephrotic syndrome with brain and other congenital
  malformations
Minimal-change nephrotic syndrome
Focal segmental glomerulosclerosis
Membranous glomerulopathy
Secondary
Syphilis
Toxoplasmosis
Rubella
Cytomegalovirus
Hepatitis B
Hepatitis C
HIV infection
Malaria
Collagen-vascular diseases (as lupus)
Toxins: lead, other heavy metals

---

than 10 years of age. In this age group, the consequences of *obstructive uropathy, chronic high-grade vesicoureteral reflux, chronic pyelonephritis, nephronophthisis–medullary cystic disease, tubulopathies,* and *chronic tubulointerstitial nephritis* increasingly compromise the GFR, and patients become more symptomatic with chronic kidney diseases.

Acquired renal disease starts to become more frequent, particularly those affecting the glomerulus, such as the *hemolytic-uremic syndrome,* acute glomerulonephritis, and glomerular diseases associated with the nephrotic syndrome. In addition, vasculitis affecting the kidney, such as *Henoch-Schönlein purpura nephritis* and *lupus nephritis,* becomes more common at this age. Infections of the kidney continue to be an important cause of renal diseases in this age group. Common clinical features of renal diseases in children from 2 to 12 year of age are listed in TABLE 14–22.

The diagnosis of renal disorders in children and adolescents is quite similar. We consider them as a single group but specify in the text any problems that may be unique to either group.

Renal diseases affecting patients 12 to 21 years of age represent a transition in the spectrum of problems seen at younger ages to those seen in adults. Structural abnormalities of the kidneys and urinary tract represent 40 percent of patients with renal and urologic diseases at this age, whereas glomerular diseases increase to 40 percent. Focal segmental glomerulosclerosis is the most common form of glomerular disease affecting African-American adolescents and young men. Essential systemic arterial hypertension is more frequent than secondary forms of *hypertension.* The problem of obesity associated with hypertension is quite prevalent. *UTIs* involving the kidneys are less common than lower UTIs involving the bladder and urethra.

TABLE 14–22 *Clinical Manifestations of Renal Diseases for Those 2 to 12 Years of Age*

Key Problems		Key Findings	
Nonspecific	Specific	Physical Examination	Urine
Poor appetite	Dysuria	Abdominal mass	Malodor
Vomiting	Abdominal	Poor abdominal	Hematuria
Constipation	pain	musculature	Proteinuria
Growth failure	Flank pain	CVA tenderness	WBCs
Excessive thirst	Enuresis	Pelvic mass	
Seizures	Incontinence	Hypertension	
Dehydration	Frequency	Edema	
Pallor	Oliguria/		
Fever	polyuria		
	Weak urinary		
	stream		

▆ KEY SYNDROME

▼ **Nephrotic Syndrome** The nephrotic syndrome may present at any age, from the newborn period to the elderly individual. TABLE 14–23 provides a definition of the *nephrotic syndrome* in the adult and pediatric populations.

In children from 6 months to 12 years of age, the most common form of nephrotic syndrome is the classic steroid-sensitive nephrotic syndrome, particularly before 10 years of age (85 percent of cases) with a significant peak at age 2. At presentation, physical examination reveals generalized edema, more prominent around the face in the early hours of the day and in the legs and ankles in the afternoon. Percussion of the flanks and the palmar side of the fingers palpating the other flank will demonstrate ascites. Demonstrate shifting dullness by placing the patient on his or her side, and as one percusses that side, the dullness disappears. Scrotal and labial edema can occur in children with severe edema. Pitting edema occurs in the ankles after the patient has been out of bed for several hours. The ungual angle, normally present at the base of the fingernails, is lost in active nephrotic syndrome owing to edema but reappears when the nephrotic syndrome is in remission. The aural cartilage feels flabby in children with active nephrotic syndrome and returns to normal consistency when the nephrotic syndrome is in remission. Blood pressure is usually normal in these children, but hypertension may occur in up to 10 percent of cases, particularly after initiation of steroid therapy. Gross hematuria is rare, but microscopic hematuria may occur in 10 percent of children with steroid-sensitive nephrotic syndrome.

13 to 18 Years of Age and Young Adults

In North America, the nephrotic syndrome in patients 13 to 18 years of age and in young adults is due to *focal segmental glomerulosclerosis*. One finds this in particular in African-American young men and other minorities (such as Native Americans and Mexican-Americans). Other causes of nephrotic syndrome in adolescents include *minimal-change disease, membranous nephropathy,* and *membranoproliferative glomerulonephritis. Lupus nephritis* also occurs at this age, affecting mainly African-American adolescent females. The physical examination reveals edema, more

---

TABLE 14–23 *Nephrotic Syndrome Definitions*

Adult
Massive proteinuria > than $3.5 \text{ g}/1.73 \text{ m}^2$ in 24 hours
Pediatric age
Massive proteinuria > than $40 \text{ mg}/\text{m}^2$ per hour or $50 \text{ mg}/\text{kg}$ per day, associated with
    Hypoalbuminemia of < than 3 grams/dl
    Hyperlipidemia
    Edema

---

prominent in the lower extremities. Muscle wasting is more likely in the chronic nephrotic syndrome. Hypertension is common, and hematuria is a frequent finding in the urinalysis.

S KEY SYNDROME

▼ **Urolithiasis** The association of renal colic and hematuria always should call to mind *urolithiasis*. It is becoming increasingly common in the pediatric population from premature infants and young children to adolescents, as well as young adults, often a consequence of modern therapeutic modalities in the NICU and PICU. Between 2 and 3 percent of kidney stones occur in children. Urolithiasis is more common in Caucasian than in African American children. There are multiple factors that predispose pediatric patients to urolithiasis (TABLE 14–24).

Clinical presentation of urolithiasis from birth to 5 years of age is gross hematuria and pain in 56 percent of cases. In young children, urolithiasis seldom presents with renal colic but rather with vague symptoms, failure to thrive, tachypnea owing to metabolic acidosis, UTIs, and as an incidental finding in 44 percent of cases. Pain may occur with palpation of the abdominal upper quadrants or percussion of the flanks. Urinalysis may reveal crystals and eumorphic red blood cells. If fever is present, look for acute pyelonephritis.

In children between 5 and 12 years of age, the presentation of urolithiasis is with gross hematuria and abdominal or flank pain in 72 percent of cases. Chronic urolithiasis may be associated with recurrent UTIs, alkaline urine, and a urea-splitting organism. These children also may present with poor growth, particularly if malabsorption or *metabolic diseases* (such as *cystinuria* or *hyperoxaluria*) are present. RTA type 1 may present with failure to grow, tachypnea, weakness, polyuria, hypokalemia, nephrocalcinosis, and nephrolithiasis. An abdominal mass may be palpable if nephrolithiasis has caused *obstruction* and *hydronephrosis*.

TABLE 14–24 *Factors Predisposing to Urolithiasis*

Preterm
Loop diuretics
Parenteral nutrition
Children
Metabolic diseases (as hypercalciuria, hyperoxalurias)
Distal renal tubular acidosis
Cystinuria
Urinary tract infections
Adolescents
Metabolic diseases (as hypercalciuria, cystinuria)
Chronic urinary tract infections
Chronic inflammatory bowel diseases
Obesity (uric acid stones)

In adolescents (ages 12 and over), the clinic presentation is similar to that in adults with abdominal pain, flank pain, and/or gross hematuria as the presenting symptoms in 90 percent of urolithiasis cases. An abdominal mass may be present if hydronephrosis has developed, and flank or abdominal pain may appear with palpation and percussion. All pediatric patients with urolithiasis require a comprehensive metabolic evaluation to elucidate the cause of urolithiasis and establish appropriate treatment to prevent recurrence of the problem and prevent permanent renal damage and chronic kidney disease. TABLE 14–25 lists disorders associated with urolithiasis.

S KEY SYNDROME

▼ **Acute Renal Failure** *Acute renal failure* is the hallmark of a decline in GFR of at least 50 percent, accumulation of nitrogen waste as well as blood urea nitrogen (BUN) and creatinine, alterations in water and electrolyte metabolism, and changes in the amount and composition of the urine. There are several categories of acute renal failure: *prerenal, postrenal,* and *intrinsic renal failure.*

Prerenal acute renal failure is due to intravascular volume depletion, decreased effective arterial blood flow, and altered renal hemodynamics. *Postrenal* acute renal failure results from obstruction of the urine flow and involves both UPJs, either ureter, or the urethra. The obstructions are of sudden onset. *Intrinsic* acute renal failure may have multiple etiologies that induce acute tubular necrosis, including ischemia, nephrotoxins, acute interstitial nephritis, and acute vascular syndromes. Ischemia may result from trauma with bleeding, hypotension, and hypovolemic shock. Ischemia also may result from *septic shock, cardiopulmonary arrest,* and *cardiopulmonary bypass.*

Nephrotoxins are numerous, including drugs (such as aminoglycoside, amphotericin B, cisplatin, and other anticancer drugs) and diagnostic agents (such as contrast media, inducing contrast nephropathy). Pigment nephropathy causing acute tubular necrosis may result from hemoglobinuria (resulting from massive hemolysis induced by toxins or mismatched RBC transfusion) and myoglobinuria (from crush muscular injury). Acute interstitial nephritis can be a consequence of factors listed in TABLE 14–26. Various types of *glomerulonephritides* include acute proliferative glomerulonephritis of multiple causes. These include *postinfectious, membranoproliferative, Henoch-Shönlein purpura nephritis,* and *rapid progressive glomerulonephritis.* Acute vascular syndrome can be due to renal artery thrombosis or renal vein thrombosis. TABLE 14–27 lists causes of acute renal failure by age parameters.

Pathophysiology of Intrinsic Acute Renal Failure (ARF)

Ischemia-reperfusion injury and exposure to toxins at the tubuloepithelial cell level result in severe depletion of high-energy chemical stores such as ATP and accumulation of degradation products and oxidants.

TABLE 14-25 *Clinical Disorders Associated with Urolithiasis in Pediatric Patients*

Hypercalciurias
Hypercalciuria with normocalcemia
Idiopathic
Inherited
Secondary hypercalciurias
Dietary calcium excess
Dietary salt excess
Vitamin D excess
Ketogenic diet
Corticosteroids
Loop diuretics
Immobilization
Phosphate depletion
Prematurity
Prostaglandin E_2
Hypercalcemia
Hyper- or hypothyroidism
Renal tubular transporter disorders or inborn errors of metabolism
Distal renal tubular acidosis type 1
Hereditary
Complete
Incomplete
Dent disease
Familial hypomagnesemia with hypercalciuria
Infantile hyperoxaluria type 1
Hyperoxaluria type 2
Idiopathic hyperoxaluria
Secondary hyperoxaluria
Dietary oxalate excess
Enteric hyperoxaluria
Parenteral nutrition in preterm infants
Cystinuria
Hyperuricosuria
Idiopathic
Mild associated with idiopathic stone disease
Familial forms
Secondary
Tumor lysis syndrome
Myeloproliferative/lymphoproliferative disorders
Syndrome of inappropriate antidiuretic hormone secretion (SIADH)
High dose pancreatic enzyme therapy
Lesch-Nyhan syndrome
Hypocitraturia
Idiopathic
Secondary
Distal renal tubular acidosis
Ketogenic diet
Hypokalemia
Bacteriuria

TABLE 14-26 *Causes of Acute Interstitial Nephritis*

Medications
Antibiotics (including methicillin and cephalosporins)
Nonsteroidal anti-inflammatory drugs (NSAIDs)
Rifampin
Phenytoin
Sulfonamides
Diuretics
Infections
Mononucleosis (Ebstein-Barr virus)
Rubella
Hanta virus
HIV
E. coli (and other bacterial infections)
Pyelonephritis
Tuberculosis
Systemic diseases
SLE (systemic lupus erythematosus)
Sarcoidosis
Sjögren's syndrome

These factors cause loss of cellular polarity, mislocalization of cellular transports, cellular swelling, increase in intracellular free calcium, activation of phospholipases and proteases, plasma and subcellular membrane injury, alteration of the cytoskeleton, cellular detachment from the basolateral matrix and from other epithelial cells, and cell death or apoptosis. At the level of the entire kidney, the consequences are

TABLE 14-27 *Causes of Acute Renal Failure by Age*

Ages 2 to 12 years
Hemolytic-uremic syndrome
Multiple organ dysfunction syndrome due to sepsis
Drug toxicity
Surgery for congenital heart diseases
Primary renal diseases
Malignancies
Tumor lysis syndrome
Post bone marrow transplantation (including kidney transplantation)
Ages 13 to 21 years
Multiple organ dysfunction syndrome due to sepsis
Trauma
Ingestion of nephrotoxic agents
Drugs
Malignancies
Solid organ transplantation
Post bone marrow transplantation

decreased glomerular filtration, tubular obstruction, back leakage, and stimulation of epithelial cell regeneration as well as differentiation.

Diagnostic Approach to ARF

The starting point is a comprehensive history, including recent illnesses such as bloody diarrhea, ingestion of specific foods (such as hamburgers), visits to animals farms, swimming in lakes, medications, febrile illnesses, skin rashes, and arthralgias. A comprehensive physical examination includes such questions as: How sick does the child look? Is he or she acutely ill? What is the status of alertness and cardiovascular function and presence of tachycardia, gallop, weak pulses, or pallor? What is the nature of the blood pressure (normal, low, or elevated)? Assess respiratory status for tachypnea, shallow respirations, and auscultation sounds (clear or wet sounds). Is the patient oliguric or polyuric? Is the urine reddish smoky in color?

S KEY SYNDROME
▼ **Chronic Kidney Disease and Chronic Renal Failure** Table 14–28 lists the definition and classification of chronic kidney disease. The distinction between acute renal failure and chronic renal failure is often ambiguous. An elevation of plasma creatinine concentration and abnormal urine of a few days or few weeks' duration represent an *acute* process. *Chronic renal failure,* on the other hand, denotes a reduction of GFR below normal lasting for several months or even years; however, this chronic process may contain acute exacerbations. Chronic renal failure is fundamentally different from acute renal failure in that chronic renal failure represents permanent loss of nephrons that is irreversible. One definition of *chronic kidney disease* is either kidney damage or GFR of less than 60 ml/1.73 m^2 per minute for 3 months or longer; *kidney damage* is defined as abnormalities in blood, urine test, or imaging studies.

All individuals with kidney damage have chronic kidney disease (CKD) irrespective of the GFR level. The rationale for including individuals with a GFR greater or equal to 60 ml/1.73 m^2 per minute is that GFR may be normal or increased despite substantial kidney damage and that patients with kidney damage are at increased risk for progressive kidney disease and cardiovascular events.

TABLE 14–28 *Definition and Classification of Chronic Kidney Disease Stages*

Stage	Description	GFR (ml/min/1.73 m^2)
1	Kidney damage with normal or elevated GFR	>90
2	Kidney damage with mild decreased GFR	60–89
3	Moderate decrease in GFR	30–50
4	Severe	15–29
5	Kidney failure	<15 or dialysis

TABLE 14–29 Causes of Chronic Renal Disease in Those Aged 10 Years through Adolescence

Glomerular disorders
Focal segmental glomerulosclerosis
Membranous nephropathy
Membranoproliferative glomerulonephritis
IgA nephropathy
Small blood vessel vasculitis
Lupus nephritis
Hereditary nephritis (Alport syndrome)
Renal tubular diseases
Bartter syndrome
Gitelman syndrome
Diabetic nephropathy

Causes of Chronic Renal Failure: 2 Years to 10 Years of Age

Causes of chronic kidney disease and chronic renal insufficiency include *hypoplastic/dysplastic kidneys, autosomal recessive polycystic kidney disease,* and *hemolytic-uremic syndrome and its sequels* (hypertension and proteinuria). *Juvenile nephronophthisis/medullary cystic disease complex* is one of the most important causes of ESRD in children around 10 years of age or early adolescence. Others include reflux nephropathy and sickle cell disease causing chronic interstitial nephritis and glomerulosclerosis. Tubular diseases (including *hyperoxaluria type 2, Bartter syndrome,* and *cystinuria*), are associated with chronic kidney disease.

TABLE 14–29 lists causes of chronic renal disease in those aged 10 years through adolescence. The most important causes of chronic kidney disease that may advance to chronic renal insufficiency and ESRD are the glomerular diseases. Focal segmental glomerulosclerosis is the most common glomerular disease causing chronic kidney disease and ESRD in adolescents, particularly in African-American adolescent boys and young men. *Diabetic nephropathy* starts to develop in older adolescents who have acquired diabetes mellitus type 1 in early childhood.

Laboratory and Imaging Studies

Laboratory and imaging studies are helpful after the differential diagnoses are formulated on clinical grounds. We list selected conditions in which the laboratory and imaging departments may be of significant value to narrow down diagnostic possibilities.

Neonatal Hypertension

The laboratory investigation of the hypertensive neonate includes serum electrolytes, CO_2, blood urea nitrogen (BUN), and creatinine levels. Severe hypertension may induce polyuria and hyponatremia owing to salt wasting induced by pressure natriuresis. It is important to keep in mind the changing normal values of creatinine in the newborn. Urinalysis and urine culture with sensitivities are necessary in newborns suspected to be infected or having congenital abnormalities of the urinary tract. The presence of oliguria, proteinuria, and hematuria favors the existence of renal parenchymal disease.

Coagulation studies are important in hypertensive septic infants, in those suspected of having renal vein or renal artery thrombosis, or in those with other coagulation abnormalities. Renal artery stenosis as a cause of hypertension in newborns is rare. The interpretation of peripheral plasma renin levels is difficult owing to the variability with gestational and postgestational age, as well as the effects of medications and different physiologic factors that influence its production. Perform appropriate laboratory studies in infants suspected of having endocrine causes of hypertension (such as 11β- or 21β-hydroxylase deficiency). Obtain plasma and urinary catecholamine metabolite levels in suspected cases of catecholamine-producing tumors, whereas thyroid hormone determinations are useful for suspected cases of *neonatal hyperthyroidism.*

Imaging studies of the kidneys and urinary tract of the hypertensive infant are important if *renal artery stenosis* is under consideration, but direct arteriography is seldom necessary at this age. Imaging studies are also critical in the presence of an abdominal mass, unilateral or bilateral enlarged kidneys, abnormal urinary sediment, hematuria, proteinuria, UTI, or absence of a clear extrarenal cause of hypertension. Ultrasonography is the least invasive of the currently available techniques. Doppler sonography adds information, although it is highly operator-dependent. Nuclear medicine renal scans are very useful for evaluating flow and function in these newborns.

Acute Renal Failure in the Neonate

The presence of hematuria or proteinuria (moderate) may be a manifestation of acute renal injury. Elevated creatinine levels, as well as BUN, hyponatremia, hyperkalemia, and anemia, may be present. An abnormally elevated fractional excretion of sodium (FENa) in the urine is the most reliable laboratory parameter that indicates acute renal failure. The formula for the determination of FENa is FENa = [(urine sodium/plasma sodium)/(urine creatinine/plasma creatinine)] × 100. In term infants, the normal value should be less than than 3 percent; FENa greater than 3 percent indicates intrinsic renal failure. These calculations should be available before administration of diuretics.

Renal ultrasonography may reveal the number and size of the kidneys, normal or abnormal echogenicity, and the presence or absence of hydronephrosis or bladder distension that suggests *bladder outlet obstruction.* A voiding cystourethrogram is necessary in male infants to confirm or exclude posterior urethral valves. Radionuclide scans are useful to assess renal flow and function. Intravenous pyelography is now seldom used.

Urinary Tract Infection

Once the infant has been stabilized, it is necessary to perform imagining studies of the kidneys and urinary tract to evaluate for congenital abnormalities such as *vesicoureteral reflux, UPJ obstruction, neurogenic bladder, ureterocele,* or *hydronephrosis.* Genitourinary tract abnormalities occur in approximately 20 percent of infants with a documented UTI. These imagining studies include bilateral renal and bladder ultrasound. After this study is completed, the next most important step is to demonstrate the presence or absence of vesicoureteral reflux. A voiding cystourethrogram (VCUG) should be done as soon the patient is stable and afebrile. Other studies, such as MRI of the kidneys or dimercaptosuccinic acid (DMSA) scan, may be indicated in some cases. They are most useful in assessment of renal scarring.

Renal Tubular Acidosis

Hyperchloremic normal-ion-gap metabolic acidosis is noted, and blood gas determinations confirm metabolic acidosis (TABLE 14–30). Extrarenal losses of bicarbonate, such as that owing to diarrhea, need to be excluded by history and laboratory data. The administration of chloride, such as with parenteral nutrition, needs investigation. In RTA, electrolytes will demonstrate hyperchloremic metabolic acidosis with a normal ion gap. Urine pH measured by pH electrode for accuracy should be used. In the presence of acidosis, the urine pH remains 5.5 or greater and will not decrease further even if the acidosis becomes more severe. In proximal RTA, urine pH will be 5.5 or less in the presence of acidosis. In hyperkalemic type 4 RTA the pH may be variable. Urinalysis may indicate the presence of substances such as glucose and amino acids, suggesting proximal tubular involvement, as seen in cases of proximal RTA.

Urine ammonium excretion should be directly measured if possible or calculated by determining the urine anion gap (UAG). The practical approach to calculate the urine anion gap is $UAG = (Na^+ + K^+)u - (Cl^-)$. NH_4^+ is present if the sum of Na^+ plus K^+ is less than the concentration of Cl^-. This situation will be the normal response in the presence of acidosis and in classic type 2 RTA; ammonium excretion is low in type 2. In type 4 hyperkalemic distal RTA, the ammonium excretion is also low. Serum potassium level determinations are important in the classification of the RTAs; hypokalemia is typically present in proximal type 2 RTA and in classic type 1 distal RTA; it is elevated in distal type 4 RTA.

Proteinuria

Qualitative methods to measure proteinuria include dipstick methods such as Albustix and Multistix (TABLE 14–31); these products contain reagents impregnated with tetrabromophenol blue buffered with citrate.

TABLE 14–30 RTA Diagnostic Studies

	Type of RTA		
Finding	Proximal [II]	Classic Distal Type [I]	Generalized Distal Dysfunction Distal Type [IV]
Plasma [K⁺]	Low	Low	High
Urinary pH with acidosis	<5.5	>5.5	<5.5 or >5.5
Urine net charge	Negative (normal)	Positive	Positive
Fractional bicarbonate excretion	>10–15 percent	<5 percent	<5–10 percent
(Urine-Blood)P_{CO_2} normal > 20	Normal	Decrease < 15	Decrease < 15
Nephrocalcinosis kidney stones	Negative	Positive ++	Negative
Fanconi syndrome	Positive in many types	Negative	Negative
Rickets renal insufficiency	Positive	Positive in some	Negative, renal insufficiency, mild

TABLE 14–31   *Definition of Significant Proteinuria by Dipstix*

1. 1+ is equal to 30 mg/dl on dipstick examination in 2 of 3 random urine samples collected 1 week apart, if urine specific gravity is 1.015 or more
2. 2+ is equal to 100 mg/dl on similarly collected urine specimen if urine specific gravity is 1.015 or more

The binding of albumin causes a color change from yellow to green by displacement of the transformation range of the indicator. The intensity of the change is related to the albumin concentration. The test does not detect small molecular weight proteins, tubular proteins, and positively charged proteins. Sulfosalicylic acid is another good method for the qualitative determination of urine protein in the ambulatory setting. Semiquantitative methods for measurement of proteinuria are the *urine protein to urine creatinine ratio in milligrams per milligram* (in children it is age-dependent) (TABLE 14–32).

Urolithiasis

TABLE 14–33 lists the laboratory and imaging studies used for urolithiasis.

Acute Renal Failure

Laboratory studies should include a complete blood count (CBC, with RBC morphology and platelet count); other tests include BUN, creatinine, electrolytes, calcium, phosphorus, magnesium, uric acid, total proteins, albumin, prothrombin time (PT), partial thromboplastin time (PTT), and complement C_3.

TABLE 14–32   *Methods to Measure Proteinuria*

Age, yrs.	mg of Protein/mg of Creatinine
0.1–0.5	0.7
0.5–1	0.55
1–2	0.40
2–3	0.30
3–5	0.2
5–7	0.15
7–17	0.15

Quantitative
1. Normal: ≤4 mg/m^2 per hour in a timed 12- to 24-hour collection
2. Abnormal: 4 to 40 mg/m^2 per hour in a timed 12- to 24-hour urine collection
3. Nephrotic range proteinuria: ≥ 40 mg/m^2 per hour in a timed 12- to 24-hours urine collection

Semiquantitative
1. After 5–7 years of age, the urine protein to urine creatinine ratio is the same in children, adolescents, and adults.

TABLE 14–33 *Initial Evaluation for Urolithiasis* *

Blood
Complete blood count (CBC)
Electrolytes, blood urea nitrogen, creatinine
Calcium, phosphorus, alkaline phosphatase, uric acid
Total protein, albumin, parathyroid hormone level
Urine
Urinalysis with urine culture and sensitivity
Fasting early morning urine for urine calcium to urine creatinine ratio
24-hour urine collection (calcium, phosphorus, magnesium, oxalate,
    uric acid, citrate, cystine, creatinine excretion)
Imaging studies
Renal and bladder ultrasound
Spiral CT is the most sensitive method for evaluation of urolithiasis
Hand x rays
Chemistry
Chemical analysis of calculi or gravel

---

*This table indicates that in the initial evaluation for urolithiasis, it is necessary to obtain
plasma as well as urinary values of different substances and other factors responsible
for the formation of urinary tract stones. Often an initial screening test is followed by
more comprehensive evaluation.
Source: From Greydanus DE, Torres AD, Wan JH: Genitourinary and renal disorders.
In: Greydanus et al. (ed.): Essential Adolescent Medicine, Eds: Greydanus DE, Patel DR,
Pratt HD. New York: McGraw-Hill, Chap. 16, pp. 329–369.

The urinalysis should include specific gravity, osmolality, pH, protein, hemoglobin, glucose, and sediment. In acute intrinsic renal failure, the urinary sediment is typically "muddy," with abundant brownish granular casts; RBC casts, white blood cell (WBC) casts, and casts containing renal epithelial cells are easily apparent to the experienced clinician.

Various indices identify renal failure (TABLE 14–34). Fractional excretion of sodium (FENa) is an age-dependent test that measures the nephron reabsorption function and is useful to differentiate prerenal failure from acute tubular necrosis. In prerenal acute renal failure, FENa is normally less than 1 percent. In term healthy newborns it is less than 1 percent (see formula above), whereas in preterm infants it is as high as 2.5 percent. In children up to 18 years of age it is less than 1 percent, and in healthy adults it is less than 1 percent. Use of diuretics and the syndrome of inappropriate antidiuretic hormone secretion (SIADH) both alter FENa.

TABLE 14–34 *Renal Failure Indices*

Fractional excretion of sodium (FENa)
Fractional excretion of urea nitrogen (FEUN)
BUN to creatinine ratio
Urine-to- plasma creatinine ratio
Urine sodium concentration
Urine determination of neutrophil gelatinase–associated lipocalcine
    (NGAL).

A more sensitive test for tubular function is the *fractional excretion of urea nitrogen* (FEUN) to differentiate prerenal failure from acute tubular necrosis in adults; it is useful even when patients have received diuretics. The formula is FEUN = $[(UUN/U_{Cr})/(BUN/P_{Cr})] \times 100$. An FEUN value of less than 35 percent typically signifies prerenal azotemia, and FEUN value of more than 50 percent indicates acute tubular necrosis.

Another index is the *BUN to creatinine ratio*, with a normal of 10 to 15:1. A BUN: creatinine ratio greater than 20:1 is seen in prerenal azotemia, gastrointestinal tract bleeding, drugs (as with steroids and tetracycline), muscle wasting, and end-stage chronic kidney disease. Also, there is the *urine to plasma creatinine ratio,* which is greater than 40 in prerenal azotemia and less than than 20 in intrinsic renal failure. Another index is *urine sodium concentration in milliequivalents per liter;* in prerenal azotemia, it is less than than 20 mEq/liter and greater than 40 mEq/liter in acute tubular necrosis.

Finally, a novel marker of acute renal injury is the *urine determination of neutrophil gelatinase–associated lipocalcine* (NGAL). This is a biomarker for acute renal injury owing to ischemia. NGAL is a renoprotective substance seen after ischemic injury that reduces apoptosis, increases normal proliferation of renal tubular cells, and enhances production of hemoxygenase 1. It enhances iron uptake by siderophores and protects the cell from injury. The urine basal concentration of NGAL is 1.6 µg/liter; it rises to 147 µg/liter 2 hours after ischemia. In the serum, the baseline mean value is 3.2 µg/liter and rises to 61 µg/liter 2 hours after ischemic injury.

The most important role for imaging studies in acute renal failure is for evaluation of acute urinary obstruction. *Renal ultrasound* is useful to determine the number, size, and echogenicity of the kidneys and the presence or absence of obstruction. A *nuclear renal scan* will evaluate blood flow and function of each kidney.

A renal biopsy in acute renal failure is the "gold standard" to establish a specific histopathologic diagnosis, consider therapeutic options, and determine prognosis.

Chronic Renal Failure

Methods to Assess Chronic Renal Disease Severity and Progression

Several methods are available to assess the severity and progression of renal disease, such as measurement of GFR. In clinical practice, most nephrologists use the measurement of plasma creatinine. Another method is calculation of GFR based on creatinine clearance. These methods are imprecise but work well in clinical practice to guide therapy and to determine renal disease progression. In the pediatric population, the *Schwartz equation* (TABLE 14–35) is appropriate in this clinical situation. This method is practical and recommended in the assessment of renal function of infants, children, adolescents, and young adults.

TABLE 14–35 *Schwartz Equation*

1. **Formula:**
   Length in cm
   GFR = K(length, cm/plasma creatinine, mg/dl) = ml/1.73 m^2
   Plasma creatinine in mg/dl.
   (K is a constant that changes with the age and gender of the patient.)
2. $K = 0.33$ for preterm infants (males and females); the normal creatinine clearance at this age is 40.6 ± 14.8 ml/1.73 m^2.
3. Between 2 and 8 weeks of age, the value of K is 0.45 for both genders; the average value of the creatinine clearance is 65.8 ± 24.8 ml/1.73 m^2.
4. After 8 weeks of age to 2 years of age, the value of is $K = 0.45$; the calculated normal clearance is 95.7 ± 21.7 ml/1.73 m^2 for both genders.
5. Between 2 and 12 years of age, K value is 0.55 for males and females; the calculated creatinine clearance is 133.0 ± 27 ml/1.73 m^2 per minute.
6. For adolescent males 13 to 21 years of age, K value is 0.70; the calculated creatinine clearance is 140.0 ± 30 ml/1.73 m^2 per minute.
7. For adolescent females 13 to 21 years of age, K value is 0.55; the calculated creatinine clearance is 126 ± 22 ml/1.73 m^2 per minute.

Clinical manifestations of chronic disease evolve slowly as renal function declines. Early, in stage 1 and 2 of chronic kidney disease, when the GFR is normal or only minimally impaired, there are no symptoms, and homeostasis is preserved. Fluid, electrolyte, and acid-base abnormalities start to manifest when chronic kidney disease reaches stage 3, in which fluid overload may manifest with edema, heart failure, or hypertension, and metabolic acidosis may result in failure to thrive. Alterations in vitamin D metabolism may predispose to bone disease.

As the chronic kidney disease advances to stage 4, anemia, hyperphosphatemia, hypocalcemia, secondary hyperparathyroidism, and renal osteodystrophy with skeletal pain develop. The risk of hyperkalemia becomes a serious problem in the management of these patients at any age. In infants and young children, malnutrition may result in serious impairment of intellectual development. Failure to grow is prominent if not treated.

In chronic kidney disease stage 5 with a GFR of less than 15 ml/1.73 m^2 per minute, the patient develops the syndrome of uremia, characterized by neurologic changes, including poor concentration, lethargy, seizures, and coma. There is anorexia, nausea, vomiting, and peripheral neuropathy. At this stage the patient needs renal replacement treatment.

Laboratory manifestations of stages 4 and 5 of chronic kidney disease are listed in TABLE 14–36.

TABLE 14–36   *Laboratory Manifestations of Stages 4 and 5 Chronic Kidney Disease*

Elevated creatinine and BUN
Hypocalcemia
Hyperphosphatemia
Hyperparathyroidism
Hyponatremia
Metabolic acidosis
Hyperkalemia
Normocytic anemia
Hypercholesterolemia and hypoalbuminemia (as seen in those with
   the nephrotic syndrome)

When to Refer

Table 14–37 notes some reasons for pediatric nephrology referral. Indications for urology referral appear in Chapter 19.

TABLE 14–37   *When to Refer to the Pediatric Nephrologist (Partial List)*

Infants and children with multicystic dysplastic kidney
Neonatal hypertension
Hypercalciuria
Hyperkalemia
Hypokalemia
Solitary functioning kidney
Small kidneys
Enlarged kidneys
Autosomal recessive polycystic kidney disease (ARPKD)
Congenital nephrotic syndrome
Bartter syndrome
Beckwith-Wiedemann syndrome
Obstructive uropathy
Steroid resistant nephrotic syndrome
Nephrotic syndrome in children 8 years of age or older and those
   with relapses
Acute nephrotic syndrome not associated with infection
Metabolic acidosis and failure to thrive
Infants with recurrent febrile urinary tract infections
Renal artery thrombosis
Renal vein thrombosis
Proteinuria
Secondary hypertension
Renal failure

15 The Hematology-Oncology System

Elna N. Saah, Renuka Gera,
Ajovi B. Scott-Emuakpor,
and Roshni Kulkarni

HEMATOLOGY

The goals of this section are

1. To outline the physiology and mechanics of the hematopoietic system and the hemostatic system
2. To describe the functional anatomy of the hematopoietic system and the hemostatic system
3. To describe the signs and symptoms associated with perturbations in the hematologic and hemostatic systems
4. To use the information derived from the preceding to develop a list of diagnostic possibilities and prioritize them
5. To define the age and gender differences in hematologic parameters and diseases
6. To develop a plan for appropriate laboratory and imaging studies that may aid in the diagnosis
7. To discuss appropriate and timely referrals for subspecialty consultation

Physiology and Mechanics

The hematopoeitic system consists of cellular elements—red blood cells (RBCs), white blood cells (WBCs), and platelets—suspended in a liquid medium called *plasma*. The latter contains coagulation proteins and enzymes that are essential for hemostasis. Endothelium and subendothelial elements such as collagen are also an essential part of the hemostatic system.

In the fetus, the mesoderm of the yolk sac initially produces blood. From the second to the seventh intrauterine period, the liver and spleen perform this function. Subsequently, the bone marrow, in all the bones, becomes the predominant site of blood production. Since fat replaces the marrow in long bones by early childhood, flat bones (such as the sternum, vertebrae, pelvis, cranium, etc.) become the predominant sites of bone marrow formation that persists throughout life.

All blood cells derive from pluripotent stem cells that become "committed" to a particular cell line. They undergo a series of differentiation steps, under the influence of "growth factor" or regulatory molecules, to give rise to mature blood cells. The stem cells retain their capacity for self-renewal, and the stromal cells and microvasculature of the marrow provide a microenvironment for sustained growth.

The purpose of the hemostatic system is to preserve vascular integrity, maintain blood in a fluid state, and prevent blood loss. The various components of the hemostatic system are cellular elements such as the endothelium and platelets, plasma coagulation factors, the fibrinolytic system, and regulators of hemostasis.

When a blood vessel is injured, it undergoes vasoconstriction that decreases blood loss. Platelets adhere to the exposed subendothelium at the site of injury (platelet adhesion), change shape, and release chemicals that recruit more platelets. The platelets attach to each other (*platelet aggregation*), forming a "platelet plug" that is usually sufficient to stop minor bleeding. The von Willebrand factor (VWF) released by the platelets serves as a tethering protein in conditions of high-flow shear.

While the intrinsic and extrinsic pathways are laboratory phenomena to explain the prothombin time (PT) and the activated partial thromboplastin time (aPTT), "cell-based" coagulation more accurately mirrors the interaction of cellular and coagulation factors. The PT measures factors VII, X, V, and II and fibrinogen.

Following injury, tissue factor (TF) is exposed and forms a complex with factor VIIa. The TF-factor VIIa complex activates factor IX to factor IXa (which moves to the platelet surface) and factor X to factor Xa. The latter generates small amounts of thrombin (factor IIa) from prothrombin (factor II) that (1) activate platelets, (2) activate factor XI to factor XIa, (3) release factor VIII from VWF and activate it, and (4) activate platelet factor V to factor Va. The factor XIa activates plasma factor IX to factor IXa on the platelet surface. Factor VIII is a cofactor for factor IXa and forms a "tenase" complex (factor VIIIa-factor IXa) that converts large amounts of factor X to factor Xa on the platelet surface. The factor Xa forms a "prothrombinase" complex with factor Va that converts large amounts of prothrombin to thrombin, the so-called thrombin burst. This results in the conversion of sufficient fibrinogen to fibrin to form a firm and stable hemostatic clot. In hemophilia, deficiency of factor VIII or factor IX results in insufficient thrombin generation owing to the lack of formation of the "tenase" complex. Primary platelet plug formation owing to platelet activation and initiation phases of coagulation is normal in hemophilia. However, any clot, owing to small amounts of thrombin in the initiation phase, is friable and porous.

Functional Anatomy

The hematopoietic system consists of RBCs, WBCs (neutrophils, lymphocytes, monocytes, eosinophils, and basophils), and platelets. All these cellular elements derive from stem cells that undergo various stages of differentiation. Numerous growth factors regulate the process of differentiation and maturation. The WBCs derive from the myeloid cell line, the T and B lymphocytes from the lymphoid, the RBCs from the erythroid, and the platelets from megakaryocytes. As the RBCs mature, they shed their nuclei and contain increasing amounts of hemoglobin that helps to transport oxygen.

The hemostatic system consists of coagulation factors. For the most part, these are enzymes that circulate as precursors (zymogen) that convert to the active enzyme called *serine protease* or as cofactors. Factor XIII is a transglutaminase, and fibrinogen is a soluble protein. The platelet, along with the endothelium, is an integral part of the hemostatic system containing granules that participate actively in coagulation.

I. HEMATOPOIETIC SYSTEM

It is important to understand that signs and symptoms of hematologic disorders are based on derangements in the normal function of one or more of the cellular elements of blood. Therefore, the goals of the chapter are to enhance understanding of these disorders by taking a rather simplified approach with pathophysiology based on excessive destruction (loss), utilization (consumption), or abnormal production (excessive or inefficient).

Obtaining a complete history is very important in any pediatric patient with a suspected hematopoietic disorder. More than most pediatric conditions, hematologic disorders have significant associated genetic and hereditary factors.

Therefore, the interviewer must have the skills of eliciting a good family history, including ethnic background. It is important to obtain a history of unusual exposures, such as exposure to chemicals, foods, medications, and nonconventional drugs, because blood cells are very sensitive to toxins in the environment.

Red Blood Cells

Anemia (Greek: "Without Blood")

The production of red blood cells (RBCs) is under the control of a feedback loop between the hematopoietic organs and the rest of the body. This feedback system assumes that hemoglobin availability for oxygen transport and delivery matches the body's needs and that production and destruction of RBCs are intricately balanced. Anemia results when there is a disruption of this relationship that originates from a primary production defect and/or increased loss or destruction outside the production factory (bone marrow).

History and Physical Examination

An attempt to distinguish between signs and symptoms is difficult with respect to hematologic diseases. The terms are often used interchangeably.

Since infants cannot express subjective symptoms per se, these often come as presenting complaints based on parental observations. Thus we refer to a *presenting complaint,* whether a patient's subjective feeling or a parental observation as a "problem."

History

Infants

The signs and symptoms listed here can apply to any pediatric age group, except the newborn. In the newborn period, anemia manifests as pallor and floppiness, contributing to low Apgar scores. Later in the neonatal period it will manifest as tachypnea, tachycardia, poor suck, and poor reflexes. Pallor is seen universally in all cases of anemia.

Children

In this age group and older, the predominant signs and symptoms will depend on the time of onset and the etiology of the anemia. Anemia that develops within hours or a few days is usually as a result of acute blood loss. In these instances, pallor may not be an important sign. Signs of volume depletion such as dizziness, hypotension, and cardiac strain may be more profound.

Rapid blood loss also may be the result of massive hemolysis. In such cases, signs of volume depletion may not be as apparent as signs of toxicity (arthralgia, fever, discolored urine, and severe abdominal pain) caused by metabolites of hemoglobin.

For slowly developing anemias, symptoms are related primarily to tissue hypoxia, listed previously.

Adolescents

Everything said about children (ages 2 to 12 years) also applies to adolescents. The only difference will be in the relative frequencies of the events. Rapid blood loss from trauma is more likely in an adolescent than in a child. Girls of this age are more likely to have anemia than boys owing to increased blood loss from menstruation. Key problems are for all age groups.

KEY PROBLEM

Fatigue The patient either feels "tired" or "weak," or the caretaker portrays the patient as such. The cause is primarily low energy owing to low oxygen supply from anemia. It is more noticeable in adolescents and children.

KEY PROBLEM

Lethargy This is a lack of interest in the environment and is often a result of long-standing anemia. It applies to all age groups and may manifest more as fatigue in infants.

KEY PROBLEM

Poor Feeding This occurs mostly in infants; it manifests as refusal of food or loss of interest during feeding.

● KEY PROBLEM

Irritability There is often restlessness and inconsolability, and it occurs mostly in infants and sometimes in children.

● KEY PROBLEM

Abdominal Pain This is often due to hepatosplenomegaly in all age groups. It may be associated with constipation in *lead intoxication.*

● KEY PROBLEM

Headache This is a nonspecific finding in all age groups.

● KEY PROBLEM

Dizziness This can be nonspecific in adolescence but also may be due to a lack of cerebral oxygenation.

● KEY PROBLEM

Shortness of Breath This relates to tachycardia and can be seen in all age groups, especially adolescents.

● KEY PROBLEM

Arthralgias Findings of joint pain occur in rapid hemolysis, mainly in children and adolescents.

Physical Examination

Key findings are for all age groups.

▼ KEY FINDING

Tachycardia This occurs with acute blood loss and volume depletion in all age groups.

▼ KEY FINDING

Postural Hypotension Similar to tachycardia, this occurs in adolescents and children.

▼ KEY FINDING

Jaundice Yellow discoloration of eyes and skin with increased RBC breakdown occurs at all ages.

▼ KEY FINDING

Pallor Low hemoglobin causes pale skin color, mucous membranes, or the subungual region in all age groups.

Synthesizing a Diagnosis

The diagnosis of anemia requires an understanding of normal hematologic values and their interpretation, as well as a basic knowledge of peripheral blood smears. These are important diagnostic tools in anemia, but they are also of paramount importance in other systemic diseases. Knowledge of normal hematologic values is necessary to make a diagnosis of anemia. These values exhibit gender differences as well as geographic and racial differences.

There are three key diagnostic tests necessary in the workup of anemia. They are examination of a peripheral blood smear, complete blood count (CBC), and the reticulocyte count. Armed with these three pieces of information, one can deduce underlying processes. In some laboratories a CBC includes the review of blood smears. TABLE 15–1 gives the conventionally accepted mean values of RBCs at various ages. The RBC values represented in the table are now generated by electronic counters as opposed to the old manual measurements. The RBC number and the mean corpuscular volume (MCV) are direct measurements; the hemoglobin concentration is the product of a chromatographic quantification, and from these values, one calculates the mean corpuscular hemoglobin (MCH) and mean corpuscular hemoglobin concentration (MCHC). The RBCs, WBCs, and platelets (Pl) are direct measurements by the same method (gated-window pool).

Laboratory

The blood smear and indices are essential for hematologic evaluation. We apply them below to the differential diagnosis of anemia.

Examination of the Blood Smear

There are many features of abnormal blood that are not detectable from electronic counters. For instance, the counters will count nucleated RBCs as WBCs. Unless one looks at the blood smear, there may be errors in diagnosis. When ordering a CBC, be sure to interpret the smears. The key features of a peripheral blood smear that may aid in the diagnosis of anemia appear in TABLE 15–2.

Types of Anemia

Anemia with Low MCV and Low Reticulocytes

The most common causes of anemia with low MCV and low reticulocytes in pediatrics are

- *Iron-deficiency anemia*
- *Anemia of chronic disease*
- *Sideroblastic anemias*

Diagnostic evaluation, aside from the three key diagnostic tests, includes iron studies (serum iron, iron-binding capacity, and ferritin), hemoglobin electrophoresis, and bone marrow aspirate.

INFANTS

Except for the hereditary sideroblastic anemias, it is rare to find this in the newborn. However, one may see this anemia, and then it is mostly due to *iron deficiency.*

TABLE 15–1 *Normal RBC Measurements for Different Age Groups and Genders*

Age	Hemoglobin (g/dl)		Hematocrit (%)		Red Cell Count (10^{12}/liter)	
	Mean	<–2SD	Mean	<–2SD	Mean	<–2SD
Birth (cord blood)	16.5	<13.5	51	<42	4.7	<3.9
1–3 days	18.5	<14.5	56	<45	5.3	<4.0
1 week	17.5	<13.5	54	<42	5.4	<3.9
2 weeks	16.5	<12.5	51	<39	4.9	<3.6
1 month	14.0	<10.0	43	<31	4.2	<3.0
2 months	11.5	<9.0	35	<28	3.8	<2.7
3–6 months	11.5	<9.5	35	<29	3.8	<3.1
6 months–2 years	12.0	<11.0	36	<33	4.5	<3.7
2–6 years	12.5	<11.5	37	<34	4.6	<3.9
6–12 years	13.5	<11.5	40	<35	4.6	<4.0
12–21 years						
Females	14.0	<12.0	41	<36	4.6	<4.1
Males	14.5	<13.0	43	<37	4.9	<4.5

TABLE 15–2 *Key Features of the Peripheral Blood Smear*

RBC	Interpretation
Nucleated RBC	Normal in newborns; associated with high reticulocyte count, acute blood loss, massive hemolysis
Normal size/normal color	Normocytic, normochromic: acute inflammation
Small, pale cells	Microcytic hypochromic: iron deficiency, thalassemia, lead poisoning, vitamin B deficiency
Large cells	Macrocytic: normal newborn; folate, B_{12} deficiency
Target cells	HbS, C, E, thalassemia, liver disease, asplenia
Basophilic stippling	Hemolytic anemias, iron deficiency, lead poisoning, thalassemia
Howell-Jolly bodies	Absence or hypofunction of spleen, megaloblastic anemia
Spherocytes	Hereditary spherocytosis, congenital hemolytic anemias (e.g., ABO incompatibility; RBC enzymopathies)
Schistocytes	DIC, thalassemia

Abbreviations: DIC=disseminated intravascular coagulopathy; Hg=hemoglobin.

CHILDREN

Iron-deficiency anemia is quite common in this age group. Any of the intrinsic causes, such as hemoglobinopathies, may become quite evident here.

ADOLESCENTS

Sometimes, but rarely, we do see anemia of chronic disease in this group. However, anemia of iron deficiency remains the most prevalent, particularly in females.

Anemia with High MCV and Low Reticulocytes

This occurs in the following disorders:

- *Megaloblastic anemia— deficiency of vitamin B_{12} and/or folic acid, drug-induced anemia, and myelodysplastic syndrome*
- *Nonmegaloblastic anemia— liver disease, hypothyroidism*

Aside from the three key diagnostic tests, the evaluation of this anemia should include serum levels of vitamin B_{12} and folic acid, thyroid function, liver function tests, and bone marrow aspirate/biopsy. This anemia is seen in all age groups.

Anemia with Normal MCV and Low Reticulocytes

This is seen in the following disorders:

- *Aplastic anemia*
- *Constitutional red cell aplasia (Diamond-Blackfan syndrome)*
- *Acquired red cell aplasia (drugs, e.g., cytotoxic antineoplastic drugs)*

- *Transient red cell aplasia [e.g., transient erythroblastopenia of childhood (TEC)]*
- *Uremia*
- *Human immunodeficiency virus (HIV) and other viruses (e.g., parvo virus)*
- *Anemia of chronic disease*
- *Kidney disease*

Combine the three key diagnostic tests for anemia with iron studies, renal function tests such as creatinine, thyroid function tests, liver function tests, erythropoietin level, and bone marrow aspirate/biopsy.

INFANTS

Primary bone marrow failure may be seen in this age group. HIV and other viral infections also may occur. TEC is a strong consideration whenever this anemia is identified, especially in infants 6 to 12 months of age.

CHILDREN

Usually by this age the primary bone marrow failures would have been diagnosed. Therefore, pay attention to the secondary bone marrow failures.

ADOLESCENTS

Aside from secondary *bone marrow failure, anemia of chronic disease* is more likely to become apparent in this group.

Anemia with Normal MCV and High Reticulocyte Count

The most common causes of anemia with elevated reticulocyte count are

- *Acute blood loss*
- *Organ sequestration (e.g., spleen or liver)*
- *Hemolysis*
  - *Immune* hemolysis (maternal-fetal compatibility, e.g., *ABO, Rh*, and other minor blood groups)
  - Mechanical hemolysis [e.g., *artificial heart valve* and *disseminated intravascular coagulopathy (DIC)*]
  - *Hereditary* hemolytic anemia [hemoglobinopathies, enzymopathies (such as *G6PD deficiency*)]
  - Hereditary membrane defects (such as *elliptocytosis* and *spherocytosis*)
  - Acquired membrane defects (such as *paroxysmal nocturnal hemoglobinemia*)
  - *Infection*-related (such as malaria parasitemia or clostridial infection)

The evaluation of hemolytic anemia involves the three key diagnostic tests and, in addition, direct and indirect Coombs' tests, cold and hot reacting antibody titers, RBC enzyme assays, hemoglobin electrophoresis, and urinalysis for *hemoglobinuria*, osmotic fragility, blood cultures, and examination of thick blood smears *for malaria parasites.*

INFANTS

Acute blood loss is mostly due to trauma. In the newborn period it might ~e a result of accidental fetal placental transfusion or an unrecognized ~eeding disorder that becomes manifest after circumcision. *Organ sequestration* may become a problem after the newborn period in this age group. This is rare but may occur in sickle cell disease. Hemolysis in this age group is mostly due to hereditary defects.

CHILDREN
In this age group, as in infants, acute blood loss is usually from trauma. Sequestration is usually from *hemoglobinopathy*, specifically *sickle cell disease*, and hemolysis from all causes may occur.

ADOLESCENTS
This age group does not differ appreciably from children.

Erythrocytosis (Polycythemia)

This is excess production of RBCs. The red cell mass is usually in a state of equilibrium in which the amount of RBCs lost through senescence (i.e., >120 days) is replaced with new cells from the bone marrow. A glycoprotein hormone, erythropoietin, which is produced in the kidney, regulates this equilibrium.

History and Physical Examination

Erythrocytosis has nonspecific signs and symptoms, including plethora and, in severe cases, central nervous system (CNS) manifestations. Therefore, the first clue of this condition may be a fortuitous finding of a high hemoglobin, high hematocrit, or high RBC count during routine blood work. There are no significant age variations in the manifestation of this disorder.

Synthesizing a Diagnosis

The following causes of high hematocrit should help in carrying out a differential diagnosis:

- Spurious erythrocytosis (e.g., *hemoconcentration* secondary to *dehydration* from all causes)
- Absolute erythrocytosis (*hypoxia, carbon monoxide poisoning, high oxygen affinity, hemoglobinopathy, high altitude, pulmonary disease, sleep apnea syndrome,* and *cyanotic congenital heart disease*)
- Renal disease (*polycystic kidneys, hydronephrosis, renal artery stenosis, glomerulonephritis, renal transplantation,* and *renal tumors*)
- Other *tumors* (*hepatoma, cerebellar hemangioblastoma, uterine fibromyoma, adrenal tumor, meningioma,* and *pheochromocytoma*)
- *Familial* erythrocytosis (e.g., *diphosphoglycerate mutase deficiency*)
- *Polycythemia vera* (a myeloproliferative syndrome with pancytosis)

Laboratory

The three key diagnostic tests used for anemia are also important here. These are review of peripheral blood smear, CBC, and reticulocyte count. In addition, the following investigations are necessary:

- Erythropoietin level
- Arterial blood gases
- Pulmonary function test
- Echocardiogram
- Hemoglobin electrophoresis
- Renal ultrasound

Platelets

History and Physical Examination

We outline below key problems and findings related to thrombocytopenia (low platelets). There are few specific problems and findings for thrombocytosis (increased platelets) except for hypercoagulability and CNS symptoms in extreme cases. However, it is important to consider problems and findings related to etiologies of thrombocytosis.

Key Findings

These symptoms are found in all ages, except in neonates. In the neonatal period, severe congenital thrombocytopenia is associated with increased incidence of intracranial hemorrhage.

- Mucous membrane bleeding
- Epistaxis
- Gastrointestinal bleed
- Spontaneous bleed

Key Problems

- Petechiae
- Purpura

Thrombocytopenia

Synthesizing a Diagnosis

As in the case of RBCs, low platelets could be a result of an increased destruction or consumption or of a production defect. A production defect may be acquired or congenital.

Acquired production defects can be a result of the following key conditions:

- Marrow infiltration (in *leukemia, metastatic cancer,* or *infection*)
- Direct destruction of megakaryocytes (radiation therapy and chemotherapy)
- *Infection:* Viruses (a variety of viral agents can cause mild to severe thrombocytopenia, such as measles, rubella, mumps, varicella, cytomegaloviruses, HIV, Epstein-Barr virus, parvo virus, hepatitis, and herpes)

- Drugs (*cytotoxic* drugs and other classes of drugs are implicated in thrombocytopenia)
- *Metabolic* causes such as folate and B_{12} deficiency
- *Cyclic thrombocytopenia* (associated with menstrual cycles)

Congenital production defects include the following key conditions:

- Aplastic anemia syndrome (e.g., Fanconi syndrome)
- Amegakaryocytic thrombocytopenia
- Thrombocytopenia with absent radius (TAR)
- Autosomal dominant thrombocytopenias (May-Hegglin anomaly, Alport syndrome)
- Autosomal recessive thrombocytopenias (Bernard-Soulier syndrome).
- X-linked thrombocytopenia (Wiskott-Aldrich syndrome)

Increased Platelet Destruction

This kind of thrombocytopenia develops when the rate of destruction is greater than the production ability of the bone marrow. Destruction can either be nonimmune or immune. Key nonimmune conditions in which thrombocytopenia occur include

- *Disseminated intravascular coagulopathy (DIC)*
- *Hemolytic-uremic syndrome (HUS)*

Key immune conditions associated with thrombocytopenia include

- Autoantibodies (*lupus, rheumatoid arthritis*, etc.)
- Alloantibody (*neonatal autoimmune thrombocytopenia, post transfusion, purpura,* and *drug-induced thrombocytopenia*).
- *Immune thrombocytopenia* (ITP)

Laboratory

Epistaxis and gastrointestinal (GI) bleed are usually signs of more serious bleeding problems. Usually these symptoms are not seen with platelet counts greater than $50,000/mm^3$. Other helpful tests include a peripheral smear for megakaryocytes (ITP), RBC morphology (HUS and DIC), autoantibodies, and alloantibodies.

Thrombocytosis

Key Points

- This is defined as a platelet count greater than $500,000/mm^3$.
- In the pediatric group, the majority of thrombocytosis is an acute-phase reaction to infection.
- The incidence is particularly high in patients with *Hemophilus influenzae* infection, where nearly half the patients have had thrombocytosis at some point in the course of the disease.
- Counts greater than 1 million/mm^3 have been recorded in some cases.
- Inflammatory cytokines, such as interleukin 1 (IL-1), may play a role in the etiology of thrombocytosis in children.

Synthesizing a Diagnosis

INFANTS
All neonates with a platelet count of greater than 500,000/mm^3 should have a presumptive diagnosis of infection. All older infants with a platelet count of greater than 600,000/mm^3 also should have a presumptive diagnosis of infection.

CHILDREN
All children with platelet counts of greater than 700,000/mm^3 should have a presumptive diagnosis of infection. Consideration also must be given to other causes of inflammation (e.g., iron deficiency and asplenia, as in sickle cell disease).

ADOLESCENTS
In this age group, the differential diagnosis becomes more extensive and includes

- Primary thrombocythemia, which is a *myeloproliferative* disorder
- Noninfectious inflammatory processes, such as *inflammatory bowel disease (Crohn disease)*
- Nonhematologic malignancies
- *Sickle cell disease* with functional asplenia
- *Splenectomized* patients
- *Iron-deficiency anemia*

Sickle Cell Disease
The sickle cell hemoglobinopathies are defects due to a single gene mutation. Sickle cell anemia is a hemoglobinopathy resulting from one amino acid substitution in which glutamic acid (an acidic amino acid) is replaced by valine (a neutral amino acid) at the sixth position of the Beta-globin chain. The sickle cell defect (HgS) is the most significant of the several known globin chain defects. The prevalence of sickle cell disease is 1 in every 375 African Americans, 1 in 1000 Spanish Americans, and 1 in 70 West Africans. It is one of the most common genetic disorders and is inherited in a basic Mendelian manner. Table 15-3 reviews major clinical features of sickle cell disease. See Essential Adolescent Medicine (Editors: DE Greydanus, DR Patel, HD Pratt), NY: McGraw-Hill; 2006:383–390.

White Blood Cells

Leukopenia

- *Leukopenia* refers to low WBC counts that are more than two standard deviations lower than the mean. WBC count is so sensitive to external influences that absolute normal values are difficult to establish.
- However, the clinically most important component of the WBC, neutrophils, plays the greatest role in determining leukopenia.

TABLE 15-3 Major Clinical Features of Sickle Cell Disease at Various Ages

	Features		
	Infancy	Childhood	Adolescent
A. Impairment of circulation	Pain, hand and foot syndrome	Pain, stroke, arthralgia, hematuria, hyposthenuria	Chronic pain, stroke, autosplenectomy, renal insufficiency, avascular necrosis
B. Red Blood Cell Destruction (hemolysis)	Pallor, jaundice, lethargy	Pallor, jaundice, lethargy, splenomegaly, cardiomegaly, shortness of breath	Exercise intolerance, pallor, jaundice, gallstones, chronic lung disease, chronic transfusion and iron overload
C. Stagnation of blood in organs	Sequestration	Sequestration	Priapism, hepatomegaly, chronic leg ulcers
Combination of A, B and C	Fever, pneumonia, osteomyelitis, susceptibility to infections (*pneumococcus* and *Haemophilus influenzae*)	Fever, pneumonia, osteomyelitis, susceptibility to infections (*pneumococcus* and *Haemophilus influenzae*)	Fever, osteomyelitis (*salmonella spp.*), acute chest syndrome, pulmonary hypertension, retinopathy, delayed sexual maturation, pregnancy complications, depression, pain intolerance, narcotic dependence, increased school absenteeism

Source: Used with permission: Kulkarni R, Gera R, Scott-Emuakpor AB: Adolescent hematology. In: Greydanus DE, Patel DR, Pratt HD, eds. *Essential Adolescent Medicine.* New York: McGraw-Hill, p. 388, 2006.

TABLE 15–4 *Normal White Blood Cell Counts by Age*

| Age | Neutrophil Count/mm^3 | |
	Mean	Range
At birth	11,000	6000–26,000
At 1 week	5500	1500–10,000
>1 week	4400	1500–7700

- Even neutrophil counts vary widely and have a wide range of normal, as shown in TABLE 15–4.

Neutropenia

This is defined as an absolute neutrophil count (ANC) of less than 1500/mm^3. Although newborn infants have higher neutrophil counts during the first few days of life and African-Americans have lower neutrophil counts, the following definition of neutropenia applies to all ages and ethnic groups.

Calculate ANC by multiplying the total WBC count by the percentage of bands and neutrophils. Any granulocytic cells less mature than bands do not figure in the estimation. TABLE 15–5 demonstrates ANCs with their relative infection risk.

History and Physical Examination

There are no specific problems or findings for neutropenia per se. Consider those associated with the etiologies discussed below.

Synthesizing a Diagnosis

The clinical presentation of neutropenia is the same regardless of age. Infection is the most common clinical feature of neutropenia. There are intrinsic causes and acquired causes.

Intrinsic Causes

- *Severe infantile agranulocytosis.* Probably inherited as an autosomal dominant condition, although autosomal recessive forms have been reported. Presents in early infancy with severe recurrent infections.

TABLE 15–5 *Absolute Neutrophil Count and Relative Infection Risk*

Neutrophil Count/mm^3	Clinical Significance
1500	Normal
1000 to <1500	No significant infection risk
500 to <1000	Some increased infection risk
<500	Significant infection risk

- *Cyclic neutropenia.* Appears to be inherited as an autosomal dominant condition. Characterized by neutropenia that occurs every 2 to 6 weeks. Presents in early infancy with recurrent fevers, pharyngitis, stomatitis, and various bacterial infections.
- *Combined neutropenia, metaphyseal dysplasia, and pancreatic insufficiency.* This is known as *Schwachman-Diamond-Oski syndrome.* Presumed to be inherited as an autosomal recessive condition. Children with this condition present with steatorrhea and infection.
- *Chédiak-Higashi syndrome.* Rare inherited disorder characterized by oculocutaneous albinism, progressive neurologic impairments, and severe neutropenia.

Acquired Causes

- *Postinfectious neutropenia.* This is usually after a viral infection or infection with certain bacteria.
- *Chronic benign neutropenia of infancy and childhood.* Chronic state of depleted mature neutrophils in the peripheral blood associated with a compensatory bone marrow myeloid hyperplasia. In over 90 percent of the patients, antineutrophil antibodies have been detected.
- *Drug-induced neutropenia.* Aside from cytotoxic drugs, phenothiazines, nonsteroidal anti-inflammatory drugs (NSAIDs), and synthetic penicillin have been implicated.
- *Chronic idiopathic neutropenia.* It is in this group that the bone marrow shows arrest of myeloid maturation.
- *Autoimmune neutropenia.* Usually associated with other known autoimmune diseases such as lupus and juvenile rheumatoid arthritis (JRA).
- *Isoimmune neutropenia.* This is seen mostly in newborn infants secondary to IgG antibodies transferred from a sensitized mother to the infant.
- *Pure white cell aplasia (PWCA).* Rare syndrome characterized by severe pyogenic infections and neutropenia, with a large majority of the patients having thymoma.
- *Neutropenia due to increased marginations.* Activation of certain complements (e.g., C_5) can result in increased adherence and entrapment of neutrophils in the endothelium, particularly that of the pulmonary vasculature.
- *Hypersplenism.* This is usually associated with pancytopenia but may lead to severe neutropenia.

Lymphocytopenia

- This is defined as an absolute lymphocyte count that is less than $1000/mm^3$.
- This is common in acute infections, particularly when the ANC is high.
- *Tuberculosis* and *certain fungal infections* frequently cause lymphocytopenia in children of all ages.
- *HIV infection* often is associated with absolute lymphocytopenia because of depletion of the population of a subset of T lymphocytes.

Leukocytosis

- There are several causes of leukocytosis in the pediatric age group, the most commonly encountered being *leukemoid reaction.*
- *Leukemoid reaction* is a WBC count exceeding 50,000/mm^3 and is an increase in circulatory myelocytes and metamyelocytes (early neutrophil precursors).
- Leukocyte alkaline phosphatase (LAP) score is always very high.

Neutrophilia

History and Physical Examination

There are no specific problems or findings owing to neutrophilia per se. Evaluate all problems and findings associated with varying etiologies.

Synthesizing a Diagnosis

Most leukocytosis is as a result of neutrophilia. Cases of neutrophilia also can be intrinsic or acquired.

Intrinsic Causes

- *Hereditary neutrophilia.* Very rare condition described in only four families with ANCs ranging between 20,000 and 70,000/mm^3 with no other symptoms or signs.
- *Chronic idiopathic neutrophilia.* Chronic leukocytosis in otherwise healthy patients.
- *Familial myeloproliferative disease.* Syndrome of leukocytosis, anemia, hepatosplenomegaly, and varying degrees of growth retardation.
- *Down syndrome.* All infants with Down syndrome will have at birth transient leukocytosis that may be mistaken for *congenital leukemia.*

Acquired Causes

- *Infections.* Moderate leukocytosis with a left shift usually occurs with acute infections.
- *Chronic inflammation.* This is possibly due to emptying of the marginal storage pool of neutrophils.
- *Stress neutrophilia.* Possibly due to epinephrine release during acute stress that mobilizes marginal pool of neutrophils.
- *Drug-induced neutrophilia.* Steroids will stimulate the release of neutrophils from bone marrow. Other classes of *drugs,* such as *beta-agonists* and *lithium,* have similar effects.
- *Asplenia.* Moderate leukocytosis is a consequence of removal of the spleen or of functional asplenia.

Lymphocytosis

- Absolute lymphocyte count greater than 1000/mm^3 is usually seen in a variety of infections, both acute and chronic.
- The following acute infections can cause lymphocytosis in children of all ages:

- *Pertussis*
- *Infectious mononucleosis*
- *Infectious hepatitis*
- *Toxoplamosis*
- *Cytomegalovirus*

- The following chronic infections can be associated with lymphocytosis in children of all ages:
  - *Tuberculosis*
  - *Brucellosis*
  - *Syphilis*
  - *Rickettsia*

II. HEMOSTATIC SYSTEM

Taking a History

An assessment of history and an evaluation of physical findings are crucial in any infant, child, or adolescent who presents with a suspected hemostatic disorder. A thorough history may be the first step toward a genetic diagnosis.

Presenting Complaint

Bleeding Disorders

In taking a comprehensive history, the key questions should include how the bleeding/bruising occurred and whether it is consistent with the explanation given. Below are listed additional questions that may be helpful in arriving at a differential diagnosis.

- What was the age of presentation? Severe *hemophilia* may present at birth either as postcircumcision bleeding or as CNS bleeding if the delivery was difficult, necessitating vacuum or forceps. Bleeding from other iatrogenic causes such as venipuncture, heel sticks, and surgical procedures also may occur. Hemarthrosis and hematomas occur typically in the older child and adolescent. Mild bleeding disorders may present with symptoms following trauma or surgery.
- Was the bleeding spontaneous or induced by trauma? Bruising in the legs and arms is common in toddlers, children, and adolescent as a result of mobility and unintentional trauma. Spontaneous bruises at sites such as the abdomen, back, chest, and axillae should raise suspicion of a bleeding disorder or intentional trauma (*child abuse*). Key questions should focus on bleeding or bruising with minimal trauma, postdental extraction bleeding, and postcircumcision bleeding.
- Is the bleeding local or diffuse? Generalized bleeding is more indicative of low platelets or, in a sick child, DIC. A generalized red rash may indicate platelet quantitative or qualitative abnormalities or *hereditary hemorrhagic telangiectasia* (HHT). A symmetric rash on the

TABLE 15-6 *Glossary of Terms*

Petechiae: pinpoint hemorrhages <2 mm in diameter
Purpura: 2 to 10 mm in diameter
Ecchymosis: >10 mm in diameter
Telangiectasias: pinpoint erythematous dots that blanch when
   compressed
Bleeding sites
   Hemarthroses: joint
   Hemoptysis: coughing blood from respiratory tract
   Hematochezia: fresh blood in stools
   Hematemesis: vomiting blood
   Melena: dark or black, tarry stools; blood from upper GI
   Menorrhagia: excess menstrual blood loss

gluteal area and extremities is more suggestive of *Henoch-Schönlein vasculitis.* Localized bleeding in a muscle or joint or following trauma is more suspicious of a coagulation disorder.

- What are the site(s), severity, and duration of bleeding (TABLE 15–6)? Prolonged bleeding, especially from mucosal hemorrhages such as epistaxis, *dental bleeding, bruises,* and *menorrhagia,* is more suggestive of *platelet disorders* or *von Willebrand disease.* Muscle, joint, and post-traumatic bleeding indicates hemophilia. In some cases, patients may complain of recurrent bleeding or passing clots. In females, a detailed menstrual history is important.
- Is the child well, ill, or critically ill? Is there a history of recent viral infections or viral immunizations? Bleeding in an otherwise well child is often due to a hereditary coagulation disorder such as *hemophilia A* or *B. Immune thrombocytopenia* (ITP) can present acutely in childhood. *Alloimmune thrombocytopenia* (NAIT) usually manifests in the newborn period. Bleeding in sick children is usually due to acquired causes.
- Did the child receive any transfusion? Any bleeding episode serious enough to warrant transfusions of blood or components should raise suspicion of bleeding disorders.
- Was there any skin rash, lymph node enlargement, or swelling of the abdomen? Rashes can result from allergies or medications or low platelet counts.
- The history should include current *medication(s)* such as aspirin, Coumadin, or anticonvulsants that may present with bleeding.

Clotting Disorders

- Note history of pain, swelling, or discoloration of extremities. Older children may present with muscle cramping. Other symptoms include redness of the extremities and shortness of breath. The site of the clot is also important. Strokes, although uncommon, can occur in children *and are usually arterial in origin. Venous thrombosis includes deep vein thrombosis* (DVT), *pulmonary embolism* (PE), and *cerebral sinovenous thrombosis* (SVT).
- Has the patient had any central venous access devices (CVADs) or arterial or venous lines that were clotted or difficult to draw?

- *SVT* may occur in states of dehydration; hence it is important to ask about frequency of urination and fluid intake.
- *Stroke* at young age or blood clots at unusual locations such as abdominal (renal, mesenteric, or portal) or cerebral vessels should prompt an investigation for thrombophilia.

Past History

In the past history, one should ask the following:

Bleeding Disorders

- History of excess bleeding with significant hemostatic challenges such as trauma or surgery (such as dental extractions, tonsillectomy, circumcision, etc.). One should inquire whether the child received a blood or plasma transfusion for the excess bleeding. The likelihood of a *congenital* bleeding disorder is remote if a patient has undergone a major surgery without any excess bleeding.
- Bleeding while brushing teeth may be due to thrombocytopenia or platelet dysfunction. In girls, excess menstrual blood loss may indicate a bleeding diathesis.
- Does the patient have an underlying medical disorder that may contribute to the bleeding? The liver synthesizes a majority of the clotting factors. Factors II, VII, IX, and X are vitamin K-dependent factors; hence liver dysfunction or malabsorption plays an important role in bleeding disorders. Platelet functions may be a consequence of uremia in renal disease. Patients with congenital heart disease and polycythemia (high hematocrit) may present with thrombocytopenia and low fibrinogen secondary to liver hypoxia and hemostasis. Patients with *malignant* disorders such as leukemia or bone marrow failure syndromes such as aplastic anemia may present with low platelets owing to replacement of marrow megakaryocytes by abnormal cells or failure of production of platelets. Patients with collagen disease such as *Ehlers-Danlos syndrome* also can present with bruises, joint disease, and menorrhagia.
- Knowledge of blood groups is also important because individuals with blood group O may have low levels of von Willebrand factor. There may be racial differences in the causes of menorrhagia.

Clotting Disorders

Since clots are a complication of central or peripheral lines, a history of recent placement of lines is significant. Does the patient have an underlying medical disorder such as leukemia with a high WBC count? Thrombosis may be associated with infections. A history of recurrent blood clots may indicate *thrombophilia* (an inherited tendency to clot).

Birth History

Bleeding Disorders

The birth history should include the type of delivery, trauma from use of vacuum or forceps during delivery, enlarged head (cephalohematoma), jaundice, bleeding, and history of transfusions. Excess bleeding with trauma such as circumcision, heel sticks, and intramuscular injections (for vaccinations and vitamin K administration) may indicate a bleeding disorder. Vacuum delivery and forceps are often associated with cephalohematoma and in some instances intracranial hemorrhage that enlarges when an underlying bleeding disorder is also present. Failure of administration of vitamin K at birth sometimes may lead to *vitamin K-deficiency bleeding* (VKBD) that is associated with low levels of vitamin K-dependent factors.

Clotting Disorders

A history of seizures and paralysis at birth, discoloration of the extremities, lack of urine, and blood in the urine may indicate a thrombotic disorder.

Family History

Bleeding Disorders

A family history of bleeding is often present in X-linked diseases such as *hemophilia A and B* (although approximately 30 percent of the cases are due to spontaneous mutation and lack family history). An autosomal pattern is more suggestive of *von Willebrand disease*, other factor deficiencies, or *hereditary hemorrhagic telangiectasia* (HHT); factor XI deficiency occurs mostly in Ashkenazi Jews.

Clotting Disorders

Thrombotic disorders are rare in childhood. In the case of a *deep vein thrombosis* (DVT), *pulmonary embolism* (PE), or *stroke*, a detailed family history of thrombosis at a young age (<50 years of age) and a history of recurrent thromboses should prompt an investigation for thrombophilia.

Social History

It is important to consider nonaccidental injury (NAI, child abuse) as a cause of bruising, most often revealed through a detailed social history.

Developmental History

It is very important to determine that the child has reached developmental milestones at the appropriate age. Intracranial hemorrhage or stroke may have profound effect on child development.

Infants

Manifestations of hemostatic disorders in newborns and infants are distinctly different from those in older children and adolescents. Delivery has an impact on bleeding manifestations in newborns. Vacuum and forceps delivery and traumatic delivery often result in cranial bleeding (cephalhematomas and intracranial hemorrhages). Bleeding episodes in newborns are often iatrogenic (heel sticks and circumcision bleeds). As toddlers become more mobile, trauma often leads to bruising. Newborns also can present with *stroke* and *renal vein thrombosis* or *sinovenous thrombosis*.

● KEY PROBLEM
◾ **Excess Bruising or Ecchymoses** Bruising manifests as discoloration of skin. Note should be made of the distribution and size of the bruises. TABLE 15–6 gives a glossary of terms that pertain to bruising and bleeding. One cannot make an accurate assessment of the bruise by color alone because it is often misleading, especially in children with dark skin. Excessive bruising or hematomas may occur following venipunctures, injections, with trivial trauma, or even spontaneously. Bruising around the head may be suggestive of a fall or *traumatic* delivery. Generalized bruising may be suggestive of platelet disorders (quantitative and qualitative), whereas localized bruising may be suggestive of an underlying muscle hematoma. Symmetric bruising accompanied by papular rash may be suggestive of *Henoch-Schönlein purpura*. The social history is important in considering *nonaccidental injury* (NAI) as a reason for bruising.

● KEY PROBLEM
◾ **Excessive Bleeding** In cases of hemophilia and other *inherited* coagulation deficiencies, the severity determines the site and type of bleeding. For example, severe hemophiliacs (factor VIII or factor IX <1 percent) may have spontaneous bleeding and may manifest at birth. Moderate (1 to 5 percent) and mild (>5 percent) hemophiliacs may manifest at an older age and following trauma.

In newborns, *cranial or intracerebral bleeding* may occur because of *trauma* of delivery. Other sites of bleeding in newborns include circumcision bleed or bleeding following venipuncture or intramuscular injections. Symptoms include apnea, abnormal movements, vomiting, etc. Jaundice may occur owing to breakdown of RBCs in the event of closed bleeding. Newborns with platelet disorders can develop petechiae at sites of injury.

In toddlers, bleeding may be spontaneous or occur especially after minor *trauma*. Oral bleeding (tongue bleed or dental bleed) owing to trauma or after shedding of deciduous teeth may be common. Bleeding into a joint may result in refusal of movement (toddlers may refuse to walk) owing to pain or limping. Swelling may or may not accompany joint or muscle bleeding (particularly if the latter is deep). The most common sites of joint bleeding are the knees and ankles. Sudden occurrence of generalized petechiae is suggestive of ITP.

Blood in the urine may be indicative of a bleeding disorder or may occur with *renal vein thrombosis* in a newborn as a result of *purpura fulminans* owing to homozygous *protein C deficiency*. DIC also may present with excessive bleeding from skin and mucous membranes and blood in the urine or stools.

KEY PROBLEM

Swelling Swelling may occur as a result of bleeding or as a result of edema owing to thrombosis. Swelling of the muscle may occur because of bleeding. Swelling of the scalp may indicate *cephalhematoma*. Swollen joints are frequent in hemophilia and other bleeding disorders, as well as *HSP* or *leukemia* and other cancers such as *neuroblastoma*.

KEY PROBLEM

Pain Unexplained crying may indicate pain as a result of bleeding or clotting. It is often associated with restriction of movement. *Arterial thrombosis* can present with painful, cold, white extremities.

KEY PROBLEM

Rash or Discoloration A red, swollen joint may be an indication of fresh bleeding. A generalized purpuric rash indicates platelet disorders (congenital and acquired). A dark, almost purplish black discoloration of the extremities may indicate gangrene as a result of thrombosis.

Children

The key symptoms of bleeding disorders in children are the same as those in infants and consist of bruising and bleeding. Cranial or CNS bleeding is rare and often due to trauma or recurrent bleeding. Bleeding in the joints is the hallmark of *hemophilia* and presents with decreased joint mobility and swelling. The symptoms of thrombosis include pain, swelling, and redness. *ITP* is fairly common in children and can present with petechiae or purpura.

An older child may be able to express pain and localize it better. A tingling sensation may precede a joint bleed.

Adolescents

Adolescents with bleeding disorders may present with painless joint swelling. This occurs because of joint destruction secondary to repetitive bleeding resulting in synovial proliferation and leading to chronic arthropathy. Patients with iliopsoas bleeding can present with pain in the abdomen and limping. In addition to bruising, mucous membrane bleeding such as epistaxis and oral bleeding may occur. Girls with bleeding disorders may present with symptoms of excess menstrual blood loss. Nonspecific symptoms of blood loss such as jaundice and anemia may occur. In adolescent girls, menorrhagia may be the first symptom of a bleeding disorder such as *VWD* or *platelet function defect*.

Adolescents with thrombosis can present with pain and leg swelling. Symptoms of pulmonary embolism include chest pain, anxiety, dyspnea, hemoptysis, and cyanosis.

Physical Examination

We summarize pertinent physical findings in TABLE 15–7.

Synthesizing a Diagnosis

TABLE 15–8 presents bleeding and clotting disorders correlated with key history and physical findings with pertinent clinical comments. We specifically do not include all possible diagnoses but rather create a framework on which the primary care physician can build on his or her thought processes.

Confirmatory Laboratory Tests

FIGURE 15–1 is an algorithm for a coagulation disorder evaluation. A combination of clinical history and clinical examination coupled with screening laboratory tests will diagnose coagulation disorders. One should, however, be aware that screening laboratory tests in mild bleeding disorders may be normal and that test results should take into account the age-related norms. All newborns have normal platelet counts (150,000 to 200,000/mm^3). Clotting factor assays are age-dependent and, with the exception of factor VIII, are low in the newborn period and reach adult values by approximately 6 months of age.

Initial screening laboratory tests should include the following:

- *CBC, including examination of the smear.* Patients with a platelet count above 50,000/mm^3 rarely have significant bleeding.
- *Platelet function analysis (PFA).* This test has essentially replaced the bleeding time and may detect VWD and platelet function abnormalities. Order this only when the platelet count is normal or greater than 100,000/mm^3. Norms vary with age.
- *Screening tests for coagulation disorders.* If possible, one must always freeze a sample of citrated plasma for the future and more specific tests such as coagulation factor assays, including VWD workup. Please note that newborns may have prolonged PT and aPTT that are normal. The commonly used tests are
  - *Prothrombin time* (PT), range 10 to 14 seconds; prolonged in deficiencies of factors VII, X, V, and II, fibrinogen, and liver disease.
  - *Activated partial thromboplastin time* (aPTT), range 30–40 seconds; prolonged in deficiencies of factors XII, XI, IX, VIII, X,V, II, and I (fibrinogen) and liver disease (factor VIII is usually normal).
  - *Fibrinogen.* A low fibrinogen is indicative of congenital deficiency or liver disease.

TABLE 15–7 *Summary of Pertinent Physical Findings in the Evaluation for Hemostatic Disorders*

Age	Inspection	Palpation	Percussion	Auscultation
Infants	Bruises, petechiae, purpura, crusted blood in nares, megalocephaly, edema of extremities, loss of consciousness, pallor, jaundice, lethargy	Newborns; oozing site of circumcision, swollen and tender joints, tenderness and swelling of muscles, liver and spleen enlargement, decreased range of motion of extremities, papular symmetric rash on the gluteal area and extremities indicative of HSP	Dullness in the right and left upper quadrants	Hear murmur owing to anemia
Children	Bruises, petechiae, purpura, megalocephaly, edema of extremities, loss of consciousness	Swollen and tender joints, tenderness and swelling of muscles, liver and spleen enlargement, decreased range of motion of extremities, papular symmetric rash on the gluteal area and extremities indicative of HSP		Hear murmur owing to anemia
Adolescents	Bruises, petechiae, purpura, megalocephaly, edema of extremities, loss of consciousness	Bruises, petechiae, purpura, megalocephaly, edema of extremities, loss of consciousness		Hear murmur owing to anemia

TABLE 15-8 Synthesizing a Diagnosis of Hemostatic Disorders

	Key History	Key Finding	Age	Comments
I. Coagulation disorder				
a. Congenital				
1. Hemophilias and other congenital coagulation factor deficiencies	Swelling, pain in the joints or muscle; inability to walk or limp; excess bleeding may be reported following surgery trauma; bleeding in urine/stools; newborns may present with circumcision bleeds or head bleeds following delivery.	Spontaneous hemarthroses and hematomas are the most common presenting features in severe hemophilia; newborns may present with circumcision bleed or signs of intracranial hemorrhage (ICH) such as apnea, abnormal movements, seizures, and vomiting; ICH due to trauma may occur in the older child and adolescent; laboratory diagnosis obtained by determining aPTT, PT, platelet function analysis (PFA that has replaced bleeding time), and fibrinogen level;	I > C > A	Hemophilia A and B are the most common X-linked inherited bleeding disorders; the presentation is identical, and the diagnosis is confirmed by specific factor assay; hemophilias are classified as mild, moderate, or severe based on plasma levels of factor VIII or IX; the other factor deficiencies are autosomal recessive.

		newborns have low levels of all clotting factors except factor VIII; levels reach adult values by 6 months of age; patients may present with anemia if blood loss is severe or chronic.		
2. von Willebrand disease (VWD)	Easy bruising, mucocutaneous bleeding such as nose bleeds, bleeding following dental extraction, rarely bleeding in joints, GI, menorrhagia	Bruises, menorrhagia, anemia Lab: Low or abnormal von Willebrand factor (VWF), VWF antigen, and ristocetin cofactor assay, prolonged bleeding time or platelet function assay	I > C > A (menor-rhagia)	Patients with blood group O have low levels of VWF
b. Acquired coagulation disorders	Liver diseases, malabsorption syndromes, vitamin K deficiency bleeding, drug induced (anticoagulants such as heparin, Coumadin, etc.)	Coagulation defect corrects with correction of underlying disorder.	I > C > A	

(Continued)

TABLE 15-8 Synthesizing a Diagnosis of Hemostatic Disorders (Continued)

	Key History	Key Finding	Age	Comments
II. Platelet disorders		Purpura or petechiae, prolonged oozing from wounds; anemia reflects blood loss.	I > C > A	
Congenital a. Qualitative disorders: Glanzmann thrombasthenia, Bernard-Soulier syndrome b. Quantitative disorders	Epistaxis, GI bleeding, postoperative or posttraumatic bleeding, menorrhagia, rarely intracranial hemorrhage or hemarthrosis	In qualitative disorders the platelet count is normal, whereas it is low in quantitative disorders; some congenital platelet disorders may be associated with bone abnormalities such as absent radii; abnormal platelet aggregation studies in patients with normal platelet counts.	I > C > A	In qualitative disorders the platelet count may be normal; examination of the blood smear may show abnormalities such as giant platelets or platelets without granules; tests of platelet function such as platelet function analysis and aggregation are indicated only when the platelet counts are normal.
Acquired disorders: Quantitative: Immune Thrombocytopenic purpura (ITP), hypersplenism, massive transfusion, myeloproliferative, myelodysplastic, and infiltrative disorders	ITP can be acute or chronic; acute ITP presents with sudden onset of purpura following a viral infection or bleeding from mucosa, kidney, oral, etc.; neonatal alloimmune thrombocytopenia (NAIT)	Petechiae, purpura, low platelet count; mucosal bleeding is common; CBC otherwise normal; in NAIT, maternal antibodies directed against antigens on baby's platelets.	I > C > A	Myeloproliferative disorders include leukemias and lymphomas; infiltrative disorders include metastatic tumors and metabolic storage diseases; myelodysplasias are commonly the aplastic anemias.

Qualitative: Drug induced (aspirin), uremia	(NAIT) is seen in healthy newborns.		
III. Vascular disorders	Rash or spots on the body	I > C > A	Henoch-Schönlein purpura classically presents with a raised purpuric rash on the buttocks and extremities; HHT can present with GI, pulmonary, or cerebral arteriovenous malformation.
	Purpuric rash, arteriovenous malformations, rash that blanches on pressure (HHT), abdominal pain, GI/CNS or renal bleeding		
III. Thrombotic disorders Arterial thrombosis, venous thrombosis, sinovenous thrombosis	Pain, swelling, discoloration, loss of consciousness, altered sensorium, seizures, shortness of breath	I > C > A	Thrombophilias include factor V Leiden, prothrombin gene mutation, elevated levels of fibrinogen, factor VIII, PA-I-1, deficiency of proteins C and S; arterial thrombi are generally platelet and fibrin clots, whereas venous clots are due to slowing of blood flow and hypercoagulability; a history of recurrent thrombi may be suggestive of inherited thrombophilia; anatomic abnormalities of arteries and veins should be ruled out by imaging studies.
	Edema, tenderness of the infarcted area, cramping; organ dysfunction such as stroke, myocardial infarction, pulmonary embolism etc. may occur; discoloration and ulceration also may occur; imaging studies such as MRI and CT scan are helpful in determining location of the clot; prolonged immobilization as may occur with trauma and surgery; antiphospholipid antibodies (APLAs) are an acquired cause of thrombosis.		

(Continued)

517

TABLE 15-8 *Synthesizing a Diagnosis of Hemostatic Disorders (Continued)*

	Key History	Key Finding	Age	Comments
Thrombohemorrhagic disorders: DIC, hemolytic-uremic syndrome, thrombotic thrombocytopenic purpura	Bleeding, rash, pain discoloration, organ dysfunction (renal failure, seizures, etc.)	Hemolytic anemia, low platelets, low clotting factors, prolonged PT, aPTT, low fibrinogen and platelets, signs of underlying causes such as infection, trauma, etc.; key findings include generalized bleeding, signs of kidney failure, anemia.	I > C > A	These patients are generally very sick and show evidence of generalized bleeding.

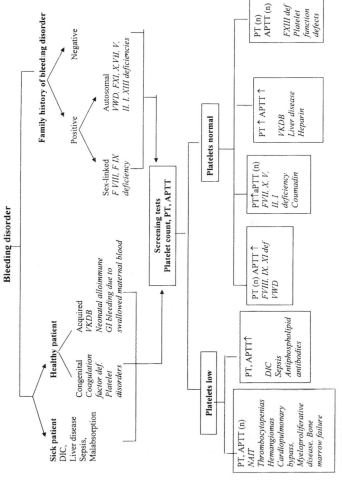

FIGURE 15-1 *Algorithm for Evaluation for Clotting Disorders.*

Bleeding disorder

Sick patient
DIC,
Liver disease
Sepsis,
Malabsorption

Healthy patient

Acquired
VKDB
Neonatal alloimmune
GI bleeding due to
swallowed maternal blood

Congenital
Coagulation
factor def:
Platelet
disorders

Family history of bleeding disorder

Positive

Negative

Sex-linked
F VIII, F IX
deficiency

Autosomal
VWD, FXI, X,VII, V,
II, I, XIII deficiencies

Screening tests
Platelet count, PT, APTT

Platelets low

PT, APTT (n)
*NAIT
Thrombocytopenias
Hemangiomas
Cardiopulmonary
bypass,
Myeloproliferative
disease. Bone
marrow failure*

PT, APTT↑
*DIC
Sepsis
Antiphospholipid
antibodies*

Platelets normal

PT (n) APTT↑
*FVIII, IX, XI def
VWD*

PT↑aPTT (n)
*FVII, X, V,
II, I
deficiency
Coumadin*

PT↑ APTT↑
*VKDB
Liver disease
Heparin*

PT (n)
APTT (n)
*FXIII def
Platelet
function
defects*

519

- For thrombotic disorders one should include D-dimers and antiphospholipid antibody assays. D-Dimers are a breakdown product of fibrin and may be elevated in individuals with thrombosis.

Confirmatory Imaging Studies

Imaging studies in coagulation disorders depend on the site of the bleeding or clotting. Radiologic evaluation [plain x-ray or magnetic resonance imaging (MRI)] of the joint is often helpful to determine the extent of joint damage in hemophilia. For example, suspicion of CNS bleeding or infarct should prompt MRI or an MR angiogram.

For evaluation of *deep vein thrombosis,* a Doppler flow study (duplex ultrasonography) is important. Failure to compress the lumen and absence of normal signals are indicative of a thrombus. MRI or CT scan is necessary to determine thrombosis of the vessels in the brain or abdomen. For patients with suspected pulmonary embolism, a spiral CT scan is helpful. A transthoracic echocardiogram with a bubble study (injection of saline into the vein with subsequent ultrasound image) determines if there are any cardiac septal defects because venous clots may traverse through such defects into the arterial system.

Angiography with the injection of a radiopaque dye will help to determine patency of arteries or veins (coronary or cerebral, renal, etc.).

When to Refer

1. Obtain a hematology consultation on all patients suspected of bleeding or clotting disorders. A personal call to the hematologist is helpful because ordering specific tests in advance can hasten a diagnosis.
2. Make referrals *prior* to administering blood or blood products because clotting factors in the blood products will interfere with the laboratory tests, thereby delaying diagnosis and institution of appropriate treatment.
3. Any prolonged bleeding episode that does not respond to usual treatment such as compression, packing, etc. should be an indication for help in evaluation.
4. Nontraumatic intracranial hemorrhages and unusual bleeding episodes such as urinary hemorrhage or gastrointestinal bleeding warrant a hematology consultation.
5. Obtain consultation if the screening teats are normal but the patient's history or physical examination warrants further specialized coagulation studies.
6. Any suspected thrombotic disorder in a young person necessitates a hematology consultation.
7. For special coagulation tests for bleeding and clotting disorders (such as tests for thrombophilia, platelet aggregation, factor assays, and VWD workup), refer the patient to a hematologists for proper testing and interpretation.

ONCOLOGY

The goals of this section are

1. To outline the molecular and genetic basis of childhood cancer
2. To describe the signs and symptoms associated with childhood cancer
3. To use the information from the preceding to develop a list of diagnostic possibilities and priorities
4. To develop a plan for appropriate laboratory and imaging studies that may aid in the diagnosis
5. To discuss appropriate and timely referrals for subspecialty consultation

Cancer is the leading cause of mortality in children younger than 15 years of age. The cancer may develop from any organ system. Leukemia, the cancer of the hematopoietic system (anatomy described earlier in this chapter) is the most common cancer seen in children. No routine screening tests are available. A high index of suspicion is the best screening tool that helps with timely diagnosis and treatment.

History

A thorough general history may reveal key underlying risks:

- Children with Down syndrome, Fanconi anemia, ataxia-telangiectasia, and Bloom syndrome.
- HIV infection in addition to lymphma predisposes children to Kaposi sarcoma and leiomyosarcoma.
- Children with hepatitis B and C are at risk for hepatocellular carcinoma.
- Survivors of childhood cancer are at increased risk for leukemia, thyroid tumor, and brain tumor.
- Organ transplant recipients who receive prolonged immunosuppressive therapy are also at high risk for malignancy.

Key Problems

An assessment of history and an evaluation of physical findings are crucial in any infant, child, or adolescent who presents with a suspected cancer; a thorough history may be the first step toward a diagnosis. It is usual for a patient to have many visits to a physician's office before arriving at a diagnosis of cancer. If the signs and symptoms persist or progress despite the treatment, suspect a malignancy. Cancer that may mimic common childhood illnesses and the key elements of their history appear in TABLE 15–9.

The cancer may arise from any organ system and could mimic various illnesses. It is helpful to remember common symptoms of

TABLE 15-9 Problems and Findings Associated with Childhood Cancer

Symptoms/Signs	Possible Malignancy	History
Adenopathy, persistent or progressive	Lymphoma, leukemia, metastatic cancer	Adenopathy develops suddenly without any signs of infection
Abdominal mass	Lymphoma, Wilms tumor, neuroblastoma, hepatoblastoma, germ cell tumor	Abdominal pain with nausea, vomiting, decreased appetite, weight loss
Bruises (persistent)	Leukemia, lymphoma, neuroblastoma	Easy bruising, bleeding owing to thrombocytopenia or a bruise owing to skin infiltration that develops without trauma and persists
Bony mass	Osteosarcoma, Ewing sarcoma, neuroblastoma	The pain is often attributed to a trivial fall, pain out of proportion to the fall
Black eye	Neuroblastoma, rhabdomyosarcoma (RMS)	No history of trauma
Diarrhea (watery, persistent)	Neuroblastoma	Diarrhea, all tests for infections negative, no change in pattern with diet
Ear drainage/earache	Rhabdomyosarcoma, Langerhans cell histiocytosis	Long duration, absence of associated cold symptoms
Fever of unknown origin	Leukemia, lymphoma, neuroblastoma	Fever intermittent, usually low grade, present for days to weeks
Headache, nausea, vomiting	Brain tumor, leukemia	Irritability, early morning, but may occur any time in the day
Hematuria	Wilms tumor	Usually painless, may have abdominal pain
Soft-tissue mass	STS, PNET, RMS	Slowly progressive mass, usually painless, no sign of inflammation
Voiding difficulty	Bladder or prostate RMS	Difficulty in voiding, no increase in frequency, no burning
Vaginitis	RMS	Bloody discharge

Abbreviations: STS = soft tissue sarcoma; PNET = primitive neurectodermal tumor.

TABLE 15-10 The CHILDCANCER Mnemonic

Continued, unexplained weight loss
Headaches, often with early morning vomiting
Increased swelling or persistent pain in bones, joints, back, or legs
Lump or mass, especially in the abdomen, neck, chest, pelvis, or armpits
Development of excessive bruising, bleeding, or rash
Constant infections
A whitish color behind the pupil
Nausea that persists or vomiting without nausea
Constant tiredness or noticeable paleness
Eye or vision changes that occur suddenly and persist
Recurrent or persistent fevers of unknow origin

childhood cancer using an acronym *CHILDCANCER* (www.acor.org/ped-onc/diseases/SOCC) as listed in TABLE 15–10.

Key Points

- Symptoms depend on the type and location of the cancer.
- An unusual constellation of symptoms that is not consistent with common childhood illness should prompt further evaluation for cancer.

Laboratory Evaluation

CBC. Anemia is a common finding in children with cancer. Neutropenia and thrombocytopenia may be the presenting symptoms of leukemia.
Comprehensive chemistry. Lymphoma/leukemia may present with electrolyte imbalance or signs of renal failure.
Lactate dehydrogenase (LDH). This is a useful surrogate test for many childhood malignancies, such as lymphoma, leukemia, neuroblastoma, and Ewing sarcoma.
Uric acid. This may be elevated because of increased cell turnover.
Alkaline phosphatase. Elevated in some cases of osteosarcoma.
Alpha-fetoprotein (AFP). Elevated in children with hepatoblastoma and germ cell tumors.
Beta-human chorionic gonadotropin (β-hCG). Elevated in gonadal tumors.

Imaging Studies

Conventional radiographs. These are easy, available, quick, and do not require sedation. Chest x-ray may provide useful information for the evaluation of lymphoma/leukemia, primary or metastatic. CT scan, ultrasound, and MRI have replaced abdominal x-rays. Intravenous excretory urography is of very limited use for the evaluation of childhood renal tumors.

Ultrasound. Because of inferior resolution compared with CT scan and MRI, ultrasound has a limited role in the evaluation of a child with cancer.

CT scan. The most valuable modality for evaluation of tumors of neck, chest, and abdomen. Water-soluble oral contrast material is necessary for a CT scan of the abdomen when suspecting perforation. Neutropenia is a contraindication for rectal contrast material administration.

Magnetic resonance imaging (MRI). Superior identification of most tumors. The soft-tissue contrast differentiation of MRI permits identification of most tumors without intravenously administered gadolinium chelate contrast material. Intravenous contrast material makes the tumor more conspicuous and allows evaluation of tumor vascularity and necrosis. MRI is the modality of choice for evaluation of brain, spinal cord, and musculoskeletal tumors and tumors of the body wall. It is complementary in the evaluation of some thoracic, abdominal, and pelvic malignancies.

Nuclear medicine scans. These are helpful for routine evaluation of musculoskeletal tumors, lymphoma, neuroblastoma, and thyroid tumors.

Immunophenotype by flow cytometry. This is available in most routine laboratories. This modality helps to recognize subtypes of lymphoma and leukemia.

Cytogenetics and molecular biology. This is performed on tumor tissue.

Synthesizing a Diagnosis

Diseases other than cancer may produce similar symptoms. To make the diagnosis of the cancer promptly, it is important to consider it in the right context. With a high index of suspicion and judicious use of laboratory and imaging techniques, there could be minimal delay in diagnosing the majority of cases. TABLE 15–11 lists laboratory and imaging studies that help to detect cancer in a child with subtle clinical findings.

Because leukemia and lymphoma are the most prevalent cancers involving the hematopoietic system, we devote special attention to these two conditions below.

Leukemia

This is the most common childhood cancer. Dysregulated proliferation of immature hematopoietic precursors results in leukemia. Acute lymphoblastic leukemia is the most common type of leukemia seen in children. Chronic leukemias are rare. Symptoms owing to lymphoblastic and myeloid leukemia are similar and divide into two broad categories shown in TABLE 15–12.

Leukemia is a systemic malignancy involving multiple organ systems. A thorough physical examination is paramount.

TABLE 15-11 *Synthesizing a Diagnosis of Childhood Cancer*

Symptom	Associations	Investigations	Possible Malignancy
Fever	Bone pain, weight loss, pallor	CBC, LDH, ESR, uric acid	Leukemia, lymphoma NBL, Ewing sarcoma
Headache	Vomiting, change behavior or school performance, gait change, vision change	MRI of the brain, CBC	Brain tumor, leukemia, lymphoma
Lymphadenopathy	Large size >2.5 cm; firm, rubbery or fixed nodes; supraclavicular location; chronic, persistent, or progressive nodes	CBC, LDH, uric acid, chest x-ray, lymph node biopsy	Lymphoma, leukemia, metastatic tumor
Bone and joint pain	May interfere with sleep	CBC, uric acid, LDH, x-ray	Leukemia, NHL, NBL, EWS, others
Anemia, thrombocytopenia, leukopenia, or leukocytosis	Significant suppression of one or more cell lines, circulating blasts, leukoerythroblastic reaction, lymphadenopathy, hepatomegaly, or splenomegaly	CBC, LDH, uric acid, bone marrow aspiration and biopsy	Leukemia, NHL, NBL
Bleeding	Bone pain, fever, adenopathy, organomegaly	CBC, LDH, uric acid, PT, aPTT, fibrinogen, bone marrow	Promyelocytic leukemia, T-cell ALL

Abbreviations: NBL = neuroblastoma; NHL = non-Hodgkin lymphoma; EWS = Ewing sarcoma.

TABLE 15-12 *Clinical High Points of Childhood Leukemia*

Bone marrow's inability to produce RBCs, WBCs, platelets (anemia, neutropenia, thrombocytopenia)	Infiltration of organ systems by leukemic blasts
	Bone pain
	Bone infiltrates
	Refusal to walk
Fatigue	Arthralgia
Lethargy	Joint effusions
Pallor	Backache
Infections	Paralysis/paresis
Mouth sores	Headaches
Fever of unknown origin	Nausea, vomiting
Bruises	Cranial nerve palsy
Hematoma	Lymphadenopathy (persistent or progressive)
Epistaxis	
Hemorrhage	Mediastinal mass
	Hepatomegaly
	Splenomegaly
	Bruises that do not go away
	Gum swelling and bleeding
	Painless testicular swelling

▼ KEY FINDING

◢Inspection In addition to the vital signs, careful inspection helps to assess the imminent threats. A common finding is pallor. The patient might appear well or acutely ill in the presence of an infection. Swelling of the face or labored breathing may be present owing to a mediastinal mass. The patient may have crusted blood in the nose or mouth. White pupil reflex may be present owing to involvement of the eye by leukemic blasts. Scattered bruises, petechiae, and purpura are common findings. Visible joint swelling or gait abnormality owing to pain occurs in some cases.

▼ KEY FINDING

◢Palpation Adenopathy involving one or more anatomic region is common. Liver and spleen may be enlarged, firm, and nontender. Leukemic infiltrates in the skin may be palpable in some cases.

▼ KEY FINDING

◢Percussion Percussion of the abdomen will help to determine the exact size of the liver and spleen.

▼ KEY FINDING

◢Auscultation Wheezes may be audible in a patient with a mediastinal mass. Patients with severe anemia often have tachycardia and a flow murmur.

▼ KEY FINDING
◤ Musculoskeletal Examination
Variable findings from normal to swelling of the digits and joints of the extremities resembling rheumatoid arthritis may occur in patients with leukemia.

▼ KEY FINDING
◤ Neurologic Examination
A thorough neurologic examination to evaluate cranial nerves and including fundus examination is paramount. Check for isolated cranial nerve deficits, papilledema, and altered vision owing to retinal hemorrhage or leukemic infiltrate in the retina.

▼ KEY FINDING
◤ Genital Examination
Vulva, vagina, and perirectal area should be examined for cellulitis or infection. Leukemic involvement of the testis causes uniform painless enlargement.

Reviewing Key Points
- The clinical presentation is variable.
- A head-to-toe examination including genital examination is important in a child suspected of leukemia.
- Absence of adenopathy or organomegaly does not exclude leukemia.

Differential Diagnosis
- *Aplastic anemia*
- *Immune thrombocytopenia (ITP)*
- *Infectious mononucleosis*
- *Rheumatoid arthritis, osteomyelitis*

Confirmatory Tests

Glossary of Terms
Anemia. Hemoglobin below normal range for age.
Thrombocytopenia. Platelet count less than $150,000/mm^3$.
Neutropenia. Absolute neutrophil count of less than $1500/mm^3$ in children older than 1 year of age and less than $1000/mm^3$ in infants.
CBC hemoglobin and platelet count. These may be normal or low. WBCs may be normal, low, or elevated. Although a majority of blast cells occur on the peripheral smear in most patients with leukemia, some patients with a normal WBC count may not have circulating blasts. Despite a normal WBC count, the patient is neutropenic. A patient with a decrease in more than one cell line on CBC with or without circulating blasts should undergo a bone marrow aspiration and biopsy.
LDH and uric acid. These are elevated in the majority of cases.
Chest x-ray. Used to evaluate for mediastinal masses.
CT scan. CT scan of the chest and abdomen is not necessary. Patients with an abnormal neurologic examination should have MRI.

Reviewing Key Points

- Abnormality of more than one cell line on CBC warrants a bone marrow examination.
- WBC count and differential for neutropenia is equally important.
- The bone marrow examination confirms the diagnosis.
- CT or MRI has a limited role.

Presenting signs and symptoms of both acute lymphoblastic leukemias, *acute lymphocytic leukemia* (ALL) and *acute myelogenous leukemia* (AML), are very similar; however, gum swelling, chloroma, and a DIC-like picture are more common in AML. AML is more common in infants and adolescents, whereas ALL is more common in children 1 to 9 years of age. Although morphologic characteristics of lymphoblasts and myeloblasts are specific enough to make the diagnosis in most cases, identification of the true origin of a leukemic blast by flow cytometry is required before starting the treatment in all cases of leukemia. Immunophenotype is also more sensitive in identifying small amounts of residual disease called *minimal residual disease* (MRD) and thus may help monitor response to therapy. Information about the exact antigenic makeup of the leukemic blast is necessary to use novel targeted biologic therapies.

Synthesizing a Diagnosis

Depending on the number of cell lines involved, the patient may present with myriad symptoms mimicking a variety of childhood illnesses such as *ITP, infectious mononucleosis, rheumatoid arthritis, osteomyelitis,* and *aplastic anemia.*

Lymphoma

Lymphoma, both *Hodgkin and non-Hodgkin* (NHL), is a malignancy originating in the organs of the immune system. NHL in a child or adolescent is a very rapidly growing, aggressive tumor, whereas Hodgkin disease usually has a slow, indolent course. Be suspicious of lymphoma in a child with persistent, progressive lymphadenopathy. A lymph node that measures greater than 1 cm in the cervical region or greater than 1.5 cm in the inguinal region is abnormal. In the absence of any signs of inflammation, the evaluation should include careful examination of local areas for infection, scratches, or bites. Lymph nodes that are nontender, rubbery, firm, fixed, rapidly enlarging, or located in the supraclavicular region are very suspicious for malignancy and merit prompt evaluation. The routine evaluation should include a CBC, LDH determination, uric acid determination, serology, and a chest x-ray. LDH is a nonspecific tumor marker for childhood cancer such as lymphoma, leukemia, neuroblastoma, and Ewing sarcoma. Patients with lymphoma who have very high levels of LDH have large tumors. Consider a lymph node biopsy in patients with persistent lymphadenopathy and a negative workup but who display:

- An enlarged lymph node that persists beyond 6 weeks in the absence of obvious infectious etiology
- Any lymph node greater than 2.5 cm in the absence of an obvious sign of infection
- Supraclavicular adenopathy
- Adenopathy with associated systemic symptoms

Non-Hodgkin Lymphoma

NHL in children is an aggressive malignancy. The patients present with lymphadenopathy most often mediastinal or abdominal and occasionally peripheral that develops in a matter of days. The American variety of Burkitt lymphoma usually presents with abdominal masses or lymphadenopathy. The rapid cell turnover often may present with signs of electrolyte imbalance, tumor lysis, and renal failure. NHL located above the diaphragm is usually of T-cell origin and may present with signs and symptoms of croup, stridor, and respiratory difficulty. Compression of the superior vena cava by a large mass may cause facial edema, facial plethora, and easy bleeding from the upper extremities. The American type of *Burkitt lymphoma* usually presents as a large abdominal mass with signs and symptoms of GI or urinary obstruction. Peripheral lymphadenopathy, although rare, may occur with either type of NHL. The evaluation for NHL includes a CBC, liver function tests, blood urea nitrogen (BUN), creatinine, uric acid, LDH, chest x-ray, and CT scans of the neck, chest, abdomen, and pelvis. Depending on the location, a CT-guided needle, laparoscopic, or excisional lymph node biopsy often will establish the diagnosis.

On physical examination, NHL, like leukemia, may involve any organ system. A complete physical examination will ascertain the acuity and extent of involvement.

Physical Examination

Respiratory. Increased respiratory rates, nasal flaring, intercostal retractions, and irritability on lying flat are signs of airway compromise. Pleural friction rub and decreased breath sounds are signs of pleural effusion.

Cardiovascular. Pericardial involvement may present as a pericardial effusion that may progress rapidly. Look for signs such as pulsus paradoxicus, pericardial friction rub, and muffled heart tones suggestive of cardiac tamponade. Facial edema and plethora are signs of superior vena cava compression.

Abdominal. There may be masses of varying size. Look for ascites and hepatosplenomegaly.

Lymph nodes. Peripheral lymph node enlargement occurs mainly in the cervical or inguinal areas but may involve any lymph node region.

Genitalia. NHL of the testes presents as unilateral painless testicular enlargement either alone or in association with other organ enlargement.

Musculoskeletal. NHL of bone usually presents with localized pain and tenderness. Occasionally, pathologic fracture may develop at the site. Bone masses are unusual.

CNS. There may be intracranial involvement or sensory, motor, or cranial nerve weakness similar to leukemia.

Hematologic. There may be anemia, leukopenia, and thrombocytopenia owing to bone marrow involvement.

Confirmatory Tests

CBC, LDH, uric acid, comprehensive blood chemistry, chest x-ray, and CT scan of neck, chest, and abdomen are mandatory. A patient with a large chest mass should have an echocardiogram and pulmonary function testing prior to general anesthesia.

Reviewing Key Points

Like leukemia, NHL may involve any organ system of the body. A thorough physical examination is mandatory. NHL is a rapidly growing tumor that requires prompt evaluation by a pediatric oncologist. Needle aspirate or biopsy will establish the diagnosis and should occur immediately on suspicion of NHL. In patients with imminent airway obstruction or signs of spinal cord compression, treatment with steroids and/or radiation may be necessary before performing the biopsy.

Hodgkin Disease

Hodgkin disease is the most common cancer in adolescents 15 to 19 years of age.

History

This usually presents with painless progressive supraclavicular, cervical, axillary, or inguinal lymphadenopathy that develops over weeks to months. The nodes feel rubbery and firm. Two-thirds of patients have mediastinal involvement and may have a nonproductive cough. Systemic symptoms associated with Hodgkin disease are fever, weight loss, and night sweats. Unusual symptoms of Hodgkin disease include pruritus and alcohol-induced pain. The pain appears within minutes of alcohol ingestion in the areas of nodal enlargement.

Physical Examination

Fever of 38°C or higher and weight loss of 10 percent or greater within the last 3 months are common. Lymph nodes are usually large, firm, rubbery, and matted. Record the largest diameter of each palpable node. In rare cases there may be hepatosplenomegaly. Genital or CNS involvement is very rare. A large chest mass may extend posteriorly and cause spinal cord compression.

Confirmatory Tests

CBC, sedimentation rate, serum copper, chest x-ray, lymph node biopsy, and a CT scan are essential. A positron emission tomographic (PET) scan is useful for further staging.

Reviewing Key Points

Adenopathy owing to Hodgkin disease develops over a period of weeks to months. Chest involvement is common. CNS and genital involvement is rare.

Tumors of the Central Nervous System (Brain Tumors)

Brain tumors as a whole represent the second most common pediatric malignancy. As compared with CNS malignancies in adults, they are predominantly (~90 percent) primary brain lesions. (i.e., do not represent metastatic lesions).

The common pediatric brain tumors include

- Infratentorial/posterior fossa: cerebellum or brain stem
  - *Medulloblastoma*
  - *Cerebellar astrocytoma*
  - *Brain stem glioma*
  - *Ependymoma*
- Supratentorial: cerebrum, basal ganglia, thalamus, hypothalamus, optic chiasm
  - *Supratentorial astrocytoma*
  - *Primitive neuroectodermal tumors (PNETs)*
  - *Craniopharyngioma*
  - *Pineal tumors*
- Others include *optic pathway gliomas, choroid plexus carcinoma,* and *atypical teratoid-rhabdoid tumors.*

The presenting symptoms and signs depend on the location of the tumor, the age at presentation of the child, and the developmental stage of the child. In general, the findings are related to increased intracranial pressure (ICP) and localizing and nonlocalizing signs.

The incidence peaks in the first decade of life. Ninety percent of these tumors occur in otherwise healthy children, with the remaining 10 percent associated with syndromes such as *neurofibromatosis types 1 and 2* (NF-1 and NF-2), *Li-Fraumeni syndrome, tuberous sclerosis,* and *von Hippel–Lindau syndrome* (VHL).

History

KEY PROBLEM

Nonspecific Many problems are nonspecific and include irritability, failure to thrive, and developmental regression.

KEY PROBLEM

Headache Headache is a principal complaint (see Chapter 12). Headaches are very common in clinical practice and generally do not require evaluation by CT scan or MRI. Ninety-five percent of children with brain tumors are screened effectively through a history and physical examination. There are important red flags associated with headache that should lead the clinician toward imaging studies. These are recurrent and worsening headaches; early-morning headaches or headaches that awaken the child from sleep; headaches associated with early-morning vomiting, especially not preceded by nausea; occurrence in a child younger than 3 years of age; headache with an associated neurologic abnormality; headache with a known history of *neurofibromatosis;* and headache with a previous history of malignancy or irradiation for *diabetes insipidus* and visual field loss.

KEY PROBLEM
Vomiting Note the preceding associations with headache and the temporal relationships. Also be suspicious of vomiting that does not respond to the usual medical treatments.

KEY PROBLEM
High-Pitched Cry This is typical for increased intracranial pressure.

KEY PROBLEM
Head Tilt This occurs with posterior fossa tumors.

KEY PROBLEM
Early Hand Preference Astute parents often will note this, and it usually suggests supratentorial lesions.

KEY PROBLEM
Seizures Change in character of previous seizure, focal deficits, prolonged postictal paralysis, and status epilepticus with first unprovoked seizure and seizures not amenable to medical management with antiepileptic drugs (AEDs).

Physical Examination

KEY FINDING
Ophthalmologic Strabismus, optic disk pallor in infants and papilledema in the older child, "setting sun" sign, Parinaud syndrome, decreased visual acuity, visual field defects and diplopia (double vision), and cranial nerve IV and trochlear nerve palsy with resultant upward and lateral deviation of the affected eye.

KEY FINDING
Sensorimotor These include hemiparesis, hyperreflexia, strabismus, and sensory deficits.

Infratentorial Tumors

These usually present with ataxia, long-tract signs, and cranial nerve palsies.

KEY FINDING
Cerebellar Signs Cerebellar signs include clumsiness (ataxia), worsening hand writing, difficulty with balance evidenced by inability to run or hop, staccato speech, dysdiadochokinesis, past-pointing, and nystagmus. These are associated with infratentorial tumors.

▼ Cranial Neuropathies

Cranial Neuropathies These are usually associated with brain stem lesions. They usually start with one nerve, and as the tumor increases in size, multiple cranial nerves become involved. Diplopia, abducens palsy, gaze palsy (inability to deviate both eyes conjugately), swallowing difficulties (which could manifest only as drooling), and Horner syndrome (ipsilateral ptosis, miosis, and anhidrosis) and peripheral facial nerve palsy (weakness in the whole half of the face).

Laboratory and Imaging

CT scan. A non-contrast-enhanced CT scan of the brain is usually the first imaging study obtained. It is readily available and delineates the location of the tumor, ventriculomegaly, or hydrocephalus.

MRI of the brain. A contrast MRI study with gadolinium has become the diagnostic modality of choice. It better delineates the tumor and determines enhancement, white matter extension, and subarachnoid spread. However, MRI may not be readily and emergently available.

MRI of the spine. Frequently evaluation of the spine is warranted for "drop metastases."

Reviewing Key Points

Presenting symptoms and signs of brain tumors are varied and depend on the site, size, and patient's age.

Headache is a common complaint in clinical practice and should prompt imaging if there is a change in its character or severity or association with unprovoked or early-morning vomiting or neurologic signs or occurs in a young child.

MRI is the diagnostic modality of choice.

Neuroblastoma

Neuroblastomas are the most common extracranial solid tumors in children, accounting for 8 to 10 percent of all childhood malignancies. They arise from primordial neural crest cells that ultimately populate the sympathetic ganglia and adrenal medulla. The site of origin therefore can be the adrenal gland or any other point along the sympathetic chain. See TABLE 15–13 for presentation by primary site. Clinical presentation depends on the primary site and if there is spread to distant

TABLE 15–13 *Clinical Presentation by Primary Site*

Abdominal	C > I
Adrenal	C > I
Thoracic	I > C
Cervical	I > C
Organ of Zuckerkandl	C > I
No primary (1 percent)	

sites (metastases) such as bone, bone marrow, liver, skin, and lymph nodes. It is a pediatric malignancy with 40 percent diagnosed in infancy and 90 percent diagnosed by age 5. It is extremely rare above the age of 10 years.

History

Neuroblastoma may be entirely asymptomatic and present as an incidental finding during investigation of a GI complaint.

KEY PROBLEM
■ **Abdominal Fullness or Discomfort**   This is a common complaint in a child able to articulate it.

KEY PROBLEM
■ **Bone Pain**   This manifests as irritability, limping, or refusal to bear weight.

KEY PROBLEM
■ **Radicular Pain**   This occurs with spinal lesions associated with compression by or spread of a primary lesion.

KEY PROBLEM
■ **Paraneoplastic Syndromes**   Opsoclonus-myoclonus, myoclonic jerking, and random eye movement (with or without ataxia) are the most common paraneoplastic syndromes associated with neuroblastoma. They are thought to be due an immunologic phenomenon.

KEY PROBLEM
■ **Bone Pain**   This manifests as irritability, refusal to bear weight in a young child, or limping in an older child. It is consistent with spread of the tumor.

Physical Examination

A regional approach is best.

KEY PROBLEM
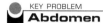
■ **Abdomen**

INSPECTION
The abdomen may be full or protuberant. If the tumor is massive, there may be obvious scrotal edema owing to venous congestion. Gross abdominal distension causing airway compromise is secondary to liver involvement in infants.

PALPATION
Fixed, hard abdominal mass. It may be in the midline, extending laterally, or it may be in the flank if arising from the adrenal gland. Hepatomegaly usually occurs in infants younger than 1 year of age with small adrenal primaries and bone marrow involvement.

▼ KEY FINDING
◤◢ **Thorax** Thoracic primaries are usually diagnosed as an incidental finding when a chest radiograph is obtained for respiratory symptoms. If massive, the tumor may be associated with *superior vena cava syndrome* with suffusion of the face, chest, and upper extremities.

▼ KEY FINDING
◤◢ **Spine** Cervical (as well as high thoracic) primary lesions may present as swelling and may be associated with *Horner syndrome* (ipsilateral ptosis, miosis, and anhidrosis).

INTRASPINAL
Extension from a paraspinal primary into the neural foramina of the vertebral bodies may lead to signs of spinal cord compression. These include paraplegia and bladder or bowel dysfunction. Perform a rectal examination to assess sphincter tone.

Findings Related to Distant Spread

▼ KEY FINDING
◤◢ **Eye** Proptosis and periorbital ecchymoses ("raccoon eyes") occur from tumor infiltration of periorbital bones.

▼ KEY FINDING
◤◢ **Skin** This presents in infant neuroblastoma as bluish, nontender, subcutaneous nodules.

Laboratory and Imaging

- A CBC may reveal a normochromic, normocytic anemia if there is bone marrow involvement.
- Blood chemistry, LDH, and ferritin.
- Do a 24-hour urine collection for catecholamines, homovanillic acid (HVA), and vanillylmandelic acid (VMA).
- Ultrasound of the abdomen is a quick and readily available tool to assess abdominal primaries. It can provide information about site of origin (adrenal versus paraspinal), lymph node involvement, and liver enlargement.
- CT scan can be used for any site and is readily available.
- MRI has replaced CT scanning as the imaging modality of choice for lesions arising from any site. It is also the best study to assess spinal involvement. MRI of the brain is very useful for orbital or skull involvement.
- Radiolabeled meta-iodobenzylguanidine (MIBG) scintigraphy is important for primary and metastatic disease. It is important for both diagnosis and monitoring.

Reviewing Key Points

- Neuroblastoma can arise anywhere along the sympathetic chain and adrenal medulla.

- In infants (younger than 1 year of age), distinct clinical features include massive hepatomegaly (causing respiratory compromise) and bone marrow involvement (Stage IVS).
- Periorbital spread could present as "raccoon eyes," leading patients to be worked up for child abuse.

Wilms Tumor (Nephroblastoma)

Wilms tumor is the most common primary renal neoplasm in children. It accounts for approximately 6 percent of all childhood cancers, with a mean age of diagnosis of 3 $1/2$ to 4 years. It occurs in otherwise healthy children, and about 10 percent are found in children with syndromic disorders such as *Wilms tumor, aniridia, genitourinary malformation,* and *mental retardation* (WAGR) and *Beckwith-Wiedemann* and *Denys-Drash syndromes.* Wilms tumor also has associations with other sporadic findings such as *hemihypertrophy, hypospadias,* and *cryptorchidism.*

History

Caregivers often will observe increasing abdominal girth or actually will palpate the tumor themselves. Wilms tumor may be asymptomatic.

Physical Examination

KEY FINDING
Hypertension This is secondary to increased renin activity found at presentation in approximately 25 percent of cases. Does the patient have a previously diagnosed syndrome?

KEY FINDING
Inspection Pay attention to observe any dysmorphic features such as hemihypertrophy, aniridia, and hypospadias. Check the abdomen for fullness, bulging flank, and varicocele that persists when the patient is placed supine, suggesting venous obstruction of the spermatic vein.

KEY FINDING
Palpation There is an immobile flank mass that does not move with respiration (as compared with the spleen). Repeated palpation of a Wilms tumor can induce spread beyond the renal capsule.

KEY FINDING
Percussion Elicit dullness from the affected flank through the full extent of the tumor.

Laboratory and Imaging

- CBC, renal function tests (BUN and creatinine), urinalysis, and calcium determination.
- Coagulation screen: PT and aPTT. Acquired *VWD* is found in as many as 8 percent of cases at presentation.

- Abdominal ultrasound. This is a useful diagnostic modality. Not only is it readily available, but it shows intrarenal location and gives information about solid versus cystic renal disease (polycystic or multicystic kidney disease).
- CT scan of the abdomen.
- Chest x-ray to check for spread to the lungs, which are a very common site for metastases.

Reviewing Key Points

- Wilms tumor is the most common renal tumor in children and presents as a painless flank mass.
- History and examination should ascertain any associated syndromes.
- Repeated palpation of a suspected lesion is discouraged.
- Abdominal ultrasound is a good diagnostic and surveillance tool.

Bone Tumors

The most common primary bone tumors in children are *osteogenic sarcoma* and *Ewing sarcoma.*

Osteogenic Sarcoma (Osteosarcoma)

Osteosarcoma is the most common primary bone tumor in children, with a peak incidence in the second decade of life. Osteosarcomas arise commonly from the metaphysis of the long bones corresponding with the periods of increased growth, but they also can affect the flat bones and the jaw. The most common site of involvement is around the knee joint (distal femur and proximal tibia). Clinical presenting symptoms are pain and swelling of the primary site in almost 90 percent of cases. Pain in other bony sites may suggest metastases. It may be intermittent initially and becomes more persistent in the absence of a history of trauma. There may be a history, however, of minor trauma and pain incongruent to the injury. This should raise suspicion of underlying pathology.

History

 KEY PROBLEM

Fever, Weight Loss, and Bone Pain Fever and weight loss are rare and are present only in advanced cases.

Physical Examination

INSPECTION AND PALPATION
The key finding is once again the swelling at the primary site. Lymph nodes are enlarged very rarely and in advanced disease only.

Laboratory and Imaging

- CBC, LDH, alkaline phosphatase.
- Plain x-ray shows bony destruction of trabeculae, Codman triangle, and "sun-burst" appearance, which results from ossification of the surrounding soft tissue in a radial pattern.

- CT scan is readily available but has been replaced by MRI.
- MRI with gadolinium contrast material is the diagnostic modality of choice because it delineates clearly the extent of tumor involvement.
- Chest x-ray and chest CT to assess pulmonary metastases, which are most common.

Ewing Sarcoma

This is a primary sarcoma of nonosseous origin in children and adolescents. It represents the second most common primary bone tumor. Tumors also can arise from extraosseous sites. Like osteosarcomas, these tumors occur predominantly in the second decade of life. The extremities are the usual site of involvement, but unlike osteosarcoma, there is involvement of other bones of the axial skeleton. These include the pelvic bones, chest wall (ribs), head and neck, and spine. The most common presenting feature is pain and swelling of the affected site. Distant pain represents metastases. Pathologic fractures are rare.

History

KEY PROBLEM
Pain, Fever

Physical Examination

KEY FINDING
Inspection   There is edema and swelling of the site.

KEY FINDING
Palpation   There is swelling of the site as well as a palpable mass, sometimes warm to the touch.

Laboratory and Imaging

- CBC, chemistry, erythrocyte sedimentation rate (ESR; may be elevated in up to 50 percent of cases at presentation), LDH, and alkaline phosphatase.
- X-ray of the primary site. "Onion skin" appearance results from multiple layers of reactive new bone formation.
- CT scan is readily available.
- MRI has become the diagnostic modality of choice because it well delineates the tumor extent and the soft-tissue involvement.
- Chest x-ray and chest CT assess for pulmonary metastases.
- Bone scan is useful for local lesions and distant metastases.

Reviewing Key Points

- Primary bone tumors occur more commonly in adolescents and present with pain and swelling. Note that the pain may be intermittent initially, and there may be brief pain-free periods.
- The lungs are a primary site of distant spread.

- Regional lymphadenopathy is uncommon, and its absence does not suggest a benign lesion.

Soft-Tissue Sarcomas (Rhabdomyosarcoma)

Rhabdomyosarcoma is the most common soft-tissue sarcoma in children. Nonrhabdomyomatous soft-tissue sarcomas (NRSTSs) do occur with similar presenting features and constitute an important differential for rhabdomyosarcoma. These are malignant tumors of mesenchymal cell origin that mature to form muscle. Therefore, they can arise from any site in the body. Primary sites of origin include the orbit, head and neck region, trunk, thorax, retroperitoneum, perineum, paratesticular region, and vagina.

History

Problems are directly related to the anatomic location of the lesion.

Key Problems

- *Orbits.* Twenty-five percent of all head and neck tumors occur in the orbit. They present with proptosis, ophthalmoplegia, and ecchymoses.
- *Nasopharynx and paranasal sinuses.* Symptoms of nasal congestion, sinusitis, and epistaxis.
- *Neck.* Swelling, dysphagia, and hoarseness.
- *Perineal/paratesticular.* Perineal lesions occur in younger children, with paratesticular lesions occurring in boys older than 10 years of age. Usually present as a painless swelling noted by parent or older child.
- *Trunk/extremities.* Painless swelling.
- *Abdomen and retroperitoneum.* By virtue of their hidden location, these usually present late when symptoms of GI obstruction become apparent (constipation). Could also present as persistent back pain.
- *Bladder/prostate.* Present with urinary symptoms, e.g., frequency and sensation of incomplete voiding.
- *Vaginal.* Botryoid tumors presenting as a cluster of grapes protruding from the vagina.

Physical Examination

Presentation depends on the site of origin; orbital tumor, by virtue of its conspicuous location, presents early.

Key Findings

Inspection. Site-specific, as above. Note swelling and ecchymoses if coincidental trauma prompted medical evaluation.

Palpation. Usually nontender swelling. Assess regional lymph node involvement because this affects the stage.

Laboratory and Imaging

- CBC, chemistry; no useful markers are available.
- Ultrasound is useful in the evaluation of tumors arising from the abdomen.

- CT scan.
- MRI is the imaging modality of choice because of its superior tissue resolution.
- Bone scan to assess bony involvement.

Reviewing Key Points

- Rhabdomyosarcomas can arise anywhere in the body.
- A high index of suspicion should prompt immediate diagnostic studies for a painless mass found incidentally by a patient or parent.

Retinoblastoma

A pediatric tumor arising from the retina, this affects predominantly young children, with a mean age of presentation of 13 to 18 months and with 90 percent diagnosed before age 5 years. They are usually unilateral, but they may be bilateral in 20 to 25 percent of cases. Bilateral involvement suggests an underlying germ line mutation. Familial cases also occur and could be either unilateral or bilateral. The most common presenting feature is a white pupillary reflex (leukokoria). Other presenting symptoms include esotropia with resulting strabismus, painful red eye with glaucoma, unilateral dilated pupil, heterochromia (different color irises), nystagmus, proptosis, and visual loss. In advanced disease, nonspecific symptoms may prompt medical evaluation. These include failure to thrive, anorexia, and lethargy.

Reviewing Key Points

- A well-child examination of the young child should include a check for red reflexes and strabismus.
- Between 70 and 75 percent of retinoblastomas are unilateral, and vision can be preserved in the majority of patients. When bilateral involvement occurs, there is a germ line mutation.

When to Refer

A pediatric oncology consultation is important for all patients suspected of having lymphoma or leukemia. A patient with persistent adenopathy and a normal CBC should have a lymph node biopsy. A pediatric oncologist must evaluate a patient suspected of lymphoma or leukemia *without delay*. Make the referral *prior* to any invasive procedures.

An abnormal red reflex or persistent or new-onset strabismus should be referred promptly to an ophthalmologist (pediatric if available). A dilated examination under anesthesia (EUA) will reveal retinal lesions.

Refer to a pediatric oncologist when findings on ultrasound show a solid intrarenal lesion. This chapter reviews symptomatology of other tumors that warrant referral.

Arthur N. Feinberg

SKIN

The goals of this section are

1. To review the physiology and function of the skin.
2. To review the anatomy of the skin
3. To review historical points in the presentation of skin disorders
4. To review physical findings of skin disorders, with particular emphasis on configuration, color, pattern, and distribution
5. To summarize in a tabular form dermatologic diagnoses with their symptoms, signs (configuration, color, pattern, and distribution), age of occurrence (infants, children, or adolescents), and systemic conditions to consider

Since dermatology is primarily anatomic and descriptive, these areas will be emphasized. The limited space of a chapter is not conducive to the typical "atlas" approach. Therefore, a limited number of illustrations are presented, but emphasis is placed on a thought process that will help to generate hypotheses that then can be narrowed down to streamline any further investigation with a more complete atlas or textbook. The tables contain clinical "high points" that should be incorporated into daily practice.

Physiology

The integument affords protection that entails physical barriers to injury and pathogens, temperature regulation, immune protection, and sensation. Protection against injury is primarily mechanical, by forming an outer layer, by containing melanocytes to mitigate solar injury, by storing fat as a cushion, by containing collagen to enhance the integrity of this barrier, and by containing sebaceous glands to lubricate the skin. Temperature regulation to conserve or dissipate heat is through eccrine gland secretion of sweat (convection), evaporation of sweat (radiation), and circulation, under autonomic regulation with varying degrees of dilation and constriction (conduction). Fat storage is also a source of energy to generate heat if necessary. Langerhans cells are the primary agents in the skin for immune protection, the function of which is to present antigens to lymph nodes. Sensory organs receive stimuli (pain, heat, light, touch, and pressure) and conduct them to the autonomic nervous system, which may then stimulate piloerection, hair movement, vasodilatation, or vasoconstriction. The sensory organs connect to sensory nerves that travel to higher centers to alert the body to avoid noxious stimuli.

Functional Anatomy

FIGURE 16–1 illustrates the anatomy of the skin layers. In more detail, the avascular epidermis, or outermost layer of the skin, consists of the stratum corneum, which the underlying layers—the stratum granulosum, spinosum, and basale—manufacture. The epidermis also contains melanocytes involved in solar protection. The dermis, underlying the epidermis, contains the support structure, such as collagen and fat, blood vessels, hair follicles with sebaceous glands attached to them, and sweat glands. The dermis contains three layers—papillary, reticular, and subcutaneous.

The hair unit, or follicle, is an invagination of the dermis and epidermis. The papilla protrudes into its base and contains its vascular supply. The base structure of the hair is the bulb, fitting over the papilla. The root consists of the bulb, which tapers into a narrower structure, up to the epidermis. Distal to that, the hair becomes even narrower and tighter as it forms the shaft. Arrector pili, or muscles, are under autonomic influence and are attached to the root. Human hair is vellus (short, soft, and colorless) or terminal (long, darker, and coarse). Vellus hair

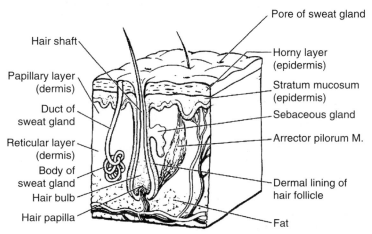

FIGURE 16–1 *Principal Skin Structures.* (*From LeBlond RF, DeGowin RL, Brown DD*: DeGowin's Diagnostic Examination. *New York: McGraw-Hill, 2004, Fig. 6-1, p. 130.*)

occurs in all age groups and is located ubiquitously except on palms, soles, dorsa of the distal phalanges, penis, and labia. Terminal hairs, which are located in the pubic region and axillae of matur(ing) individuals and on the face and body of males, are dependent on androgenic stimulation. Terminal hairs on the scalp appear in infants, children, and adolescents. Each follicle grows individually in a cyclical fashion. See section on hair below for phases of hair growth.

Problems

Gathering historical information about dermatologic conditions is not hard if limited only to the integument. Subjective patient complaints are primarily sensory and consist of three key problems: pain, temperature, and itching. Obtain a history of possible exposures to given areas of the skin. However, since numerous medical conditions, especially allergies, have dermatologic manifestations, a good, full medical history is both appropriate and necessary. Always remember the ectodermal origin of skin and central nervous system (CNS) and the importance of assessing neurodevelopment in the diagnosis of neurocutaneous syndromes.

Findings

A dermatologic examination consists primarily of observation and palpation. However, percussion and auscultation should not be a lost art to the dermatologist, who may be in the position of having to make broader medical diagnoses based on integument manifestations. The four cornerstones of the dermatologic examination are configuration, color, pattern, and distribution.

Configuration

The key primary dermatologic findings are enumerated below with illustrations (FIGURES 16–2 through 16–9).

- Macules are flat, circumscribed lesions that are visible to the eye and whose edges are not palpable. Always determine their color, pattern, and distribution. Once palpation has determined that these are macules, are there any changes in their pattern when pressure is applied to the skin? Does palpation elicit tenderness, blanching, or more surrounding erythema? An erythematous macule may extend its redness and develop a palpable edge (wheal and flare).
- Papules are raised lesions 1 cm or less in diameter. They are nonmobile and extend only up to the surface of the dermis. Vegetations are irregular papules and are verrucous if the covering is dry and hard and papillomatous if epidermis covers them. Does palpation elicit surrounding erythema and edema (Darier sign)? If palpation elicits

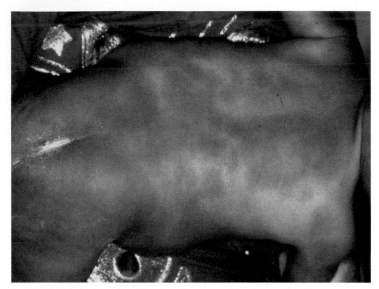

FIGURE 16-2 *Macule (Blue) as Illustrated by Mongolian Spots.*

blanching, this indicates a vascular content of the lesion. Does scratching a nearby area induce a new lesion (Koebner phenomenon)?
• Plaques are papules or collections of papules that are more than 1 cm in diameter.

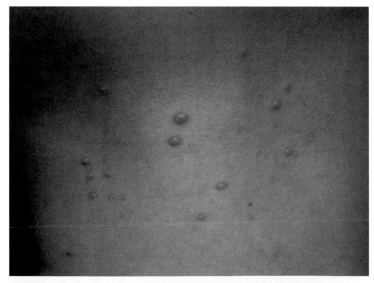

FIGURE 16-3 *Papules, as Illustrated in Molluscum Contagiosum.*

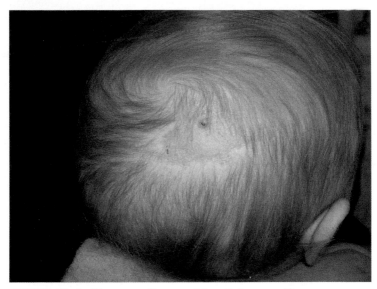

FIGURE 16-4 *Plaque, as Illustrated in a Sebaceous Nevus.*

- Nodules are elevated lesions that are located deeper than papules in the dermis and sometimes the subcutaneous fat. The overlying epidermis and superficial dermis do not attach to them and therefore move over the lesions. Larger nodules are tumors.

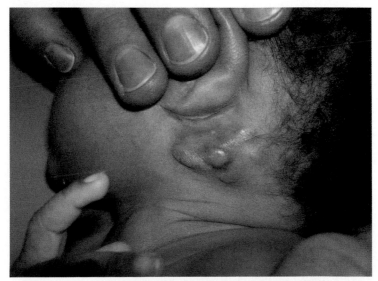

FIGURE 16-5 *Flesh-Colored Nodule or Tumor (Larger Nodule).*

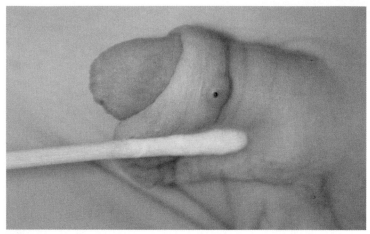

FIGURE 16–6 *Cyst, Illustrated as a Manifestation of Acne.*

- Cysts are sharply circumscribed, movable nodules containing fluid (e.g., serous fluid, pus, and sebum).
- Vesicles are sharply marginated superficial collections of clear fluid located in the epidermis and are 1 cm or less in diameter.

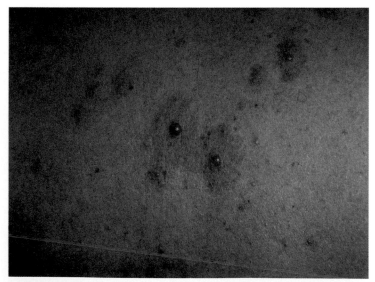

FIGURE 16–7 *Vesicles, Illustrated in Varicella.*

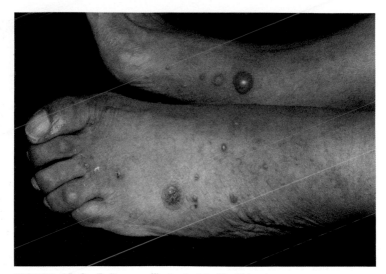

FIGURE 16-8 *Bullae, as Illustrated in Dyshidrosis.*

Does palpation on nearby normal skin elicit new vesicles (Nikolsky sign)?
- Bullae are large vesicles more than 1 cm in diameter.
- Scales are dried fragments of dead skin. Does removal of a piece of the scale induce bleeding (Auspitz sign)?

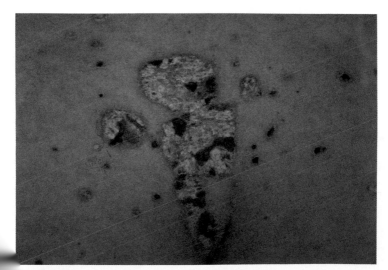

FIGURE 16-9 *Scales, as Illustrated in Psoriasis.*

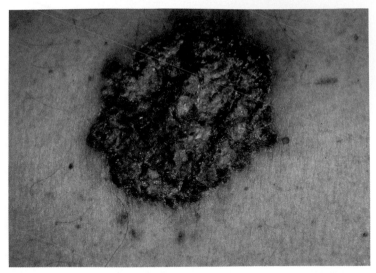

FIGURE 16-10 *Secondary Scales/crusts, Illustrated in Nummular Eczema.*

Certain dermatologic lesions are a complication of a primary lesion and therefore are termed *secondary* (FIGURES 16–10 through 16–21).

- Scales can be secondary and are dried, greasy fragments of adherent dead skin that may be due to previously infected or inflamed papular lesions.

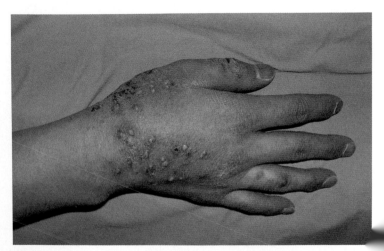

FIGURE 16-11 *Pustules from Staphylococcal Infection.*

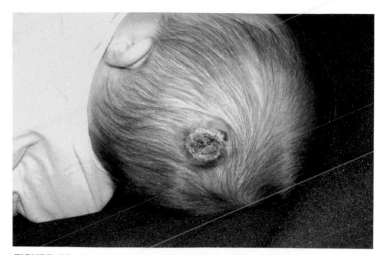

FIGURE 16–12 *Erosion and Crust Secondary to Scalp Hemangioma.*

- Pustules are papules containing white blood cells (WBCs) and serum (pus). Abscesses are larger collections of pus that run deeper into the dermis and subcutaneous tissue. Sinuses are tracts that connect an underlying structure to the skin and may be congenital or acquired as a result of an infection.

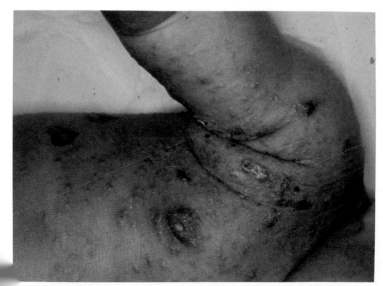

FIGURE 16–13 *Excoriations Owing to Acne.*

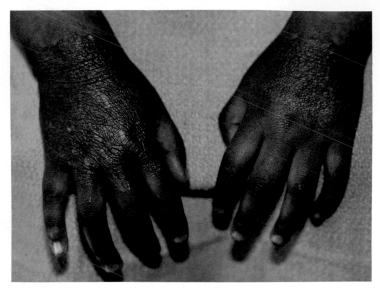

FIGURE 16–14 *Lichenification with Eczema.*

- Erosions are well-demarcated losses of superficial epidermis usually secondary to rupture of a vesicle. Excoriations are scratch marks on the skin.
- Crusts are dried exudates that can consist of serum, pus, dried blood, or scales. There is an antecedent lesion such as a vesicle, pustule, abscess, or erosion.

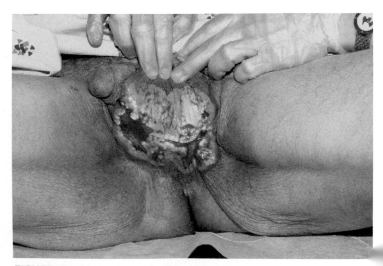

FIGURE 16–15 *Ulcer of the Scrotum.*

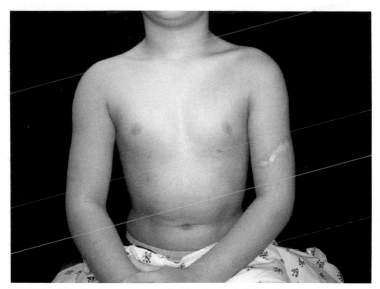

FIGURE 16-16 *Induration with Morphea of Scleroderma.*

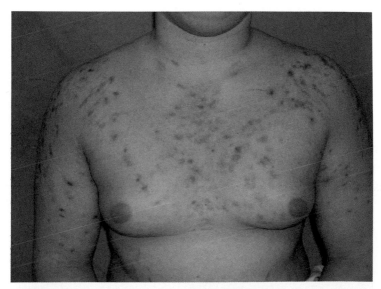

FIGURE 16-17 *Scars Secondary to Herpetic Lesion.*

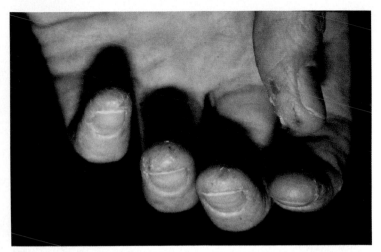

FIGURE 16-18 *Cracks and Fissures with Dyshydrosis of the Hand.*

- Lichenifications are extensive areas of dried plaques induced by repeated scratching.
- Ulcers are depressed lesions with loss of both epidermis and dermis. They may be painful or anesthetic, so it is important to palpate them. They are a consequence of infection, trauma, or malignancy.

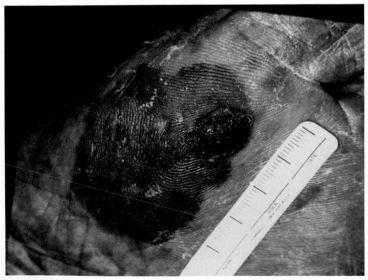

FIGURE 16-19 *Black Tumor (Malignant Melanoma).*

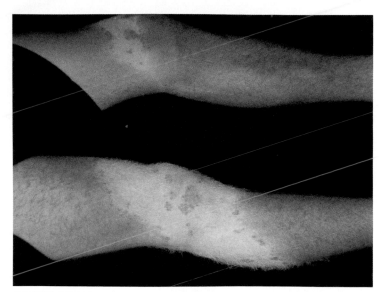

FIGURE 16–20 *White Macule (Vitiligo).*

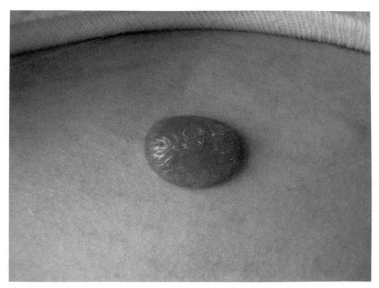

FIGURE 16–21 *Yellow Papule.*

- Indurations and scleroses are hardening of the skin characterized by thickening and are often a consequence of previous inflammation or trauma.
- Scars are due to formation of new connective tissue after destruction of the epidermis, dermis, and subcutaneous areas.
- Fissures are painful cracks in the skin owing to inflammation.

Color

Skin lesions have many different colors to them, each with clinical significance.

- Red points to increased blood flow and is a result of inflammation or vascular collections.
- Purple is a result of increased blood flow in a vascular collection, perhaps with more venous content, or a result of ruptured blood vessels with extravasation. Palpation of vascular collections will cause blanching, whereas palpation of extravasated blood will not.
- Brown or black indicates pigment deposit.
- Blue also indicates pigment deposit or a vascular collection with more venous content.
- Green also may indicate pigment deposit and also may result from a resolving hematoma.
- Yellow lesions may contain fat or sebum.
- Flesh color indicates a lesion with normal overlying skin.
- White may indicate depigmentation or keratin deposits in lesions.

Pattern

Individual lesions may be linear, annular, reticular, oval, burrowed, serpiginous, or variable in size and shape (e.g., *erythema multiforme*). Examine the lesion for uniformity. Some may have areas of clearing, often central, or lack uniformity diffusely. Examine borders of lesions for irregularity and definition. Progressive irregular borders and pigmentation always raise concern for *malignancy*. Some lesions may appear on a stalk (filiform, or threadlike). How does the lesion behave? Is it consistent or evanescent? Evanescence is typical of *urticaria, rheumatic fever,* and *rheumatoid arthritis*. Does it change size or shape? This will occur in *urticaria, erythema multiforme,* and *erythema chronicum migrans* of *Lyme disease.*

Distribution

The distribution of skin lesions is often helpful in dermatologic diagnosis. Key types of distribution are

- Flexural distribution is located in the antecubital and popliteal fossae, the neck, and behind the ears. This is typical of *eczema* (FIGURE 16–22)
- Dermatomal distribution follows a pattern similar to that of innervation emanating from the spinal cord (see Chapter 12 for an illustration). This is typical of *herpes zoster* (FIGURE 16–23).

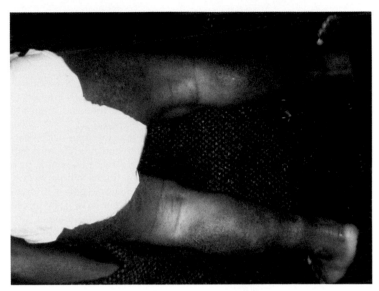

FIGURE 16–22 Flexural Distribution of Eczema.

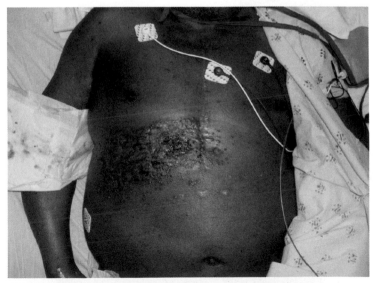

FIGURE 16–23 Dermatomal Distribution of Herpes Zoster.

- Acrodermatitis is similar to sun-exposed sites and is located additionally on the palms, soles, fingers, and toes and perhaps periorally, perianally, and the tip of the nose (FIGURE 16–24). Examples are *hand-foot-mouth disease* (coxsackie virus), *acrodermatitis enteropathica,* and *Gianotti-Crosti syndrome.*
- Acneiform rashes typically distribute on the face, upper chest, shoulders, and back. *Rosacea,* which looks similar to acne, is limited to central portions of the face, particularly the nose, forehead, chin, and cheeks.
- Lines of Blaschko reflect the embryologic development of the dermis. Normally, the dermal cells differentiate and migrate in a pattern somewhat similar to dermatomes. Abnormal genes may turn off this process. In autosomally inherited conditions, a homozygote usually dies in utero or soon after birth. A heterozygote will demonstrate lesions following Blaschko's lines. Similarly, in a sex-linked trait, the female with the extra functioning X chromosome may survive with lesions following Blaschko's lines, whereas the male will not survive. This occurs in *linear epidermal nevi, sebaceous nevi, incontinentia pigmenti* ("whorl" pattern), *focal dermal hypoplasia,* and other genetic syndromes (FIGURE 16–25).

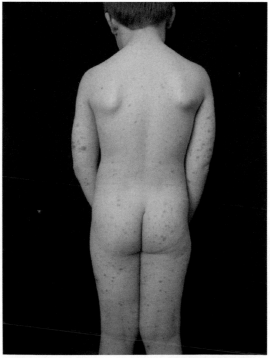

FIGURE 16–24   *Acropustulosis Distribution in Gianotti-Crosti Syndrome.*

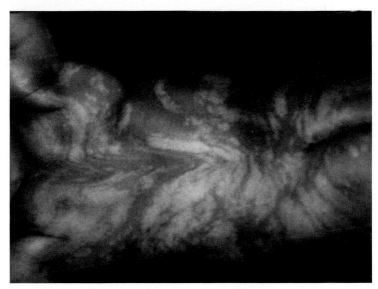

FIGURE 16–25 *Blaschko's Lines in Hypomelanosis of Ito.*

- Sun-exposed sites are the arms and legs distal to where short sleeves and short pants end. Consider *lupus* and *drug eruptions.*
- Clothing-covered sites are generally opposite to the sun-exposed sites but may be more extensive if the patient wears long shirtsleeves and pants. This is common with *diaper rashes.*
- Unique patterns. Several conditions have their own distributions, as illustrated below:
- *Scarlatiniform rashes (streptococcal)* demonstrate erythema of the cheeks that spares the circumoral region, antecubital regions, axillae, and groin.
- Collagen-vascular diseases have unique distributions. Note the "butterfly" pattern in *lupus erythematosus* and the heliotrope and extensor surface distribution of *dermatomyositis.*
- *Erythema nodosum* presents with painful nodules that are associated with *streptococcal infection, sarcoid, inflammatory bowel disease,* and other conditions and are located pretibially.
- *Henoch-Schönlein purpura* presents as nonblanching red and blue macules located primarily on the buttocks and lower extremities, concentrated at the ankles.
- *Rocky Mountain spotted* fever starts at the wrists and ankles and spreads centripetally toward the midline.
- *Varicella* begins centrally and spreads centrifugally to the periphery.
- *Erythema infectiosum* (fifth disease) presents with the "slapped cheek" appearance as well as a reticulated rash more over the extremities but in more pronounced cases on the trunk as well.

- *Pityriasis rosea* presents with a unique "herald patch" followed by multiple oval salmon-pink lesions over the trunk, back, and front in a "Christmas tree" pattern. It usually spares the extremities, but in darker-skinned individuals it may take on the "reverse" pattern (FIGURE 16–26).
- *Monilial* rashes are typically over the penis and scrotum or labia in girls. It may extend into the crural region and inner thigh and have satellite lesions around the edges.
- *Tinea versicolor* distributes about the shoulders and back.
- *Scabies* distributes in the webs of the fingers, particularly between the thumb and index finger, and in the groin area. Burrowing lesions also occur over the trunk.
- *Kawasaki disease* rashes are over the trunk and proximal extremities but also accentuate in the groin, perianally, and periurethrally. There is also marked erythema of the palms and soles, as well as mucus membrane involvement.
- *Granuloma annulare* is circular with rubbery edges and is located mainly on the dorsum of the hands and feet or sometimes on extensor joint surfaces.
- *Acanthosis nigricans,* associated with *obesity, polycystic ovary syndrome,* and *insulin resistance,* is dark, rough pigmentation located on the neck, axillae, knuckles, and elbows.
- *Lichen planus* is located on flexural areas and at mucus membranes.
- *Lichen sclerosus et atrophicus* is located on the genitalia and perianally in both sexes.

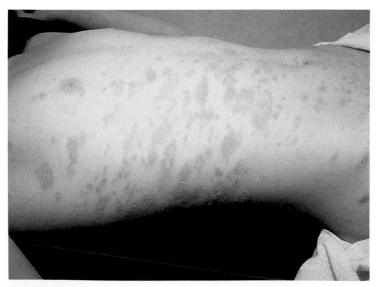

FIGURE 16–26 *Pityriasis Rosea.*

- *Seborrhea* is located on the face, scalp, and eyebrows and in the intertriginous areas.
- *Dyshidrosis* is located on the hands and feet, more on the digits.

A long tabular summary of dermatologic diagnoses ensues, based on configuration and color and then broken down further into pattern distribution, age of occurrence, and associations with systemic disorders. Refer to Chapter 5 for neonatal dermatology. An organizational framework is presented for approaching dermatologic conditions. It is by no means complete and should serve to stimulate further investigation.

Synthesizing a Diagnosis

TABLES 16–1 through 16–5 illustrate macules, papules, nodules and cysts, blisters and bullae, and primary scales. They include secondary complications such as excoriations, erosions, pustules, lichenifications, abscesses, and sinuses when applicable. TABLE 16–6 outlines induration, sclerosis, and atrophy, and TABLE 16–7 illustrates ulcers.

HAIR

The goals of this section are

1. To review anatomy and development of hair follicles
2. To review cycles of hair growth
3. To enumerate the symptoms and signs of abnormalities of hair
4. To develop differential diagnoses related to hair abnormalities

Developmental Anatomy

Hair follicles begin to develop at the end of the first trimester. They originate from ectoderm with an invagination of the epidermis and mesenchyme, the mesoderm, which forms the dermal papilla. FIGURE 16–25 provides an anatomic illustration.

The follicles develop first on the face and by 18 weeks cover the scalp. They then proceed in a cephalad to caudad direction to cover the entire body with lanugo, thin, dark hairs, around 7 months of gestation. Newborns have shed lanugo by birth and replaced it with shorter, finer vellus hairs, although there may be residual lanugo present, often on the newborn's back and ears. Newborns have terminal hairs, darker and thicker, on the scalp, eyelashes, and eyebrows. Newborns may have shed their scalp hair by birth or soon thereafter, but will regrow. At puberty, more terminal hair develops in the axillary and pubic regions.

TABLE 16-1 *Macules*

Configuration and Color	Pattern and Clinical Characteristics	Distribution	Age Incidence	Etiology and Associated Systemic Diagnoses, Comments
I. Red macules:				
A. Exanthems				
1. Measles	Morbilliform, fever, cough, Koplik spots	Face → neck → downward	Unimmunized, all ages	Rubeola virus
2. German measles	Morbilliform, occip. nodes, fever, arthralgia	Face → neck → downward	Unimmunized, all ages	Rubella virus
3. Roseola	Fever, fussy, rash after fever ↓, occip. nodes	Face → neck → downward		Herpes 6 virus
4. Fifth disease (erythema infectiosum)	"Slapped cheek," reticular rash, arthralgia, ↓ RBC production	Cheeks, extremities	Infants (I), children (C), and adolescents (A)	Parvovirus B-19
5. Mononucleosis	Also papules, fatigue, sore throat	Diffuse	I, C, A	Epstein-Barr virus
6. CMV, toxo.	Hepatosplenomegaly (HSM)	Diffuse	C, A	CMV, Toxo
7. Hand-foot-mouth	Also papules and vesicles, throat, palms, soles	Diffuse		Enterovirus
8. Rocky Mt. spotted fever (RMSF)	Tick bite, fever, arthralgia, headache, rash may be petechial → vasculitis	Wrist and ankles, then proximally	C, A	*R. rickettsii*
9. Ehrlichiosis	Similar to RMSF + HSM, meningitis, WBC involvement	More diffuse than RMSF	I, C, A	Ehrlichia sp.

B. Allergies				
1. Urticaria	Itch, wheal, and flare, flat with borders, evanescent	Ubiquitous, blanches	I, C, A	Viral, allergic causes
2. Drug eruption	May be papular, morbiliform, minimal itch	Ubiquitous, blanches	I, C, A	Drug exposure hx
3. Urticaria pigmentosa	Also, papular, vesicular → pigmented (brown) + Darier sign initially	Ubiquitous, blanches initially	I, C, A	Mastocytosis
C. Bacterial infections				
1. Cellulitis	Erythema, ? entry point, lymphangitis, painful	Localized, spreads	I, C, A	Usually strep., staph.
2. Erysipelas	Similar to cellulitis w/ sharp, palpable border	Localized, spreads	I, C, A	Strep. > staph.
3. Toxic shock syndrome	Diffuse erythema, mucosa, desquamates later	High fever, hypotension	A, C	Staph., strep., multisystem, TSST, tampon use, nasal packing
D. Telangiectasias (tel.)	Linear net-like pattern; may bleed in mucous membrane areas; ataxia-tel. with immune and CNS disorder	Single or multiple Reticular or stellate	I, C, A	Ataxia-tel., Weber-Osler-Rendu, collagen-vasc. dis., pregnancy Hepatic disease

(Continued)

TABLE 16-1 Macules (Continued)

Configuration and Color	Pattern and Clinical Characteristics	Distribution	Age Incidence	Etiology and Associated Systemic Diagnoses, Comments
E. Petechiae from abnormal bleeding	Pinpoint, red, nonblanching	Areas of trauma, or diffuse if spontaneous bleeding, HSP located on buttocks and legs	I, C, A	Thrombocytopenia (ITP), malignancy, HUS, collagenvasc.) Vasculitis (HSP, collagenvascular disorders) Sepsis, DIC
F. Inflammatory disorders	Erythema marginatum, urticarial-appearing, evanescent, arciform	Ubiquitous	C, A	Rheumatic fever
	Fleeting, sometimes painful, fever, HSM, arthritis	Truncal, but ubiquitous	I, C, A,	Juvenile rheumatoid arthritis
	Malar butterfly rash, telangiectasias (often periungual), arthritis, hepatic, renal, others	Face, sun-exposed areas, palms and soles	C, A	Lupus erythematosus
	Heliotrope, telangiectasias, may be scaly and atrophic, proximal weakness	Symmetric, extensor joint surfaces	C, A	Dermatomyositis
G. Traumatic 1. First-degree burns	Demarcated, painful; pattern depends on nature of injury (sunburn in exposed areas)	Localized to injury	I, C	Consider child abuse (cigarette burns, submersion, others)

2. Intertrigo	Bright red, some scaling or erosions	Obese pts., rubbing of intertriginous skin	A, C	Mistaken for monilia
3. Petechiae	Location of trauma, "factitious," ruptured capillaries; facial petechiae with severe coughing or vomiting	Pt. generally healthy	A, C, I	Accidental, self-inflicted, abuse, cultural practices (coining)
II. Blue macules				
1. Blue nevus	Sharply circumscribed, may be papular	Anywhere	I, C, A	Benign
2. Melanoma	Irregular borders, nonuniform pigment, variegated color, >4 cm in diameter	Sun-exposed areas	A, C	Fair-skin, + family history
3. Tattoo	Artistic pattern, but may be secondary to foreign body	Anywhere	A, C	History of trauma, FB (e.g., pencil).
III. Purple macules Ecchymoses/purpura	Traumatic in normal patient, but also consider all causes under "Petechiae" above	Anywhere	I, C, A	Review "Petechiae" above

(Continued)

TABLE 16-1 Macules (Continued)

Configuration and Color	Pattern and Clinical Characteristics	Distribution	Age Incidence	Etiology and Associated Systemic Diagnoses, Comments
I. Brown macules				
A. Diffuse hyperpigmentation	Generalized			
1. Endocrine disease	Stria (Cushing), oral hyperpigmentation (Addison), vitiligo, proptosis, goiter (↑ thyroid)	Anywhere, more in sun-exposed areas	A, C, I	Addison, Cushing, hyperthyroidism
2. Metabolic disease	Kayser-Fleischer ring, CNS sx (Wilson), hair and nail changes (hemochromatosis)		A, C	Wilson, hemochromatosis
3. Hepatic disease	Pruritus, jaundice, xanthomata		A, rarely C	Biliary cirrhosis
4. Drug-induced	Hx of malignancy, malaria, cardiac arrhythmia		A, C, I	Antimalarial, anticancer, and antiarrhythmic medications
B. Localized hyperpigmentation				
1. Acanthosis nigricans	Brown to black; may be papular; associated with obesity and insulin resistance; amenorrhea, hirsuitism	Axillae, neck, knuckles and elbows	A, C, I	Insulin resistance, polycystic ovary syndrome (PCOS)

2. Nevi	Uniform, regular border, round	Anywhere	A, C, rarely I	Watch for malignant change
3. Lentigo syndromes	Nevi, atrial myxoma, myx. fibroma, ephelides Lentigo, ECG abn, ocular hypertelorism, pulm. stenosis, abnormal genitalia, retardation, deafness	Anywhere	A, C, I	NAME syndrome LEOPARD syndrome
	Lentigo, GI polyps, premature puberty			Peutz-Jeghers syndrome
4. Becker nevus	Brown to black, irregular pigmentation, satellites, contains hairs	Shoulder and trunk	A, C	
5. Café-au-lait spot	Tan, regular, >0.5 cm, >five, axillary freckles, Lisch nodules, optic gliomas, neurofibromas	Diffuse	A, C	Neurofibromatosis type I
	Tan, irregular, unilateral, precocious puberty, bone dysplasia	Unilateral, single or multiple		McCune-Albright syndrome
6. Postinflammatory hyperpigmentation	Any inflammatory lesion; more in darker-skinned individuals	Location of original lesions	A, C, I	Eczema, drug rash, excoriations

(Continued)

TABLE 16-1 Macules [Continued]

Configuration and Color	Pattern and Clinical Characteristics	Distribution	Age Incidence	Etiology and Associated Systemic Diagnoses, Comments
7. Fungal infection.	Brown, circular, some scaling, clear center; may be red; hair loss	Anywhere, more on thighs, crural area, and trunk	I, C, A	Tinea corporis, cruris, or capitis (ringworm)
	Diaper rash, red to brown	Penis, scrotum labial with satellite lesions		Monilial diaper rash
	Streaky rash, lightly to hypopigmented, occasional scales	Shoulder, neck	C, A	Tinea versicolor
V. White macules				
A. Diffuse (total)	Total body pigment loss	Diffuse	I, C, A	Eye findings: nystagmus, photophobia, ↑ skin ca, Retardation (MR), seizures
1. Albinism	Melanin loss, eczematous rash Albinism	Diffuse	I, C, A	
2. Phenylketonuria				
3. Hematologic problems Hermansky-Pudlak Chediak-Higashi	Total pigment loss, sharply demarcated	Diffuse	I, C, A	Platelet dysfunction, bleeding WBC abnormality, infection
B. Localized				
1. Piebaldism		Face, trunk, back, proximal extremities and symmetrical	I, C, A	Genetic testing available May be associated with deafness (e.g., Waardenburg with white forelock, heterotropia of iris)

566

2. Tuberous sclerosis	Multiple small hypopigmented lesions, +Wood light, Shagreen patches (raised plaques), Angiofibromas on face (formerly Adenoma Sebaceum)	Face, nasolabial folds	C, A, often not detected in infancy	Seizures, MR
3. Incontinentia pigmenti	Diffuse, preceded by vesicular lesions	Swirling pattern (Blaschko)	I, C, A	Developmental delay, usually lethal in males, ectodermal abn.
4. Nevus depigmentosus	Large areas of hypopigmentation	Linear pattern (dermatomal)	C, A, rarely I	Usually isolated, but rarely assoc. with neurologic abn.
5. Halo nevus	Pigmented center, surrounding depigmentation	Anywhere	C, A	Benign, depigmented area of lymphocytic infiltration
6. Pityriasis alba	Discrete, may be scaling	Face and neck	A, C, rarely I	Associated with atopy
7. Postinflammatory hypopigmentation	Localized to areas of original inflammation	Anywhere	A, C, I	Multiple causes, allergic, toxic, infectious/inflammatory
8. Tinea versicolor	See above under postinflammatory hyperpigmentation	Neck, back	C, A	Fungal
9. Vitiligo	Diffuse, sharp, milk-white	Anywhere, nonsymmetric	A, C, I	Absent melanocytes, may be secondary to endocrine or immune disorder

Abbreviations: HSM = hepatosplenomegaly; CMV = cytomegalovirus; TSST = toxic shock syndrome toxin; DIC = disseminated intravascular coagulation; Pts = patients; Assoc. = associated; Abn = abnormal.

TABLE 16–2 *Papules*

Configuration and Color	Pattern and Clinical Characteristics	Distribution	Age Incidence	Etiology and Associated Systemic Diagnoses, Comments
I. Red papules A. Infectious				
1. Folliculitis	Pinpoint, in hair follicles, may form pustules, abscess	Hair location, esp. upper body	A, C, rarely I	Staph. *Pseudomonas* from pools and hot tubs; ↑ in immunocompromised pt.
2. Scarlet fever	Pinpoint "sandpapery", red cheeks, circumoral pallor	Diffuse, ↑ in axilla and groin	C, A	Group A strep. rarely viral (scarlatiniform) Strawberry tongue, Pastia's lines antecubital fossa area
3. Lyme disease	Eryth. chronicum migrans, ring (railroad track edges)	Location of tick bite	A, C	*Borrelia burgdorferi*, assoc. cardiac, neurol., and arthritis
4. Fungal infection	See Table 16–1. Scales Pustules, abscess	Anywhere, abscess more on hands, feet, and scalp	A, C	Tinea cruris (groin), barbis (beard), versicolor, others
5. Secondary syphilis	Maculopapular, scaly	Anywhere, palms and soles	A	Adenopathy, HSM, Treponema pallidum
6. Warts	Pink, scaly, or keratotic; hypopigmented; may be flesh	Anywhere, plantar, periungual	C, A	Papilloma virus
7. Gianotti-Crosti	Small red papules	Face, extremities, buttocks	C, occ I	Viral prodrome, HSM, subsequent hepatitis
8. Scabies	Papules with burrows, may form vesicles	Web of fingers, groin more diffuse in infants	A, C less in I	Sarcoptes scabii, pruritus

B. Allergic				
1. Papular urticaria	Small raised papules, blanches	Anywhere	C, A, I	Pruritic, self-limited, also may be viral; may be larger, polymorphous w/clear centers (E. multiforme)
2. Insect bites	Similar to pap. urt., entry site, excoriations from scratching	Exposed areas	C, A, I	Pruritic, self-limited
3. Drug eruption	Pink-red, may be scaly	Symmetric, oral lesions	A, C, I	Occ. pruritic, unrelated to duration of medication
4. Eczema	Pink, scaly plaque, secondary to weeping, excoriation, ↑ or ↓ pigment with healing; may be nummular (coin-like), pin point follicular in dark skin pt.	Antecubital and popliteal fossae; behind ears, neck, hands; more diffuse and on cheeks in infants	I, C, A	Pruritic, remissions and flares, associated with asthma; nummular eczema more in adolescents
5. Contact dermatitis	Papules initially, may form crusts, plaques & vesicles. May be excoriated	Exposed areas; pattern of contact (streaks for poison ivy, patch below umbilicus for nickel from belt buckle)	C, A, I	Very pruritic, does not spread by scratching unless antigen is present, e.g., rhus oil from poison ivy

(Continued)

TABLE 16-2 *Papules (Continued)*

Configuration and Color	Pattern and Clinical Characteristics	Distribution	Age Incidence	Etiology and Associated Systemic Diagnoses, Comments
C. Inflammatory				
1. Miliaria	Tiny red papules; occ. vesicle	Neck and back; sweat-exposed	I, C, A	Red-miliaria rubra, vesicle-miliaria crystallina
2. Acne	Red or flesh papules (comedones) black papules (open comedones), may be pustular	Face, forehead, back	A, C	Plugged oil glands (whiteheads) become inflamed (blackheads) or infected (pustules)
3. Vasculitis				
a. Blanching				
1. Juvenile rheum. arthritis (JRA)	Discrete red evanescent macules and papules w/fever	Anywhere	I, C, A	Arthritis, lymphadenopathy, hepatosplenomegaly (HSM)
2. Lupus erythematosus	Red papules with scale; over time get pigment change, atrophy, telangiectasia	Sun-exposed or malar area	A, C	Multisystem disease, psych problems, renal, arthritis
3. Kawasaki disease	Papular/macular	Anywhere; erythema of palms and soles; mucus membrane involvement	I, C	Persistent fever, lymphadenopathy, arthritis, coronary aneurysm.
b. Petechial	See "Petechiae," TABLE 16–1	See "Petechiae," TABLE 16–1		See "Petechiae," TABLE 16–1

4. Granulomatous disease				
a. Common				
1. Granuloma annulare	Ring, clear center, rubbery papules on edge.	Dorsum hands and, feet extensor surfaces	A, C	Often mistaken for ringworm. Self-limiting
2. Pyogenic granuloma	Red, vascular, friable	Anywhere, often of face and hands	C, A	Bleed easily. Needs excision.
3. Foreign body (FB)	Red brown papules	Location of FB	I, C, A	Remove foreign body
b. Rare	Red brown papules	Anywhere		Consider leprosy, sarcoidosis, TB and atypical mycobacteria. leishmaniasis, fungal disease
D. Other				
1. Seborrhea	Scaly, greasy, occ crusts and plaques	Scalp, eyebrows, eyelids, cheeks, intertriginous areas	I, C, A	"Cradle cap" in infants
2. Keratosis pilaris	Perifollicular, pinpoint, pink, horny papules	Extensor surface of arms and thighs	A, C, I	Assoc. with dry skin (eczema, ichthyosis)
3. Pityriasis, rosea	Large herald patch, salmon color oval small patches in "Christmas tree" pattern, scaly	Trunk, proximal extremities	A, C	Mild itching, self-limiting (up to 3 months), mistaken for tinea
4. Psoriasis	Red plaques, may be pustular, sharp margins, white-silvery scale; may have guttate (droplike) pattern, nail pitting	Anywhere, but often extensor surfaces, scalp	A, C	Chronic or recurrent, mild itch, often mistaken for eczema, tinea, or seborrhea; guttate-type assoc. with strep. and is self-limited Often mistaken for eczema

(Continued)

TABLE 16-2 *Papules (Continued)*

Configuration and Color	Pattern and Clinical Characteristics	Distribution	Age Incidence	Etiology and Associated Systemic Diagnoses, Comments
5. Eczematoid rashes				
a. Dyshidrosis	Papules, peeling, burning	Hands, feet, big toes	A, C, I	Areas of sweating, excessive
b. Eczema herpeticum	Umbilicated vesicles	Preexisting eczema → spreads	C, I, A	Herpes simplex present aka Kaposi's varicelliform eruption
c. Lip-smacking dermatitis	Irritated, scale, fissure, crust	Perioral, cheilitis	C, A	History of lip licking
d. Wiskott-Aldrich syndrome	Eczematous or seborrheic, petechiae	Anywhere	I, C, A	Immunodeficiency, draining ears, thrombocytopenia
e. Acrodermatitis enteropathica	Patches with crusting, weeping, excoriations, pustules	Acral areas, tip of nose perioral hands and feet, diaper area	I	Zinc deficiency
f. Metabolic disorders				Consider PKU, biotin deficiency, urea cycle defects
7. Strawberry hemangioma	Deep red, blanching	Any location	I	Absent or small at birth, maximize by 9 mos., then regress; turn gray when resolving

II. Flesh-colored papules

	Description	Location		Notes
1. Acne, warts	See under "Red Papules"			
2. Molluscum contagiosum	Smooth, domed, umbilicated, white plug	Anywhere	C, A	Poxvirus, contain eosinophils
3. Neurofibromatosis	See under "Brown Macules"	Anywhere	C, A, I	Fleshy neurofibromas
4. Tuberous sclerosis	See under "White Macules"	Angiofibromas of face	C, A, I	
5. Nevi	See under "Brown Macules"	Anywhere	A, C, fewer in I	Watch for malignant change
6. Keloids	Shiny, bulging, sharp border	Area of injury	A, C	Dark-skinned pts, female > male
7. Lichen sclerosus et atrophicus	May be macular, scaly, in plaques or atrophic	Anywhere, often genitalia	A, C	
8. Lichen striatus	Linear, scaly, sometimes erythematous	Blaschko's lines	A, C	Self-limiting, may be genetic, lethal in males
9. Lichen nitidus	Pinpoint, may coalesce, non scaling	Arms, genitalia, dorsal hand	A, C	Koebner phenomenon, male > female

III. Brown papules
A. Single

	Description	Location		Notes
1. Mastocytosis	See "Red Macules/Allergies"			
2. Melanoma	Changing mole, spreading, irregular border, pigment variability	Sun-exposed areas	A, C (rarely)	"ABCD" mnemonic, asymmetry, border, color, and diameter

(Continued)

TABLE 16-2 *Papules (Continued)*

Configuration and Color	Pattern and Clinical Characteristics	Distribution	Age Incidence	Etiology and Associated Systemic Diagnoses, Comments
B. Multiple				
1. Multiple atypical nevi	May be macular, some color and border variation	Sun-exposed areas, fair-skinned patients	A, C	Watch for malignant changes
2. Langerhans histiocytosis	May be yellow or macular, seborrhea-like	Trunk, axilla, groin	A, C, I	Systemic involvement, bone marrow infiltration, diabetes insipidus
3. Acanthosis nigricans	See "Brown Macules"			
IV. Blue-black papules				
A. Single				
1. Melanoma	See "Brown Papules" and "Blue Macules"			
2. Ecthyma gangrenosum	Blue to black center; may be multiple	Anywhere, often axillary or genital area	I, C, A	Malignancy or immunosuppression *Pseudomonas aeruginosa*
3. Blue nevi	See "Blue Macules"			
4. Foreign body	See "Blue Macules"			

B. Multiple				
1. Lichen planus	Some scales, hyperkeratosis, hyper/hypopigmentation, See "Red Papules"	Flexural surfaces, mucosa, genitalia	A, rarely C	"Four p's" purple, pruritic polygonal papules
2. Acne				Blackheads
V. Purple papules	See "Purple Macules"			
1. Subacute bacterial endocarditis	Osler's nodes (tender), Janeway lesions (nontender) Splinter hemorrhages	Fingers and toes Palms Subungual	A, C, I	Fever, changing heart murmur
VI. Yellow papules				
1. Xanthomas	May be eruptive (surrounding erythema), noneruptive, or tubular	Eruptive, anywhere. Noneruptive, extensor areas, over tendons eyelids (xanthelasma)	A, C	Severe hyperlipidemia, liver disease, nephrotic syndrome, thyroid disorders
2. Pseudoxanthoma elasticum	Pale, grouped, interspersed with normal skin	Flexural areas, neck	A, C	Diffuse arterial disease, premature myocardial infarction

Abbreviations: HSM = hepatosplenomegaly; PKU = phenylketonuria; mos = months; TB = tuberculosis; w/ = with; occ. = occasional; psych = psychological; Pt = patient; E = erythema; esp = especially; neurol = neurological.

TABLE 16–3 Nodules and Cysts

Configuration and Color	Pattern Characteristics	Distribution	Age Incidence	Etiology and Associated Systemic Diagnoses, Comments
I. Cysts				
A. Epidermal				
1. Epidermoid cyst	Single or multiple, white keratin	Face, scalp, neck, trunk	C, A, milia in infants	Gardner syndrome (polyps, desmoid tumors)
2. Vellus hair cyst	Small, 1–2 mm, from vellus follicle	Anywhere	C, A	May be genetic
3. Steatocystoma	1–3 cm, yellowish, sebaceous glands and hair follicles	Chest, arms, face	C, A	Autosomal dominant type (multiple)
4. Syringomas	1–2 mm; flesh to brown, numerous	Face, eyelids, cheeks, genitalia	A	Females > males; ↑ in Down syndrome
5. Trichoepithelioma	Skin-colored up to 8 mm diameter	Cheeks, lips, labial fold	C, A	large and multiple = autosomal dominant, disfiguring
B. Dermal				
1. Dermoid cyst	Congenital, firm, attached to bone	Eyes, head, neck over bony ridges	I, C, A	Contains dermal structures
C. Subdermal cysts				
1. Synovial (ganglion)	Over tendon, feels tense	Wrist, anywhere, one or more	A, C	Enlarge after trauma or bleeding

II. Nodules
A. Flesh and red color

1. Dermatofibroma	0.3–1-cm diameter; may be dimpled	Trauma or amputation	A, C	
2 Angiofibroma	"White macules," tuberous sclerosis	Anywhere + mucosa	C, A	
3. Neurofibroma	"White macules," neurofibromatosis but may be sporadic and solitary	Face, lips, oral mucosa	A, C I, C, A	
4. Neuromas	Solitary traumatic Multiple—idiopathic Multiple—Multiple endocrine neoplasia	Anywhere	C, A A, C C, A	Autosomal dominant, medullary cancer of thyroid and pheochromocytoma
5. Cowden disease	Multiple hamartomas		A, C	Autosomal dominant, multiple hamartomas of ecto-, endo-, and mesodermal origin; assoc, with cancer of breast and thyroid

B. Juxtaarticular

1. Rheumatoid arthritis	Multiple, symmetric	Elbow, hand, ankle, knee	A, C	
2. Rheumatic fever	Multiple, symmetric	Elbow, hand	A, C	Major criterion for rheumatic fever
3. Xanthoma	See "yellow papules"		A, C	

(Continued)

TABLE 16-3 *Nodules and Cysts (Continued)*

Configuration and Color	Pattern Characteristics	Distribution	Age Incidence	Etiology and Associated Systemic Diagnoses, Comments
C. Inflamed red nodules				
1. Carbuncle	Red, warm, fluctuant	Areas with hair	A, C, I	Pus, culture for bacterial etiology
2. Hydradenitis suppurativa	Develops from pustules, abscesses	Groin, axilla	A, occ. C	Inflammation of apocrine gland; may develop sinus as complication
3. Erythema nodosum	Red-blue, tender 1–5 cm diameter, varying stages, may be recurrent	Pretibial area	A, C,	Associated with strep., sarcoidosis, tuberculosis (TB), inflammatory bowel disease, allergy, oral contraception, collagen-vascular disease
4. Panniculitis				
a. Cold	Red, indurated, nontender, may have plaques	Cheeks, or other areas if cold-exposed	I, C	Crystallization and rupture of fat cells, self-limiting
b. Subcutaneous fat necrosis	Similar to cold panniculitis, spontaneous	Anywhere	I	Self-limiting
c. Lupus panniculitis	Purplish, painless, 1–5 cm	Face, extremities, buttocks	A, C	Resistant to treatment, may be disfiguring

TABLE 16–4 *Blisters (Vesicles) and Bullae*

Configuration and Color	Pattern Clinical Characteristics	Distribution	Age Incidence	Etiology and Associated Systemic Diagnoses, Comments
I. Vesicles and bullae				
A. Vesicles				
1. Miliaria crystallina	Tiny (see "Papules")		I, C, A	"Prickly heat"
2. Dyshidrosis	Tiny (see "Papules")		C, A, I	
3. Insect bites (flea, scabies)	May vesiculate (see "Papules")		C, A, I	
4. Contact dermatitis/ eczema	See "Papules"			
5. Hand-foot-mouth disease	Vesicles with red base	Palms, soles, throat (posterior)	C, A, I	Enterovirus (coxsackie A types)
6. Varicella (chickenpox)	Umbilicated, red base, eventually form crusts	Proximal → distal, centrifugal, mucosal surfaces		Fever, pruritus
7. Eczema herpeticum	See "Papules"			
8. Herpes simplex I, primary	Vesicles → crusts	Oral mucosa, gingivae, tongue	I, C	Fever, → diminished intake, painful
9. HSV I recurrent	"Cold sores"	Oral mucosa, face "whitlow" on finger	C, A	Recur same location, stings initially, associated with illness or stress
10. Herpes zoster	Umbilicated vesicles → crusts	Dermatomal, also eye and face	A, C	Sting or burn initially, mistaken for impetigo
11. HSV II	Groups of vesicles	Genitalia	A	STD, burning, may be primary or secondary; observe for transmission to newborn

(Continued)

TABLE 16–4 *Blisters (Vesicles) and Bullae [Continued]*

Configuration and Color	Pattern Clinical Characteristics	Distribution	Age Incidence	Etiology and Associated Systemic Diagnoses, Comments
B. Bullae, traumatic				
1. Second-degree Burns	See "Macules" for first-degree burns	Dependent pressure areas	I, C, A	Consider abuse based on distribution
2. Pressure sores	Associated w/plaque (rubbing)		I, C, A	Severe disability
C. Bullae, infectious				
1. Impetigo	Yellow crust, weeping, satellite lesions, erosions, yellow crusts, pustules	Anywhere, esp. face mouth, nose	I, C, A	Bullae most likely staph. infection
2. Staph.-scalded skin syndrome	Diffuse erythema, exfoliation	Generalized +Nikolsky sign	I ,C, A	SSSS toxin
3. Dermatophyte infection	Red erosion, scale and crust	Palms, soles, fingers and toes	A, C	Originally a blister
D. Bullae-immunologic				
1. Pemphigus vulgaris (PV)	Severe, large bullae, erosions Intraepidermal	Start on scalp, oral mucosa, then spread all over	A, C	Severely ill, can be fatal, due to secondary sepsis, +Nikolsky sign, IgG antibody to desmoglein

2. Pemphigus foliaceus	Similar in appearance, more superficial on biopsy	Similar to PV	A, C	Not as ill as PV, may be self-limited or persistent. IgG antibody to desmoglein
3. Linear IgA bullous dermatosis, CBDC (chronic bullous dermatosis of childhood)	Tense small bullae, may be linear or annular "string of pearls," subepidermal	Lower trunk, legs, but may spread anywhere	C, A	Varying degree of illness. Biopsy with PMN and eosinophils. IgA antibodies, local and circulating
4. Bullous pemphigoid	Tense blisters >2 cm, subepidermal	Similar to CBDC, occasional oral mucosa involvement	C, A	Subepidermal bullae, IgG and C3 deposits on roof of blister, eosinophils
5. Epidermolysis bullosa acquisita	Similar to BP; more mucous membrane involvement	Acral initially, but may spread	A, C	IgG deposits at base of blister; defect in collagen VII; assoc. with IBD and collagen-vascular disease
E. Bullae, other				
1. Epidermolysis bullosa simplex	Mild, recurrent	Acral, elbows, knees	I, C	Autosomal dominant. Superficial, intraepidermal, improves with age
2. Epidermolysis bullosa letalis	Severe associated with atrophy and dystrophy; subepidermal	At birth, anywhere, but generally spares acral areas except for nails	I, C	Autosomal recessive may be lethal, severe mucous membrane and nail involvement

(Continued)

TABLE 16-4 Blisters (Vesicles) and Bullae (Continued)

Configuration and Color	Pattern Clinical Characteristics	Distribution	Age Incidence	Etiology and Associated Systemic Diagnoses, Comments
3. Stevens-Johnson syndrome (SJS)	Severe mucous membrane involvement, extensive, confluent blisters, thin-walled, + Nikolsky sign, split at epidermal-dermal junction with necrosis	Starts as red macules on head, spreading down and forming blisters after 1–3 days	A, C	Prodrome of fever, flulike symptoms, severely ill, may get secondary sepsis, scarring, and permanent damage to eyes (keratitis); associated with drugs such as phenobarbital, antibiotics
4. Toxic epidermal necrolysis (TEN)	Severe end of spectrum for SJS	See SJS above	A, C	More severe than SJS, higher morbidity and mortality
5. Erythema multiforme	Formally thought as mild end of SJS spectrum; hivelike lesions with some target formation, may form blisters	Anywhere, mild mucous membrane involvement	A, C	Infectious causes, mycoplasma, recurrent herpes

Abbreviations: STD = sexually transmitted disease; IBD = inflammatory bowel disease; assoc. = associated; PMN = polymorphonuclear neutrophils; esp = especially; w/ = with.

TABLE 16-5 *Primary Scales*

Configuration and Color	Pattern and Clinical Characteristics	Distribution	Age Incidence	Etiology and Associated Systemic Diagnoses, Comments
I. Ichthyoses				
A. Lamellar ichthyosis	Collodion baby, large thick brown scales after collodion clears, scars	More on legs and scalp; facial involvement → ectropion	I, C, A	↑ water loss, temp. instability, autosomal recessive, 1:100,000 incidence
B. Ichthyosiform erythroderma	Similar to lamellar ichthyosis, erythematous, bullous and nonbullous forms	Similar to lamellar ichthyosis; flexural and intertriginous areas	I, C, A	Autosomal recessive 1:100,000 incidence
C. Ichthyosis vulgaris	Mild scaling	Diffuse, spares flexural areas	I, C, A	Starts around 3 mos., improves over time; autosomal dominant, incidence 1:250; association with atopic dermatitis
D. X-linked ichthyosis	Large "dirty" scales, mild	Similar to ichthyosis vulgaris	I, C, A	Starts around 3 mos., improves with age, incidence 1 to 2:6000 males, assoc. with cryptorchidism, Kallmann and Poland syndromes

(*Continued*

TABLE 16-5 *Primary Scales (Continued)*

Configuration and Color	Pattern and Clinical Characteristics	Distribution	Age Incidence	Etiology and Associated Systemic Diagnoses, Comments
E. Epidermolytic hyperkeratosis	Diffuse scaling, blisters at birth	Generalized, esp intertriginous areas, palms and soles	I, C, A	Autosomal dominant or sporadic, worsens with age, foul odor due to skin to bacterial overgrowth
II. Syndromes with ichthyosis				
A. Netherton syndrome	Hair shaft abnormality, linear pattern, lamellar	Anywhere	I, C, A	Autosomal recessive, failure to thrive
B. Refsum disease	Similar to ichthyosis vulgaris	Similar to ichthyosis vulgaris	A	Blindness, deafness, ataxia, polyneuritis, disorder of phytanic acid metabolism
C. Sjögren-Larsson syndrome	Lamellar ichthyosis	Similar to lamellar ichthyosis	I, C, A	Spasticity, MR, seizures, tooth defects
D. KID syndrome	Keratosis, ichthyosis, deafness	Extremities, head	I, C, A	Keratoconjunctivitis
E. CHILD syndrome	Ichthyosiform nevi	Anywhere	I, C, A	X-linked recessive, congenital hemidysplasia, ichthyosiform nevi, limb defects; also heart and renal defects
F. Conradi syndrome	Ichthyosis, erythroderma, alopecia	See "Ichthyosiform. erythroderma"	I, C, A	Chondrodysplasia punctata, eye and bone defects

TABLE 16-6 *Induration, Sclerosis, Atrophy*

Configuration and Color	Pattern and Clinical Characteristics	Distribution	Age Incidence	Etiology and Associated Systemic Diagnoses, Comments
I. Induration and sclerosis				
A. More common				
1. Urticaria pigmentosa	See "Red macules"	Generalized, more groin and axillae	I, C, A	More severe cases
2. Scleredema	Induration, diffuse, red	Chest and back	A, C	Post strep. infection
3. Scleroderma	Poorly defined, variable thickening, pigmentation, calcifications	Acral → proximal	A, C	Ulceration of fingertips; calcincosis circumscripta
B. Rare				Amyloidosis, ataxia-telangiectasia, porphyria, graft-vs.-host, leprosy, mucopolysaccharidosis, hypothyroidism (myxedema), PKU, progeria
II. Atrophy				
A. More common				
1. Lichen sclerosus et atrophicus	See "Flesh-colored papules"			
2. Lupus erythematosus	Red, scaly, telangiectasia, variable pigmentation, hair loss, plaques	Sun-exposed areas, scalp	A, C, I	Females > males, multisystem involvement, renal hematologic, CNS, others

(Continued)

585

TABLE 16-6 *Induration, Sclerosis, Atrophy (Continued)*

Configuration and Color	Pattern and Clinical Characteristics	Distribution	Age Incidence	Etiology and Associated Systemic Diagnoses, Comments
3. Morphea	White-yellow, circumscribed plaque	Trunk, proximal extremities, face	A, C	Females > males, nonprogressive form of scleroderma
4. Poikiloderma	Atrophic, scaly, mottled, wrinkly	Face, neck, trunk	I, C	Associated with malignancies
5. Ehlers-Danlos syndrome	Wrinkly, "cigarette-paper," purpuric	Areas of trauma	C, A	Hyperextensibility, collagen deficiency, 10 clinical forms
6. Striae	Linear, usually vertical; colored red, white, purple	Areas of growth and stretch	A, C	Females > males, assoc. with pregnancy, weightlifting, obesity, Cushing syndrome, steroid toxicity
7. Necrobiosis lipoidica diabeticorum	Red-yellow plaques, ulcer	Anywhere, especially shins	A	Long-standing diabetes, can be painful
8. Trauma	Depressed areas	Trauma or injection site	A, C	Insulin, steroid, or other injection sites
9. Scarring (atrophic)	Depressed, hypopigmented	Site of inflammation	A, C, I	Varicella, shingles, smallpox, rickettsial pox
B. Rarer				
1. Progeria	Induration, sclerosis, atrophy	Diffuse	I, C, A	Alopecia, birdlike, early atherosclerosis
2. Lawrence-Seip syndrome	Dystrophy, acanthosis nigricans, hirsutism	Generalized, severe	I, C, A	Multiple endocrine abnormalities, insulin resistance
3. Werner syndrome	Scleroderma-like, calcifying	More on face	A	Diabetes, hypogonadism, early atherosclerosis

Abbreviations: PKU = phenylketonuria; CNS = central nervous system; assoc. = associated; esp. = especially; mos. = months; MR = mental retardation; Temp = temperature.

TABLE 16-7 *Ulcers*

Configuration and Color	Pattern and Clinical Characteristics	Distribution	Age Incidence	Etiology and Associated Systemic Diagnoses, Comments
I. Painless				
A. Neuropathic	Sharp, heaped edges	Areas of trauma, pressure	A, C, I	Sensation loss (spina bifida, neuropathy, toxic metal ingestion, diabetes)
II. Painful				
A. Ischemic				
1. Vasculitis	Small, sharp edges, purpura, possible gangrene	Acral, but spread anywhere	A, C, I	Consumptive coagulopathy (e.g., DIC), septic emboli, collagen-vascular diseases, calcinosis cutis, Behçet's, cryoglobulinemia, Hgb SS, ergotism
B. Granulomas	Similar to ischemic, may be assoc. with vasculitis	Midline, nasal, oral, mucous membraines	A, C	Inflammatory bowel disease, TB (lupus vulgaris), Wegener (older adolescents)
C. Mechanical				
1. Decubital	Undermined, spread in diameter and depth	Pressure areas, bony prominences	A, C, I	Bedridden patients, e. g., profound impairment
2. Traumatic	Configuration of area of trauma, possible gangrene	Location of trauma		Burns, cold, corrosives

(Continued)

TABLE 16-7 *Ulcers (Continued)*

Configuration and Color	Pattern and Clinical Characteristics	Distribution	Age Incidence	Etiology and Associated Systemic Diagnoses, Comments
3. Radiation	Bullae → shaggy ulcers → sharp ulcers if chronic, variable pigmentation, telangiectasia	Location of radiation therapy	A, C, I	Cancer patients
4. Factitious	Odd shape, scarring	Arms, face	A, C	Self-mutilation (Lesch-Nyhan synd.), adolescents with psychiatric problems (rubbing, cutting)
D. Infectious				
1. Puncture wounds	Indurated and yellow, white, or brown base, satellites, occ. sinus	Area of bite, abscess	A, C, I	Determine bacterial etiology (staph, MRSA, strep., TB, *Pasturella multocida* for animal bite, others)
2. Multiple rarer causes	Indurated and yellow, white, or brown base, satellites, occ. sinus			Anthrax, atypical *mycobacteria*, *Cryptococcus*, blastomycosis, coccidioidomycosis, Pseudomonas (ecthyma gangrenosum)
3. Ulcer + adenopathy a. Cat scratch fever	Nodes ± painful May present only as large node	Arm, hand, face, axillary node	A, C	*Bartonella henselae*, cat scratch, bite, or lick
b. Tularemia	Oculoglandular type	Face, eyes, and limbs	A, C, I	*Pasturella tularensis*, rodent or tick from rodent

588

c. Sporotrichosis	Ulcer, nodules along lymphatics	Finger, hand	A, C	*Sporothrix schenckii*, roses, timber, other plants
d. Rarer types				Plague, amebiasis, leishmaniasis, leprosy, yaws
4. Genital ulcers				
a. Aphthous	Painful, small, sharp margins	± Nodes	A	Behçet's, viral etiologies
b. Balan(oposth)itis	Erythema, pain	Glans penis and prepuce	A, C	Bacterial (strep., staph.), monilial
c. Primary syphilis	Chancre, single, punched-out, indurated base, ± pain, nodes	Male and female (often missed)	A	If in child, sexual abuse until proven otherwise, *Treponema pallidum* on darkfield exam
d. Gonorrhea	Mild erosions → small ulcer, marked exudate	Male and female (often missed)	A	If in child, sexual abuse until proven otherwise; *Neisseria gonorrhoeae*
e. Herpes simplex	Vesicles → erosions → ulcer, stinging		A, C	Think abuse in children Herpes simplex, +Tzanck smear, PCR; in child, think sexual abuse but not always
f. Genital warts	Heaped up, cauliflower-like, but may be flat	± Nodes	A	Condyloma acuminata: +HPV, possible sexual abuse (about 50 percent)
			A, C, I	Condyloma lata, secondary syphilis, sexual abuse in children until proven otherwise

Abbreviations: DIC = disseminated intravascular coagulation; Hgb SS = sickle cell anemia; MRSA = methicillin-resistant *Staphylococcus aureus*; PCR = polymerase chain reaction; HPV = human papilloma virus; synd = syndrome; TB = tuberculosis.

Physiology

The normal hair cycle consists of the following phases:

Anagen. This represents active growth, where the hair follicle begins in the deep dermis and wraps itself around the dermal papilla. The loose previous hair of that follicle is pushed out. This phase generally lasts 2 to 3 years.

Catagen. This is a transitional phase lasting about 3 weeks. Hair growth ceases, and the hair bulb dislodges itself from the dermal papilla. The end of the hair now has a blunt club shape to it.

Telogen. This is the resting phase, which lasts 3 to 4 months. The hair now assumes a mace-like shape at the base and dislodges itself with the onset of the new anagen phase.

At any given time 70 percent or more of hair is in the anagen phase, so ongoing hair loss is not noticeable.

Problems

Although most of dermatology is morphology-driven, there are still key historical points to cover:

- Time of onset? Congenital or acquired?
- How does the condition progress? Does it wax and wane? Is it becoming steadily worse?
- Is there a patient history of systemic illness that may explain the problem?
- Is there a family history of a similar condition?
- Are there associated systemic symptoms and signs with the present condition?
- Is the patient exposed to medications or toxins that may cause hair loss?
- Is there any pain, stinging, or pruritus?
- Is there a history of injury or underlying allergy or infection?
- How is the patient's emotional stability? Is there a history of self-mutilation or hair pulling?

Findings

Hair problems are due to hair loss (alopecia), excess hair (hypertrichosis), or abnormalities of the hair shaft. Examination of hair is by observation and palpation. Key findings related to each of the problems are enumerated below.

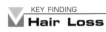
KEY FINDING
Hair Loss

Pattern

Is the hair completely or partially absent? Is the shaft intact or abnormal? Is there a differential in length of hairs that are present? Is the hair loss in patches or diffuse? What is the shape of the patch? Are there abnormalities of the skin underlying the area of hair loss such as inflammation or scarring, or is the underlying skin smooth? Are there hair stubbles present?

Distribution

Is the hair loss focal or diffuse? Did it begin focal and spread, or has it always been diffuse? What specific areas are involved?

General Physical Examination

Are there any abnormalities of other ectodermally derived structures (CNS, eyes, and teeth)? Is there difficulty with temperature control, as manifest by excessively warm skin or lack of perspiration? Does the general physical examination lead to any other systemic conditions?

Synthesizing a Diagnosis

The best approach is to use the patient history to categorize whether the condition is congenital/genetic, metabolic/toxic, infectious/inflammatory, or traumatic. We will take each category and build on it with key findings to arrive at a diagnosis.

Congenital/Genetic

Check the underlying scalp for abnormalities. Cutis aplasia and incontinentia pigmenti cause scarring. Nevi or hemangiomas will retard hair growth in the involved areas. It is helpful to examine hair shafts under magnification. In *monilethrix* the hair has a beaded appearance, whereas in *pili torti* the shaft is twisted. In *trichorrhexis invaginata* the hair appears like bamboo, and in *trichothiodystrophy* the hair appears ribbon-like. TABLE 16–8 demonstrates differential diagnoses that are congenital and/or genetic in origin.

Metabolic/Toxic

Is there a family history of metabolic disorders? *Hyperthyroidism* is associated with hair loss. Consider *homocystinuria*, often associated with Marfanoid habitus, ectopia lentis, and blood clot formation. *Johanson-Blizzard* syndrome consists of hypothyroidism, pancreatic insufficiency, genital defects, craniofacial malformations, and developmental delay. Toxins may cause hair loss by direct damage with associated scarring. Examples are alkali burns, thermal burns, radiation, surgery, allergens, and heavy metal intoxication such as thallium and arsenic.

TABLE 16-8 *Congenital Hair Loss*

Observation	Diagnoses
Localized	
I. Nonscarring	
A. Underlying skin abnormality	Nevus, sebaceous nevus, hemangioma, hamartoma
II. Scarring	Incontinentia pigmenti, cutis aplasia
Generalized	
I. No underlying skin abnormality	
A. Isolated	Monilethrix
B. Syndromic	Menkes kinky hair syndrome (pili torti, severe retardation), woolly hair syndrome (pili torti), trichothiodystrophy (retardation, hypogonadism, progeria-like), progeria (thinning of skin, senile pigmentary changes), cartilage-hair hypoplasia syndrome (leg bowing, wide metaphyses, short stature), trichorhino phalangeal syndrome (mild loose skin, protruding ears, bulbous nose, bony abnormalities, mild retardation), Hallermann-Streiff syndrome (short stature, frontal bossing, thin nose, parrot-like, eye defects)
II. Underlying skin abnormality (syndromic)	Ectodermal dysplasia syndromes associated with eye, CNS, hypohidrosis; dyskeratosis congenita (poikiloderma, reticulate pigmentation, telangiectasia, atrophy), CHILD syndrome (hemidysplasia, ichthyosis, limb defects)

Hair loss from *chemotherapy* is nonscarring and results from cessation of the anagen phase of hair growth.

Infectious/Inflammatory

Tinea capitis, or scalp fungus, is endemic among African-American children. It starts with mild, red, scaly patches of the scalp, and hair loss ensues. The pattern is typically with stubble formation owing to hair breakage. Lesions are annular but also can be diffuse. The scalp lesions may become inflamed, forming pustules that often are misconstrued for impetigo. Occasionally, the inflammation becomes more intense and forms raised, boggy plaques (kerions).

Alopecia areata presents as localized round patches of hair loss with perfectly smooth skin. They vary in size and on rare occasions will progress to *alopecia totalis* (entire scalp) or *alopecia universalis* (entire body). Hairs from the periphery of the area of loss will resemble exclamation points under magnification. Although there is no outward evidence of inflammation, skin biopsies do indicate evidence of lymphocytic infiltration and antigen-antibody complexes.

Telogen and anagen effluvium results from the arrest of the hair cycle at either stage. This is often a consequence of a high fever, infection, stress such as surgery, and certain drugs. There is loss of hair over a 3- to 5-month period. Although distressing, the hair invariably grows back over several months. Presence of club-shaped hairs supports this diagnosis. *Anagen effluvium* is the result of chemotherapy and heavy metal intoxication.

Traumatic

Traumatic hair loss is common in children and usually manifests in bizarre patterns. Traction alopecia results from devices such as barrettes and bands that pull hair out over time. Hair pulling (*trichotillomania*) is not uncommon in children. In toddlers, this may be a normal means of self-stimulation to induce sleep (often with hair twirling and thumb sucking), but in older children and adolescents, it may be a manifestation of an obsessive-compulsive disorder. Typically, there is not complete hair loss in the patches, and the length of each hair is variable.

In small infants, particularly with the present "back to sleep" movement, many have a large occipital patch of hair loss owing to constant exertion of pressure on that area. This is a self-limiting condition that resolves as the infant sits and spends less time on his or her back.

Hypertrichosis or Hirsutism

Hypertrichosis refers to localized patches of increased hair growth. Examples in children are *nevi* and *hamartomas.* It also may be a consequence of localized application of steroids, particular androgenic, or become more extensive owing to *hypothyroidism, porphyria,* or exposure to other *drugs* such as phenytoin, cyclosporine, and minoxidil.

Hirsutism refers to excessive hair growth in a child or a woman in a male pattern. This often results from endocrine dysfunction, examples of which are *Cushing, adrenogenital,* and *polycystic ovary syndromes.*

Hirsutism may be congenital and can be either genetic (syndromic) or the result of exposure to toxins such as phenytoin and alcohol. Examples of syndromes include *Coffin-Siris syndrome, mucopolysaccharidoses, leprechaunism, trisomy 18, Marshall-Smith syndrome,* and others. Consult a text on dysmorphology for further detail.

NAILS

The goals of this section are

1. To review developmental anatomy of the nails
2. To enumerate key historical and physical findings
3. To develop differential diagnoses for nail abnormalities

Developmental Anatomy

The nails begin development at 10 to 11 weeks of gestation with a skin fold, out of which develops the nail matrix. The matrix is the area of growth, producing the more visible distal nail plate. The white crescent at the base of the nail (lunula) is the distal end of the nail matrix. A normal newborn has fully developed nails.

Problems

Nail disorders are either congenital or acquired. Thus a full history is paramount to arriving at a diagnosis. Key historical points are

- When did the patient or caregiver first notice this abnormality?
- Is there a family history of any dermatologic or nail disorders?
- Are there any exposures to infections, medications, or toxins (include travels)?
- Is there a past history of any dermatologic illness, including but not limited to psoriasis, alopecia areata, lichen planus, and atopy?
- Is there a past history of systemic illness such as lupus erythematosus, immunodeficiency, uremia, or endocrine disorder?
- Is there any history of trauma?

Findings

Descriptions of key nail abnormalities are as follows:

- Absence, atrophy, or dysplasia
- Hypertrophy of nail bed (onychauxis, pachyonychia)
- Spoon nail (koilonychia)
- Clubbing (angle between nail bed and plate greater than 20 degrees)
- Nail pitting (psoriasis, alopecia areata)
- Brittle nail plates (onychorrhexis)
- Separation of the nail (onycholysis)
- Discolored nail plates (yellow, red, blue, white)
- Subungual hemorrhage or hematoma
- Nail ridging (transverse of longitudinal)
- Transverse lines or ridges (Mees lines, Beau lines)

Synthesizing a Diagnosis

Nail disorders are divided into congenital/genetic and acquired. Acquired disorders may be metabolic/toxic/nutritional, infectious/ inflammatory, traumatic, or associated with many chronic illnesses. Sometimes they are idiopathic. Diagnoses below and their key historical points and findings are discussed below.

Congenital

See TABLE 16–9.

Acquired

- *Metabolic/toxic/nutritional.* Congenital metabolic disorders such as Lesch-Nyhan syndrome manifest hypoplasia of nails owing to hyperuricemia and nail abnormalities owing to self-inflicted trauma. Nail dystrophy is prominent in *acrodermatitis enteropathica* (zinc deficiency) and diabetes. Also, *uremia* produces whitening of the proximal nail bed. Always be mindful of nail hypoplasia caused by *in utero exposure* to anticonvulsants, warfarin, and alcohol. *Malnutrition* and specific deficiencies manifest as nail abnormalities. The nails of generalized malnutrition are dry and brittle and may contain transverse ridges. They are also friable and appear laminated (onychorrhexis). *Iron deficiency* or *hemachromatosis* may cause koilonychia. *Chronic poisoning* by heavy metals such as thallium, and arsenic or fluoride, may cause transverse white bands *(Mees nails)*. Chronic tetracycline exposure, more likely in adolescents, may cause onycholysis. Changes in nail color may be due to tetracycline exposure

TABLE 16-9 *Congenital/Genetic Disorders of Nails*

Diagnosis	Key Historical Points	Key Findings and Comments
I. Isolated		
A. Koilonychia	No other abnormalities	Spooning, clubbing, autosomal dominant, benign
B. Ingrown nails		Self-limiting, benign in infants
C. Congenital clubbing	No cardiac or pulmonary problems	Isolated and benign
II. Ectodermal dysplasias		
Pachyonychia congenita	Deafness, blindness, keratoses	Nail thickening, yellow-brown discoloration
Dyskeratosis congenita	See TABLE 16-8	Similar to pachyonychia congenita
III. Hereditary disorders w/systemic involvement		
A. Nail-patella syndrome	Not limited to nails, +family history	Autosomal dominant, absence or hypoplasia of nail and patella
B. Tuberous sclerosis	Retardation, +family history	Periungual fibromas; see "White macules," "Flesh-colored papules," and "Cysts" above.
C. Ichthyosis	See primary scales table	Hyperplastic nails
D. Chromosomal abn.	Retardation, multiple anomalies	13, 18, 21, 3q, 7q, 8p, and 9p (aplastic, hypoplastic), Turner,
1. Trisomies		Noonan (hypoplastic, koilonychia), Coffin-Siris,
2. Others		Hallermann-Streiff, others, koilonychia in trichothiodystrophy,
E. Rarer syndromes		incontinentia pigmenti

(yellow), chlorine or bromine exposure (green), carbon monoxide exposure (deep red), and phenothiazine or antimalarial exposure (blue-gray).

- *Infectious.* The most common condition seen in childhood and adolescence is a *paronychia,* which is usually acute and appears as a painful red swelling of the proximal or lateral nail folds. *Staphylococcus aureus* is the most common cause. The condition may be chronic, caused by Monilia, or may be a manifestation of an underlying immunodeficiency. Chronic fungal infections *(onychomycoses)* may appear more frequently in adolescence.
- *Neoplastic.* These conditions are rare in children and adolescents. *Melanoma* will cause brown-black discolorations. Sometimes benign lentigienes, isolated or syndromic (e.g., *Peutz-Jeghers syndrome*), will cause this discoloration.
- *Traumatic.* The most common nail trauma seen in day-to-day practice involves *subungual hematomas*: blue, painful accumulation of blood under the nail; avulsions and fragility (onychorrhexis, onycholysis); and fraying or dystrophy from picking and chronic biting. *Subungual hemorrhages* may be spontaneous or induced by minimal trauma and often are due to *embolic phenomena, endocarditis, sepsis,* and *vasculitis.*
- *Chronic disease.* Recovery from any severe illness, e.g., sickle cell crisis, may produce transverse ridges (*Beau lines*). Look for clubbing and cyanosis associated with chronic cardiac or pulmonary disease. *Half-and-half (Lindsay) nails* and white proximal nails present in *uremia* and *chronic liver* and *heart disease. Telangiectasia* and *splinter hemorrhages* with or without trauma always should raise suspicion for *endocarditis.* Chronic conditions may produce significant changes in nail color. Brown discoloration is due to *Addison disease.* Yellow nails are associated with *jaundice* and *carotenemia,* and blue or gray nails occur in *Wilson disease.*
- *Idiopathic.* Sometimes nail abnormalities will be diffuse but not associated with any underlying condition. Examples include *twenty-nail dystrophy,* characterized by yellow, dystrophic, friable nails (all of them). This condition may last several years but usually resolves. Frequently, *onychorrhexis* may be idiopathic or benign and familial. Reedy nails and longitudinal striations appear as an exaggeration of a normal nail and rarely have any significant cause.

Confirmatory Laboratory Studies

After making a diagnosis, the following laboratory aids are often useful to confirm or negate the hypothesis. These should be available in a primary care office setting.

- *Gram stain.* This is helpful to determine the content of lesions such as polymorphonuclear cells, eosinophils, and bacteria.

- *KOH (potassium hydroxide) preparation for fungi.* Look for hyphae for fungal infections, budding yeast for *Candida,* or a "meatballs and spaghetti" pattern of *tinea versicolor.* A KOH prep will demonstrate oval opalescent bodies of *molluscum contagiosum.*
- *Low-power microscopy* to identify *lice,* eggs.
- *Tzanck smear* to identify *varicella* and *herpes simplex.* Note the presence of multinucleated giant cells.
- *Wood's lamp.* This is helpful for diagnosis of certain *fungal infections,* specifically *Microsporum.* Unfortunately, this accounts for only about 10 percent of fungal skin infections. *Tinea versicolor* yields a yellow-green fluorescence, as will *Pseudomonas* infections. Pigmented skin absorbs ultraviolet light; nonpigmented skin reflects it. Thus the Wood's lamp is often helpful to detect *vitiligo* in a fair-skinned individual or *tuberous sclerosis* in infants with earliest onset of depigmentation.

The Psychodiagnostic Examination

Joseph L. Calles

The goals of this chapter are

1. To learn the key elements of the psychiatric history and mental status examination and how they may be modified to match the developmental level of the patient
2. To classify the psychiatric disorders encountered in younger patients by the major domains of impairment, i.e., disturbances of thought, feeling, and/or behavior
3. To outline the criteria used in arriving at specific psychiatric diagnoses
4. To learn when to pursue medical, neurologic, and/or psychological evaluations/consultations in order to clarify or confirm diagnoses

Psychiatric History and Mental Status Examination

Psychiatric History

For several generations, a medical adage has stated that "80 percent of diagnosis is made by the history," and this has certainly held true in the field of psychiatry. Although we may observe certain physical *signs* of illness in our patients (e.g., the characteristic tics of Tourette disorder), it is generally the *symptoms* elicited during the clinical interview that guide the diagnostic process.

In order to obtain information (from patients and their caregivers) that is relevant, useful, and complete, it is helpful to follow a consistent format for data gathering. This can and will be modified to correspond to the quality and quantity of the information received, the source of information (e.g., patient versus parent), and the chronological and developmental age of the patient.

Here are the elements that should be included in a standard psychiatric history:

1. *Source of information.* Is the patient able to describe his or her symptoms, or does the caregiver have to provide the information? Has the caregiver known the patient all of his or her life, or has there been limited (e.g., in a foster-care setting) or sporadic (e.g., changes

in custody) contact? Is the information reliable, i.e., is it provided out of concern for the child, or is there another agenda, such as getting medications to "quiet" the patient or to qualify for disability compensation? Is the information intelligible, or are there speech/language impediments to the process, including having to conduct the interview through an interpreter?

2. *Identifying information.* What is the name (including preferred name, such as a nickname), age (in years and months), gender, race/ethnicity, school name and grade (if applicable), and living situation (e.g., where and with whom) of the patient? Who referred the patient for the evaluation?

3. *Chief complaint.* What is the referring person, the caregiver (if different from the referrer), and (if possible) the patient himself or herself concerned about? This important issue will appear in the next section.

4. *History of present illness (HPI).* All good stories involve a timeline, and this one—the patient's story—is no different. The sequence of how problems developed is the frame onto which to attach other details. The purpose of this section is not only to document symptoms to make a diagnosis but also—and more important—to get a sense of how illness has affected that patient and those around him or her. Important elements in this section, to be addressed for each problem, include

   • *Temporal factors.* When did the problem begin? Has it been continuous or episodic? How often does it occur? When does it occur (e.g., time of day, day of week, time of year)? How long does it last? What is the longest period of time that the problem was absent before it recurred?

   • *Spatial factors.* Where did the problem begin? Where does it commonly occur now? Are there any settings in which the problem does not occur?

   • *Modifying factors.* What initially precipitated the problem? Does it still trigger an episode? Does anything make the problem worse? Does anything make it better? How do people in the immediate environment respond when the problem is evident?

   • *Severity.* What is the most serious thing that the patient ever did during an episode? Compared with when the problem first started, is it better, worse, or about the same?

   • *Quality.* If worse, in what ways? If better, in what ways?
     The general and specific symptoms to inquire about appear in the sections on classification and diagnosis.

5. *Past psychiatric history.* Has the patient ever had formal psychiatric or psychological evaluations? If yes, when, where, and by whom? What were the diagnoses, and were recommendations made? Did the patient follow them? If so, what were the responses? Is the patient currently in therapy, or was the patient in therapy in the past? If yes, what type, how often, for how long, and with whom? Did the therapy help? If yes, in what ways? Is the patient taking psychotropic medications? Has the patient ever been in a psychiatric in-patient unit? Day (partial) hospital program? Residential treatment center? Respite program? Runaway shelter? Any other treatment setting? If yes to any of these, what were the circumstances?

TABLE 17–1 is a guide to get details about the medication history, and the caregiver or patient, as part of the preappointment paperwork, can fill it out.

6. *Past medical history.* Is the patient currently in treatment for any acute or chronic medical conditions? Who is the primary care physician? Are there any medical specialists involved in his or her care? Is there any history of hospitalizations? Surgeries? Trauma (especially head injury)? Seizure activity (especially nonfebrile)? Serious infections (especially of the CNS)? Are immunizations up to date? Any adverse reactions to vaccinations? Any adverse reactions to medications? Any allergies? If currently on any nonpsychotropic medications, list the names, dosages, indications, and responses. Has the patient been sexually active (including oral and anal intercourse)? Did he or she use contraception? Is there concern about or history of sexually transmitted diseases?

7. *For females, obstetric and gynecologic history.* At what age was menarche? Are menses regular? When was the last menstrual period? Are they painful to the point of being unable to function? Does mood change before menses to the point of being less able to function? In what way does mood change? Has the patient ever been pregnant? If yes, how many times? What were the outcomes?

8. *Substance use history.* Does the patient use tobacco or alcohol? Does the patient use illicit substances, such as marijuana, cocaine, heroin, etc.? If so, what are the routes of use (including intravenous)? Does the patient misuse licit substances, such as prescription medications, over-the-counter medications, weight-gain or weight-loss products, nutritional products, herbal products, or "energy" beverages (including coffee and other caffeinated drinks)? Does the patient ever inhale volatile compounds (such as gasoline, paint thinner, correction fluid, various sprays, etc.) to get "high?" (This practice is sometimes referred to as *huffing.*)

   If the patient answers "Yes" to any of these items, at what age did the activity start? When was the last use? How often does the patient use it? How much? Any adverse consequences, such as "blackouts," memory loss, withdrawal, or other physical symptoms? How about behavioral consequences, such as engaging in unwanted and/or unprotected sex?

9. *Developmental history.* Was it a planned pregnancy? Was the patient wanted? Were there any complications during the pregnancy? Were there exposures to any drugs (licit or illicit), alcohol, nicotine, toxins, or radiation? Was the baby born at term, prematurely, or postdates? Were there any complications at the time of birth or shortly thereafter? What were the Apgar scores? Did the baby require bilirubin lights? Were any neonatal screening test results abnormal? Breast-fed, bottle-fed, or both? For how long? How was the feeding experience for both mother and child? Did the child's growth (length, weight, and head circumference) follow standardized curves, or were there significant deviations? Were developmental milestones on time, early, or late? At any point were there concerns about the patient's development? At what age was the patient able to sleep

TABLE 17-1 *Psychotropic Medication History*

Medication Name	Highest Dosage	For How Long?	Helpful? Yes/No	If Yes, for How Long?	Why Stopped?	If for Side Effects, Which Ones?
Fluoxetine	30 mg.	2 weeks	Yes, before the increase	2 mos. at 20 mg., then stopped working	Side effects	Became angry and irritable, then destructive
Medication 2						

through the night? At what age was the patient able to separate from caregivers and not experience intense anxiety?

10. *Social history.* The purpose of this section is to assess the quality and quantity of past and present relationships, as well as to document losses, traumas, transitions, and any other events that may have had a negative effect on the patient. It also identifies positive elements in the patient's life. Categories include

- *Current living situation.* With whom does the patient live? What are their sexes, ages, and relationships to the patient? With whom does he or she relate the best? With whom does he or she have the most conflicts? What type of dwelling do they reside in? What are the sleeping arrangements? In what sort of setting (e.g., rural, city, etc.) is it in? Is the area safe? How quickly can law enforcement and fire safety officers get to the residence?

- *Losses.* Has the patient lost a close relative, neighbor, friend, or significant other through death? Have any important people moved away and broken contact with the patient? How old was he or she when those things happened? How well do they remember the person or event? How do they feel about the person or event?

- *Traumas.* Has the patient experienced any neglect? Was it emotional, physical, or both? Has the patient experienced any abuse? Was it verbal, emotional, physical, and/or sexual? Was there protective services involvement? Did they remove the child from the home? How did the child respond to that? Was there court involvement? Did the child have to testify? How did the child respond to that? Was parental contact limited or discontinued? Did the parents have their rights terminated? How did the child respond to that?

- *Transitions.* Was the child ever placed in a shelter, group home, or foster home? At what age(s), with whom, and for how long? How did the child respond to that? Was the child adopted? At what age and by whom? What does the child know or remember about the adoption? How well has the child adapted to his or her new family? Does the child feel wanted, loved, and cared for? In how many homes, in how many cities, has the child lived in? If moves were frequent and/or numerous, what were the reasons?

- *School.* Did the patient participate in day care, Head Start, preschool, Montessori, or any other enrichment experience? At what age did it start, for how long did it last, and was it helpful? In what way(s)? Did the patient begin kindergarten earlier, on time, or later? If later, did the patient participate in a "young fives" program? Was the patient ever advanced or retained a grade? How has the patient performed academically? Have grades been consistent? Any recent declines? How has the patient performed on standardized tests? Are the scores consistent with classroom grades? Does the patient have any learning difficulties? In what areas? Is there documentation of them? Was any formal psychoeducational testing administered? Did the patient go through the Individualized Educational Plan (IEP) process? If he or she did not qualify for special educational services, was a Section 504 plan instituted? Does the patient receive any type of tutoring? How about vocational training? Have there been any detentions, suspensions (in school or out of school), or expulsions? For what reasons were those actions taken?

- *Peer relationships.* Does the patient have friends? A best friend? Where does he or she usually make friends (e.g., school or neighborhood)? How easily? How long do friendships tend to last? If briefly, why? What aged peers—younger, older, or same—does he or she do best with? What type of peers—"nice kids" versus "troublemakers"—does he or she tend to associate with? Have there been romantic relationships? If so, did his or her behavior or functioning change? If yes, were the changes positive or negative? How did the patient react to breakups in those relationships?

- *Interests and activities.* What sorts of things does the patient enjoy doing? Does he or she have hobbies? Is there participation in sports? Is the activity solitary (e.g., swimming or tennis) or team-oriented (e.g., soccer or baseball)? Is there participation in clubs or organizations, either in school (e.g., drama or student government) or in the community (e.g., scouting or 4-H)? Does the patient do any volunteer work? Do the patient and his or her family attend any religious services?

- *Work.* Has the patient ever had a job? If yes, at what age did he or she start working? What kind of work was it? If currently employed, how many hours a week are involved? Are any during school hours? Is the work to earn money, school credits, or both? What does the patient do with the money earned?

- *Legal.* Has the patient ever been involved in the legal system as a result of participating in illegal activity? Have there been status offenses (e.g., violating curfew)? Have there been misdemeanor charges (e.g., minor shoplifting or vandalism)? Have there been any felony charges (e.g., robbery or aggravated assault)? Have there been any drug-related charges? Has any time been served in a juvenile home, jail, or any other court-ordered correctional facility? Has the patient ever been on house arrest, probation, or a tether? Has there been any court-ordered treatment, e.g., anger-management classes?

11. *Family history.* Are there any family members, who are blood-related, who have had any of the following:
    - Problems similar to the patient's?
    - Developmental delays or learning problems?
    - A seizure disorder?
    - A mood disorder, such as depression or bipolar disorder?
    - A psychotic disorder, such as schizophrenia?
    - An anxiety disorder, such as panic disorder or social anxiety disorder?
    - A disruptive behavior disorder, such as attention-deficit/hyperractivity disorder or conduct disorder?
    - A substance-use disorder, either abuse or dependence?
    - An eating disorder, such as anorexia nervosa or bulimia nervosa?

- A problem with inappropriate or excessive anger, especially if associated with physical aggression?
- A history of legal incarceration (especially if the index episode was in early life or if episodes were repetitive)?
- A history of psychiatric treatment, hospitalizations, or the taking of psychotropic medications?
- A history of suicide attempts or completed suicide?

The Mental Status Examination (MSE)

After a complete history, the *subjective* (or patient-reported) portion of the evaluation is complete. The second, complementary part of the evaluation is the *objective* or examiner-observed and -administered portion. The goal of performing an MSE is to determine the patient's current state of affective, cognitive, and psychomotor functioning.

The initial step in conducting an MSE relies on the examiner's observational skills. This is important in all patients but especially so in younger patients who are preverbal. If you have ever watched a show on TV from a distance or in a noisy room such that the dialogue couldn't be heard, you may have noticed that at times you could figure out what was happening *just by watching facial expressions, bodily movements, and the people's reactions to each other.* This is the same process used in the MSE.

The traditional MSE is reported using the following format:

1. *Appearance.* Compared to the average for chronologic age, is the patient shorter than, taller than, or at the expected height? Is weight appropriate for the height? Does the patient look younger than, older than, or consistent with the chronologic age? Does the patient appear to be well nourished and healthy or sickly? How is the patient's hygiene and grooming? (Use the nose as well as the eyes!) Is the patient's clothing well fitted, clean, and appropriate to the weather? Describe the patient's facial expression: smiling, frowning, tense, angry, fearful, apprehensive, distressed, or neutral/bland. Does it vary? How? Describe the patient's eye contact: staring, full, intermittent, absent, or avoidant? What is the patient's motor activity like? Does he or she resist holding? Is there any crawling, creeping, walking, running, climbing, and/or jumping? Is it age-appropriate? Can the patient's activity be redirected? Can the patient stay seated when requested to do so? Are any abnormal motor movements such as tics or tremors? Are any abnormalities of gait? Is the patient clumsy?
2. *Speech.* Are speech sounds produced spontaneously, in response to questions, or both? Is the *quality* of speech appropriate for chronologic age? If not, is it intelligible to the examiner? If not, is it intelligible to the caretaker? Is there any slurring, lisping, or stuttering? Are any letters missing from words, or are any extra letters added to words? Is there any jargon, i.e., made-up words? Is the rate of speech normal-paced, rapid, or slow? Is there a latency (delay) of response? Is the *quantity* of speech appropriate to the questions or circumstances, i.e., are verbal productions single words, phrases, or full

sentences? Is the number of words minimally sufficient, or are responses elaborated? Is there too much information?

3. *Mood.* This describes the *subjective,* or internally experienced, emotional state of the patient. In children who are preverbal or nonverbal, the examiner must surmise mood from visual information (as described previously). In verbal patients, this can be obtained directly by asking them, "How do you feel?" Internal state, however, can be complex and confusing, and patients may have trouble putting them into words. Facilitate this by giving the patient a menu of emotional words from which to choose, e.g., *happy, sad, mad, anxious, nervous, worried, scared, numb,* or *empty.*

4. *Affect.* This describes the examiner's perception of the patient's internal emotional state based on the *objective* information derived from all the examiner's senses and interpreted through the interpersonal interaction with the patient and his or her caregiver. The affect should be *mood-congruent;* i.e., it should match the mood. For example, a patient who says that he or she feels sad should look, sound, and act sad. If mood and affect don't match (e.g., a patient endorses sadness but is smiling and laughing, energetic, etc.), affect would be described as *mood-incongruent.*

5. *Thought process.* This describes *how* the patient thinks. Thought patterns should be coherent, logical, and goal-directed, even in younger children. For example, toddlers usually can communicate (using only a few words) their needs and desires such that most adults can understand what they are. If the listener is having difficulty following the flow and intent of the patient's conversation, it may suggest that his or her thought processing is incoherent, illogical, or random. Further evaluation would be indicated to rule out an actual thought disorder (see the section "Disturbances of Thought").

6. *Thought content.* This describes *what* the patient thinks. Whether the mental content is reality-oriented (e.g., deciding which chore to do first) or fantasy-oriented (e.g., thinking about what vacation might be like), it should always be under the patient's conscious control. Disturbances of thought content *quality* are perceived as intrusive, unwanted, distressing, foreign, and/or difficult to control. Disturbances of thought content *quantity* can run the gamut from minimal (or *impoverished*) thoughts to multiple, competing thoughts that are overwhelming to the patient.

7. *Cognition.* In its most basic definition, this function is comprised of *level of consciousness, attention and concentration, memory, orientation,* and other higher-level mental processes. Is the patient's level of consciousness alert, somnolent, stuporous, or absent? Is the patient attentive and focused, distractible and variably attentive, or inattentive? Can the patient interrupt his or her activity? Can the patient switch tasks when requested to do so? Can the patient remember information that is historical (i.e., obtained before coming to see you)? Can the patient remember new information (i.e., presented during the visit with you)? Is the patient oriented to *time* (e.g., day of the week), *place* (e.g., city lived in), *person* (e.g., names of people in the home), and *situation* (i.e., the reason that he or she is being

seen by you)? (*Note:* It is not uncommon for children and adolescents to answer "I don't know" when asked why they were brought in to the doctor or what kinds of problems they are having.)

8. *Insight.* Insight—or the patient's explanation of *why* he or she is having problems—is important to assess implications for change. The more fully and accurately a person can identify the factors that are contributing to his or her distress, the better is the prognosis for resolution of those problems. However, the younger the person, the less likely it is that he or she will have insight. Therefore, when working with children and adolescents, insight—although desirable— is not a necessary component of positive change.

9. *Judgment.* Far more important than insight is judgment—or the patient's *ability to make good decisions.* As was described with insight, the younger the person, the less likely it is that he or she will have judgment. Unfortunately, the passage of time does not guarantee the acquisition of judgment; one only has to read or see the news to find plenty of examples of adolescents and adults who have made bad decisions. The consequence of poor judgment (e.g., legal problems) is one of the most common reasons for younger people to be referred for a psychodiagnostic evaluation.

10. *Impulse control.* The term *impulsivity* can be defined as a person's tendency *to act before thinking about possible consequences.* To have impulse control, therefore, implies that a person is able to control the expression of his or her feelings and urges, keeping in mind the possible negative effects that his or her actions could have on self and/or others. Just as with insight and judgment, the younger the person, the less likely it is that he or she will have impulse control. There is often a connection between poor judgment and poor impulse control, but this is not always the case (e.g., the person who plans a bank robbery has the former but not the latter).

Once all the data have been obtained through a thorough psychiatric history and careful mental status examination, the next step is to determine in which major area(s) of impairment the patient's symptoms and problems are represented.

Domains of Impairment

Disturbances of Thought

As mentioned previously, thought disturbances can occur in both process and content. In order to better appreciate what the patient's inner life is like, it is important to explore and characterize both aspects.

Thought Process

Conceptualize this as referring either to the *quantity* or *density* of thoughts or to the *coherence* or *flow* of thinking. Commonly used terms include

- *Poverty of thought,* i.e., a paucity or seeming absence of thoughts.
- *Thought blocking,* i.e., the sudden interruption of a line of thought, usually associated with the patient's inability to recapture it (much like a light bulb burning out).
- *Vagueness,* i.e., thoughts that are unclear or ambiguous such that the listener cannot understand the patient's intended message. An example would be a response to a question that doesn't really say anything.
- *Circumstantiality,* i.e., the presence of excessive but unimportant details such that the the patient misses the "big picture."
- *Tangentiality,* i.e., the veering away from a topic with no subsequent return to it without prompting.
- *Flight of ideas,* i.e., the usually rapid shifting from topic to topic with only minimal connectedness from one topic to the next. An example (from my practice years ago): An adolescent at a hospital in Lansing, Michigan, which is in Ingham County, received a letter on which appeared the word Ingham. In rapid succession, he stated "Ingham, ham, that's pork, I'm a pig."
- *Looseness of associations,* i.e., thoughts or ideas that generate with no interconnectedness from one to the next. Most people hearing this would consider it "crazy."

Thought Content

As the term implies, this describes the actual mental content of the patient's thinking. Commonly used terms include

- *Rumination,* i.e., the "chewing over and over" of the same topic. An example would be an adolescent girl who repeatedly asks herself "Why did I go there?" after a sexual assault at a party.
- *Obsessions,* i.e., thoughts that are intrusive, unwanted, distressing, repetitive, but difficult to eliminate. There is a common, associated question that patients ask themselves that begins with "What if . . . ?" (e.g., "What if I didn't lock the door?").
- *Compulsions.* These are most commonly physical actions (see the section "Disturbances of Behavior"), but they also can be mental in nature. Unlike obsessions, these mental actions can be controllable to some extent, are used to reduce distress in some way, and therefore may be desirable and voluntarily repetitive. The problem lies in the increased distress whenever the actions stop, thus reinforcing and increasing the amount of time spent performing the actions. They may interfere with other thoughts and behaviors such that functioning declines. An example might be someone who repeatedly performs math calculations in his or her head.
- *Phobias,* i.e., irrational fears of objects, people, or situations. Common phobias include fears of heights, enclosed spaces, the dark, storms, various animals, crowds, strangers, and being alone.
- *Illusions,* i.e., the misperception of an object or person that exists in reality. This is fairly common and can occur at any age. An example is the young child who sees a "monster" in the tree outside the bedroom window.

- *Hallucinations,* i.e., the perception of something that does not exist in reality. They can be experienced in any sensory modality, i.e., hearing (auditory), vision (visual), smell (olfactory), taste (gustatory), and/or touch (tactile). The younger the child, the more likely it is that he or she will normally experience some hallucinations, most commonly auditory (such as hearing his or her name called). One way to explore this is to ask, "Do you ever hear/see/smell/taste/feel things that other people don't?"
- *Delusions,* i.e., false, fixed beliefs. The most common types are paranoid (e.g., thinking that he or she is being watched, followed, plotted against, etc.), grandiose (e.g., thinking that he or she is the smartest student, best athlete, best looking, etc.), religious (e.g., thinking that he or she can absolve all sins or that he or she is on a special mission from God), jealous (e.g., people resent the patient for what he or she has and want it), and erotomanic (e.g., a famous actor or musician is in love with the patient). Not surprisingly, there can be overlapping and combining of types.
- *Thought insertion and deletion,* i.e., believing that thoughts are put into and out of the head. He or she will attribute this to some outside agent or force, so it can be associated with delusional thinking.
- *Referential thinking,* i.e., the patient believing that certain utterances— from the media, in overheard conversations, etc.—are specifically for him or her and also have some sort of special significance. For example, a TV commercial that says "Change your life today!" could prompt the person to drop out of school, quit his or her job, etc.
- *Suicidal ideation,* i.e., the thoughts associated with the desire to die. In active suicidal ideation, the patient can imagine the means to kill himself or herself. Of concern is when the person has plans to put those thoughts into action. In passive suicidal ideation, the patient wishes to be dead but has no clear thought about how it might happen and no intention to make it so. Patients sometimes will say that they wish that they would go to sleep and "never wake up." *Always take suicidal ideation seriously.*
- *Homicidal ideation,* i.e., thoughts of killing another person. These can be vague or can be quite specific, including the means by which they would carry out the act(s). *Always take homicidal ideation seriously,* and depending on the laws of the local jurisdiction, it may be reportable to law enforcement personnel.
- *Low self-esteem,* i.e., a negative self-appraisal. This can be a patient's perception of unsatisfactory aspects of his or her appearance, abilities, and/or desirability. Common self-derogatory descriptors include "stupid," "ugly," "fat," "no good," and "unlovable."

Disturbances of Feeling

As mentioned earlier, the evaluation of a patient's emotional state includes the patient's subjective experience of feelings (or *mood*) and the objective but indirect experience (or *affect*) of that patient by the examiner.

Mood

The more sustained emotional states that the patient may experience include

- *Euthymia,* i.e., a general sense of evenness, normality, contentment, or happiness. This is the healthy, nonpathologic mood state that patients should aspire to.
- *Euphoria,* i.e., the presence of an exaggerated feeling of happiness or well-being, as if one is "high." Sometimes interchanged with the term elation.
- *Depression,* i.e., the feeling of being sad, down, low, or unhappy. Sometimes patients describe this as "bored" or "empty."
- *Anhedonia,* i.e., the absence of pleasure, no matter the circumstances.
- *Anxiety,* i.e., a sense of tension or nervousness. In children, this can manifest as worry.
- *Irritability,* i.e., being easily annoyed or upset, even by "little things."
- *Anger,* i.e., being mad, irate, or furious. In its most extreme form it can lead to rage.
- *Fear,* i.e., a sense of dread or apprehension that something bad will happen. The concern can be for the self and/or for others.

Affect

As mentioned in the section on the MSE, assessment of the patient's facial expressions, speech characteristics, bodily movements, etc. determines his or her *affect.* Comparing the affect with the patient's mood will reveal either congruence or incongruence. Affect also can be described in terms of range and reactivity, such as

- *Broad,* i.e., a full range of emotional expression, usually implying that the emotions displayed are appropriate to the setting, topic, etc.
- *Labile,* i.e., a variety of emotional expressions that are rapidly shifting, minimally provoked, exaggerated, and usually inappropriate. Very young children can switch from tearfulness to laughter in literally seconds; the older the person, the less normal and more pathologic lability becomes.
- *Silly,* i.e., excessive and inappropriate smiling and laughter.
- *Constricted* (or *restricted*), i.e., a limited, minimally reactive emotional display. For example, a child who looks sad or mad throughout the interview, although he or she might be able to smile or laugh appropriately at a humorous comment.
- *Blunted,* i.e., a limited emotional display and no reaction to surrounding events.
- *Flat,* i.e., the absence of emotional display and reactivity. This presentation makes it impossible to know what the patient is experiencing if he or she is also not talking.

Disturbances of Behavior

Given that one cannot perceive the thoughts and feelings directly, disruptions in behavior are the most obvious indicators that something i "not right" with the patient; they are also the most common reason for referral for mental health evaluation. Behavioral disturbances include

- *Homicidal acts,* i.e., the deliberate attempt to take the life of another person. This can occur for many different reasons, from paranoia, to retribution, to financial gain.
- *Suicidal acts,* i.e., the deliberate attempt to take one's own life. This also can derive from multiple different etiologies but is most commonly associated with depression and hopelessness.
- *Destructive behavior,* i.e., the damaging of property, either inadvertently or deliberately. An example of intentional damage would be spray painting buildings (a.k.a. tagging). An example of unintentional damage would be someone driving off in anger and getting into a motor vehicle accident.
- *Self-injurious behavior* (SIB) [a.k.a. *deliberate self-harm* (DSH)]. This refers to the intentional infliction of bodily harm. An all-too-common form of contemporary SIB is cutting; SIB also can include burning, scratching to bleed, picking of scabs (to prevent healing), pulling of hair, poking with pins, piercing of body parts, self-made tattoos, punching oneself, rubbing to the point of inflammation (e.g., with a pencil eraser), and head banging. In extreme cases, fractures and concussions may occur, and body parts can be severely damaged or lost.
- *Compulsions* (also called *rituals*), i.e., actions that are generally irresistible (although they can be controllable to some extent), are used to reduce distress in some way, and therefore may be desirable and voluntarily repetitive. The problem lies in the increased distress (a buildup of tension) whenever the actions stop, thus reinforcing and increasing the amount of time spent performing the actions. It may interfere with other thoughts and behaviors such that functioning declines. It is usually associated with a feeling or belief that "something bad will happen" if the actions are not carried out. An example might be someone who repeatedly washes his or her hands owing to a fear of "germs."

The Psychiatric Diagnostic Process

The diagnostic categories, clinical features, and format for the multiaxial assessment, described below are from the standard reference of psychiatry in the United States, the American Psychiatric Association's *Diagnostic and Statistical Manual of Mental Disorders,* Fourth Edition, Text Revision (Washington, DC: American Psychiatric Association, 2000) (DSM-IV-TR).

To qualify as a disorder in the DSM-IV-TR, the condition must cause a significant amount of *distress* to the individual and/or must cause a significant amount of *dysfunction.*

Despite the clarity of the diagnostic criteria, sometimes there is confusing or insufficient data in the history to make a definitive diagnosis. The DSM-IV-TR allows for two options to compensate for this. The first s the *provisional* diagnosis, which applies when there is "a strong presumption that the full criteria will ultimately be met" but that current information is insufficient to make a "firm diagnosis." The second is the *not otherwise specified* (NOS) diagnoses, which occurs in every major category. This allows the clinician to make a diagnosis, even when the available information does not support a more specific diagnosis. For example, a patient with a great deal of anger and aggression may not satisfy the criteria for any specific mood disorder; in such a case, "Mood Disorder NOS" could apply.

The Multiaxial Assessment

Very briefly, clinical information is organized into five major domains or axes; they are

Axis I: Clinical Disorders. This represents the majority of DSM-IV-TR diagnoses. Also included on this axis is a diverse group called "Other Conditions That May Be a Focus of Clinical Attention" (e.g., "Noncompliance With Treatment").

Axis II: Personality Disorders and Mental Retardation.

Axis III: General Medical Conditions. The DSM-IV-TR stipulates that medical issues on this axis should be those "that are potentially relevant to the understanding and management of the individual's mental disorder." This would exclude acute, time-limited, nonserious illnesses, e.g., the common cold. This always should include the illness that is the cause of a "Mental Disorder Due to a General Medical Condition," e.g., "Delirium Secondary to Encephalitis."

Axis IV: Psychosocial and Environmental Problems. This axis refers to life circumstances "that may affect the diagnosis, treatment, and prognosis of mental disorders." An example would be being homeless.

Axis V: Global Assessment of Functioning (GAF). This is an objective, clinician-based evaluation of the patient's current level of functioning. It is a 1- to 100-point scale (0 is reserved for "inadequate information") that divides into 10 groups of 10 points each to facilitate the determination of the GAF score. It is common to designate two GAF scores: the current GAF and the GAF that is/was the highest level in the preceding year. This latter GAF score is useful to predict prognosis.

Specific Psychiatric Diagnoses: Axis I

The DSM-IV-TR classifies the Axis I disorders into 16 major categories (TABLE 17–2), each of which contains several specific diagnostic criteria sets (see the DSM-IV-TR for details).

Although almost any DSM-IV-TR diagnosis can apply to children or adolescents, only the most common and clinically relevant disorders will appear in the following sections (NOS diagnoses will not be mentioned). The DSM-IV-TR stipulates to rule out medical and substance-related disorders before proceeding with the psychiatric diagnostic process (see the section "Further Evaluations").

- *Disorders Usually First Diagnosed in Infancy, Childhood, or Adolescence.* Excluding mental retardation (which is coded on Axis II), the Axis I disorders in this section are represented in the following categories

TABLE 17–2 *Axis I Clinical Disorders*

Disorders usually first diagnosed in infancy, childhood, or
  adolescence
Delirium, dementia, and amnestic and other cognitive disorders
Mental disorders due to a general medical condition
Substance-related disorders
Schizophrenia and other psychotic disorders
Mood disorders
Anxiety disorders
Somatoform disorders
Factitious disorders
Dissociative disorders
Sexual and gender identity disorders
Eating disorders
Sleep disorders
Impulse-control disorders not elsewhere classified
Adjustment disorders
Other conditions that may be a focus of clinical attention

- *Learning disorders.* These usually present when a student is having difficulty keeping up in class or especially when he or she is falling behind despite making an honest effort. Students often will say that they "don't understand" the material. Time spent completing homework literally can take hours, and battles over assignments are not uncommon. Students, teachers, and parents become very frustrated. When formally evaluated, scores on standardized psychoeducational testing will be less than 2 standard deviations below those expected for the person's chronologic age, intellectual level (IQ), and current grade level.
  - *Reading disorder.* In addition to poor comprehension, this can manifest as difficulties with the mechanics of reading (the student will read very slowly) or with reading accuracy (misreading letters, words, or phrases; sometimes called *dyslexia*). This disorder tends to run in families.
  - *Mathematics disorder.* The student with this problem may have difficulties in grasping concepts, understanding operations, or remembering sequences (e.g., not being able to learn multiplication tables). The student may not manifest any difficulties until he or she attempts to learn more complicated functions (e.g., doing okay with addition and subtraction but struggling with multiplication).
  - *Disorder of written expression.* Although poor spelling or handwriting can be part of this disorder. Do not diagnose this if the problem is misspelling or illegible handwriting. A more important sign of this disorder is poor communication of information owing to errors in grammar, punctuation, and/or sentence structure.
- **Key Point:** *Academic decline despite good efforts.*
- *Motor skills disorders*

- Developmental coordination disorder. Caregivers notice this as "clumsiness" in the child who may have difficulties in gross and/or fine motor functioning. He or she may sustain injuries through frequent tripping or falling. In the clinical setting it may appear as delays in achieving motor milestones at the appropriate times.

Key Point: *Delayed motor development.*

- *Communication disorders.* These are usually apparent when the child or adolescent is unable to effectively and efficiently communicate his or her ideas or needs to others. The problem can be due to disordered language (i.e., the symbolic or mental component of communication) or disordered speech (i.e., the mechanical component of communication, which is usually talking but also includes signing).
  - *Expressive language disorder.* There are two basic forms of this disorder: developmental (congenital) and acquired (secondary to a medical condition affecting the CNS; also called *acquired aphasia*). Both present similarly, with abnormalities in the quality and/or quantity of communication sufficient to impair functioning. The developmental type first usually appears by the preschool years but can be subtle and missed until later. The acquired type has an abrupt onset coincident with the onset of the medical illness.
  - *Mixed receptive-expressive language disorder.* Very similar to the expressive language disorder, this disorder has the additional burden of abnormal receptive language abilities. Patients misunderstand or misinterpret verbal input, which the clinician may misconstrue for a hearing deficit, inattention, mental retardation, or a diffuse developmental disorder. Expressive language is concomitantly impaired (think "garbage in, garbage out").
  - *Phonological disorder.* This involves the misarticulation of speech that is inconsistent with age and cultural influences. The patient omits sounds (letters or combinations) and substitutes others or mispronounces them (e.g., lisping). Severity ranges from mild to severe (i.e., unintelligible, even to family members).
  - *Stuttering.* Sometimes called *stammering,* in this disorder, speech is quite dysfluent, with delays and/or repetitions of sounds (especially the first letters of words) or even whole words. The problem creates tension in the speaker and often impatience in the listener. The patient may practice words mentally before speaking (scripting). He or she may substitute easier words for the originally intended word. Some will avoid speaking to reduce embarrassment.

Key Point: *Impaired ability to effectively comprehend and/or produce spoken language.*

- *Pervasive developmental disorders* (PDDs). These conditions demonstrate fairly global impairments in communication, socialization, cognition, and behavior. No two people with the same diagnosis are exactly alike and can vary widely in how impaired they are in any given functional area. They may excel in some skill areas, even approaching genius levels (*savant* skills).

- *Autistic disorder.* By definition, there must be qualitative deficits in social skills, communication skills, and interests, activities, and behaviors. Language development is delayed or even absent. About three-quarters will function in the mentally retarded range. People with this disorder often appear "odd" or "different." The onset is before 3 years of age, although in milder forms recognition may occur later.
- *Asperger disorder.* This shares many of the features of autistic disorder, but there are no significant language delays, nor major impairments in cognitive abilities or in adaptive behaviors, with the exception of social skills. There is no specified age of onset.

Key Point: *Poor social skills and limited interests.*

- *Attention-deficit and disruptive behavior disorders*
  - *Attention-deficit/hyperactivity disorder.* One of the most common psychiatric disorders in young people; its hallmarks are the triad of inattention, hyperactivity, and impulsivity. There are three subtypes: (1) combined type, (2) predominantly inattentive type, and (3) predominantly hyperactive-impulsive type. The relative ratios of symptoms that are present determine the differentiation. Some maladaptive symptoms (such as not being able to sit still and complete a task) should be present before the age of 7 years and should occur in at least two settings, such as at school and at home.
  - *Conduct disorder.* This is a serious behavioral disorder in which there are repetitive acts of aggression, destructiveness, lying, stealing, or violating major rules (e.g., truancy). Many of these behaviors will lead to legal involvement. At least one behavior should be present for 6 months and at least three for 1 year. The dividing line between childhood-onset and adolescent-onset types is age 10 years.
  - *Oppositional defiant disorder.* Although not as severe as conduct disorder, this disorder still can be quite disruptive of the home and school environments. Patients are angry, argumentative, challenging, provocative, and do not take responsibility for their actions nor accept their consequences. The behaviors should be present for at least 6 months.

Key Point: *Behaviors that interfere with the patient's functioning and that are disruptive to the surrounding environment.*

- *Feeding and eating disorders of infancy or early childhood*
  - *Pica.* The ingestion of nonfood items (e.g., sand) for at least 1 month. Attraction to food is intact. The behavior is not part of a particular cultural practice (e.g., eating soil "for health"), nor is it appropriate for developmental level (as in toddlers). It may occur in association with various developmental disabilities or psychosis.
  - *Rumination disorder.* The repetitive regurgitation and spitting out, chewing, and/or swallowing of previously ingested food. This disorder usually occurs within the first year of life (later in mental retardation), lasts at least a month, follows a period of normal functioning, and may be more common in males.

Appears to be a response to understimulation or stress or related to developmental delays. Often remits spontaneously.

Key Point: *Abnormal oral ingestion or regurgitation; look for environmental and developmental disturbances.*

- *Tic disorders*
  - *Tourette disorder.* This disorder is characterized by the presence of tics (sudden, rapid, repetitive but nonrhythmic, stereotyped movements or vocalizations) with more than one motor and at least one vocal type present at some time during the illness. The tics do not have to occur together. Common motor tics include exaggerated eye blinking and head jerking. Common vocal tics include excessive throat clearing and sniffing; uncommonly, verbal profanities may be blurted out (this is called *coprolalia*). Tics are variably present for more than 1 year with no quiescent period of more than 3 months. Onset occurs before age 18 years of age.
  - *Chronic motor or vocal tic disorder.* The only major difference from Tourette is that the motor and vocal tics are mutually exclusive.
  - *Transient tic disorder.* Similar to the tic disorders just noted, except that the tics are present for at least 4 weeks but for no longer than 12 consecutive months.

Key Point: *Motor and vocal tics alone or together, acute or chronic.*

- *Elimination disorders*
  - *Encopresis.* The repetitive defecating—involuntary or intentional—in inappropriate places (e.g., soiling clothing). It can occur with or without constipation and overflow incontinence. This occurs at least monthly for at least 3 months. Chronologic (or developmental) age is at least 4 years.
  - *Enuresis.* The repetitive urinating—involuntary or intentional—in inappropriate places (most commonly wetting the bed). It occurs twice a week for at least 3 consecutive months, but any pattern that causes distress may warrant the diagnosis. It can occur at night (nocturnal), during the day (diurnal), or both. Chronologic (or developmental) age is at least 5 years.

Key Point: *Repetitive and inappropriate defecating and urinating.*

- *Other disorders of infancy, childhood, or adolescence*
  - *Separation anxiety disorder.* The presence of excessive anxiety (not appropriate for developmental age) related to or in anticipation of separation from home or from attachment figures. The anxiety is both psychic (worry) and somatic (headaches, gastrointestinal complaints). Onset is before age 18 years, and symptoms are present for at least 4 weeks.
  - *Selective mutism.* Speaking does not occur in social settings but variably occurs in more familiar and intimate settings. There is some overlap with social phobia. Duration is at least 1 month.
  - *Reactive attachment disorder of infancy or early childhood.* A reaction to pathologic care (insufficient satisfaction of emotional, physical, and/or attachment needs), the disturbance in social relatedness manifests in two forms. The inhibited type demonstrates social avoidance, resistance, ambivalence, or vigilance. The disinhibited type shows a lack of social discrimination and

appropriate interpersonal boundaries (e.g., being overly friendly with strangers). This disorder begins before age 5 years.

Key Point: *The disorders described here arguably could be included in the anxiety disorders section because anxiety related to social discomfort is common to all three.*

* *Delirium, Dementia, and Amnestic and Other Cognitive Disorders.* These disorders often occur only in adults, especially the elderly. However, in children and adolescents, anytime there is a "clinically significant deficit in cognition or memory that represents a significant change from a previous level of functioning," seek a medical or substance-related explanation. The three main acquired disorders of cognition are

  * *Delirium.* Defined as a relatively rapid onset of altered consciousness and cognitive functioning (often inaccurately termed *confusion*). Disturbances of visual perception (illusions, hallucinations) can develop and be misinterpreted as psychosis. There tends to be a waxing and waning of symptoms; serial evaluations, therefore, are essential.

  * *Dementia.* Sometimes referred to as an *encephalopathy,* dementia is characterized by multiple cognitive deficits in the areas of memory (*amnesia*), language (*aphasia*), motor functioning (*apraxia*), recognition (*agnosia*), and/or executive functions (such as planning and organizing). There are two main types of dementia based on temporal course: progressive and static. The progressive dementias tend to be gradual in onset and unrelenting in their course, sometimes to the point of death. In younger people, many of these are due to genetic (especially metabolic) or infectious (e.g., HIV, prions, measles) etiologies. The static dementias tend to have a more rapid onset following a clearly defined insult to the CNS, e.g., head trauma or stroke. The deficits do not progress unless there is another acute insult. Fortunately, some recovery of functions is possible.

  * *Amnestic disorder.* This denotes a significant memory disturbance without other cognitive impairments that occur with delirium and dementia. The patient has difficulty recalling old and learning new information.

  Key Point: *Any significant decline in cognitive functioning requires a comprehensive medical evaluation.*

* *Substance-Related Disorders.* Since almost any substance (during intoxication or withdrawal) can cause or mimic almost any psychiatric disorder, we will not discuss specific syndromes. It is important, however, to distinguish between substance dependence and substance abuse.

  * *Substance dependence.* By definition, the substance-dependent person should manifest at least three of the following characteristics within the same 1-year period of time:

    * Tolerance, i.e., need for more of the substance(s) or diminished effects from the same amounts.

    * Withdrawal, i.e., distressing physical and psychological symptoms when use is reduced or stopped or using to abate or avoid those symptoms.

- Increasing amounts and/or time of use of the substance(s).
- Unsuccessful attempts to cut down or control use despite the desire to do so.
- Excessive time spent acquiring, using, and recovering from the substance(s).
- Diminished or discarded important activities in favor of using.
- Continued use despite the known presence of physical or psychological sequelae.
- *Substance abuse.* This is also defined as occurring within a 12-month period. The criteria for abuse focus solely on the negative effects of the substance on
  - Academic, occupational, domestic, social, or other interpersonal functioning
  - Legal status
  - Judgment that places the person in dangerous situations, e.g., driving while intoxicated

Key Point: *One should consider or rule out substance-use disorders in patients from preadolescence on.*

- *Schizophrenia and Other Psychotic Disorders.* The onset of schizophrenia before adolescence fortunately is rare. However, it is not uncommon to see the first evidence of this illness in late adolescence or early adulthood. The classic symptoms of psychosis—present for a significant portion of a 1-month period—include two (or more) of the following: hallucinations, delusions, disorganized speech, greatly disorganized or catatonic behavior, or negative symptoms (e.g., blunt affect or absence of motivation). It may be difficult to identify early on in younger patients because they do not express or characterize symptoms well. Nonpsychotic hallucinations (e.g., hearing one's name called) are also common in younger people.

Key Point: *Careful observations and questioning may be required to identify psychotic symptoms.*

- *Mood Disorders.* These clinical conditions are either depressive disorders or bipolar disorders. Mood disturbances from substances or medical conditions can have either presentation.
  - *Depressive disorders.* The defining mood state here is that of depression, a sustained feeling of being sad, low, or down. In younger people, however, depression can be experienced as anger or irritability.
    - *Major depressive disorder* (MDD). Episodes are either single or recurrent (interval at least 2 months). Symptoms must be present for at least 2 weeks, must include either the sad/mad mood or loss of interest/pleasure, and must include four other DSM-IV-TR symptoms. A common mnemonic to use is SIGECAPS (TABLE 17–3).
    - *Dysthymic disorder.* Symptoms are similar to those of MDD but also include low self-esteem and hopelessness. Duration is at least 1 year in children and adolescents. May coexist with MDD (double depression).

Key Point: *Even young children can reliably report about mood, sleep, appetite, etc.*

TABLE 17–3 SIGECAPS: Mnemonic for Depressive Episode

Sleep, which is either increased or decreased
Interests, which are greatly decreased or absent
Guilt, which is inappropriate; feeling worthless
Energy, which is low; easily fatigued
Concentration, which is poor; inattentive, indecisive
Appetite up or down; weight gain or loss
Psychomotor agitation or retardation (observed, not reported)
Suicidal thoughts (passive or active) or actual attempts

- *Bipolar disorders.* At some point in the course of these illnesses there must be either a manic or a hypomanic episode. The criteria for a manic episode include an excessively elated, expansive, or irritable mood for at least 1 week (or less if hospitalized) and at least three other DSM-IV-TR symptoms (four if mood is only irritable); a helpful mnemonic is DIGFAST (TABLE 17–4). A hypomanic episode is nearly identical, except that symptoms need only be present for 4 or more days, and the degree of impairment is less severe. The DSM-IV-TR describes some subtypes of bipolar disorder that vary by symptom profile and course (TABLE 17–5).

  Key Point: *There is currently some controversy regarding the diagnosis of bipolar disorder in younger people, especially prepubertal children. Until and if they are changed, the clinician should adhere to the DSM-IV-TR criteria.*

- *Anxiety disorders.* One of the basic human emotions, *anxiety,* can be synonymous with other terms such as *nervousness, tension, unease,* or *worry.* Its autonomic effects (e.g., increases in heart and breathing rates) and psychic effects (e.g., feeling that something "bad" will happen) are nearly identical to those caused by *fear.* The major difference is that the trigger for fear is an external factor that is potentially harmful or fatal in fact (e.g., an approaching street gang at night) versus a relatively harmless external factor (e.g., rejection) or an ill-defined internal sensation (e.g., feeling that something is "not right") that triggers anxiety.

TABLE 17–4 DIGFAST: Mnemonic for Manic Episode

Distractibility, focusing on irrelevant external details
Indiscretion, i.e., involvement in pleasurable but potentially harmful activities
Grandiosity, i.e., an overly inflated sense of self or one's accomplishments
Flight of ideas, racing thoughts
Activity that is greatly increased, psychomotor agitation
Sleep greatly reduced but felt not to be needed
Talking greatly increased, pressured

TABLE 17–5   *Types of Bipolar Disorder*

Bipolar I disorder (BPD-I): Think *mania with/without MDD.*
Can also have:
    Hypomanic episodes
    Mixed episodes (i.e., concurrent depressive and manic symptoms)
    Rapid cycling (more than four episodes in one year)
Bipolar II disorder (BPD-II): Think *hypomania with MDD.*
Cyclothymic disorder: Think *hypomania with dysthymic disorder*

- *Panic disorder.* Recurrence of spontaneous panic attacks and a history, for at least 1 month, of fear of another attack, concern about an adverse consequence (such as dying), and/or a change in behavior (such as avoiding places where attacks have occurred). The attacks are short-lived (peaking within 10 minutes), during which at least four symptoms of panic are present (TABLE 17–6). Panic disorder may or may not accompany *agoraphobia,* the fear of abandonment or entrapment without possible escape.
- *Specific phobias.* The exaggerated fears in these disorders are triggered by well-defined external cues such as *animals* (e.g., spiders), *natural factors* (e.g., heights, storms), *blood* or *needles,* or *situations* (e.g., driving). The symptoms (which can be identical to a panic attack) must be present for at least 6 months.
- *Social phobia* (also commonly known as *social anxiety disorder*). Very similar to specific phobias, except that the trigger is a social situation in which the person is fearful of saying or doing something that will draw unwanted attention, opinions, or criticism.
- *Obsessive-compulsive disorder.* Obsessions (see the section "Disturbances of Thought") and/or compulsions (see the section "Disturbances of Behavior") are unwanted, distressing, and interfere with normal behavior. Unlike with adults, children may not perceive or appreciate the irrational nature of the symptoms.

TABLE 17–6   *Symptoms of Panic Attacks*

Palpitations, pounding heart, or accelerated heart rate
Sweating
Trembling or shaking
Sensations of shortness of breath or smothering
Feeling of choking
Chest pain or discomfort
Nausea or abdominal distress
Feeling dizzy, unsteady, lightheaded, or faint
Derealization (feelings of unreality) or
Depersonalization (being detached from oneself)
Fear of losing control or going crazy
Fear of dying
Paresthesias (numbness or tingling sensations)
Chills or hot flushes

- *Posttraumatic stress disorder (PTSD).* After exposure to some intensely distressing event (e.g., a motor vehicle accident), children may manifest repetitive play with trauma themes, recurrent nightmares, physical symptoms, physical avoidance of reminders, emotional blunting, or autonomic arousal. Symptoms are present for more than 1 month. There may be a delay in onset (more than 6 months after the event).

- *Acute stress disorder.* Symptoms are similar to those of PTSD except that they last for at least 2 days and no more than 4 weeks. They also occur within 4 weeks of the traumatic event.

- *Generalized anxiety disorder (GAD).* The hallmark of this disorder is *excessive worry* that generates a lot of anxiety. It occurs almost daily for 6 or more months, and patients feel restless, easily tired, unfocused, irritable, tense, or poorly rested (only one of these is required in children). Sometimes the concerns that younger patients with GAD have are more adult-like, such as worrying about unpaid bills, that they won't get into college, that they'll end up homeless, etc.

Key Point: *Since anxiety can present in varied ways, its symptoms must be elicited by direct questioning.*

- *Somatoform Disorders.* These disorders have in common unconscious physical symptoms that are suspicious for but not diagnostic of a specific medical condition. It is not uncommon—even in children and adolescents—for patients with these disorders to have had multiple medical evaluations before entertaining or making a psychiatric diagnosis.

  - *Conversion disorder.* The hallmark of conversion disorder is the production of *neurologic* symptoms, either motor, sensory, or seizure-like (one of the most common presentations). The onset or exacerbation of the problem is usually associated with an identifiable psychosocial stressor.

  - *Pain disorder.* As the name implies, *pain* is the presenting problem. In children, the most common anatomic pain sites are the head and the abdomen. Psychosocial factors—with or without a general medical condition—predispose to, precipitate, or perpetuate the painful condition.

Key Point: *All patients who present with physical symptoms should be asked about current life stressors.*

- *Factitious Disorders.* These disorders differ from the somatoform disorders in that the patient produces physical and mental symptoms intentionally, presumably to get attention from caregivers. The patient assumes the "sick role." There is a bizarre—and potentially dangerous—variant of this called factitious disorder by proxy, wherein the caregiver does something to the child to intentionally make him or her ill. The caregiver garners attention indirectly through the care of the child.

Key Point: *These can be missed in the absence of a high index of suspicion.*

- *Dissociative Disorders.* All these disorders have in common dissociation, a psychological defense mechanism that protects a person from intense negative thoughts and emotions, usually in connection with some trauma or stressful situation. It is more common in younger people but can persist into adulthood. It presents as a "tuning out" emotionally and cognitively either at the time of the event or later on as amnesia for the event.

Key Point: Should be included in the differential diagnosis of memory loss.

- *Sexual and Gender Identity Disorders.*
  - *Paraphilias.* These disorders share the preoccupation with fantasies or behaviors that are intensely sexually stimulating, and objects, people, or situations that society finds inappropriate, abnormal, and often illegal will trigger them (TABLE 17–7). Although onset of some features can begin in childhood, the fully defined syndrome usually does not appear until adolescence. It occurs almost exclusively in males.
  - *Gender identity disorder (GID).* Often beginning at a very young age, people with GID experience the thoughts, feelings, and fantasies usually associated with the opposite biologic sex. They also desire to live as if they were that other sex. Concurrently, there is a lack of acceptance of one's anatomy, including genitalia.

  Key Point: *The paraphilias are unusual sexual fantasies and behaviors. People with GID feel that they are in the "wrong body."*

- *Eating Disorders.* Owing in large part to the popular media, most people are aware of eating disorders and the high rates of morbidity and mortality associated with them.
  - *Anorexia nervosa (AN).* Fueled by an intense fear of being fat (even when thin), patients with AN (mostly females) will starve themselves or binge and purge to the point of weighing less than 85 percent of expected weight for age. After menarche, there is the absence of three or more consecutive periods.

TABLE 17–7 *Paraphilias*

Exhibitionism—exposing one's genitals to an unsuspecting stranger ("flashing")
Fetishism—using nonliving objects (e.g., female underwear)
Frotteurism—touching/rubbing against a nonconsenting person (such as on a bus)
Pedophilia—sexual activity with prepubescent children (generally aged 13 years or younger)
Sexual masochism—being humiliated, beaten, tied up, or otherwise made to suffer. Sexual sadism—inflicting pain, suffering, or humiliation onto others
Transvestic fetishism—cross-dressing in a heterosexual male
Voyeurism—observing an unsuspecting person who is naked, disrobing, or engaging in sexual activity ("peeping Tom")
Paraphilia NOS—others, including necrophilia (corpses) and zoophilia (bestiality)

- *Bulimia nervosa.* Bulimic patients engage in bingeing, with or without purging (vomiting or using laxatives, diuretics, or enemas). The binges demonstrate rapid, out-of-control ingestion of large amounts of food and occur about twice weekly for 3 months.

  Key Point: *There can be a lot of overlap between these two eating disorders.*
- *Sleep Disorders.* There has been an increasing awareness that disrupted and inadequate sleep in children and adolescents is much more common than previously thought.
  - *Dyssomnias.* These are abnormalities in *quantity, quality,* or *temporal aspects* of sleep.
    - *Primary insomnia.* Difficulty with falling or staying asleep or sleep that is not refreshing for at least 1 month. This diagnosis holds only when the clinician has eliminated all other medical, psychiatric, and substance-related disorders.
    - *Primary hypersomnia.* Similar to primary insomnia, except that patients sleep excessively, night or day.
    - *Narcolepsy.* Patients with this condition have, for at least 3 months, the irresistible urge to sleep on a daily basis. They also experience *cataplexy* (generalized loss of body tone) and/or REM-sleep related events during sleep-wake transitions. Those events are *hypnagogic* (at sleep onset) or *hypnopompic* (at sleep termination) hallucinations, or *sleep paralysis.*
  - *Parasomnias.* These are defined by *abnormal behaviors or physiological events* associated with sleep, certain sleep stages, or the transitions between sleep and being awake.
    - *Nightmare disorder.* The repetitive occurrence of scary dreams that awaken the child, who alerts and orients quickly and seeks out reassurance. Tends to occur in the latter half of the night or nap period (when REM sleep is more frequent). The child may avoid going to sleep secondary to fear of recurrence.
    - *Sleep terror disorder.* This is distinguished from nightmare disorder in important respects: The child doesn't alert or awaken; reassurance doesn't abate the episode; it tends to occur in the first third of sleep (when delta sleep is more common); there is no memory for the event; and there are signs of intense autonomic arousal (e.g., diaphoresis, tachypnea, and tachycardia). The episode typically begins with the child yelling out, which alerts the caregiver.
    - *Sleepwalking disorder.* This shares some features with sleep terror disorder (e.g., phase of sleep, no awareness, no recall), but instead of the autonomic signs, there is motor activity. Children get out of bed and, if not monitored, can engage in potentially dangerous behavior (e.g., going outside).

  Key Point: *All these sleep problems can cause functional impairment in the child but also can have a negative impact on the caregiver's sleep.*
- *Impulse-Control Disorders Not Elsewhere Classified*
  - *Intermittent explosive disorder (IED).* The classic episodes of IED are recurrent outbursts of damaging aggression toward persons or

property. They tend to be overreactions to even minor stressors or trivial events. As other disorders—psychiatric, substance-related, or medical—can present with aggression. Consider IED a diagnosis of exclusion.

- *Kleptomania.* The impulsive and recurrent stealing associated with this disorder serves to relieve emotional tension. There is no financial gain (e.g., the patient gives away or discards stolen items).
- *Pyromania.* In this disorder, fire setting serves the same purpose that stealing does in kleptomania.
- *Pathological gambling.* This disorder is different from the others in this section; in that it has many of the characteristics of an addiction, including need for greater activity over time, difficulty stopping, irritability when cutting back, hiding the behavior or lying about it, engaging in illegal activities to secure money, and financial problems.
- *Trichotillomania.* The relief behavior here is repetitive hair pulling, with noticeable hair loss. The hair can be pulled from anywhere on the body, but the scalp area is the most common. It can be severe enough to lead to baldness.

Key Point: *All these disorders have in common the irresistible urge to engage in a behavior that relieves tension.*

- *Adjustment Disorders.* Emotional or behavioral symptoms that develop in response to identifiable stressor(s) within 3 months after onset of the stressor(s). The symptoms cause distress and/or functional impairment. Common examples include a transient decline in mood and school performance after moving to a new city or losing sleep/appetite and feeling suicidal after a breakup with a significant other. The disturbances are not better explained by other Axis I disorders.

Key Point: *Do not use this diagnosis if the issue is bereavement, which is a normal response to loss.*

Specific Psychiatric Diagnoses: Axis II

As mentioned much earlier in this chapter, Axis II is reserved for mental retardation and personality disorders.

- *Mental Retardation (MR).* The diagnosis of MR requires that there be a below-normal score (intelligence quotient, or IQ) on a standardized test of intellectual functioning and also impairments in at least two areas of adaptive functioning, such as self-care and social skills. There are four levels of MR severity based on IQ scores (TABLE 17–8).

TABLE 17–8 *Degrees of MR Severity*

Mild mental retardation: IQ level 50–55 to about 70
Moderate retardation: IQ level 35–40 to 50–55
Severe mental retardation: IQ level 20–25 to 35–40
Profound mental retardation: IQ level below 20–25

Key Point: *There must be a good correlation between lower IQ and lower functional level to justify the MR diagnosis.*

• *Personality Disorders.* The concept of *personality* implies a relatively fixed constellation of thoughts, affective patterns, behavioral repertoires, and interpersonal negotiations that are highly individualized. In people with *personality disorders,* all areas of internal and external functioning deviate from the cultural norm, causing them to appear as inflexible, unstable, impulsive, and poorly tolerant of stress. They have poor insight into how others perceive them and how they affect other people. They have a tendency to blame others for their distress and failures.

If this in some way sounds like how a young child would think and act, it is no coincidence. Personality disorders arise from an unfortunate combination of a certain temperament (that is already predisposed to hypersensitivity) and a caregiving environment that is abusive, neglectful, ambivalent, and/or unpredictable. Think of this as a developmental arrest, and as such, signs of the personality disorder are usually evident by adolescence.

There are many types of personality disorders (TABLE 17–9), and the reader should refer to the DSM-IV-TR for details. If a clinician suspects a personality disorder in a child or adolescent, obtain specialty psychiatric consultation.

Key Point: *Personality disorder diagnoses can be made cautiously in children and adolescents, with the exception of antisocial personality disorder, which can only be made when the person is at least 18 years of age.*

TABLE 17–9 DSM-IV-TR Personality Disorders (PD)

Cluster A: A pattern of "odd or eccentric" characteristics

Paranoid PD—mistrust, suspiciousness, interpretation of others' motives as malevolent

Schizoid PD—social detachment, restricted emotional range

Schizotypal PD—discomfort in intimate relationships, cognitive or perceptual distortions, eccentric behaviors

Cluster B: A pattern of "dramatic, emotional, or erratic" characteristics

Antisocial PD—disregard for the rights of others and violation of those rights

Borderline PD—unstable interpersonal relationships, self-concept, emotions, and impulse control

Histrionic PD—excessively emotional and attention seeking

Narcissistic PD—grandiose, requiring admiration, lacking empathy

Cluster C: A pattern of "anxious or fearful" characteristics

Avoidant PD—inhibition, inadequacy, and hypersensitivity in social settings

Dependent PD—submissive, clinging, excessive need to be nurtured

Obsessive-Compulsive PD—overly orderly, perfectionistic, and controlled

---

Further Evaluations

Since the DSM-IV-TR requires that medical and substance-use disorders be ruled out before considering making formal psychiatric diagnoses, the first step in all patients must be to obtain a thorough medical and substance-use history (see the first part of this chapter), as well as performing a complete physical examination, even in the absence of somatic complaints. Depending on the findings from the history and physical examination, other investigations could include

- *Routine laboratory studies.* This includes checking the patient's blood for hematologic, hepatic, metabolic, and nutritional abnormalities and checking the blood and urine for renal abnormalities. Urine screens for drugs of abuse are also currently routine tests, even in younger children, because intentional or inadvertent exposure is becoming more common in our society.
  Key Point: *It is important to use the pediatric normal ranges for these tests because many laboratories report only normal ranges for adults.*
- *Special laboratory studies.* Consider genetic testing to help identify a developmental disorder or intellectual deficits. This can involve karyotyping, testing for fragile-X syndrome, or any number of sophisticated and syndrome-specific tests.
- *Specialty consultation.* Although physicians diagnose most medical conditions in a primary care setting, pediatric subspecialty consultation is necessary when diagnosis is unclear or when it requires more specialized evaluation. It is also a good idea if the actual management of the condition will require more specialized and comprehensive care not found in the primary care setting.
- *Electrophysiologic studies.* The use of the electroencephalogram (EEG) to look for seizure activity can be very helpful at times. For example, some patients with IED actually derive their aggressive outburst from nonconvulsive seizure activity. Likewise, a child who presents with inattentive-type ADHD actually could be experiencing absence seizure activity.
  Key Point: *The EEG should not be considered a routine test in all patients.*
- *Neuroimaging studies.* The main reason to perform neuroimaging in younger patients is to rule out hemorrhages and mass lesions. Occasionally, malformed or absent brain structures will appear incidentally. Patients who have an altered level of consciousness, non-tensiontype headaches, visual and auditory deficits, or focal sensorimotor deficits should undergo neuroimaging. Patients who demonstrate asymmetric abnormalities on the EEG also should undergo neuroimaging.
- *Psychological testing.* Given the overlap of some symptoms in the DSM-IV-TR, as well as the sometimes poor quality of historical information, making a psychiatric diagnosis can be difficult. Psychological testing can provide much needed data to help clarify diagnostic confusion. Many tests are self-report instruments, so they can

be especially useful in patients who have difficulty with verbal expression or who become anxious during face-to-face encounters. Depending on the types of tests available to the evaluating psychologist, ability to read or write may limit what is useful.

Key Point: *The younger the patient, the less reliable are the results of the testing.*

- *Neuropsychological testing.* This type of testing is highly specialized, and the person who is qualified to conduct a neuropsychological evaluation requires years of extra training and experience. It is invaluable in cases where there are intellectual delays or declines or where there are cognitive impairments that do not fit neatly into specific diagnostic categories.

Conclusion

This chapter should prove useful in your work with younger patients who are demonstrating disturbances of thought, feeling, or behavior. As previously alluded to, the reader is encouraged to refer to the DSM-IV-TR for more detailed information. There are many other resources available, either through your local medical library or via the Internet.

18 Principles of Developmental Diagnosis

Dilip R. Patel

The goals of this chapter are

1. To review the basic concepts and definitions applied in the study of developmental problems
2. To review the main features of common conditions considered in the differential diagnoses of developmental disorders
3. To describe signs that should prompt further developmental evaluation

Basic Concepts

Key Principles

- Gross motor development progresses in a cephalocaudal sequence, whereas fine motor development progresses from midline to lateral.
- The primitive reflex patterns have to be lost or integrated into evolving complex motor patterns for later (sequential) voluntary motor development to proceed.
- Not all children attain developmental milestones at the same rate or at the same time; there is a range of normal variation.
- Not all typically developing children progress at the same rate in all developmental domains.
- The sequence of typical development is the same in all children.
- Development progresses from generalized and reflexive responses to more specific and purposeful responses.

Definitions

Domains of Development

Development generally follows four domains and has a "typical" progression when it is proceeding as expected:

1. *Motor* development consists of fine motor and gross motor domains.
2. *Speech and language* development has both receptive and expressive domains.

629

3. *Social-emotional* development is a reflection of or a combination of development in other domains that includes fine motor adaptive abilities, overall communication abilities, and cognitive abilities.
4. *Cognitive* development generally refers to visual perceptual, visual motor, and problem-solving skills and abilities. Language development is a good indicator of overall cognitive development.

Speech and Language

Speech is the production of sounds for words. *Prosody* is the pattern of rhythm, stress, and intonation of the speech. *Language* is a system of symbolic knowledge represented in the brain and used for meaningful communication. The English language has 44 phonemes. A *phoneme* is a unit of sound in speech. Airflow obstruction accompanies the production of consonant sounds, whereas it does not in the case of vowel sounds. A *morpheme* (word) refers to the smallest meaningful unit of language. The basic components of the language appear in TABLE 18–1.

TABLE 18–1 *Basic Components of Language*

Structure or form of language

Phonology	Sound system of the language that is made of phonemes; use of phonemes and conventions for their combinations	
Grammar	Morphology	Rules or conventions for constructing meaningful words, e.g., adding *-s* or *-es* to a word to indicate plural (duck/ducks)
	Syntax	Rules or conventions for constructing meaningful phrases or sentences and their relationship, e.g., word order: "Daddy go there." But "There Daddy go" is not typical English structure.

Content of the language

Lexicon	Vocabulary
Semantics	Relationship among words; symbols representing universal concepts; meaning of words (e.g., in relation to objects, agents, an action, states, attributes or locations); meaning and relationship of abstract concepts (e.g., idioms and proverbs).

Use of the language

Pragmatics	Rules or conventions for use of language in a socially and culturally appropriate manner and in the appropriate context, e.g., turn taking, eye contact, maintaining a topic in conversation.

Developmental Quotient (DQ)

DQ is a measure of rate of developmental progression in a given developmental domain. It is calculated as follows:

$$DQ = (DA/CA) \times 100$$

where DA is development age and CA is chronologic age. A significant delay is a DQ that is equal to or less than 70 in a given domain.

Intelligence Quotient (IQ)

IQ is a measure of cognition or intelligence and is calculated as follows:

$$IQ = (MA/CA) \times 100$$

where MA is mental age. Standardized tests of intelligence, individually administered, measure IQ.

Developmental Delay

Developmental delay refers to the significantly delayed attainment of milestones or skills in one or more domains but in a correct sequence compared with that of typically developing children.

Developmental Deviation

Developmental deviation, or *atypical development,* refers to the attainment of developmental skills in a given domain that is out of sequence, e.g., when an infant rolls from supine to prone before prone to supine.

Developmental Dissociation

Developmental dissociation refers to the attainment of developmental skills at significantly different rates between two or more domains of development, e.g., when there is delayed motor development relative to other domains in cerebral palsy.

Developmental Regression

Developmental regression refers to loss of previously acquired developmental milestones or skills or failure to acquire new skills.

Global Developmental Delay

Global developmental delay refers to significant developmental delay in two or more developmental domains in children younger than 5 years of age. It is difficult to measure IQ reliably before age 5 or 6 years of age.

Mental Retardation

Mental retardation (MR) is significantly subaverage intellectual functioning (IQ of 70 or less with a standard error of measurement of 5 on an individually administered standardized intelligence test) with limitations in adaptive behavior as expressed in conceptual, social, and practical adaptive skills.

Developmental Surveillance

Developmental surveillance refers to gathering and synthesizing information about the developmental progress of a child based on history and observations by parents or other caretakers and health care practitioners and during periodic visits on a longitudinal and continuous basis over time. The goal of the developmental surveillance is to identify children who *may have* developmental problems.

Developmental Screening

Developmental screening refers to the administration of a brief standardized screening test in order to identify children *at risk* of a developmental disorder.

Developmental Evaluation

Developmental evaluation is essentially a diagnostic process that may involve appropriate laboratory testing, genetic testing, metabolic testing, neuroimaging studies, and psychological testing, as well as specialist consultations. The goal of the evaluation is to *identify a specific developmental disorder* and its etiology, if known.

History

A thorough developmental history should include the following information with obvious age-appropriate considerations. Obtain the information from parents and other caretakers and school and other professionals when appropriate.

Past History

Prenatal

Mother's age at birth of the child/father's age at birth of the child/ prenatal care/gravida (number of pregnancies)/parity (term/preterm/ abortions/living)/prenatal infections/multiple gestation/previous pregnancy loses/maternal weight gain/fetal activity/maternal medical and obstetric problems/eclampsia/prenatal monitoring and tests/medications/ smoking/drugs/alcohol/radiation exposure/at-risk sexual behaviors.

Perinatal

Hospital or home delivery details/length of gestation/labor (induced/ spontaneous)/vaginal/forceps/cesarean section/intrapartum monitoring/ use of analgesia or anesthesia (epidural)/prolapsed cord/ breech/polyhydramnios/oligohydramnios/prolonged rupture of membrane/maternal fever/toxemia/abnormal bleeding/abnormalities of placenta/ meconium or foul-smelling amniotic fluid.

Neonatal

Birth weight/height/head circumference/Dubowitz/small for gestational age (SGA)/large for gestational age (LGA)/Apgar scores/ need for resuscitation/duration of stay/respiratory distress/assisted ventilation/apnea/cyanosis/seizures/infections/jaundice/blood type/Coombs'/congenital anomalies/feeding problems/brain imaging/ laboratory tests.

Developmental

Initial parental concerns about development/previous developmental evaluations/specific developmental diagnosis if any and at what age/ early major milestones.

Medical/Surgical

Major illnesses/injuries/hospitalizations/procedures or investigations/ surgeries (e.g., congenital heart disease).

Family History

Fetal wastage/unexplained infant or childhood deaths/parental and sibling health/medical conditions in family members (congenital/genetic/ neurologic/psychiatric/medical)/learning disorders/speech and language disorders.

Personal/Social History

Parent occupation/socioeconomic status/parental level of education/ primary caregiver/living situation/school functioning/any current services or therapies (occupational therapy/physical therapy/ speech therapy/ other)/any current early intervention or special health care services or plans (individualized family service plan/individualized education plan/individualized transition plan)/extracurricular activities/family adjustment/school adjustment/use of medications (some have adverse effects on cognition and behavior).

Review of Systems (Based on Presenting Symptoms as in Any Medical Evaluation)

Infants

KEY PROBLEM

■ Predominant Delay in Motor Milestones Generally, delayed or atypical motor development manifests earlier than other domains of development. Because there is a range of periods during which infants achieve typical milestones, the most common cause of apparent motor delay is a normal variation or maturational lag. The most significant cause of motor delay in infancy is cerebral palsy, which consists of motor delay, abnormal tone, and posture.

Clinical presentation and features of infants and children with *cerebral palsy* may vary depending on its type and severity. A child older than 2 months of age with cerebral palsy may have poor head control, stiff legs, and scissoring. A child older than 6 months of age still may not have head control, may not sit unsupported, and may preferentially use only one extremity. A child older than 10 months of age may crawl by pushing off with one hand and leg while dragging the opposite hand and leg and may not sit without support. A child older than 12 months of age may not be crawling and may not stand with support. A child older than 24 months of age may not be walking yet or able to push a toy with wheels. Other causes of predominantly motor delay include *traumatic* insults to the central nervous system (CNS) (kernicterus, birth injury, stroke, *metabolic* insults, and congenital infections), *spinal cord disorders* (myelomeningocele, Werdnig-Hoffmann disease), myopathies, muscular dystrophies, and benign congenital hypotonia.

KEY PROBLEM
Atypical Development Predominantly Affecting Social, Cognitive, and Language Milestones
A full evaluation for autism, significant cognitive delay, or language impairment is mandatory in infants with the following: no babbling, pointing, or other gestures by 12 months of age; no single words by 16 months; no two-word spontaneous phrases by 24 months of age; and any loss of previously acquired language or social skills. A deficiency in joint attention, i.e., the ability to attend to both an object and a person at the same time (e.g., when the infant or child points to or shows an object to his or her mother and simultaneously looks at her), is often an early sign in infants and toddlers with autism.

Other conditions to consider in infants with predominantly language, cognitive, and social delays include hearing impairment, severe cognitive deficits, genetic disorders, inborn errors of metabolism (including hypothyroidism), and severe nutritional or environmental deprivation.

Developmental regression may occur in autism between 18 and 24 months. Some of the less common conditions associated with progressive encephalopathy with onset before age 2 years include *metabolic* conditions such as *amino acid metabolism, lysosomal storage disease, hypothyroidism, mitochondrial diseases, tuberous sclerosis, Lesch-Nyhan syndrome, Rett syndrome, Canavan disease,* and *Pelizaeus-Merzbacher disease.*

Children

KEY PROBLEM
Atypical Language Development
Speech and language problems may present as any number of symptoms, including poor intelligibility (normal 25 percent by age 1, 50 percent by age 2; 75 percent by age 3, and 100 percent by age 4), persistent baby talk, mispronunciations of words, or lack of spontaneous speech.

Main causes of atypical development in pre-school-age children are *autism spectrum disorders, mental retardation,* and *developmental language disorders.*

Children with autism have qualitative impairment in communication skills, qualitative impairment in social relatedness, and a range of atypical stereotypical behaviors. Motor development is normal. *Autism spectrum disorders* typically develop by age 3 years, some as early as

18 months. Parents usually first notice unusual behaviors and language difficulties in the child. They may describe the child as not socially responsive to others or as intensely focusing on one item for a long period of time. The child may demonstrate withdrawn, aggressive, or self-abusive behavior; have poor eye contact, become attached to a particular toy; and excessively line up toys or other objects. A child with autism spectrum disorder may not play pretend games, may want others to leave him alone, may have trouble understanding other people's feelings, and may demonstrate echolalia. Children with *Asperger syndrome* demonstrate normal cognitive and language abilities and predominant deficits in social development.

Children with *mental retardation* have predominant deficits in cognitive and language abilities. Their social development is consistent with their mental age, and they have no motor deficits. Some of the signs of mental retardation that parents may observe include that the child is late to sit, crawl, walk, or learn to talk and that the child has trouble speaking, finds it hard to remember things, has trouble understanding social roles, has trouble seeing the results of his or her actions, or has trouble solving problems. There is no identifiable specific cause in most children with mild mental retardation. The likelihood of identifying a specific etiology increases as the severity of mental retardation increases. Some of the known causes of mental retardation include *fragile-X syndrome*, *fetal alcohol syndrome*, *other genetic syndromes*, *lead toxicity*, *iron deficiency*, *brain malformations* or *dysgenesis*, and *tuberous sclerosis*. *Fragile-X syndrome* is the most common inherited form of mental retardation.

Children with *developmental language disorders* have predominant deficits in various aspects of language development, whereas their social, motor, and cognitive development is normal. Differential diagnosis of speech and language delay/disorders includes speech and voice disorders, hearing impairment, developmental language disorders, mental retardation, autism spectrum disorders, maturational language delay, and lack of environmental stimulation for language learning and literacy. A bilingual home environment is not a cause for language delay. The basic components of the language are presented in TABLE 18–1.

The various subtypes of *developmental language disorders* have been described and are based on particular aspects of the language that are affected. *Expressive language disorders* predominantly affect speech production. In *verbal dyspraxia* (also called *developmental apraxia of speech*), the child will have difficulty in planning, sequencing, and executing voluntary speech sounds. The speech is dysfluent, unintelligible, and significantly delayed with inconsistent articulation errors. *Speech programming deficit disorder* is characterized by fluent, unintelligible, jargon and is considered by most speech-language pathologists to be similar to verbal dyspraxia, and both largely lead to be speech production problems.

Mixed receptive-expressive language disorders are characterized by deficits in both comprehension and expression of speech. *Verbal auditory agnosia*, or *word deafness*, is characterized by profound impairment in comprehension of spoken words. Children are mostly nonverbal or have very limited verbal expression. This is a rare condition in children. In *phonologic* or *syntactic deficit disorder*, the comprehension or the ability to recognize phonological rules, receptively, is mostly preserved or is relatively better (in most children) than expression. It is characterized by significant omissions, distortions, and substitutions of words, and the speech is telegraphic, with limited vocabulary and grammatical errors. The child tends to use short sentences and has difficulty in repetition of words or sentences.

Higher-order processing disorders of language are more complex. *Lexical deficit disorder,* or *lexical-syntactic deficit,* is characterized by severe deficits in word finding and paraphrasing, jargon, and pseudostuttering. There is significant deficiency in understanding of connected speech, impoverished syntax, and syntactic distortions. Spontaneous language is relatively better than language on demand. The child may respond to simple commands, and his or her ability to decode *wh-* questions is limited. *Semantic-pragmatic deficit disorder* is characterized by poor discourse of connected speech, although the child may be talkative. The phonology and syntax (often simplified syntax) are preserved. Other characteristics of this disorder include atypical choices of words, word-finding deficits, significant deficits in comprehension and verbal reasoning, and tangential and stereotyped speech, often with echolalia. Children manifest deficiencies in conversational skills characterized by speaking aloud to no one in particular, poor maintenance of the topic, and responding inaccurately or out of context to commands and questions. This is a rare condition in children. *Developmental speech disorders* are described in TABLE 18–2.

Selective mutism is failure to speak in specific social situations, such as in school, whereas the child is able to speak in other situations, such as at home. Between 20 and 30 percent of children with selective mutism have associated articulation problems and language delays. Some children may use gestures to communicate in specific situations. The child may manifest shyness, clinging, temper tantrums, or oppositional behaviors.

KEY PROBLEM
◄ Regression of Previously Acquired Developmental Skills or Lack of Acquisition of New Skills

Main causes of developmental regression include *autistic regression, Rett syndrome, childhood disintegrative disorder,* and *Landau-Kleffner syndrome. Rett syndrome* demonstrates loss of developmental milestones after a period of normal development, autistic behaviors, characteristic abnormal wringing hand movements, and a deceleration in head circumference. Following early regression, there is some recovery, but then stagnation and late motor deterioration ensue. Some of the other features in children with Rett syndrome include hyperventilation, breath holding, air swallowing, bruxism, gait dyspraxia, neurogenic scoliosis, autonomic dysfunction, inappropriate laughing and screaming spells, and intense eye communication.

Childhood disintegrative disorder (CDD) is a rare condition characterized by loss of previously acquired motor, language, and social skills. It has a very high male predominance, and the typical onset is between 3 and 4 years of age. The much later onset of loss of skills after a period

TABLE 18-2 *Developmental Speech Disorders*

Speech sound disorder

Also described as functional articulation disorder or phonological disorder. Characterized by errors in articulation and speech sounds, consistent substitution of simple sounds for complex sounds or single consonants for blended consonants, dropped consonants, and errors within words. Problem may not be recognized until preschool.

Stuttering

Disturbed speech fluency with atypical rate and rhythm and repetitions of sounds, syllables, words, and phrases generally accompanied by evidence of stress or physical tension. There may be sound prolongations, interjections, pauses within words, and blocking of words. Typical onset between 2 and 7 years with peak at age 5 years.

Resonance disorders

Can be either hypernasal or hyponasal voice owing to anatomic factors. Hypernasality may be due to dysfunction of the velopharyngeal mechanism, seen, for example, in cleft palate. Hyponasality is seen, for example, in nasal congestion, upper respiratory infections, nasal anomalies, and hypertrophied adenoids.

Dysarthria

Due to dysfunction of the neuromuscular or motor mechanism for speech production (e.g., cerebral palsy). Characterized mainly by inconsistent misarticulations of speech sounds and words, poor intelligibility, and slow speech.

Verbal dyspraxia and speech programming deficit disorder

Both terms describe similar types of largely speech production problems. These disorders may significantly influence expressive language as well (see text).

---

of normal development differentiates it from Rett syndrome. Children with CDD have a very low IQ and often develop seizures. These children also lose bowel and bladder control.

Landau-Kleffner syndrome (LKS) typically occurs between the ages of 3 and 8 years. After the first 3 years of normal development, the child loses language skills. Nonverbal cognitive abilities and social skills are not affected. Abnormal pattern of sleep electroencephalography and seizures, especially during night, are characteristic of LKS.

Less common causes of progressive encephalopathy with developmental regression with onset after 2 years of age include *genetic/metabolic* lysosomal *storage disease, disorders of gray matter* such as *ceroid lipofuscinosis* and *mitochondrial disorders, white matter diseases* such as *adrenoleukodystrophy* and *Alexander disease, acquired human immunodeficiency syndrome (AIDS) encephalopathy,* and postinfectious *subacute sclerosing panencephalitis.*

KEY PROBLEM

◗ Early Learning Difficulties and Behavioral Symptoms

Early (about third grade) academic or learning difficulties can present as poor grades, delay in completing assignments, inattention, delay in learning new skills, and difficulties in comprehending or reading. These children also may be shy and withdrawn and have behavioral problems at school. Differential diagnosis should include *attention deficit/hyperactivity disorder (ADHD), sensory impairments, specific learning disability, developmental coordination disorder,* and *mental retardation* or *borderline intellectual functioning.*

Vision and hearing impairment may be associated with other developmental disabilities. A child with *visual impairment* might close or cover one eye, squint the eyes or frown, complain that things are blurry or hard to see, have trouble reading or doing other close-up work or hold objects close to eyes, and blink more than usual or seem cranky when doing close-up work such as looking at a book.

A child with *hearing impairment,* complete or partial, might not turn to the source of a sound from birth to 3 or 4 months of age, may not say single words such as *dada* or *mama* by 1 year of age, and may turn his or her head when he or she sees you but not if you only call out his or her name. This often is mistaken for not paying attention or just ignoring.

Developmental coordination disorder affects school-age children and persists into adolescent years. Difficulties in motor coordination will cause substantial impairment in academic function or activities of daily living. Earliest manifestations may include difficulty sucking and swallowing, drooling during infancy, and speech difficulties and delayed motor milestones during early childhood. Parents may observe that the child has difficulties with many of the fine motor tasks such as using scissors, tying shoe laces, or buttoning or unbuttoning. The child also may drop objects, have poor handwriting, or frequently bump into furniture or other people. Differential diagnosis includes ADHD, visual impairment, and MR.

Adolescents

KEY PROBLEM

◗ Academic Difficulties

Developmental learning disabilities or disorders are the main consideration in older children and adolescents with difficulties with school work. In addition to specific signs associated with learning disorders, these children may present with behavioral problems. The differential diagnoses also should include *anxiety disorders, ADHD, pervasive developmental disorders,* and *disruptive behavior disorders.* In adolescents, also consider *substance abuse* and *depressive disorders.*

Developmental learning disorder is diagnosed when the child's or adolescent's scores on an individually administered standardized achievement test (in reading, mathematics, or written expression) are substantially below those expected based on his or her age, education, and level of intelligence (on individually administered standardized tests).

Reading disorder may not be apparent until the fourth grade, especially if mild and in a child with a high IQ. Some of the clinical features of reading disorder include delayed language, problems with rhyming words or words that sound alike, difficulty learning letters of the alphabet, spelling errors, difficulty reading (decoding) unfamiliar or nonsense words or single words, and slow reading.

Children with *mathematics disorder* will demonstrate problems with skills in arithmetic by the end of second or third grade. Some of the features include difficulties understanding or naming mathematical terms, operations, or concepts; difficulties decoding or recognizing mathematical symbols or signs; and difficulties copying numbers or figures and following sequences of mathematical steps, counting, and multiplication tables.

Disorder of written expression is apparent by the end of the fifth grade and manifests problems with writing skills, which include grammatical errors, punctuation errors, poor paragraph organization, spelling errors, and very poor handwriting.

Nonverbal learning disability demonstrates difficulties with problem solving and visuospatial and visuoperceptual deficits, whereas the language-based skills and intelligence are normal.

Physical Examination

In infants, examination should focus on neurologic and developmental assessment (see Chapter 12). The examination should document serial measurements of height, weight, and head circumference on appropriate graphs. Also, a meticulous search for dysmorphic features or congenital anomalies should be an integral component of the examination (see Chapter 6). In addition, in adolescents, the examination should include assessment of Tanner stage (see Chapter 13) and mental status examination (see Chapter 12).

Synthesizing a Diagnosis

Any parental concern about development, hearing, or vision is an indication for further evaluation for developmental or sensory problems. Ask certain key questions (TABLE 18–3) at the outset in the process of synthesizing a developmental diagnosis. We present an algorithm for evaluation of the child with global developmental delay in FIGURE 18–1.

TABLE 18–3   *Suspected Developmental Delay: Key Questions*

Developmental assessment
Is a developmental delay present?
Is the delay global or selective?

History (problem context, developmental, family, medical, review of
   systems)
Do caretakers perceive development to be a problem?
Was there a distinct onset to the developmental problem?
Has developmental regression been noted?
Does the history suggest a potential etiology?

Psychological/ behavioral assessment
What is the nature of the caretaking environment?
Are significant emotional/behavioral problems present?

Physical examination
Is there physical evidence of a potential etiology?
Are growth retardation and/or microcephaly present?

Sensory evaluation
Is hearing or visual deficit present?

Laboratory evaluation
Are specific diagnostic testes warranted?

Source: From Rudolph CD, et al (eds): *Rudolph's Pediatrics*, 21st ed. New York: McGraw-Hill, 2003, p. 16, with permission.

Laboratory and Other Diagnostic Tests

- Hearing evaluation is mandatory in all children with symptoms or signs of a developmental disorder. Current guidelines recommend universal hearing screening by 1 month of age, with subsequent further diagnostic audiologic testing completed by 3 months of age. For infants identified as having a hearing impairment treatment intervention should start by age 6 months. Hearing screening is also part of periodic health maintenance examinations.
- Vision screening should be part of periodic health maintenance examinations in all children.
- Developmental screening with appropriate standardized screening instruments (TABLE 18–4) is part of the periodic health maintenance examinations in the primary care setting at 9, 12, and 30 months of age. If there is no periodic health maintenance examination at 30 months, then perform it at 24 months of age.
- Similarly screening for autism (FIGURE 18–2) with standardized autism screening tools should be routine at the 18- and 24-month visits.
- If office screening yields suspicion for a developmental disorder, a more formal and advanced testing is necessary. Clinical psychologists with special expertise in the diagnostic testing of children with developmental disorders should perform this.

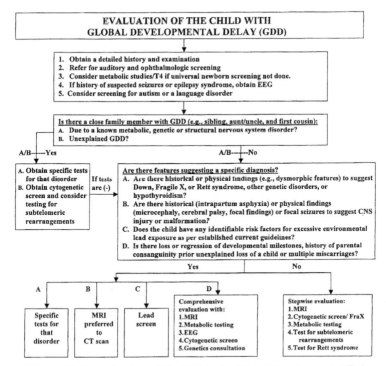

FIGURE 18–1 *Evaluation of the Child with Global Developmental Delay.*
Note: Audiologic and ophthalmologic screening is recommended in all children with global developmental delay. Metabolic studies usually consist of obtaining a urine organic acid screen, quantitative serum amino acids, serum lactate and ammonia levels, capillary or arterial blood gas, and thyroid function studies. (From Shevell M, et al: Practice parameter: Evaluation of the child with global developmental delay. Neurology *60;376, 2003, with permission from the American Academy of Neurology.)*

- Consider neuroimaging, electroencephalography, tests for genetic disorders, and specific laboratory tests for metabolic disorders based on history and examination and in consultation with appropriate medical specialists (TABLE 18–5).

When to Refer

- Children identified as being at risk for developmental problems based on developmental screening should have a referral for more formal diagnostic testing by a clinical psychologist. All children with significant developmental delay—with a DQ of 70 or less—should have formal psychological testing.

TABLE 18–4   *Examples of Developmental Screening Instruments*

General developmental screening
Ages and stages questionnaires
Battelle Developmental Inventory Screening Tool, 2d ed.
Bayley Infant Neurodevelopmental Screen
Brigance Screens II
Child Development Inventory
Child Development Review—Parent Questionnaire
Denver II Developmental Screening Test
Infant Development Inventory
Parents' Evaluation of Developmental Status

Gross motor screening
Early Motor Pattern Profile (EMPP)
Motor Quotient

Language and cognitive screening
Capute Scales
Communication and Symbolic Behavioral Scales Developmental
   Profile: Infant, Toddler Checklist
Early Language Milestone Scale 2

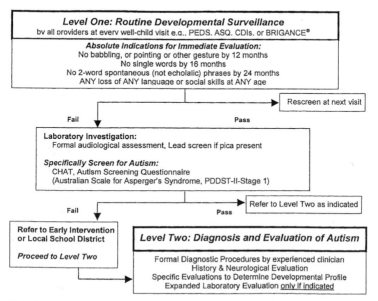

FIGURE 18–2 *Autism Practice Parameter Algorithm. (From Filipek PA, et al: Practice parameter: Screening and diagnosis of autism.* Neurology *55:468–479, 2000, with permission of the American Academy of Neurology.)*

TABLE 18-5 *Laboratory Studies Recommended for the Child with Developmental Delay and Specific Signs and Symptoms*

Sign or Symptom	Laboratory Studies
Neurologic regression Sensory abnormalities Unexplained new or progressive neurologic finding Failure to thrive accompanied by neurologic findings	Urine for organic acids Serum amino acids, lactate, pyruvate, and very long chain fatty acid concentrations (peroxisomal disorders)
Cranial abnormalities (e.g., microcephaly)	Viral titers for congenital infection Urine for cytomegalovirus Cranial CT scan or MRI
Gross motor delay with associated hypotonia, weakness, and hyporeflexia	Serum creatine phosphokinase Aldolase concentrations Electromyography Nerve conduction velocity
Congenital malformations Many atypical physical features	Chromosomal karyotype
Family history of unexplained mental retardation	Cytogenetic studies for fragile-X syndrome
Language delay	Audiologic evaluation

Source: From Rudolph CD, et al (eds): *Rudolph's Pediatrics*, 21st ed. New York: McGraw-Hill, 2003, p. 440, with permission.

- All infants and children with developmental regression should come to the attention of a pediatric neurologist. These children also may need an evaluation by a clinical geneticist, specialist in metabolic diseases, or other experts as indicated.
- Refer children with disorders of speech and language because such disorders are complex. All children suspected of such disorders demand evaluation by a speech-language pathologist for formal diagnosis.
- Refer infants and children with symptoms and signs suggestive of autism spectrum disorders to specialists with special expertise in their evaluation.
- Specialty consultations with a pediatric neurologist, neurodevelopmental disabilities physician, endocrinologist, geneticist, and other specialists may be necessary based on history, signs and symptoms, and initial psychological and laboratory testing.

19 The Male Genitourinary System

Julian Wan

The goals of this chapter are

1. To outline the normal physiology and anatomy of the pediatric male genitourinary (GU) system
2. To outline the pathophysiology that produces the symptoms and signs referable to the pediatric male GU system
3. To catalogue the major common problems in infants, children, and adolescents
4. To explain how to perform a complete physical examination referable to GU symptoms and signs
5. To synthesize a list of GU diagnoses in tabular form
6. To outline confirmatory laboratory, imaging, and investigative procedures and when to refer to a specialist

Anatomy, Physiology, and Mechanics

Normal

The male genitourinary (GU) system constitutes the union of two major physiologic organizations: the urinary system and the male reproductive system. They join at the lower urinary tract, where the bladder empties into the prostatic urethra. At this point the vas deferens meets the ejaculatory ducts emptying into the verumontanum at the prostatic urethra just above the external urinary sphincter. They share a common pathway thereafter down the bulbous and pendulous urethra and fossa navicularis, which exit the penis at the urethra meatus. FIGURE 19–1 illustrates the gross anatomy.

The urinary system consists of the kidney, collecting system of the renal pelvis and ureter, the bladder, and the urethra. The kidneys lie behind the eleventh and twelfth ribs in the retroperitoneum. The kidneys filter blood continuously at the glomerulus. As the filtrate progresses down the collecting system, the renal tubules reabsorb and secrete other solutes and fluids. As the filtrate enters the collecting ducts, it becomes more concentrated in the medulla to become urine. The urine then gathers into calyces, which drain into a central collecting space, the renal pelvis. From there the urine actively continues via peristalsis down long

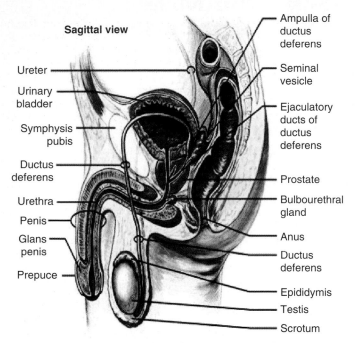

FIGURE 19-1 *Gross Anatomy of the Male Genitourinary Tract (Antero-Posterior View).* *(From Van De Graaff KM:* Human Anatomy. *New York: McGraw Hill, 2002, Fig. 20(a).1, p. 699.)*

muscular tubes, the ureters, that connect the pelvis to the bladder. This peristaltic action is independent of gravity and activity and occurs regardless of posture, movement, or exercise. The ureters course down the retroperitoneum, over the psoas muscles, and enter the bladder. There are three points of narrowing in the course of the ureter that are of clinical importance. They are (1) the point where the ureter meets the renal pelvis, the ureteropelvic junction (UPJ), (2) where the ureters pass over the iliac vessels at the lower brim of the bony pelvis, and (3) where the ureter enters the bladder, the ureterovesical junction (UVJ). The ureter does not enter directly into the bladder. It passes obliquely so that it runs within the muscular wall for a considerable distance (4 to 7 cm) before entering the interior. These narrowing points are important because they are areas where urinary calculi can obstruct and cause subsequent hydronephrosis. The bladder is a spheroid-shaped hollow organ that sits in the bony pelvis just behind the pubic symphysis. It has an epithelial lining that is normally impermeable to urine and its solutes. The body of the bladder consists of several layers of smooth muscle that wind over the epithelium, forming a concentric flexible layer called the *detrusor muscle.* This layer normally can relax and expand to accommodate large volumes of urine with little or no change in internal pressure. The muscle also can contract and rapidly shrink the volume of the bladder, thereby emptying it in a few seconds. At the base of the bladder is a triangular region, the trigone. The ureteral orifices comprise two of the vertices, with the opening of the urethra at the bladder neck completing the triangle. The trigone is a particularly sensitive part of the bladder, and the presence of calculi, foreign bodies, or lesions can result in irritating urinary symptoms. The urethra is the tube that carries the urine from the bladder to the outside world. Its mucosa consists of the same transitional epithelium that covers the inside of the bladder and ureter. At the junction with the bladder, the urethra courses through the middle of the prostate gland, where it becomes the prostatic urethra. This part of the urethra is the important junction point where the vas deferens connect to the urethra. The vas deferens insert on either side of the verumontanum, a small mound at the floor of the prostatic urethra. The prostatic urethra and bladder neck have layers of smooth muscle on the outside that normally keep the urethra lining closed against each other in an adherent fashion termed *coaptation*. Just distal to the prostatic urethra is the external urinary sphincter, which is composed primarily of strands of skeletal muscle from the pelvic floor. At rest, the detrusor is in a state of inhibition, allowing for further filling, during which time the bladder neck is closed, the proximal urethra is sealed, and the external sphincter muscles are active. During voiding, a coordinated process occurs that relaxes the sphincter just before the bladder contracts. Initially, the bladder neck and proximal urethra open. The external sphincter muscles then relax, which further helps to open the urethra. The detrusor muscle then contracts, and urination occurs. The urinary reflex is under control of the autonomic nervous system, with the sequence of events at urination stimulated by parasympathetic input and urinary retention in between voiding as a sympathetic function. The pontine micturition center in the brain stem mediates this reflex. Coincident with the time of toilet training, neural maturation allows input from higher centers for more conscious control of urination. Bladder capacity gradually increases from birth, with the "rule of thumb" being ounces of capacity = age in years +2, applicable up to age 14. The urethra, which carries the urine outward, turns to head up into the penis. This point of curvature is the bulb or bulbous urethra. The urethra then enters into the body of the penis and becomes the pendulous urethra. Finally, the urethra ends on the surface of the glans penis at the fossa navicularis, which emerges at the meatus.

Male genitalia arise from a common embryologic reproductive tract. Male sex differentiation occurs because of the activity of the *SRY* gene on the Y chromosome. The gene leads to masculinization of the reproductive tract. This occurs because of the hormonal activity of testosterone, dihydrotestosterone, and Müllerian inhibiting substance (MIS). Absence or incomplete activity of these hormones will lead to a feminization of the reproductive tract or some state in between, also known as *intersex* or *ambiguous genitalia*. The male reproductive tract consists of the testes, epididymis, vas deferens, seminal vesicles, prostate, and penis. The testes form inside the abdomen and during the last trimester descend through the inguinal canals into the scrotum. The cooler scrotal location is critical to later spermatogenesis. The testes are ovoid and have a homogeneous texture. There is a tough outer capsule, the tunica albuginea, that encapsulates each testicle. The testes have three major structures: (1) seminiferous tubules, which produce spermatozoa, (2) Leydig cells, which produce testosterone, and (3) Sertoli cells, which produce MIS. The Leydig cells and seminiferous tubules are part of an endocrine loop controlled by the pituitary gland via luteinizing hormone (LH) and follicle-stimulating hormone (FSH). At puberty, testes produce spermatozoa, which collect in the epididymis. They are then transported up the vas deferens into the spermatic cord, which travels back up the inguinal canal and then around behind the bladder, where it joins the duct of the seminal vesicle to form the ejaculatory duct. This duct, in turn, inserts into the prostatic urethra at the verumontanum. There it mixes with secretions from the prostate and seminal vesicles to form the ejaculate. The head of the epididymis caps the upper pole of the testicle. The body of the epididymis curves along the posterolateral border of the testicle, and at the lower pole or tail it joins the vas deferens, a muscular tube, that courses back up to the inguinal canal as part of the spermatic cord.

The penis consists of three cylindrical structures (FIGURE 19–2). There are two corpora cavernosa, which comprise the bulk of the penis. They anchor against the pubic bones and rise to end beneath the glans penis. The third structure is the corpus spongiosum, and it passes ventrally to the corpora cavernosa and carries within it the urethra. As it nears the tip of the penis, it expands and forms a cone-shaped cap, the glans penis. The urethra exits the glans either at the tip or on the ventral surface. The point of exit is the meatus. A concentric flap of skin covers the glans and is the foreskin or prepuce (FIGURE 19–3). At rest, the penis is flaccid, but under psychosexual stimulation, involving the parasympathetic nervous system, the corpora cavernosa becomes engorged with

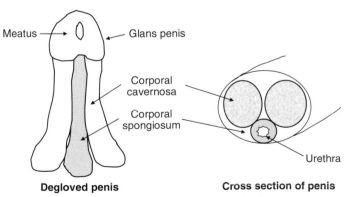

Meatus — Glans penis

Corporal cavernosa

Corporal spongiosum

Urethra

Degloved penis　　　　**Cross section of penis**

FIGURE 19–2 Basic Structure of the Penis. Two views of the penis degloved, showing the relationship between the corporal bodies and the urethra.

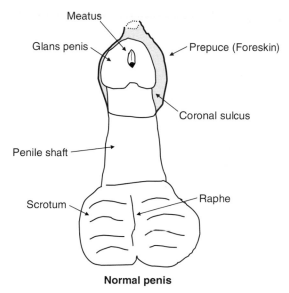

Normal penis

FIGURE 19–3 *The Foreskin and Its Relationship to the Other Parts of the Penis.*

blood, creating an erection. Stimulation under the control of the sympathetic nervous system leads to the sequential contraction of the epididymis, bulbous urethra, and ejaculation, which leads to the forceful expulsion of semen. *Priapism* is persistent painful erection not related to psychosexual arousal.

The scrotum is a sac with two parallel compartments in which sit the testicles. The scrotal wall has a thin layer of muscle, the dartos muscle, over which lies a layer of wrinkled skin. The dartos muscle can cause the scrotum to shrink or expand, and the testicles are usually freely mobile within their compartments. The testicles maintain their connection with the body via the spermatic cord, which consists of arterial, venous, and lymphatic conduits. The lymphatics of the testicles drain into the retroperitoneal lymph nodes along the vena cava and aorta. The lymphatics of the scrotum and penis drain into the inguinal and pelvic lymph nodes.

During the third trimester of gestation, the testicles begin to descend from the abdomen into the scrotum. The testicle descends down a prescribed path through the internal ring and the inguinal canal. The gubernaculum shortens and becomes the lowest point of fixation of the testicle in the scrotum. Part of the peritoneum can drape over the testicle, comes down the inguinal canal, and even reaches the scrotum. Usually this extension naturally atrophies and seals up completely, but if it remains patent, it becomes a persistent processus vaginalis. This can lead to the development of hydroceles or hernias.

The prostate is a gland that sits beneath the bladder. The urethra passes through its center. At birth, it is quite small and underdeveloped, but with puberty it becomes larger and takes on the shape of a bell pepper with a broad base and a narrow apex. The base abuts the bladder, and the apex meets the external urinary sphincter. The posterior prostatic surface lies against the anterior rectal wall, easily palpated on rectal examination. On digital examination, the surface divides into two halves sagittally.

Pathophysiology

In general, pathology within the pediatric male GU system manifests as one or a combination of the following: (1) pain at or referred from a GU structure, (2) mass or swelling in a GU organ, (3) lower urinary tract symptoms (specifically: urgency, frequency, dysuria, or pyuria), (4) hematuria or urethral discharge, (5) change in usual voiding pattern and degree of continence, and (6) malformation or maldevelopment of a GU structure.

Pain is the most basic symptom in clinical medicine and usually spurs patients and families to seek medical attention. In some cases there is an obvious history such as trauma, but often the cause is unclear, or the discomfort is pain from another location (*referred pain*). Pain within the pediatric male GU system can result from causes such as infection and inflammation but also from obstruction of urinary flow resulting in distension of the urinary tract. There are no sensory nerves within the kidney or ureter as there are in the muscle or skin. Distension of the urinary system, for example, owing to an obstructing urinary calculus can lead to peritoneal irritation and subsequently to pain, nausea, and vomiting.

A mass or swelling in the GU system can present as a visually obvious finding such as a swollen red scrotum or can be found incidentally on a routine physical examination, such as a lump on a testicle. Common causes include neoplasia, obstruction of urinary flow, or the presence of an abnormal connection that allows fluid or solid structures to penetrate into spaces, such as with an inguinal hernia or hydrocele. Inflammation and infection also can cause swelling, such as in pyelonephritis and testicular torsion.

The lower urinary tract system includes the bladder and urethra and has innervation, which allows the sensations of urgency, frequency, pyuria, and dysuria. The quality and force of the voided stream also are discernible. Collectively, these symptoms and signs make up the *lower urinary tract symptoms* (LUTS). These can occur owing to direct irritation, such as found in a bladder infection, or indirectly owing to a narrowing of the urethra caused by a stricture. The narrowing hinders urine flow and, in turn, distends the urethra above the stricture, leading to urgency, frequency, and dysuria.

Hematuria is a finding that can be due to infection, inflammation, neoplasia, urinary calculi, or obstruction. Bleeding or inflammation can occur from anywhere in the system: kidney, ureter, bladder, or urethra. Blood in the bladder that has dwelled there will appear dark and can form clots with a consistency of gelatin or pudding. In contrast, bleeding that comes from the urethra (infravesical) or that is quite brisk will be more of a bright red color. Discoloration of the urine also can develop owing to metabolic abnormalities in the biliary system or as a result of ingestion of various foods, drugs, and substances. Urethral discharge can be the result of an active infection, a draining abscess, or an embedded calculus or foreign body.

A change in the normal storage and emptying function of the bladder can be the result of many disorders manifesting along the spectrum from total incontinence to complete retention. *Incontinence* is the unplanned and unwanted loss of urinary control. It can occur because of a leak or fistula, such as seen after trauma, or it can occur as a result of a congenital malformation. It also may occur because of delay in maturation, voiding dysfunction, or as a harbinger of more serious neurologic problems. Patients with abnormalities, injuries, or diseases of the CNS may develop problems storing and emptying urine. Urinary retention can occur owing to a child's fear of pain and discomfort during voiding, obstruction with a neoplasm at the bladder neck or a urethral stricture, or as a result of a neurologic abnormality that prevents normal voiding. Always bear in mind that anuria is not necessarily retention. Rather, it may be the result of acute renal failure, and the patient is not voiding because there is no urine.

Finally, abnormalities of normal embryogenesis and growth can lead to malformation or maldevelopment. These can range from very obvious conditions such as cloacal or bladder exstrophy to more subtle disorders such as cryptorchidism. Typically, these conditions present with a constellation of pathognomonic findings. They may be seen prenatally with gestational ultrasound.

History

Neonates and Infants

A full general history is necessary to make a proper diagnosis. This is covered in Chapter 1 and will not be repeated here. With a limited medical history in neonates and infants, much depends on the observations of the parents or guardians. Symptoms and signs below refer in particular to the pediatric male GU tract. The diagnoses are organized into etiologic groups.

Among newborns, there is a unique category of antenatally detected problems. It is now commonplace for expectant mothers to have several ultrasounds during pregnancy. The resolution of the ultrasound machines now allows scanning of the fetus through the amniotic fluid. Unfortunately, this process can be operator-dependent, and the purported diagnosis may not necessarily be accurate. A thorough evaluation to confirm the possible diagnosis is therefore a requirement. There are three major antenatal concerns that involve the GU system: antenatal *hydronephrosis, oligohydramnios,* and report of another significant malformation.

KEY PROBLEM

History of Antenatal Hydronephrosis in a Newborn
Ultrasound resolution makes it possible to detect fetuses that have hydronephrosis. This finding does not necessarily pinpoint the cause of the hydronephrosis. The spectrum of possible congenital diagnoses include *UPJ obstruction, vesicoureteral reflux (VUR), UVJ obstruction, ureteral duplication with or without an ureterocele, multicystic dysplastic kidney,* and *posterior urethral valves.* The typical systematic workup includes a renal and bladder ultrasound, voiding cystourethrogram (VCUG), and renal scintiscan (also called DRS for Dynamic Renal Scan or MAG3 with Lasix) as needed. Although it is commonplace to perform an ultrasound on the first or second day of life, often this can be misleading because the infant is adapting to extrauterine life. An initial "normal" finding requires a second confirmatory ultrasound at 4 to 6 weeks of life. Consider prophylactic antibiotics until further studies rule out VUR.

KEY PROBLEM

History of Oligohydramnios in a Newborn
Amniotic fluid is essentially fetal urine. When the volume of amniotic fluid is low, there should be concern about the renal function of the fetus and the possible presence of *posterior urethral valves* in males. After birth and once the infant is stable, a full evaluation would require a renal and bladder ultrasound and a VCUG. The lack of volume can result in the baby having *respiratory problems* because the chest and lungs do not have the opportunity to expand fully and develop prior to delivery.

KEY PROBLEM

History of Another Antenatally Detected Malformation in a Newborn
If an infant has a prenatal diagnosis of some other significant congenital malformation, it is important to confirm this immediately. For example, patients who have been diagnosed antenatally with *gastroschisis* or an *omphalocele* have turned out instead to have *prune-belly syndrome* or *bladder exstrophy.*

KEY PROBLEM

Retention of Urine
Many newborns do not void during the first 12 hours of life. Therefore, not having a wet diaper initially is not necessarily pathologic but depends on the timing. If after 12 hours there is no voiding and the neonate seems otherwise stable and well, one should consider the possibility of *congenital* obstruction (*posterior urethral valves*) or renal anomalies (*polycystic kidneys* or *bilateral UPJ obstruction*). Some newborns have other conditions that seemingly do not have a direct GU connection; thus a review of the overall medical history is important. For example, patients diagnosed with *traumatic cerebral hypoxia, sacrococcygeal teratoma,* or *spina bifida* may have urinary retention. For infants, one also must consider *urinary tract infection (UTI)* in addition to obstruction and renal abnormalities. Obstructions include undiscovered *urethral strictures, posterior urethral valves* (not discovered as a newborn), and *rhabdomyosarcoma* of the bladder neck and prostatic urethra. Once one drains the patient's bladder and he or she is stabilized, further investigation is

necessary. Regardless of whether infection is the primary cause, a thorough evaluation of the bladder and urethra by VCUG and ultrasound is essential. Other causes include obstruction (*obstructing bladder stone, obstructive swelling after a traumatic attempted urethral catheterization*), neurologic (*spinal cord injury, spina bifida, tethered spinal cord, cerebral palsy, brain tumor, stroke,* or *encephalitis*), and functional (these disorders or other causes of marked *constipation* are associated with bladder dysfunction). Infants and children who have severe constipation can be infrequent voiders and in some cases have urinary retention. *Congenital* vascular anomalies such as *arteriovenous malformation* on the spinal cord, when ruptured, can result in sudden retention. Keep in mind *vascular accidents* to the spinal cord in infants and children who present in retention after a cardiac or vascular procedure. A small *thrombus* can embolize a spinal artery, leading to ischemia of the spinal cord. This can result in transient to persistent retention. *Traumatic injuries* to the spinal cord can lead to a period of "spinal shock" where the bladder may be areflexic. After 6 to 12 months, this can change and manifest as increased urinary frequency with detrusor hyperreflexia (so-called bladder spasticity).

The major differential diagnosis to bear in mind is *acute renal failure.* There are now inexpensive ultrasound devices designed to estimate bladder capacity and quickly determine if there is a distended bladder, particularly if this is not clear on physical examination. The possible causes of acute renal failure appear elsewhere. It is important to remember that infants and children who have only a solitary functional kidney (owing to either a congenital condition such as *multicystic dysplastic kidney* or *renal agenesis*) may enter acute renal failure from unilateral events that would not normally cause a sudden and complete loss of renal function.

KEY PROBLEM
■ Hematuria or Discoloration of Urine   Urine normally has a yellowish tint because of urea. Dilution and concentration can affect the intensity of the color. The presence of other colored or pigmented substances in the urine will lead to a color change. A history of a major urine color change requires further investigation. Determine first if there is a true color change and not just the effect of dehydration or dilution. Search for possible association with activities, foods, or medications. Reddish colored urine is not necessarily due to blood. Colorless urine may be very dilute. This can occur because of *excessive fluid intake, chronic glomerulonephritis, diabetes mellitus,* and *diabetes insipidus.* Cloudy whitish urine can be due to alkaline urine, which precipitates the diluted phosphates. *Pus* and *chyle* both can produce milky cloudy urine. A dark yellowish to amber-colored urine can be due to dehydration or as a reaction of antibiotics and chemicals. *Drugs* such as tetracycline and pyridine can color the urine bright yellow. Orange urine can result from urobilinogen, pyridium (an antispasmodic that turns orange in acid urine), rhubarb, senna, and anthracyclines. Reddish urine can be due to ingestion of beets, aniline dyes used to color candy, freshly voided hemoglobin or myoglobin, porphyrin, phenolphthalein (a cathartic that turns red in alkaline urine), rifampin, and doxorubicin. Bluish green urine can be due to bilirubin, methylene blue, and *Pseudomonas* UTI.

Blackish brown urine can be due to *dehydration,* leading to a very concentrated urine, bilirubin, hemoglobin that has dwelled in acid urine,
methemoglobin, porphyrin, and tyrosine. Hematuria can be gross (visible to the unaided eye) or microscopic (detectable only on microscopy
or urine dipstick). Microscopic hematuria is greater than four red blood
cells (RBCs) per high-powered field on a spun urine specimen. Gross
hematuria can occur at the initiation of voiding (initial hematuria), at
the end of voiding (terminal hematuria), or throughout voiding (total
hematuria). Initial hematuria suggests a urethral source, whereas terminal hematuria suggests hemorrhage from the bladder or bladder neck.
Total hematuria, especially if present with formed, older, purplish black
clots, suggests bleeding from the kidneys or ureters or profuse bladder
hemorrhage. With sufficient time, blood that has pooled within the bladder will form purplish black clots with the consistency of pudding or
gelatin. In most cases the occurrence of hematuria requires a complete
workup of the GU tract, including upper tract imaging and cystoscopy.
Obtain a urine culture and sensitivity to rule out urine infection, which
is a common cause of hematuria. The full spectrum of possible diagnoses for hematuria is quite broad and can be organized into functional
groups: *hereditary* disease (*sickle cell anemia, hemophilia,* and *polycystic kidney disease*), *inflammatory* and *infectious conditions* [*bacterial cystitis, viral
cystitis* (especially among newborns), *glomerulonephritis, schistosomiasis,*
and *polyarteritis*], *metabolic conditions* [*hemorrhagic cystitis* owing to chemotherapy (cyclophosphamide and ifosfamide)], *traumatic* (blunt and
penetrating injuries, recent surgery, and instrumentation), *neoplasia*
(*Wilms tumor* and *rhabdomyosarcoma* of the bladder neck and prostatic
urethra), and *vascular* (*renal arteriovenous malformation*).

True hematuria has to be distinguished from *myoglobinuria* and *hemoglobinuria.* The latter is due to filtration of plasma-free hemoglobin or the
lysis of RBCs in the urine. The differential diagnosis includes *transfusion
reaction, high-titer cold-agglutinin disease, malaria, typhus, anthrax, enveno-
mation by snakes or spider bites, ingestion of fava beans or oxidant drugs in
patients with glucose-6-phosphate dehydrogenase (G6PD) deficiency, thrombotic thrombocytopenic purpura, hemolytic-uremia syndrome,* and *hypertension.* Myoglobinuria occurs when damaged muscles release myoglobin
into the circulation. Muscle pain and a history of injury or trauma with
prolonged muscle ischemia are common findings. Patients who have had
a major crush injury or compartment syndromes are particularly at risk.

KEY PROBLEM
◢ Discharge from the Umbilicus
In the newborn pe-
riod there is usually some degree of discharge as the umbilical cord seals
up; the stump necroses and falls off, and skin covers over the umbilical
remnant to form the base of the future "belly button." Typically, this
occurs some time in the first 2 to 3 weeks after birth. When there is persistent drainage or fluid coming from the stump, consider three conditions:
urachal sinus, urachal cyst, and *patent urachus.*

During embryogenesis, there is a direct connection between the umbilical cord and the dome of the bladder. This connection, the urachus,
should seal spontaneously after birth. A congenital *patent urachus* results

when there is persistence of the communication between the bladder and the umbilicus. Infants present with continuous or intermittent drainage from the umbilicus. Straining, crying, voiding, coughing, or rubbing over the area between the umbilicus and the bladder can accentuate the drainage. The tract can become inflamed and lead to swelling and a serous, bloody, or purulent discharge. The treatment is surgical excision and closure. A *patent urachus* also can occur with a bladder outlet obstruction such as *posterior urethral valves* and can resolve spontaneously with correction of the underlying obstruction.

A *urachal sinus* can result from partial closure of a patent urachus. The tract closes at the bladder end but remains open at the umbilical end. This can result in a long tract that can become infected and result in persistent purulent discharge, periumbilical tenderness, and an intermittently wet umbilicus. It may be mistaken for granulation tissue at the skin level and so may undergo several rounds of ineffective cauterization using silver nitrate sticks.

A *urachal cyst* results when both ends of the urachus have closed, leaving a fluid-filled structure in between the umbilicus and the bladder dome. Usually it occurs in the distal half of the urachus. In infancy, such cysts usually are asymptomatic, but they sometimes occur incidentally during other evaluations (such as workup for UTI). Usually they present in early childhood when they become symptomatic, although one finds rare cases late into adolescence. Symptoms are usually due to infection and subsequent inflammation and include fever, pain, a suprapubic mass, and occasionally irritative voiding symptoms. *Staphylococcus aureus* and *Streptococcus* species are the most common bacterial organisms. Because of the close proximity of the peritoneum, there can be abdominal discomfort. Rare cases of septic rupture leading to death have occurred.

KEY PROBLEM
■ Change in Voiding Habits
Most newborns void frequently and may wet their diapers 10 to 20 times per day. As the baby grows older, voiding frequency decreases as the functional bladder capacity increases with age, growth, and neurologic maturity. Most infants are not ready for toilet training until at least age $1\frac{1}{2}$ to 2 years. Remember that infants and children do not have the same voiding habits as adults. A typical adult may void four to five times between waking in the morning and retiring to sleep at night. Surveys of normal children found that children under age 4 years of age typically void six to ten times per day. Fewer than 10 percent of normal children 4 years of age or younger void four times or less per day.

If the infant or newborn has infrequent voiding (but not retention), consider several diagnoses. If there are associated *inflammatory and infectious conditions* such as fever, hematuria, pyuria, cloudiness of urine, listlessness, and poor feeding, consider UTI. Perform a full workup with a catheterized urine specimen. Remember that in newborns and infants there may not always be fever, so the physician must maintain a high index of suspicion. Other inflammatory conditions include *glomerulonephritis*, renal complication from systemic *lupus erythematosus,* and *sickle cell anemia.* It is also possible to have a case of *posterior urethral valves* that eluded earlier detection. Infants who had a urethral catheterization or cystoscopy early in life can develop *urethral strictures.* Other causes include bilateral UPJ narrowing, urinary calculi, and *neoplasia* at the bladder neck. Imaging is necessary to rule out obstruction within the urethra and in the upper tract. *Metabolic* reaction to *drugs* such as nonsteroidal anti-inflammatory drugs or antibiotics such as penicillin may be an issue. *Neoplasia* such as *rhabdomyosarcoma* of the lower urinary tract typically presents as retention or poor urinary flow. Usually the mass is located at the bladder neck and prostatic urethra and can be visualized on ultrasound and VCUG. Neurologic conditions such as *spinal cord injury* (traumatic), *spina bifida, syringomyelia* (congential), *myelitis, encephalitis* (infectious/inflammatory), *brain tumor* (neoplastic) and *stroke* may manifest infrequent voiding. Remember to check the bladder capacity and to look for a large postvoid residual, which suggests that the patient may not actually be voiding as much as suffering from overflow incontinence, a situation more akin to retention.

If the infant or newborn seems to have increased voiding frequency, one should first consider an increase in total urine volume, i.e., polyuria, or other cause, such as incomplete emptying or irritation of the bladder. Increased urinary volume (polyuria) can result from increased osmotic load (such as seen with *diabetes mellitus*), increased intake of *fluids, medications,* or a decrease in renal concentrating ability. The diagnoses include *congenital renal tubular acidosis type I, diabetes mellitus, inflammatory interstitial nephritis, diuretic use, hypercalcemia, hypokalemia, postobstructive diuresis, excessive fluid intake,* and *psychogenic polydipsia.*

When the urinary volume is not increased (no polyuria), the increased urinary frequency results from causes that manifest by irritating or obstructing the lower urinary tract. The diagnoses include *infectious and inflammatory* conditions such as *UTI, chemical cystitis, hemorrhagic cystitis,* and *mechanical and traumatic* conditions such as *meatal stenosis,* which can present with increased urinary frequency but classically also has splaying or deflection of the stream. It occurs nearly exclusively in boys who are circumcised or have had urethral instrumentation. Also consider *obstruction and neoplasia,* such as urinary obstruction owing to a stricture in the urethra or bladder or tumor in the lower urinary tract such as *rhabdomyosarcoma* of the bladder neck and prostatic urethra. *Neurologic* conditions such as *spinal cord injury, spina bifida, brain tumor, stroke,* and *encephalitis* may be an issue. Functional: constipation is associated with voiding dysfunction. Remember that this is a period of maturation, and it is normal for some children to go through periods of increased urinary frequency. *Extraordinary urinary frequency syndrome* is a condition that affects infants and children up to age 10 years. It presents with increased urinary frequency (12 to 30 times per day) and often causes the child to get up at night to void. There is no history of UTI or constipation, and there is no evidence of obstruction. Usually it is a self-limited condition that resolves spontaneously within 6 months, and the only associated finding is that the child often has had some recent social change, such as a new sibling, home, school, etc.

Pain and Swelling in the Penis

The foreskin cannot normally retract fully in newborns, infants, and children up to around the ages of 5 to 7 years. *Phimosis,* or the pathologic inability to retract the foreskin, therefore is not usually a problem until the child is older or if scar tissue (cicatrix) has developed at the tip resisting retraction. Typically, these patients will present with a history of the foreskin ballooning during voiding. A retracted foreskin without replacement to the normal position may form a *paraphimosis* (FIGURE 19–4). The differential diagnosis includes *infectious and inflammatory* conditions such as a reaction to an arthropod or insect *bite, reaction to medication,*or *Henoch-Schönlein purpura.*

The penis can swell pathologically owing to *priapism* (nonerotic persistent erection). A number of causes can lead to this condition but best known in children is *sickle cell anemia.* There are two forms: high flow and low flow. Low-flow priapism occurs with obstruction of venous outflow. High-flow priapism occurs when there is an arteriovenous shunt or "short circuit" resulting in more blood flowing in than can flow out normally. The differential diagnosis of low-flow priapism includes (*hereditary*) *sickle cell anemia;* (*neoplasia*) *leukemia* (especially chronic granulocytic leukemia), in which cells can block venous outflow; (*iatrogenic*) reaction to *drugs* (especially serotonin reuptake inhibitors); and (*idiopathic*) unknown cause. High-flow priapism is a result of trauma to the penis or groin; typically, a fall creates an arteriovenous shunt leading to the priapism. A blood gas sample taken from the engorged penis will differentiate between high-flow (oxygen saturation will be like arterial blood, normal blood pH) and low-flow (oxygen saturation will be like venous blood, low pH) priapism.

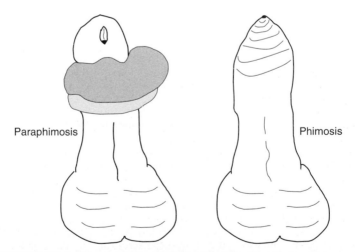

Paraphimosis

Phimosis

***FIGURE 19–4** Paraphimosis and Phimosis. The phimotic foreskin cannot be retracted. The paraphymotic foreskin, once retracted, cannot be repositioned.*

KEY PROBLEM

◾ Maldevelopment of the Penis (Hypospadias, Epispadias, Duplicated Urethra) See subsequent discussion under "Physical Examination."

KEY PROBLEM

◾ Maldevelopment of the Testicle (Undescended Testicle) The testicles normally descend from their intraabdominal position and course their way down through the inguinal canal and into the scrotum during the third trimester. In some otherwise normal infants the testicles may descend during the first year of life. If the testicles have not descended into the normal position by age 1 year, there is no benefit from continued observation. There are several important questions to answer: (1) Were the testicles present at birth? (2) Are the testicles visible or palpable at times? (3) Is the issue of a hard-to-find testicle something that has just arisen? (4) What is the condition of the other testicle? The first question is important because testicles can become lost owing to a missed torsion, or there may have been a neonatal torsion that was unrecognized. By the time of the first well-baby examination, the testicle may have atrophied. If there is an absent testicle on one side and the contralateral testicle is larger than normal, one should be suspicious of a possible missed torsion. A degree of compensatory hypertrophy of the testicle can occur during the first year of life. An undescended testicle often appears in the groin either within the inguinal canal or just beyond the external ring. Parents and physicians often note a history of "something" in the groin. During descent, testicles can develop attachments to the cremasteric muscles. When anxious, the baby or infant will tense up the groin muscles and draw the testicles out of the scrotum and into the groin. This phenomenon is called *retractile testicles.* One should consider this if the child has no prior history of an undescended testicle and suddenly has no testicle in the scrotum or one very hard-to-find testicle on a subsequent physical examination; particularly if the examiner is new and unfamiliar with the child. Bilateral *undescended testicles* should prompt the examiner to be very thorough with the rest of the genital examination. *Ambiguous genitalia* and *intersex* are present if bilateral undescended testicles are associated with an abnormal phallus and urethra. Patients with bilateral undescended testicles and otherwise normal genitalia will need evaluation to determine if the testicles are either intraabdominal, hard to find, or absent.

KEY PROBLEM

◾ Swelling of the Scrotum and Groin In newborns and infants, reports of a swelling in the scrotum can be due to several possible causes: *hernia and hydrocele, undescended or retractile testicle,* or *testicular torsion.* The testicles descend during the last trimester from the intraabdominal position and nestle down inside the scrotum. During descent, the testicles move through the internal ring, down the inguinal canal, and out the external ring into the scrotum. The testicles draw behind them long cables of blood vessels, nerves, lymphatics, and other supporting structures in the form of the spermatic cords. Usually the

muscle layers of the inguinal canal seal tight around the spermatic cord, but there can be a gap. Down this gap can pass an extension of the peritoneum, the processus vaginalis. Usually this structure atrophies and seals up spontaneously, but occasionally it can remain open and then becomes a patent processus vaginalis. This structure can extend all of the way down and swell to encompass most of the volume on that side of the scrotum. A *hydrocele* forms when fluid that lubricates the lining of the peritoneum passes down. Typically there will be reports of shifts in size and shape, which worsen with straining, such as during constipation or with coughing. Hydroceles transilluminate (FIGURE 19–5) and are not usually present with pain or scrotal skin changes. This is a *cord hydrocele*. When a solid structure such as a loop of bowel or a tongue of omentum works its way down, it becomes an indirect hernia. Occasionally, other structures such as diverticulum from the bladder also can descend into the space. Hydroceles sometimes can resolve spontaneously at less than 6 months of age. If this has not happened by the time the child is standing or walking at 1 year, it becomes very unlikely to resolve spontaneously. It will require repair to prevent it from converting to a hernia. *Hernias* need surgical correction, but unless they are associated with marked pain, vomiting, discoloration of the scrotum and groin, or obstruction suggestive of *incarceration,* repair can wait until the child is stable enough for general anesthesia. Hernias do not transilluminate. The testicle should be distinct on examination. A retractile testicle may mimic a small hydrocele if it is mobile and retracts up into the groin. Similarly, an undescended testicle that is beyond the external

FIGURE 19–5 *Transillumination of the Scrotum.*

ring or within the inguinal canal can be mistaken for a hernia. Occasionally, there may be a history of swelling that is not apparent on physical examination. Subtle hernias and hydroceles that are only present with straining may not be evident when one initially examines the child. Consider a repeat visit with examination both supine and upright to bring these out.

The major differential diagnoses are *testicular* or *paratesticular tumor* and *testicular torsion,* which appear below. Other diagnoses include *mechanical and traumatic* conditions such as *ascites,* which can descend into a patent processus vaginalis; ventriculoperitoneal shunts, which can migrate into the processus vaginalis and distend it in patients with *hydrocephalus;* blunt and penetrating *trauma* to the abdomen and *varicoceles,* albeit rare, which can occur if there is venous obstruction centrally, such as within the inferior vena cava; and *infectious and inflammatory* conditions such as *epididymitis* and *orchitis,* which can mimic a hydrocele and hernia (see below).

KEY PROBLEM

◖ Pain and Swelling of the Scrotum The contents of the scrotum can become infected and inflamed. *Infectious orchitis/ epididymitis* can cause swelling and pain and lead to a reddish discoloration of the scrotum. Usually this is associated with a positive urine culture and a tender scrotum. Possible causes to investigate include outlet obstruction, voiding dysfunction, or a *persistent mesonephric duct.* The mesonephric duct normally develops to form the ureter but can persist abnormally, linking the ejaculatory duct and ureter into a common tubule. Bacterial causes include *Escherichia coli, Mycoplasma, gonorrhea, Chlamydia, tuberculosis, brucellosis, syphilis,* and *leprosy.* Viral *orchitis* can occur due to *mumps, echovirus, lymphocytic choriomeningitis virus,* and *arbovirus group B.* The major differential diagnoses are *testicular torsion* and *neoplasm.* Other diagnoses include (*traumatic*) trauma to the testicle, (*inflammatory*) testicular torsion, and appendix testis torsion; *Henoch-Schönlein purpura* (HSP) can manifest within the testicle and can mimic orchitis, epididymitis, and torsion. In HSP there is often a characteristic purplish purpura along skin pressure points such as those along elastic waist bands and socks.

KEY PROBLEM

◖ Pain Mass and Swelling of the Scrotum and Penis Gross blunt and penetrating *trauma* to the penis, scrotum, and testicle is self-evident. Be cognizant of two important points. First, major injuries to these structures can involve the urethra, so one should be wary about placing a catheter unless the urethra is intact and patent. Second, blunt trauma to the testicle may result not only in a hematoma but also may cause testicular rupture. The hematoma from the trauma limits physical examination. If the history (typically some type of misadventure such as a fall or misjudged leap) and gross examination suggest a sizable testicular hematoma (one that has obliterated the usual contours of the testicle), then suspect testicular rupture and order a scrotal ultrasound to confirm the diagnosis. If rupture has occurred, one needs prompt intervention because of the risk of testicular atrophy and loss if left untreated.

Pain and Mass and Swelling of the Scrotum

The testicle descends into the scrotum and during childhood and into adolescence is usually only fixed at two points: at the spermatic cord and down at the gubernaculum. The testicle therefore is free to rotate and can spin on the axis of the spermatic cord. This can lead to torsion of the cord, which can spin completely around two, three, or more times. The twisting shortens the cord and occludes the lymphatics, veins, and finally, the arteries that supply the testicle. If left untreated, torsion can lead to ischemia and testicular loss in about 6 hours. There is pain and discomfort to palpation. Urine analysis is normal. Usually this twisting, intravaginal torsion (i.e., it occurs within the tunica vaginalis and not within the vagina) occurs within the scrotum and is the form that presents in children and adolescents. The treatment is surgical, to untwist the testicle. Among neonates, torsion can occur during testicular descent, and the spermatic cord twists not just within the tunica vaginalis but also in the inguinal canal. Possible associations include large babies, long labor, and breech presentation. A major differential diagnosis is torsion of an appendix testis or epididymis. There are small residual pieces of tissues that dangle off the epididymis or testicle. These are the remnants of the Müllerian duct that have not completely regressed. They are usually tear-shaped on a thin vascular stalk, and when they twist, they can become ischemic. This may mimic true testicular torsion and manifest many of the same findings in the scrotum, including swelling, pain, and reddish discoloration. In fair-skinned children, there is a classic finding called a *blue-dot sign*. The torsed necrotic appendix appears as a small purplish or bluish spot visible just under the scrotal skin and above the testicle. Other differential diagnoses include *infectious and inflammatory conditions* such as orchitis and epididymitis, HSP, and *neoplasia* such as *testicular* and *paratesticular tumors*.

Mass and Swelling of the Scrotum

Swelling within the scrotum can be due to the presence of a testicular or paratesticular *neoplasm*. Among neonates and infants, the most common diagnoses are a germ cell testicular tumor or a paratesticular *rhabdomyosarcoma*. Germ cell testicular tumors are usually hard and do not transilluminate. They are painless unless necrotic. *Teratoma* and *yolk sac tumor* are the most common histologic types. Suspect metastases in patients who have a history of another neoplasm. The testicle is immunologically privileged and has a blood-tissue barrier that can limit the effectiveness of chemotherapy. Metastases to the testicle can occur in particular with *leukemia* and *lymphoma*. Rarer variants include embryonal cell carcinoma and non-germ cell testicular tumors such as *Leydig cell tumors* and *Sertoli cell tumors*. The presence of a mass requires urgent workup and exploration to determine the diagnosis. The major differential diagnoses include *infectious and inflammatory conditions* such as *orchitis, epididymitis,* and *HSP* and *mechanical and traumatic conditions* such as trauma to the testicle or spermatic cord, testicular torsion or torsion of an *appendix testis, hernia,* and *hydrocele*.

Children

Between the ages of 2 and 12 years it becomes possible to obtain a more complete and accurate history from the child. Because of embarrassment, the child may not volunteer information about enuresis or constipation. Similarly, he or she may describe masses or lesions within the scrotum in very vague terms. Be suspicious of any reports of obscure "belly" pain, and always inquire directly about the genitalia.

KEY PROBLEM

Retention of Urine As with newborns and infants, urinary retention should lead to an investigation of possible urinary obstruction or failure of the bladder to empty normally. If this occurs suddenly, there is usually lower pelvic pain from the distended bladder. If it has developed slowly over a long period of time, there may be no pain, and the change in urination may be gradual. The patient and family may report incontinence instead of urinary retention, mistaking overflow incontinence for enuresis. Physical examination typically will show a distended bladder, and an elevated postvoid residual will appear on ultrasound or with catheterization. The differential diagnoses include (*congenital*) *posterior urethral valves;* (*infectious and inflammatory*) *UTI, sexually transmitted diseases* (STDs), particularly *herpes simplex* infection of the bladder; (*iatrogenic*) use of certain medications; (*mechanical and traumatic*) *urethral stricture, urethral calculus, bladder stone, urethral injury and extravasation,* and *bladder injury with rupture;* (*neoplasia*) *bladder neck or prostatic urethral rhabdomyosarcoma* and *bladder cancer;* (*neurologic*) *spinal cord injury, spina bifida, myelitis, multiple sclerosis, cerebral palsy,* and *encephalitis;* and (*psychosocial*) *sexual abuse.* A number of medications can affect the ability of the bladder to empty, and therefore, a careful medication history is important. Anticholinergics and tricyclic antidepressants in particular can stop bladder activity completely.

KEY PROBLEM

Hematuria or Discoloration of Urine In addition to the diagnoses listed in the newborn and infant section, there are also the following: (*mechanical and traumatic*) *exercise-related hematuria;* (*neoplasia*) *renal cell cancer and ureteral cancer;* and *ureteral polyps.*

KEY PROBLEM

Lower Urinary Tract Symptoms A history of urgency, frequency, pyuria, and dysuria initially should bring to mind a possible UTI. In addition, other possible diagnoses include (*mechanical and traumatic*) *urethral stricture* and *meatal stenosis;* (*iatrogenic*) *diuretics, lithium,* and other *drugs* that increase urine output; (*infectious and inflammatory*) *sterile pyuria,* which is strongly suggestive of GU *tuberculosis,* and *interstitial nephritis;* (*metabolic*) *diabetes mellitus, diabetes insipidus,* and *hypercalciuria;* (*neoplasia*) *bladder cancer;* (*neurologic*) *spinal cord injury, spina bifida,* and *detrusor overactivity;* and (*psychosocial*) *psychogenic polydipsia, caffeine ingestion,* and *sexual abuse.*

KEY PROBLEM

Discharge from the Umbilicus See the diagnoses listed in the preceding section.

Change in Voiding Habits (Incontinence) Any

history of incontinence should begin with an inquiry into the possibility of a UTI (*infectious*). Many children will manifest incontinence, urgency, and frequency when they have an active UTI. Once that has been ruled out, consider the nature of the incontinence. Inquire about the frequency and timing of wetting. Inquire about the usual number of voids per day and the number of bowel movements per week. Does the child wait until the last moment to void? Does the child use avoidance maneuvers such as Vincent's curtsy (squatting on the heel of their foot) or do a "potty dance" to delay going to the bathroom? Is there a history of sleep disorders? Sleep apnea, loud snoring, and sleep waking may occur with nocturnal enuresis. Most children become continent by age 5 years. Typically, daytime urine and bowel control develops first followed by nighttime bowel and finally nighttime urine control. Incontinence can take several different forms: daytime only, nighttime only, and day and night. Daytime-only incontinence should lead to further investigation into toilet habits. If the child is completely dry at night but wets during the daytime, it paradoxically suggests that the child's subconscious is doing a better job at maintaining continence than his or her conscious self. Usually the explanation lies with poor toilet habits, particularly infrequent voiding and constipation. Some children learn that it is possible to defer and delay voiding by using mental and physical tricks. This becomes a habit, and they no longer respond to earlier signals but react only to the strongest of urges. This makes them vulnerable to urge incontinence. Nighttime-only wetting or classic nocturnal enuresis has three major theoretical causes: bladder capacity and activity mismatch, failure to concentrate urine appropriately at night, and sleep disorders. Classic *nocturnal enuresis* with no history of daytime wetting, no previous infection, and a positive family history for such will obviate the need for extensive urologic evaluation or referral. Day and night wetting can be a combination of the two other states, poor daytime toilet habits and nighttime wetting. The differential diagnoses include (*mechanical and traumatic*) pelvic floor and bladder neck trauma (often seen in straddle injuries); (*neurologic*) *stroke, encephalitis, brain and spinal cord tumor, multiple sclerosis, spinal cord injury,* and *spina bifida;* (*functional*) *nonneurogenic neurogenic bladder;* and (*psychosocial*) *sexual abuse.*

History of Pain in the Abdomen, Pelvis, and

Genitalia Pain in the abdomen, pelvis, and genitalia may originate from an internal urinary organ. Urinary obstruction leading to distension of the kidney and ureter can refer pain to the costovertebral angles of the back, flank, upper abdomen, groin, and genitalia. The differential diagnoses include (*mechanical and traumatic*) kidney and ureteral trauma, obstructing kidney and ureteral stone, UPJ narrowing, ureteral stricture, and UVJ narrowing; (*iatrogenic*) *drugs;* and (*infectious and inflammatory*) *pyelonephritis* and *HSP*. Drugs can precipitate within the urinary system to form obstructive crystals. Protease inhibitors used to treat HIV infection, such as indinavir, are an example. They are also notable for being radiolucent on both plain x-ray imaging and CT scan.

KEY PROBLEM
History of Mass or Swelling in the Kidney Mass or swelling in the kidney can be due to tumor, cyst, or urinary obstruction and dilatation. The differential diagnoses include (*congenital*) *duplicated urinary system, renal anomalies such as horseshoe kidney or ectopic kidney, multicystic dysplastic kidney,* and *polycystic kidney disease;* (*neoplasia*) *kidney cancer* and *Wilms tumor;* (*mechanical*) *hydronephrosis* owing to a stone, *UPJ narrowing, ureteral fibroepithelial polyp,* and *megaureter* with UVJ narrowing; and (*infectious and inflammatory*) *pyelonephritis* and *xanthogranulomatous pyelonephritis* (classic triad: mass, kidney stone, infection).

KEY PROBLEM
Pain and Swelling in the Penis See also the diagnoses listed in the preceding section.

KEY PROBLEM
Maldevelopment of the Testicle The causes are *congenital.* The testicle should have descended by this age if it were to occur spontaneously. An *undescended testicle* will not develop normally in terms of future fertility and hormone function and poses a risk for *neoplasia.* For these reasons, when faced with an undescended testicle, it is important to establish if it is present and, if so, to try to bring it down or remove it. Likewise, if the testicle is absent, it is important to establish this definitively. One can live a normal life and develop through puberty if the other testicle is normal, but it may affect the choice of future hobbies and sports. Be sure to inquire about any history of prior episodes of scrotal pain, swelling, and redness, which makes one suspicious of a missed *testicular torsion.*

KEY PROBLEM
Swelling of the Scrotum and Groin The scrotum can swell as a result of an intrascrotal process such as *torsion, orchitis, varicocele,* or a *hydrocele or hernia.* Typically, these are unilateral processes, whereas in cases of bilateral scrotal swelling it can be due to an *inflammatory* reaction to *medications* (such as antibiotics), insect or arthropod *bites* (ticks, mites, centipedes, millipedes, spiders, and scorpions), or as a result of a systemic condition such as *HSP.* The swelling also can be part of an overall edema from cardiac (*right-sided heart failure*), vascular problems (*thrombosis* of the inferior vena cava or pelvic veins), tense *ascites,* or *nephritic syndrome.* See also the diagnoses listed in the preceding section.

KEY PROBLEM
Pain and Swelling of the Scrotum In addition to the diagnoses listed in the section for newborns and infants, include *varicocele, epididymal cysts,* and *scrotal gangrene.* Varicoceles or varicose spermatic veins of the pampiniform plexus usually manifest on the left side. They typically present as a baggy mass in the scrotum. They occur because the left spermatic vein has a longer course than the right; it inserts higher up into the left renal vein (not into the inferior vena cava)

and has fewer intravenous valve leaflets that help resist varicose vein formation. These can change in size and prominence with straining in an upright posture. When distended, they also can be painful and ache. About 90 percent of varicoceles are on the left side, with another 9 percent found bilaterally. A unilateral right-sided varicocele merits evaluation to rule out a retroperitoneal mass such as a renal tumor possibly compressing the right spermatic vein. Varicocele raises the temperature inside the scrotum, causing subfertility and infertility.

Epididymal cysts are the same as *spermatoceles*. They are small cysts that protrude from the head of the epididymis. They can range from small (1 to 4 mm in diameter) to large (5 to 10 cm). They are usually painless, benign, and transilluminate. It is necessary only to observe them unless they increase dramatically in size or if pain and discomfort supervene.

Scrotal gangrene (*Fournier* gangrene or *syndrome*) is a form of perineal infection that results from a mixture of aerobic and anaerobic bacteria often with gas formation. The infection is often a complication of diabetes mellitus and is rapidly progressive with foul-smelling necrosis. There is usually fever, pain, and redness and an area of necrosis in the scrotum. The full extent of the degree of necrosis is often obscure and more extensive on the first impression. Full wide debridement with antibiotic coverage is the preferred treatment.

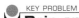
KEY PROBLEM
Pain and Mass and Swelling of the Scrotum
See also the diagnoses listed in the preceding section.

KEY PROBLEM
Mass and Swelling of the Scrotum (Testicular and Paratesticular Mass) See also the diagnoses listed in the preceding section.

Adolescents

To interview an adolescent is more difficult than other age groups because of their evolving concerns about identity, privacy, modesty, and independence. Teenage males are notorious for their minimalist form of communication, and the interviewer should make strong efforts to elicit a complete history. The interviewer should actively introduce sensitive topics such as sexual activity, incontinence, encopresis, and symptoms involving the genitals. One should never assume that the patient will bring up an issue if it concerns him or her. In this case, silence is not golden. The interviewer should avoid slang and vernacular speech unless exceptionally well versed in it. The meaning of terms in popular vernacular communication can shift rapidly and involve many subtle contextual clues that if used incorrectly can lead to at least bemusement and at worst serious misunderstanding.

When discussing serious concerns such as sexual history and activity, adopting a nonjudgmental but honest, straightforward approach is best. Pointing out the factual dangers of risky sexual practices, for example, is important and practical regardless of any potential feelings of moral or ethical disapproval.

Discharge from the Umbilicus
Body piercing and *tattooing* have become the latest way teenagers can express their independence. Piercing and tattoos of the umbilicus can cause infection. There can be allergic reactions that flare up in areas of inserted nickel-plated studs. See also the diagnoses listed in the preceding sections.

Retention of Urine
During acute flares of *UTI* and *HSV* infections, urinary retention can occur. See also the diagnoses listed in the preceding sections.

Hematuria or Discoloration of Urine, Urethral Discharge
Inflammation and infection of the urethra and the associated glands that empty into it can result in purulent secretions that seep out at or between urination. There can be associated pus or blood. Assess the quality of the discharge. Is it clear or cloudy? Is it painful or painless? Are their any associated lesions? Has the patient been sexually active recently? The differential diagnoses include (*infectious and inflammatory*) *Reiter syndrome, Behçet syndrome,* and *STDs* (*Chlamydia trachomatis, Neisseria gonorrhoeae,* and *Ureaplasma urealyticum*) and (*mechanical and traumatic*) *urethral trauma* and *foreign body.* See also the diagnoses listed in the preceding sections.

Lower Urinary Tract Symptoms
See also the diagnoses listed in the preceding sections.

Change in Voiding Habits
See also the diagnoses listed in the preceding sections.

History of Mass or Swelling in the Kidney
See also the diagnoses listed in the preceding sections.

History of Pain in the Abdomen, Pelvis, and Genitalia
See also the diagnoses listed in the preceding sections.

Pain and Swelling in the Penis
Penile lesions, masses, and swellings are most often the result of *trauma* or *infection* and *inflammation.* The differential diagnoses include (*trauma*) penile trauma such as *fracture* of the penis (this can occur if trauma occurs during erection and results in rupture of one or both corpora cavernosa, with significant

pain and swelling) and (*infectious and inflammatory*) *condyloma acuminatum* (venereal warts, papilloma), *syphilitic chancre* (flat, painless lesion), *Haemophilus ducreyi* or *chancroid* (painful lesion), *herpes simplex* (painful blisters), *penile ulcers* (*Behçet syndrome,* i.e., *aphthous ulcers* of the penis and mouth), and *lymphogranuloma venereum* (*Chlamydia trachomatis*).

● KEY PROBLEM
◢ **Pain and Swelling of the Scrotum** See also the diagnoses listed in the preceding sections.

● KEY PROBLEM
◢ **Pain, Mass, and Swelling of the Scrotum** See also the diagnoses listed in the preceding sections.

● KEY PROBLEM
◢ **Mass and Swelling of the Scrotum: Testicular and Paratesticular Mass** See also the diagnoses listed in the preceding sections.

Physical Examination

It is not critical from which side one approaches the patient. The exam room design may place the table so that it is flush against the wall, so it may be wise to be comfortable examining the patient from either side. Always wash your hands in front of the patient and family before and after the examination. Washing just before the examination in addition to blocking transmission of bacteria and viruses also helps to warm the hands, which will make the child more comfortable during the examination.

Newborns and Infants

Most babies are naturally curious, and if approached gently, they will not be apprehensive, being accustomed to diaper changes. If the baby seems anxious, it may be reassuring to have a parent keep a hand on the baby's shoulder or arm during the examination.

▼ KEY FINDING

Inspection With every physical examination, the first step is to take an overall impression, or gestalt, of the patient. Does anything strike the examiner? Does the child seem sick or ill? Are there any obvious *congenital* malformations or anomalies? Are there obvious skin findings such as jaundice, bruising, purpura, petechiae, redness, or swelling? Is the child well developed? Is the abdomen distended or flat?

Look at the child's face and head. Does anything seem irregular or odd? Does the tongue appear enlarged? If it is, consider the *Beckwith-Wiedemann syndrome,* a congenital condition that links *macroglossia, hemihypertrophy,* and the risk of *Wilms tumor.* Look at the eyes carefully for partial or full absence of the iris (*aniridia*), a congenital condition associated with *Wilms tumor.*

Does the body seem symmetric? Does the left side match the right side in development? Sagittal *hemihypertrophy* has been associated with the *Beckwith-Wiedemann syndrome.* This usually affects all or part of one side of the body, but there are cases that involve parts of both sides of the body. Sometimes hemihypertrophy is not present at birth but becomes apparent later in childhood. Look at the back. Does it appear normal, or are there irregularities? Are there any protrusions, irregular hair tufts, or odd clefts or masses, particularly those whose bottoms are not visible? This should prompt suspicion of some underlying spinal problem such as a *tethered spinal cord* or *spina bifida.*

Does the abdomen look normal? A flabby-appearing abdomen with little musculature is pathognomonic for the *prune-belly* (*Eagle-Barrett*) *syndrome.* This condition classically has a triad of a flabby abdomen lacking musculature, bilateral *hydronephrosis,* and bilateral *undescended testicles.* The lack of musculature in the anterior abdominal wall allows intraabdominal contents such as the small intestines to be visible beneath the skin, subcutaneous fat, and peritoneum. Does the skin look normal? Is there any bruising or discoloration? Abdominal ecchymosis suggests *intraperitoneal bleeding.* Among neonates, consider *adrenal hemorrhage.* For older infants, consider looking for *trauma* such as a splenic injury.

Is the abdominal wall complete? The bladder originates as a flat plate that later rolls together to form a closed volume. When this does not occur, the bladder plate remains exposed and is termed *bladder exstrophy.* The abdominal wall remains laterally displaced, and the bony pelvis is open with widening of the pubic symphysis. An extreme variation is *cloacal exstrophy.* In this case, not only is there malformation of the bladder, but the hindgut, which should form the colon, rectum, and anus, also has failed to form correctly. With exstrophy, protect and cover the bladder plate with petrolatum and a layer of plastic wrap, which is simple and inexpensive.

Is there obvious distension to the abdomen? In the upper abdomen, consider a renal mass or a dilated kidney, such as seen with an *UPJ narrowing.* In the lower abdomen and pelvis, distension should suggest an enlarged bladder, such as in *posterior urethral valves.* Is there discharge, distension, or irritation from the umbilicus? These symptoms suggest an *urachal sinus, cyst,* or *tract.* Continue down to the groin, and note if there are any obvious bulges or swelling. These can be due to an inguinal hernia or an *undescended testicle.* If the primary complaint is that of an *undescended testicle,* it is often preferable to begin the examination further up the abdomen. This helps to relax and acclimatize the child to the temperature of the examiner's hands. Rather than just reaching down into the genitalia, first undress the area and observe. Does the scrotum seem well developed? Does it have the normal rugae, i.e., that folded, refolded look? Are the testicles visible? Often babies and infants referred for *undescended testicles* actually will have *retractile testicles.* If the patient is relaxed, the testicles will bob up and down in the scrotum. A penlight or otoscope is often helpful to transilluminate a scrotum to differentiate swelling owing to fluid accumulation (hydrocele) (FIGURE 19–5) from that owing to a solid mass (hernia, tumor, torsion, etc.).

Proceed down to the genitalia. First take in a general impression. Do they seem normal? Examine lesions on the genitalia carefully. They may occur from benign and harmless causes such as *diaper rash* or chafing from a too-tight diaper or outfit. Genital *warts* warrant further investigation by social work and child protection toward possible sexual abuse, although benign causes are also not uncommon (usually in these cases a parent or a child care worker has an active or dormant wart on his or her hands). Many jurisdictions mandate reporting all suspected (not necessarily proven) cases, so each practitioner should be aware of the local requirements. Is the scrotum symmetric, and is the phallus complete and straight? Is there more swelling on one side than the other? Is one side irritated or erythematous? Does the scrotum end at the base of the phallus? Scrotal folds normally end at the base of the phallus. When they course above the level of the phallus and beyond onto the pelvis, it is called *penoscrotal transposition*. This is a condition that accompanies *hypospadias*. Does the scrotum seem relaxed? Is it red or irritated? Is it swollen? Swelling in the scrotum can be due to *hydrocele, hernia,* or underlying *inflammation* such as *testicular torsion, torsion of the appendix testis, epididymitis,* or *orchitis*. Note that in cases of larger hydroceles and fair-complexioned children, the scrotum can take on a faint light bluish cast. This is due to the scattering and reflection of the higher-frequency blue-light spectrum. Is there a fine blue spot in the upper scrotum? This can be an underlying *necrotic appendix testis* that has torsed and is termed a *blue-dot sign*. Generalized genital swelling can be a side effect of *drugs* (especially antibiotics), insect or *arthropod bites,* and *HSP*.

Look at the phallus, and examine the foreskin carefully. It should be supple and flexible. Are there any extra or unexpected openings? If the child has had previous surgery, a fistula can appear as a small reddish spot that may look moist or wet. In children who have not had operations, a second urethral opening may represent a urethral duplication. Typically, this can occur anywhere on the shaft and may or may not communicate with the bladder directly. When faced with two urethral openings, the more ventral one is typically the one that is better developed and has a natural course, whereas the dorsal one is more likely to have an irregular, ectopic course. Is the phallus the appropriate size and shape? The phallus for a typical full-term baby is at least 2.5 cm in length when fully stretched out. If the phallus is smaller and shorter, it may be a micropenis, which can be associated with an underlying endocrine abnormality such as *hypopituitarism* or *hypoadrenalism*. Note that this measurement does not include curvature owing to *chordee* or *hypospadias*.

At this age it is not possible to retract the foreskin fully. This is a natural form of *phimosis*. Redness and irritation and the presence of pus under the prepuce should raise suspicion of *balanitis*. If the child has had a circumcision, note if there is any residual foreskin. The typical circumcision today leaves the glans completely exposed, allowing an easy view of the coronal sulcus. Round, ovoid, waxy-looking deposits are smegma, which is a natural mixture of desquamated skin cells and oils and is not due to infection. Look at the ventral and dorsal penile shaft skin. Are they equal in length? Does the penis curve or bend over to one side? If so, this is a *chordee*, which can exist independently or in association with *hypospadias*. If the penis is straight, does it seem to twist or turn to one side? This is *penile torsion*. Is there a clear separation of the prepuce from the scrotum? In some cases the ventral shaft skin is less well developed, and a web of skin develops that links the foreskin to the scrotum (*webbed penis*). In a circumcised patient, sometimes the healing edge "pops" over the edge of the glans and heals in a cicatrix, thereby trapping the penis. This is a *buried penis*. The foreskin is normally too tight at this age to fully retract but is usually flexible enough to expose the tip. Often the meatus is also visible. Never attempt to retract the foreskin forcefully in uncircumcised infants. If retracted, replace it. Failure to reposition it will lead to edema because the lymphatic and later venous drainage of the foreskin is affected. This, in turn, leads to redness, swelling, and tenderness in the glans and shaft distal to the retracted foreskin. This is *paraphimosis* and requires emergent reduction to prevent permanent damage to the penis. If the prepuce is incomplete or less well developed (often misnamed as a "natural circumcision"), be suspicious of an underlying penile anomaly. In most cases the less developed foreskin is on the ventral surface. Usually this finding is associated with chordee or hypospadias.

Look at the tip of the penis carefully (FIGURES 19–6 through 19–8). In patients who are uncircumcised, the meatus is normally just visible at the tip after stretching back the prepuce carefully to reveal the top of the glans. In circumcised babies and infants, the meatus is atop the phallus or on the ventral surface of the glans. Is there a normal meatus? It is

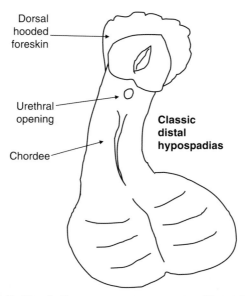

FIGURE 19–6   *Classic Components of Hypospadias (Distal). Note the three parts: incomplete foreskin present only on the dorsum, low-lying urethral opening, and less well-developed ventral shaft resulting in a chordee.*

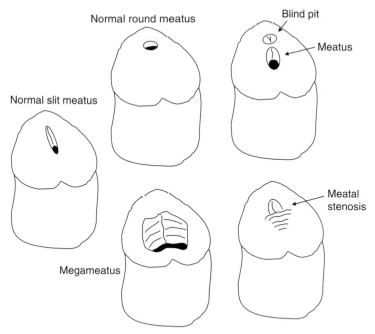

FIGURE 19-7 *Typical Shapes of Urethral Meatus and Common Anomalies: Megameatus, Blind Pit, and Meatal Stenosis.*

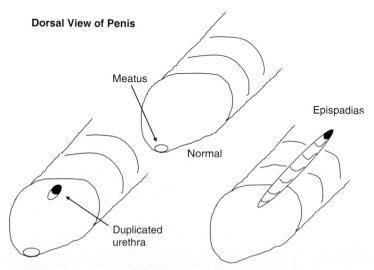

FIGURE 19-8 *Urethral Duplication and Epispadias.*

usually a round hole or ellipse. The meatus may appear moist if the child has just voided or have a glabrous mucosal sheen when compared with the glans or penile shaft. If the opening is quite small or not visible, inquire about the urinary stream because there may be a meatal stenosis. Is the meatus larger than normal or abnormal in shape? The usual opening is smooth and symmetric and has a circular or ellipsoid shape. If it seems wide-mouthed and gaping, it may be a megameatus. This is a normal variation and usually does not require intervention but needs proper diagnosis. Are there any "openings" or "pits" near the urethra? These could be openings of a duplicated urethra but more commonly are blind-ending pits that represent small congenital anomalies. They were involutions that were supposed to meet and join the urethra but did not. They often occur with hypospadias and can range from short, shallow pits to long grooves in the glans just about the meatus.

The meatus may be low and not present on the tip or ventral glans. This is *hypospadias* and usually does not occur in an isolated fashion. It is a congenital condition that typically involves the development of the whole anterior of the phallus. Therefore, it is usually found to have absent ventral foreskin (or, conversely, dorsal hooded foreskin), *chordee* owing to less ventral shaft skin, and a lower than normal urethral opening. There can be maldevelopment of the penis with an opening dorsally on the glans, shaft, or penoscrotal junction. This anomaly is an *epispadias* and often accompanies *bladder exstrophy.*

Unusual-appearing genitalia, especially with hypospadias, severe chordee, or a markedly small phallus and undescended testicles, should raise concern about the possibility of *ambiguous genitalia* or *intersex.* This is a complex situation and can be the result of abnormalities in gonad sex differentiation, underlying endocrine-metabolic disorders such as *congenital adrenal hyperplasia*, abnormalities in the enzymatic processing of testosterone to dihydrotestosterone, and abnormalities in androgen receptors.

KEY FINDING

Palpation When palpating the patient, begin on the abdomen and back. If the back has an abnormal cleft, hair tuft, or crease, carefully spread the surrounding skin to look at the base. Does the underlying spinal column feel intact and complete? If it is abnormal, be suspicious of an underlying spinal anomaly such as a *tethered spinal cord* or *spina bifida.* Is there tenderness to palpation along the costovertebral angles? This is typically the tender area in *pyelonephritis* and symptomatic *hydronephrosis* (FIGURE 19–9).

Palpate the abdomen with both hands in the typical fashion with one hand ventrally and the other supporting from underneath. The kidneys are normally not palpable even in very thin, small babies and infants. The presence of a palpable kidney may represent a renal mass or a distended kidney owing to hydronephrosis. A renal neoplasm such as *Wilms tumor* is typically quite firm and can occupy seemingly the whole abdomen. Among infants, a dilated kidney owing to *hydronephrosis* can hinder respiratory excursion and chest motion on the affected side. Other diagnoses include *polycystic kidneys* and enlarged spleen or liver, which

Anterior Abdomen and Pelvis

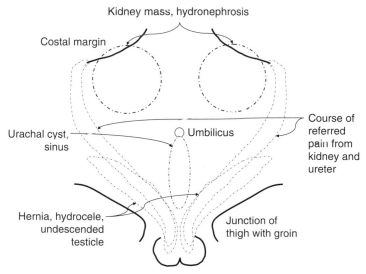

FIGURE 19–9 *Anterior Abdomen and Typical Location for Palpation and Associated Conditions.*

can mimic an enlarged kidney. The bladder in babies and infants is often higher than in older children and can extend up toward the umbilicus. A distended bladder, such as seen in urinary retention, is usually along the midline and extends downward until it disappears under the pubic symphysis. Are there any abnormalities from the umbilicus down toward the symphysis? A urachal cyst or sinus may palpate as a ridge or bump along the midline. Palpation may express urine or pus.

In cases where an *undescended testicle* is possible, after palpating the abdomen, extend the examination down along the groin, following the course of the inguinal canal. An undescended testicle, if it is palpable, will feel like a small round mass that may be mobile like a marble under a layer of cloth. One trick is to apply a thin layer of surgical lubricant along the surface. This decreases the skin friction and can allow the fingertips to glide over the groin, thereby revealing a hard-to-feel testicle. Note that groin lymph nodes are usually lower in position, at or beneath the level of the inguinal ligament, and feel like small round seedlike structures. A bulge in the groin may be a *hernia*. If it includes bowel, it may have palpable peristalsis and, if reducible, will slide back inside.

The scrotum should feel empty except for the testicles and spermatic cords (FIGURE 19–10). *Hernias* are usually distinct from the testicles on palpation. A *hydrocele* may be distinct as well or may seem to envelop the testicles. Transillumination is very useful in distinguishing between the two. Hydroceles, when transilluminated, reveal a characteristic "glow," whereas hernias, being solid, will not allow light to pass. The testicle

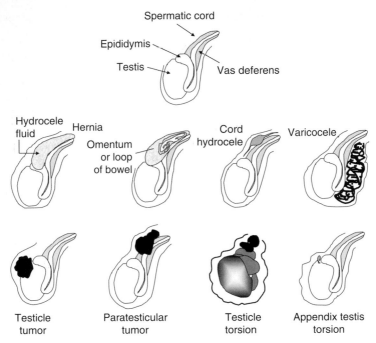

FIGURE 19-10 *Scrotal and Groin Masses and Swelling.*

should be firm but not hard. It should be smooth in contour and without protrusion. The epididymis is typically prominent above and behind the testicle. If there is a mass, determine its boundaries and nature. Is it hard? Is it distinct from the testicle or part of it? Does it transilluminate? Testicular tumors are hard (often rock hard) and protrude from the testicle or subsume the bulk of the testicle itself. Among infants and babies, *teratoma* and *yolk sac tumors* are the most common diagnoses. If the mass is small and appears to be a lesion on the surface of the testicle itself, it could be an *epidermis cyst* within the wall of the testicle, managed by local excision. If the mass presents on the spermatic cord, one must consider in addition to an *incarcerated hernia* a paratesticular mass such as a *rhabdomyosarcoma* or *varicocele*. The varicocele will have a distinctive appearance of varicose veins and will feel like a mass of individual tubules clumped together, similar to a "bag of worms" or a mass of cooked spaghetti within a plastic bag. In patients in whom there is a history of trauma, be suspicious of a testicular rupture if the contour of the testicle is not discernible on physical examination. Finally, if there is a size disparity between the two testicles, one always should be wary that often the so-called larger testicle is not actually larger but rather the contralateral is smaller and may represent a *dysplastic testicle* or an old missed *torsion.*

Palpation of the phallus should start with the flexibility and elasticity of the skin of the phallus and prepuce. Are there are bumps or nodules under the skin? Often these are smegma inclusion cysts, which are entrapped collections of smegma. In an uncircumcised baby, gently retract the foreskin to see if the meatus is visible, but do not attempt to retract the foreskin fully at this age. In the case of a circumcised penis, check to see if there is any adherent foreskin. Filmy attachments that have a good chance of breaking down spontaneously often will have a fine seam or edge. In contrast, scar tissue that has grown over from the circumcision scar to the glans will not separate without the aid of surgery. Scar tissue will have a distinct surface bridging the shaft to the glans over the coronal sulcus much like a highway overpass covers an underlying road.

In patients with *hypospadias,* take care to check the ventral penile skin. Does it seem well developed and elastic? In some cases the ventral skin is thin with almost a translucent quality. This is indicative of urethral maldevelopment underneath the skin, and the actual point where the normal urethra forms may be quite a bit lower.

KEY FINDING

Percussion Percussion is of limited use in the GU examination but has definite applications. It is particularly useful in determining the margins of an enlarged kidney mass and the extent of a distended bladder.

KEY FINDING

Auscultation Unlike the bowels or lungs, there are no organs within the GU system that auscultation can evaluate directly. In some cases, hernias with a loop of intestine may appear in the groin or scrotum, but rarely is auscultation necessary to make a diagnosis. After surgery or trauma, bowel function usually returns within a few days. If there is persistent delay, one always should be suspicious of a possible urine leak. Urine leaking into the peritoneum will prevent or delay the return of normal bowel function.

KEY FINDING

Transillumination Transillumination with a small penlight covered by a disposable glove is a very useful tool when evaluating scrotal and groin swellings. Remember to lower the room light to maximize this effect. See the preceding discussion under inspection and palpation for specific details.

Children

The physical examination of a child differs from that of the neonate and infant in several ways. First, most, if not all, of the superficially obvious congenital maldevelopments and malformations will have come to attention. Second, the child now can help by providing verbal feedback during the examination and by pointing out the areas of discomfort.

KEY FINDING

▼Inspection In addition to the discussion in the preceding section, when examining children in this age group, be cognizant of the appearance of the underwear. Children who present with complaints of dysuria, incontinence, or hematuria may leave signs within their underclothes. This observation is particularly helpful when trying to judge the severity and nature of incontinence. Urine-stained underwear usually suggest at least a daytime wetting problem. Soiled underwear from stool suggests *encopresis,* hinting at a more serious and complex voiding dysfunction. The area under elastic bands such as along the waist lines and the top of socks can be spots where the purpura of *HSP* often will appear. *Varicoceles* will engorge when the patient is upright or when asked to cough or perform a Valsalva maneuver. When the patient is supine and relaxed, the varicocele usually softens and becomes less swollen.

This is the primary age of testicular torsion. Note the appearance of the contralateral testicle. In some cases it is possible to see the position or lie of the testicle within the scrotum. A horizontal lie is a predisposing risk factor to *torsion.* Remember that the presentation may change depending on the time of examination. Early on, there may be only discomfort and faint erythema and minimal swelling. As the condition progresses, there will be more swelling, redness, and pain. The discoloration and swelling that started unilaterally may seem on cursory evaluation to involve both sides as the inflammation worsens. Finally, if untreated, the degree of discomfort may lessen as the nerve endings die from ischemia; however, the swelling and erythema usually will persist for several weeks.

KEY FINDING

▼Palpation In addition to the discussion in the preceding section, an abdominal mass encountered in this age group includes constipated bowels. Consider adding a rectal examination if the patient is markedly constipated to feel for impacted stool. Patients who present with a possible *kidney stone* may yield clues to the progress or location of the stone on palpation. There is no direct sensation of the kidney or ureter, but the overlying peritoneum can give a rough estimation of the progress of inflammation and swelling. Stones as they pass often will refer discomfort along the course of the ureter that corresponds roughly on the abdominal surface to a curve running from beneath the rib cage across the groin and down into the scrotum and penile base.

Palpation of the scrotum at this age also can yield other findings besides those discussed previously (*testicular tumor, paratesticular tumor, hernia, hydrocele, varicocele, testicular torsion,* and *torsed appendix testis*). These also include *epididymal cysts* or *spermatoceles* that are typically round, smooth, and painless just above the upper pole of the testicle or head of the epididymis. *Inclusion cysts* can present along the midline of the scrotal skin. Small, round, distinct nodules can form along the scrotal raphe. They are benign and usually do not require excision unless infected.

Priapism will present with a firm penis that is usually painful. If the patient has a history of recurrent episodes (as in cases of *sickle cell anemia*), there may be palpable plaques or hard spots in the corporal cavernosa. These may yield a "woody" feeling to the penis and are palpable even when the penis is flaccid.

▼ KEY FINDING

M Percussion See the discussion in the preceding section.

▼ KEY FINDING

M Auscultation See the discussion in the preceding section.

▼ KEY FINDING

M Transillumination See the discussion in the preceding section.

Adolescents

The examination of adolescents must be sensitive to their developing sense of independence, control, modesty, and privacy. It may be helpful to carefully outline the examination and describe what will ensue.

▼ KEY FINDING

M Inspection Tattoos and skin ornamentation with piercing are no longer uncommon in this age group and can occur in the umbilicus and even the genitalia. Look for signs of *inflammation* such as redness, discharge, or swelling owing to localized skin infections and allergy.

Genital lesions and discharge owing to *STDs* become more prevalent in this age group. *Syphilis* presents primarily as a painless round ulcer on the genitalia. *Chancroid,* in contrast, presents with a painful round lesion. *Gonorrhea* usually manifests as a creamy purulent discharge with associated dysuria and pyuria. *Chlamydia* often will have a thin and clear discharge. *Condylomata,* or genital warts, present typically with multiple sites along the genitalia and groin. Always check carefully within the scrotal folds and the perirectal region when a wart is present. Applying a thin coating of acetic acid, such as in common vinegar, is useful in highlighting the lesions. The warts develop a whitish surface appearance. Be sure to check within the meatus and under the foreskin. Be sure to retract the foreskin and spread the meatus to look for hidden lesions. *Herpes simplex virus* (HSV) *infection* usually presents as painful, clear blisters on the genitals. Bear in mind that multiple infections are not uncommon and that it is important to screen all patients with an STD for other STDs, including *HIV* and *hepatitis B*. Patients with urethritis, arthritis, and conjunctivitis should bring to mind *Reiter syndrome.*

Occasionally at this age, a patient will present because of concern about genital size. Often these older boys are prepubertal and obese.

Typically, these individuals have a normal penis length (about 5 to 7 cm stretched flaccid). The apparent smallness is because of a penis buried in a suprapubic fat pad and an infraumbilical pannus. However, if the penis does measure less than 4 cm (especially if other findings are present, such as small testes or delayed puberty), further evaluation is necessary to look for an endocrine problem. See also the discussion in the preceding section.

▼ KEY FINDING
Palpation Testicular *tumors* in this age group begin to resemble histologically those found in adults. *Seminoma* becomes more common than *teratoma* and *yolk sac tumor*. See the discussion in the preceding section.

▼ KEY FINDING
Percussion See the discussion in the preceding section.

▼ KEY FINDING
Auscultation See the discussion in the preceding section.

▼ KEY FINDING
Transillumination See the discussion in the preceding section.

Synthesizing a Diagnosis

See TABLE 19–1.

Confirmatory Laboratory

See TABLE 19–2.

Confirmatory Imaging

See TABLE 19–3.

When to Refer

TABLE 19–4 lists the conditions and findings that should prompt referral to a specialist for further evaluation and treatment.

TABLE 19–1 *Synthesizing a Diagnosis*

Site/ Involvement	Problems and Findings	Diagnosis	Age of Incidence
Abdomen	Mass	Renal or adrenal mass, hydronephrosis	I, C, A
	Malformation of abdominal wall	Prune-belly syndrome	I, C, A
	Malformation of bladder	Exstrophy, classic or cloacal	
	Hematuria/ discharge from umbilicus	Urachal sinus or persistence urachus	I, C, A
Groin	Mass	Hernia, hydrocele	I, C, A
	Mass	Undescended testicle	I, C, A
Kidney	Mass/swelling	Hydronephrosis—may be UPJ narrowing, vesicoureteral reflux, duplication, obstructing stone	I, C, A
	Mass	Tumor—malignant, Wilms tumor, in infants usually a congenital mesoblastic nephroma, in older children: renal cell cancer	I, C, A
	Mass	Tumor—benign, multicystic dysplastic kidney	I, C
	Mass	Polycystic kidneys (autosomal dominant type)	C, A
	Pain	Pyelonephritis	I, C, A
	Pain	Obstruction owing to anatomic narrowing or stone	C, A, I
	Hematuria/ discharge	Calculi, hydronephrosis— UPJ, tumor, intrinsic kidney disease	I, C, A
	Malformation	Horseshoe kidney, pelvic kidney	I, C, A
Ureter	Mass/swelling	Hydronephrosis— blockage, UPJ narrowing, UVJ narrowing, obstructing calculus	C, A, I

(Continued)

TABLE 19-1 *Synthesizing a Diagnosis (Continued)*

Site/ Involvement	Problems and Findings	Diagnosis	Age of Incidence
	Pain	Obstruction owing to anatomic narrowing or calculi	I, C, A
Bladder	Mass/swelling	Urinary retention	I, C, A
	Hematuria/ discharge	UTI	I, C, A
	Hematuria/ discharge	Bladder calculi	I, C, A
	Pain, LUTS	UTI, cystitis, vesicoureteral reflux	I, C, A
	Pain, LUTS	Bladder calculi, foreign body	I, C, A
	Retention	Tumor of bladder neck and prostatic urethra— rhabdomyosarcoma	I, C, A
	LUTS	UTI, urethral stricture, posterior urethral valves	I, C, A
	LUTS, UTI, retention	Ureterocele	I, C, rarely A
	Incontinence	Enuresis, voiding dysfunction, neurogenic bladder	C, A, I
Genitalia	Malformation	Hypospadias	I, C
	Malformation	Epispadias	I, C
	Malformation	Duplex urethra	I, C
	Malformation	Meatal stenosis	I, C, A
	Mass	Testicular tumor, paratesticular mass, hydrocele, hernia	I, C, A
	Malformation	Penile adhesion, phimosis, paraphimosis, residual foreskin	I, C, A
	Malformation	Ambiguous genitalia or intersex	I, C, A
	Scrotal swelling	Varicocele	C, A, rarely I
	Scrotal swelling	Hernia, hydrocele	I, C, A
	Scrotal swelling/ pain	Orchitis, epididymitis, HSP	A, C, I
	Scrotal swelling/ pain	Testicular torsion, neonatal variant (I), appendix testis torsion, trauma	C, A, I
	Penile mass, discharge	STD, balanitis if foreskin is phimotic (I, C)	A, C, I

Abbreviations: I = neonate and infants; C = children; A = adolescents; HSP = Henoch-Schönlein purpura; LUTS = lower urinary tract symptoms; STD = sexually transmitted disease; UPJ = ureteropelvic junction; UVJ = ureterovesical junction; UTI = urinary tract infection.

TABLE 19-2 *Confirmatory Laboratory Investigation*

Laboratory Study	Comments	When to Order
Urine		
Urine analysis	Basic evaluation	Pain, mass, LUTS, discharge/hematuria
Urine culture	Identify urine infection and determine which antibiotics are effective	LUTS, discharge/hematuria
24-hour urine	Basic evaluation once stone has been identified and confirmed	History of urinary calculi
Blood		
Hemoglobin and hematocrit		Anemia, marked gross hematuria
White blood cell count		Infection
Platelet		Bleeding, hematuria
Coagulation (PT, PTT)		Bleeding
Electrophoresis of blood	Aid in diagnosing sickle cell anemia	Priapism workup if cause of low-flow priapism is unknown
Blood gas	Blood drawn from engorged penis, differentiates between high- and low-flow forms of priapism	Priapism workup
Serum		
Basic panel		Hydration, renal function
β-hCG, AFP	Elevated levels suggest metastatic spread	Testicular tumor markers
MIS		Ambiguous genitalia and intersex
Steroid precursor and metabolites	17-Hydroxyprogesterone, progesterone, deoxycorticosterone, corticosterone	Ambiguous genitalia and intersex
LH, FSH, testosterone		Ambiguous genitalia and intersex, bilateral undescended testicles
Parathyroid hormone level		History of urinary calculi
Karyotype	Determine genotypic sex and any anomalies	Ambiguous genitalia and intersex

Abbreviations: LUTS = lower urinary tract symptoms; PT = prothrombin time; PTT = partial thromboplastin time; AFP = alpha-fetoprotein; β-hCG = beta human chorionic gonadotropin; FSH = follicle-stimulating hormone; LH = luteinizing hormone; MIS = Müllerian inhibitory substance.

TABLE 19–3 Confirmatory Imaging

Test	Comment	When to Order
Handheld bladder scanner	Quick bedside method to assess postvoid residual and fullness of bladder	Retention, decreased force of stream
Ultrasound of kidneys and bladder	General evaluation of the urinary system	Pain, mass, hematuria, UTI, hydronephrosis
VCUG	Evaluates for stricture, posterior urethral valves, and vesico-ureteral reflux	Retention, decreased force of stream, UTI, hydronephrosis, anomalies of urethra
Ultrasound of scrotum with Doppler	Useful in determining nature of scrotal mass; Doppler ultrasound can determine presence of testicular blood flow	Pain, swelling in scrotum, testicular or scrotal mass, evaluates possible testicular torsion, useful in cases of suspected testicle rupture
Ultrasound of spine	Available within the first 6 months of life to evaluate the spinal cord before spinal column becomes too calcified	Urinary retention, decreased force of stream, suspected spinal cord abnormality during infancy
KUB	80 percent of stones are radiopaque	Urinary calculi evaluation, basic evaluation of pain, mass; constipation and for radiopaque foreign bodies
CT scan of abdomen and pelvis	~99 percent of all stones will be visible on CT, even stones that are radiolucent on plain x-ray	Useful for a rapid evaluation of possible stones; stone protocol CT
IVP	Study that helps define kidney and ureteral anatomy	Hydronephrosis, hematuria, stone, renal and ureteral duplication anomaly
MRI spine	Ordered if there is a suspicion of a neurogenic bladder	Neurogenic bladder, retention, dysfunctional voiding

(Continued)

TABLE 19-3 Confirmatory Imaging *(Continued)*

Test	Comment	When to Order
MRI urogram	Useful when other standard tests are unable to adequately illustrate anatomy	Hydronephrosis, duplication, anomaly
DMSA/MAG3	Quantifies renal function	Scarring, renal function assessment
MAG3 with Lasix (also known as DRS)		Hydronephrosis, UPJ narrowing
Angiography		Vascular evaluation, high-flow priapism
Urodynamics		Neurogenic bladder, voiding dysfunction

Abbreviations: CT = computed tomography; VCUG = voiding cystourethrogram; KUB = x-ray image of abdomen from kidneys, ureters, and down to bladder; IVP = intravenous pyelogram; MRI = magnetic resonance imaging; DMSA = technetium-labeled dimercaptosuccinic acid; MAG3 = technetium-labeled mercaptoacetyltriglycine.

TABLE 19-4 When to Refer

Condition or Finding	Comment
Antenatal hydronephrosis	Initial ultrasound done during the first week of life may not fully discern degree or nature of problem.
Bladder exstrophy Cloacal exstrophy	Keep exposed bladder surface covered with clean plastic wrap and a coating of petrolatum.
Prune-belly syndrome	Has distinctive flabby abdomen.
Hypospadias Epispadias	Opening may be hard to see if there is severe chordee.
Urethral duplication	More ventral opening is usually the primary urethra.
Urachal sinus, tract, or cyst	Presents with umbilical discharge.
Chordee	Can be associated with hypospadias.
Ambiguous genitalia or intersex	Involve specialists as soon as this is suspected.
Phimosis	Note that it is a normal state not to be able to retract the foreskin until age 5 to 7 years.
Paraphimosis	Emergency referral for relief.
Undescended testicle	Check to be sure it is not retractile.
Difference in testicle size	Often the problem is one testicle is smaller or atrophic.

(Continued)

TABLE 19–4 *When to Refer (Continued)*

Condition or Finding	Comment
Urinary calculi	Children rarely experience urinary calculi, so when they do occur, they should be thoroughly evaluated.
Urinary retention	Rule out urinary tract infection; inquire about toilet habits and any other conditions.
Gross hematuria	Needs a thorough workup to rule out tumors and calculi.
Microscopic hematuria	If not due to a urinary tract infection or known nephrologic cause such as glomerulonephritis.
Poor urinary stream	Must first rule out urinary tract infection as a cause.
Splayed urinary stream	Often meatal stenosis.
Urinary tract infection	Urinary tract infections in prepubertal children should be evaluated for possible anatomic or functional causes.
Acutely painful scrotum or testicle	Emergent evaluation needed to rule out testicular torsion.
Trauma to genitals	Be wary of placing a catheter unless one is sure that the urethra is not injured. Be suspicious of testicular rupture if faced with a scrotal hematoma.
Scrotal or groin swelling	Consider hernia, hydrocele, varicocele.
Scrotal or groin solid mass	Consider testicular and paratesticular tumors.
Varicocele	Vast majority are left-sided.
Enuresis	Nocturnal enuresis that persists beyond the start of elementary school should be evaluated.
Voiding dysfunction	Abnormal day and night wetting and/or voiding problems.
Spina bifida Spinal cord injury CNS injury/disease	Injuries or malformation of the CNS may affect bladder function.

The Gynecologic System and the Child

Jennifer Johnson

The goals of this chapter are

1. To outline the normal physiology and anatomy of the pediatric female gynecologic system
2. To outline the pathophysiologic processes that produce symptoms and signs referable to the pediatric female gynecologic system
3. To list major common gynecologic problems in the prepubertal female
4. To describe how to perform a physical examination appropriate to the presenting signs and symptoms
5. To use tables to summarize major diagnoses by age group
6. To outline confirmatory laboratory, imaging, and investigative procedures and referrals to specialists with their indications

Physiology

The hypothalamic-pituitary-gonadal (HPG) axis functions actively in the fetus, neonate, and infant. Its driving force comes from neurons in the hypothalamus that secrete pulses of gonadotropin hormone–releasing hormone (GnRH). During this time, gonadotropin secretion is sufficient to stimulate maturation of primordial follicles, usually only to the stage of primary (preantral) follicles. Owing to partial inhibition by higher central nervous system (CNS) centers, the GnRH "pulse generator" functions at a low level in late infancy and early childhood. Follicle-stimulating hormone (FSH) and luteinizing hormone (LH) levels increase measurably in the first 2 to 3 years of life. Consequently, ovaries produce small amounts of estrogen until 2 to 3 years of age. From 2 to 8 years of age, there is greater, but still incomplete, suppression of the HPG axis by the CNS. Pulsatile release of small amounts of GnRH, GnRH-stimulated secretion of LH and FSH, and increased nocturnal secretion of LH occur even during this quiescent period. Disinhibition at puberty causes the amplitude and frequency of GnRH pulses to increase, stimulating the production of gonadotropins that lead to puberty and reproductive capability. The adrenal glands increase secretion of the androgens dehydroepiandrosterone (DHEA) and dehydroepiandrosterone sulfate (DHEA-S) peripubertally as well. Puberty is also discussed in Chapters 13 and 21.

Primordial follicles progress to the preantral stage independent of gonadotropal stimulation from childhood through menopause. The preantral follicles generally involute before developing an antrum that would be capable of hormone synthesis. Rarely, primordial follicles mature to the large antral stage and produce hormones. They may become large enough to develop an asymptomatic cystic structure that is visible on ultrasound examination.

Anatomy

The internal portion of the female gynecologic system is composed of the ovaries, fallopian tubes, uterus, and vagina. The uterine cervix opens into the vagina at its external os. Externally, the vulva consists of the mons pubis, clitoris, and labia majora and minora. The labia minora surround the vestibule of the vagina, which contains the hymen, vaginal orifice, and openings of the greater vestibular (Bartholin's) glands. Before puberty, the uterus has a tubular shape and is 2 to 3 cm long; the cervix is approximately twice as large as the fundus. The ovaries are 0.5 to 1 cm in the long axis. They may be located in the abdomen rather than the pelvis owing to their small size. The vagina is 4 to 6 cm long. The labia majora and minora, prominent in the newborn owing to stimulation by maternal estrogens, lose their fullness after the first 2 months of life. In particular, the labia minora seem to disappear until estrogen production stimulates their growth again at puberty. This lack of the labial fat pads causes the lower third of the vagina to be directly exposed to bacteria and external irritants when the child squats or is seated. The hymen does not lose its fullness until 18 to 24 months of age, at which time it becomes thin and translucent.

In prepubertal girls, the unestrogenized mucosa of the vestibule is thin, highly vascularized, and appears red. The vaginal mucosa is similarly thin and red-appearing, and secretions are scant. In addition to the vagina's neutral pH and lack of anatomic protection, several factors predispose prepubertal girls to vaginal infections. These include lack of glycogen and lactobacilli and low levels of antibodies. Colonization by as many as 10 species of bacteria normally occurs.

The perineal median raphe runs in the midline along the short distance between the vulva and the anus. The minimal separation between the vagina and anus in infants and young girls contributes to the risk of vaginal infection with enteric organisms. This is especially true because good hygiene may be difficult to maintain in girls who are learning to toilet independently.

History

In addition to the information acquired during a complete general history (see Chapter 1), specific questions are important in the evaluation of gynecologic complaints. In infants and younger children, all or most information is from the parents. Does the child have abdominal pain or urinary or bowel symptoms (especially constipation)? Does she have vulvar pruritus? Has she or her caretakers noticed skin changes or a mass on the perineum? Is there a history of trauma or of inserting foreign bodies into body orifices? Who takes care of the child, and are the parents concerned about possible sexual abuse?

The problems discussed in this chapter refer in particular to the gynecologic system of the prepubertal female. There is considerable overlap between gynecologic problems presenting in the first 2 years of life and those that develop later in childhood.

Infants

KEY PROBLEM
■ Ambiguous Genitalia (Intersex) in the Neonate

Individuals who are intersex (i.e., have genital ambiguity) at birth fall into several categories. They may have external genitalia of uncertain gender, hypospadias and a single palpable gonad, or bilaterally impalpable testes. Patients in the latter two groups may have otherwise normal male external genitalia but must nonetheless be evaluated for intersex conditions.

By far the most common cause of virilization of the female external genitalia is *congenital adrenal hyperplasia* (CAH). This presentation of CAH, which can be a result of a defect of one of the five genes required for cortisol synthesis, is nearly always due to 21-hydroxylase deficiency. Excess androgen levels in utero result in virilization. Mild to severe clitoromegaly and a urogenital sinus occur in varying degrees of severity. This condition traditionally is referred to as *female pseudohermaphroditism.* The presence of one or two palpable gonads, which may appear in the inguinal canal or labia, rules out CAH. If none are present, measure serum electrolytes immediately in case the infant has a salt-losing form of CAH. The length of the stretched clitoral/penile structure is an important measurement (see Chapter 13).

Other categories of intersex include *gonadal dysgenesis* (mixed gonadal dysgenesis is the second most common cause), *true hermaphroditism,* and *male pseudohermaphroditism.*

Important historical information about the pregnancy includes length of gestation, use of *exogenous hormones* (oral contraception, assisted reproduction), and results of any ultrasound or prenatal chromosomal analyses. Does the mother herself demonstrate any signs of virilization or hypercortisolism (*Cushingoid* features)? Helpful clues from the family history include consanguinity, neonatal deaths, urologic abnormalities, precocious puberty, amenorrhea, or infertility.

KEY PROBLEM
■ Vaginal Bleeding

Parents reporting vaginal bleeding may have noted blood on a diaper, toilet tissue, or underpants. They may not have examined the genital area themselves, and their knowledge of genital anatomy may be incomplete. Careful questioning about when, where, and how they noticed the blood and about the apparent frequency and duration of the bleeding will help to sort things out. It is also important to ask about factors that can be related to symptoms, such as vulvar itching (scratching may cause bleeding), constipation (associated with *rectal fissures),* and dysuria, urgency, and frequency (hematuria associated with a urinary tract infection may result in blood on toilet tissues). Etiologic considerations differ in these situations, as discussed below.

This symptom is subject to misinterpretation. Blood may come from a *prolapsed urethra* or a *rectal fissure.* Pruritic lesions of the vulva such as *atopic* and *seborrheic dermatitis, psoriasis,* and *lichen sclerosus* may become excoriated and bleed. Vertically transmitted condyloma acuminata may bleed spontaneously or after minor trauma (see discussion of vulvar masses above and of child abuse below). Blood on toilet tissue also may be due to a *urinary tract infection* (UTI).

Hormonal Causes

The drop in levels of transplacentally acquired maternal hormones occasionally causes withdrawal vaginal bleeding in newborns. Onset is within the first 10 to 14 days of life. Withdrawal bleeding after ingestion (e.g., of oral contraceptives) or absorption (via skin creams) of exogenous estrogens also can occur at any time before puberty.

Vaginal bleeding may occur in the absence of development of secondary sexual characteristics as a form of incomplete precocious puberty. Probably a transiently functional ovarian cyst secretes sufficient estrogen for growth of the uterine endometrium. Such *isolated menses* are limited to a single or several episodes that may occur in girls from 1 to 9 years of age. We discuss complete precocious puberty later in this section.

Vulvovaginal Infection

Vulvovaginal infections are generally nonspecific (see "Vulvovaginitis" later in this section) and not generally associated with bleeding. Is there a history of poor perineal hygiene, exposure to chemical irritants (as soaps), or tight clothes? However, infection with *β-hemolytic streptococci* or *Shigella* or other enteric flora may cause a hemorrhagic vaginitis. Usually there is a history of preceding diarrhea.

Vaginal Foreign Body

This is a common cause of vaginal bleeding. Just as children may place objects in their ears or nose, young girls may insert a foreign body, most commonly toilet tissue, into their vagina. The retained object breaks down the thin vaginal mucosa and incites a foul-smelling, bloody discharge.

Trauma

Trauma to the vagina or vulvar area may cause bleeding. The bleeding may due to scratching of *pruritic dermatoses,* (including those due to *Sarcoptes scabiei* or *Phthirus pubis*) witnessed or unwitnessed *accidental trauma,* or *sexual abuse.* Always consider the possibility of sexual abuse.

Straddle injuries that crush perineal tissues against the pelvic bones are a fairly common cause of injury with bleeding. These may cause *laceration* or *abrasion* of the labia or posterior fourchette. Bleeding from injuries to the vagina and hymen, however, virtually always is attributable to penetration, either accidental (fence post) or intentional (sexual abuse). See later in this chapter for further discussion of suspected sexual abuse.

Tumors

Tumors, although rare, may present with vaginal bleeding. Always consider *sarcoma botryoides* (embryonal rhabdomyosarcoma) of the hymen or vagina, a rare tumor occurring primarily in girls 2 to 5 years old, when this is the presenting complaint. It grows in grapelike clusters that may protrude from the vagina, producing a mucosanguineous discharge. In older girls, embryonal rhabdomyosarcomas are more commonly in the cervix or uterus. Rarely, a benign vaginal polyp may develop in infants.

KEY PROBLEM

Vulvar Erythema, Irritation, Pruritus, and/or Bleeding (Vulvitis) Infants and toddlers may develop diaper or candidal dermatitis that affects the vulvar area. Conditions such as psoriasis and seborrheic and atopic and contact dermatitis that appear more commonly on other areas of the body also may present on the vulva. There may be associated pain or bleeding. Pinworm infestations may cause vulvar pruritus and associated bleeding. If the mother looks, she may notice the small white worms crawling from the anus at night. Nonspecific irritation may be from commercial "diaper wipes," scented soaps, or bubble baths. The clinician should be familiar with lichen sclerosus, in which the epidermis becomes thin and white but associated with thickening of the dermis. It affects skin in a "keyhole" distribution around the vaginal and anal orifices and commonly causes pruritus and pain. Excoriation and even purpura may contribute to the appearance of trauma.

Labial adhesion is associated with chronic irritation and dermatoses. It occurs in up to one-fourth of infants and prepubertal girls, especially in the first 5 years of life. After even superficial injury, the even normally thin skin agglutinates to the opposing labial tissue.

Questions to pose to the parents include: Have similar symptoms occurred previously? What was the treatment, and was it successful? Does the child have, or has she had, other skin problems such as cradle cap *(seborrheic dermatitis)*; dry, itchy skin, particularly on the cheeks *(eczema)*; or "sensitive skin"? How and how frequently do you cleanse the genital area? Is there a family history of skin conditions such as atopic dermatitis or psoriasis?

KEY PROBLEM

Vulvar or Vulvovaginal Mass Hymenal *cysts* or *tags* may occur in neonates, infants, or young children. *Hydrocolpos,* the accumulation of mucus or other nonsanguineous fluid in the vagina owing to an imperforate hymen, may present as a bulging hymen at birth or in young girls. *Hemangiomas* may occur on the vulva, including the clitoral region. They generally involute when the child is 2 to 5 years of age.

A number of mass lesions may appear on the vulva and labia. Straddle injury may cause a vulvar *hematoma*. A gonad or gonadal remnant (as in intersex conditions such as male pseudohermaphroditism owing to *androgen insensitivity syndrome*) or *inguinal hernia* may present as a labial mass. *Cysts, lipomas*, and *fibromas* are but a few of many mass lesions that occur in the prepubertal girl. Malignant vulvar neoplasms such as squamous cell carcinoma and adenocarcinoma are rare.

Skin-tag-like protrusions on the perineal median raphe occur in about 10 percent of prepubertal girls up to age 4 years. These "infantile perineal protrusions" are most common in newborns. They are typically located in the midline just anterior to the anus. The soft-tissue protrusion is pyramidal with a tonguelike lip. The skin is normal or red-colored, smooth or velvety.

Condylomata acuminata present as small flesh-colored papules with pinpoint red spots (capillaries) in prepubertal girls. They may be located on the mucus membranes of the vulva or around the anus. Onset after 2 years of age is highly suspicious for sexual abuse.

Ask the parents who bring their daughter for evaluation of a vulvar or vulvovaginal mass when they first noticed it, whether (and how) it has changed since then, and whether there is any history of vulvar trauma or reason to suspect sexual abuse.

KEY PROBLEM
■ Breast Development
Uni- or bilateral breast development without other signs of puberty before 8 years of age defines *premature thelarche* and falls into the category of incomplete precocious puberty. It is most common in girls 6 months to 3 years of age, does not progress, and usually regresses after 2 years of age. The etiology is uncertain possibly owing to increased breast tissue sensitivity to the low concentrations of estradiol produced at this age. There is a 10 percent likelihood that early breast development will progress to central precocious puberty (see below), especially when its onset is after 2 years of age (see Chapter 13).

Premature breast development also may occur owing to *exogenous estrogen* or production of endogenous estrogens from an *ovarian cyst* or *tumor*. Under these circumstances, there is nipple development along with vaginal estrogen effects. Question parents about the onset and course of breast development, as well as about the possibility of exogenous estrogens.

KEY PROBLEM
■ Pubic and/or Axillary Hair Development
Nonprogressive development of pubic (premature pubarche) and/or axillary hair before 8 years of age without breast development, evidence of virilization, increased growth rate, or clitoral enlargement is most often due to premature adrenarche (early onset of increase in adrenal androgen

secretion). This is part of the spectrum of incomplete precocious puberty. About 20 percent of these girls later have functional ovarian hyperandrogenism *(polycystic ovary syndrome)*.

KEY PROBLEM
◖ Breast and Pubic/Axillary Hair Development (Isosexual Precocious Puberty) As in normal puberty, breast development and pubic/axillary hair occur synchronously in isosexual precocious puberty. About 50 percent of cases are classified as true central precocious puberty (CPP), in which disinhibition of the hypothalamic-pituitary-gonadal (HPG) axis occurs at a younger than normal age. In 95 percent of girls, CPP is idiopathic, although it is frequently associated with an asymptomatic hypothalamic hamartoma. Other causes of CPP include *congenital anomalies, postinflammatory changes, trauma,* and *neoplasia.*

The remaining 50 percent of cases of precocious puberty are classified as pseudoisosexual precocious puberty, in which hormones produced independent of gonadotropin control stimulate development of breast and pubic hair and occasionally cause uterine bleeding. Sources include ovarian cysts and granulosa cell and extragonadal tumors. In primary hypothyroidism, LH and FSH receptors activate by an unknown mechanism, which may lead to thelarche and uterine bleeding. The hyperprolactinemia associated with primary hypothyroidism may cause galactorrhea. In *McCune-Albright syndrome,* a germ line mutation of the LH receptor leads to granulosa cell production of estradiol. Exogenous sex hormones are always a possible etiology.

Physical Examination

Even though good hand washing suffices, always wear gloves during the female gynecologic examination. Mothers are accustomed to having their health care providers wear gloves during a genital examination and generally expect the same for their daughters, regardless of age.

Otherwise, all that is necessary for the relevant physical examination is good lighting. The overhead lighting in typical exam rooms is often barely adequate for good visualization of the genital area. The light from an otoscope, which a parent can hold, may provide adequate illumination. Some examiners prefer to don a head-mounted flashlight of the type outdoors enthusiasts like to use. If an examiner chooses to use a lamp, it should serve to provide additional indirect lighting if possible. Older children, especially, may be frightened by a big "spotlight" on their genital area.

Newborns and Infants

Older children in this age group may become anxious if the examiner proceeds directly to the genital area without first engaging in "ice-breaking" activities. These include playful conversation, auscultation (which also affords the opportunity to inspect the breasts), and a gentle abdominal examination. The examiner may accomplish these activities with the child held comfortably in the parent's lap. The parent then should place the child on the examining table, remove the diaper, and stand next to the child during the examination. Explanation of each step of the genital examination will lessen parental anxiety prior to conducting it. For example, you might say, "I'm going to use my thumbs to separate the labia." Describe and demonstrate each finding, normal or abnormal, as you proceed. Many parents will reexamine their child at home later, and they need to know what they are seeing. This also helps give parents the vocabulary and pronunciation they may need to ask questions. Say, for example, "Here are Allison's labia majora, and I notice they seem to be stuck together here at the bottom."

KEY FINDING

Inspection In this age group, inspection focuses on the breasts and genitalia. As discussed in preceding sections, neonates often have slight breast tissue development owing to maternal estrogens. Older infants and toddler girls may have breast tissue development in premature thelarche or, rarely, in precocious puberty. Subcutaneous fat in the breast area frequently gives the appearance of breast tissue. Look to see if the nipples are flat (in the same plane as the chest wall) or elevated above the surrounding tissue. The latter more strongly suggests the possibility of enlargement of actual breast tissue, but palpation is necessary to determine whether this is the case.

Inspect the genital area with the child lying on her back, legs separated in a "frog leg" position (thighs spread apart, knees bent, and soles of feet together). First, obtain an overview of the entire diaper area. Does it look generally normal in terms of anatomy and skin condition? Are there any asymmetries, such as might be due to a mass? Are there any rashes, scratches, ecchymoses, or hypo- or hyperpigmented areas? Look carefully at the mons pubis. Are there any pubic hairs (which may have minimal pigment)? Retract the clitoral hood, and inspect the clitoris. If it appears enlarged, measure the length with the hood retracted, causing slight stretching of the clitoris. Then inspect the labia majora for growth of long, downy, or pigmented hairs. Look for distinct skin folds where the labia merge into the perineum. Adhesions here are common and of no consequence in this age group. If the labia are not separable with gentle lateral tension, look for midline *labial adhesions,* which rarely may be complete enough to result in obstruction of urinary flow. After separating the labia, inspect the vulva for any asymmetries, excoriations, lesions *(condylomata acuminata, molluscum contagiosum),* masses, discolorations, hemangiomas, or lacerations. Next, identify the urethral meatus just above the vaginal opening. This can be difficult for the novice examiner to find. Is there any inflammation or swelling? Note that the thin, delicate mucosal surfaces of the vulva often appear erythematous because they are highly vascularized. Locate the hymen at the vaginal orifice. Is there a clear opening in the hymen? Slight manipulation of the tissue may be necessary to find it. If the hymen appears not to be patent, is it bulging? Is there discharge (as in *nonspecific vaginitis* due to poor perineal hygiene, chemical irritants, tight-fitting pants, others), blood, or a protruding mass (sarcoma botryoides)? Then inspect the perineum for skin tags, protrusions, hemangiomas, and other masses or lesions. Gently lift the child's legs and inspect the anus, surrounding skin, and lower buttocks. Hypopigmentation around the anus occurs in *lichen sclerosus*. Slight outward tension of the anus may reveal an *anal fissure* as the source of blood on a diaper. Test the "anal wink" reflex by gently stroking the perianal skin. This reflex may extinguish itself in a child who has repeatedly had insertion of objects into the rectum, as in sexual abuse. Finally, turn the child over so that the lower back and buttocks can be viewed. Are there rashes, excoriations, or ecchymoses?

KEY FINDING
Palpation Palpate the breasts if one or both appear enlarged. Breast tissue, which is firmer than fatty subcutaneous tissue, may be palpable only below the nipple, or it may extend to an area larger in diameter.

Palpate the inguinal lymph nodes because an infected lesion on the external genitalia may cause lymphadenopathy, especially large and tender in primary genital *herpes simplex infection*. This is very rare in children, and its diagnosis should prompt questions regarding possible sexual abuse. Examine the labia majora to rule out rare masses. Texture and tenderness will give clues to the etiology of asymmetries or masses. A painless, rubbery, clearly circumscribed lesion may be a *Gartner duct cyst*, whereas a tender, firm mass whose borders are not clearly discernible may be *cellulitis*.

KEY FINDING
Percussion Percussion does not have applications in the gynecologic examination of the prepubertal child. The uterus is located in the lower pelvis posterior to the pubic symphysis. Although the ovaries may be located in the abdominal cavity, owing to the small size of the pelvis, even functional ovarian cysts will be too small to identify by percussion.

KEY FINDING
Auscultation Auscultation has no particular use in evaluating infants' gynecologic conditions.

Children

Given the number of injections in current vaccine schedules, it is common for children through the age of 6 or 7 years to be quite apprehensive about a visit to the medical clinic or doctor's office. Anticipation of a gynecologic examination generally increases a girl's anxiety. Thus you may encounter hesitation or resistance under the best of circumstances. The following general recommendations supplement those in Chapter 2. They will help put the patient at ease, thereby facilitating the examination itself.

Even the youngest children in this age group should have an opportunity to participate in her care, allowing her to retain some sense of control. The answer to "Amy, tell me why Mommy/Daddy brought you to see me today" provides considerable information. The child who does not reply may be shy, anxious, or uninformed; the girl who spouts out "'Cuz my bottom itches" usually will need less coaching. As explained previously, a brief general physical examination should precede the genital examination. Younger children, as well as older ones, who hesitate to get on the examination table should have the opportunity to sit on the parent's lap. In preparing the child for the genital examination, inform the child that it is now time to "look at where it itches," "check down there," or "see how I can help" with the problem.

Children who have remained in a parent's lap during the general examination will prefer the same during the gynecologic examination. Accomplish this easily by asking the girl to remove her pants and underpants and then sit on the parent's lap with legs in the "frog leg" position. Girls who are old enough for an examination on the table should have the opportunity to disrobe privately from the waist down and to wear an appropriately sized drape or gown. An accompanying mother generally assists young girls with disrobing and remains during the examination; ask accompanying males to excuse themselves once the patient is 4 years of age or older. Starting at 7 or 8 years of age, ask girls if they wish their mother to remain in the room while they are disrobing and during the gynecologic examination. The mother stands next to the patient's head during the examination. Once the child is lying on the table, draped and ready for the examination, ask her to bend her knees and draw her heels "up to your bottom." Then guide the patient in putting her legs into a "frog leg" position by asking her to touch one knee to the wall next to the table and the other to your hand that is at the side of the table.

Before commencing the examination, state that you are putting on gloves to "help keep things clean" and reassure the child that you will tell her "everything I'm going to do before I do it." Depending on age and cooperativeness, invite the patient to assist by holding the otoscope ("flashlight").

Once you have examined the child in this position, you may wish to ask her to kneel on the table in knee-chest position. The hymenal orifice opens, and it is often possible to visualize the lower aspect of the vagina using the otoscope.

KEY FINDING

Inspection Prior to inspection, review the girl's growth chart, including the body mass index (BMI) curve. A jump in height percentiles may indicate an increase in height velocity associated with precocious puberty. Girls whose BMI is at or above the 95th percentile may experience pubarche at a younger age. Next, on general inspection, look and listen for signs of virilization, such as facial, axillary, and lower abdominal hair and a deep voice. This points to an external or peripheral cause of precocious puberty. Does there appear to be breast development? After preparing the patient, proceed with inspection of the genital area. In older girls, the sexual maturity rating (SMR, Tanner stage) of breasts and pubic hair allows an estimate of when menarche might be expected to occur. See Chapter 13 for the Tanner charts (Figures 13-2 and 13-3).

▼ KEY FINDING
Palpation This is similar to the preceding section. Additionally, a rectal examination is necessary if there is vaginal bleeding. You can use it to assess uterine size in suspected precocious puberty. (Remember, the uterus is only 2 to 3 cm long prior to puberty.) Vaginal bleeding or a bloody vaginal discharge may be due to a vaginal foreign body. You may be able to detect an object through the anterior wall of the rectum and even "milk" it out of the vagina.

▼ KEY FINDING
Percussion As noted previously, percussion does not provide additional information in the gynecologic examination.

▼ KEY FINDING
Auscultation Auscultation does not have a role in the gynecologic examination.

Synthesizing a Diagnosis

TABLE 20–1 offers a summary of key diagnoses related to the gynecologic system in children younger than 12 years old. Most problems and findings can be present at any time during this age range. Age predilection, if any, appears in the right-hand column.

Confirmatory Laboratory Evaluation

TABLE 20–2 lists key studies helpful either to directly confirm clinical hypotheses or to prepare for a referral to a specialist. Confirmatory diagnostic laboratory testing and/or imaging studies are not necessary for many of the conditions discussed in this chapter if an adequate history and physical examination provide enough evidence.

When to Refer

The majority of conditions discussed in this chapter fall in the purview of the primary care physician. The following conditions and findings should prompt referral to a specialist for further evaluation and treatment:

Ambiguous Genitalia. A girl who appears to have only mild clitoromegaly must have an emergent referral to a pediatric endocrinologist even if results of laboratory studies for CAH are not complete. All other forms of ambiguous genitalia require urgent referral to a pediatric urologist, geneticist, and others who will help to evaluate the child and advise the parents.

TABLE 20-1 Synthesizing a Pediatric Gynecologic Diagnosis

Location	Problem/Findings	Diagnosis	Typical Age Group, if Any
Clitoris	Clitoromegaly, no palpable gonads	CAH	Neonate
		Exogenous androgens	
		Virilizing tumor	Infant, child
	Clitoromegaly, palpable gonad(s)	Intersex disorder	Neonate
	Firm erythematous mass	Hemangioma	
Urethra	Blood stains ± dysuria	Urethral prolapse	5–9 years
	Painless urethral mass	Ureterocele	Child
Labia	Unable to completely separate	Labial adhesions	Infant, child
	Mass	Gonad or gonadal remnant, inguinal hernia, lipoma, fibroma, malignant tumor	
Vulva	Flesh-colored papules with pinpoint red spots	Condylomata acuminata (HPV); differential diagnosis: molluscum contagiosum (umbilicated papules)	
	Painless mass	Hemangioma, lipoma, fibroma, cyst, resolving hematoma	
	Tender mass	Hematoma	
	Rash, pruritus, excoriations	Atopic dermatitis	
		Candida dermatitis	
		Contact dermatitis	
		Diaper dermatitis	
		Seborrheic dermatitis	
		Pinworm (*Enterobius*) infestation	
		Lichen sclerosus et atrophicus	
		Psoriasis	

Site	Finding	Diagnosis	Age
Hymen	Skin-colored mass	Hymenal cyst or tag	Neonate-toddler
		Hydrocolpos secondary to imperforate hymen	Neonate-toddler
	Friable bleeding mass	Sarcoma botryoides	2–5 years
	Bleeding tear or laceration	Trauma, including abuse	Neonate, infant, child
	No opening in hymen	Imperforate hymen or small orifice	Neonate
Vagina	Bleeding	Withdrawal of maternal estrogens	Infant
		Vaginal polyp	
		Withdrawal of exogenous estrogens	Child
		Precocious puberty	1–9 years
		Isolated menses	2–5 years
		Sarcoma botryoides of hymen, vagina	Older children
		Sarcoma botryoides of cervix, uterus	
		Trauma, including abuse	
	Bloody discharge	Retained foreign body Hemorrhagic vaginitis due to β-hemolytic streptococci, enteric flora, *Shigella* species	
	Nonbloody discharge	Nonspecific vulvovaginitis	
	Firm erythematous mass	Hemangioma	<4 years
Perineum	Pyramidal skin-tag-like protrusion	Infantile perineal protrusion	
	Flesh-colored papules with pinpoint red spots	Condylomata acuminata (HPV); rule out molluscum contagiosum	Infant, child
Anus	Bleeding	Anal fissure	Child
	Pruritus	Pinworms	Child
	Tender, erythematous swelling of surrounding tissue	β-hemolytic streptococcal infection	

TABLE 20–2 *Helpful Laboratory Studies*

Symptom or Sign	Test or Imaging Study	Comment
Ambiguous genitalia	Serum and urine electrolytes	Emergency
	Serum 17-hydroxyprogesterone level	
	Chromosome analysis	
Breast and pubic/axillary hair	Plasma estradiol	
	Thyroid function tests	
	Prolactin	
Episodic vaginal bleeding	Plasma estradiol	
	Bone age	
Serosanguineous vaginal discharge	Vaginal culture for β-hemolytic streptococci and enteric pathogens, including *Shigella*	
Both anal and vulvar pruritus	"Scotch tape" test in early morning to identify *Enterobius vermicularis*	
Painful perianal erythema	Rectal culture for β-hemolytic streptococci	

Suspected precocious puberty. A girl who has progressive breast development after 2 years of age or who has both breast development
and pubic or axillary hair without signs of virilization may have *isosexual precocious* or *pseudoprecocious* puberty. She may or may not
have vaginal bleeding. The referral to a pediatric endocrinologist is
not urgent from a medical perspective, but this concern is associated with high level of parental anxiety.

Documented vaginal bleeding not due to trauma or infection. This may be
due to a *retained foreign object,* a vaginal or cervical *polyp* or tumor
(including *rhabdomyosarcomas*), isolated menses (presence of a functional ovarian cyst producing estrogen), or premature menarche
associated with *precocious puberty.*

Traumatic injury. Refer lacerations or other injuries requiring suturing to
a gynecologist. If the history is not consistent with the findings on
physical examination, or if the examiner otherwise suspects abuse,
reporting to local child protective service authorities is mandatory.

Virilization. Clitoromegaly, excess facial hair, a deep, husky voice, or the
appearance of pubic or axillary hair in conjunction with any of these
indicate virilization through a metabolic defect such as *congenital
adrenal hyperplasia (CAH),* an androgen-producing *tumor,* or *exogenous androgens.*

Urethral abnormalities. Urethral prolapse and prolapsed ureterocele
require evaluation by a pediatric urologist.

Dermatologic conditions. Lesions that do not respond to common therapies for the presumed diagnosis may represent an unusual condition
requiring the diagnostic acumen of the specialist. *Psoriasis* is one such
condition, and *lichen sclerosus* another. In its classic presentation, lichen
sclerosis may be easy to diagnose, but its progressive course and
potential for debilitation call for the involvement of a specialist.

Mass lesions. Any patient with an inguinal, labial, or vulvar mass of uncertain origin demands referral. A palpable foreign body in the vagina that is not easily removable or causes ongoing suspicion for a *foreign body* should generate a referral to a pediatric gynecologist. Even when the diagnosis is clear, mass lesions (e.g., *hydrocolpos*) may need treatment by a specialist.

Sexually transmitted infections. Positive tests for *gonorrhea* (culture) after the neonatal period and for *Chlamydia trachomatis* (culture or other approved test) in girls older than 3 years of age are diagnostic of sexual contact and should be referred to the local/regional child abuse investigation center or, if unavailable, to child protective services. Also make a referral for *Trichomonas vaginalis* diagnosed by wet mount or polymerase chain reaction (PCR) in girls older than 1 year old or if a patient older than 2 years has condylomata acuminata (due to human papillomavirus). These conditions are highly suggestive but not diagnostic of sexual contact.

21 The Gynecology System and the Adolescent

Donald E. Greydanus, Artemis K. Tsitsika, and Michelé J. Gains

THE ADOLESCENT BREAST

The purposes of this section are

1. To outline the relevant embryology of the female adolescent breast system
2. To outline concepts of normal adolescent breast development, history taking, and examination of the breasts
3. To understand the key problems of breast mass, breast asymmetry, and breast pain (galactorrhea is presented in Chapter 13)
4. To synthesize a list of breast diagnoses found in adolescent females
5. To outline confirmatory imaging and other procedures, as well as list disorders to refer to specialists (as gynecologists or surgeons)

Embryology

Breast tissue begins to develop in utero as epidermal cells migrate into mesenchyme during the fourth to sixth fetal weeks and develop into primitive *mammary ridges* or *milk lines* (FIGURE 21–1). This results in thickening of ectoderm that extends from the axilla to the groin with the development of upper, middle, and lower ridges. There is a normal atrophy of the upper and lower ridges during the tenth fetal week, leaving the middle ridges to develop into normal breast tissue, later consisting of lactiferous ducts and mammary glands. Failure of the upper and lower milk lines to atrophy results in the development of extra breast tissue. The surrounding mesenchyme later becomes the breast fibrous and adipose tissue. Solid cords (15 to 20) develop from secondary buds in each gland, and these cords become the future milk ducts and lobes of the breast glands. The areola (nipple) develops in the fifth fetal month.

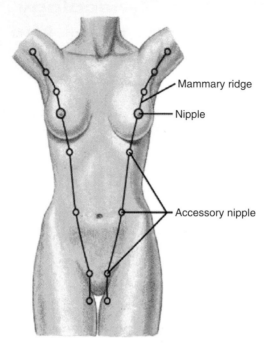

FIGURE 21–1 *The Mammary Ridges (Milk Lines). (From Van De Graaff KM:* Human Anatomy. *New York: McGraw-Hill, 2002, Fig. 2.3, p. 25.)*

Normal Adolescent Breast Development

Many hormones affect the development of breast tissue, including estrogen, progesterone, growth hormone, insulin, adrenal corticoids, and thyroxine. During childhood, the breast consists of epithelium-lined ducts with surrounding connective tissue. Puberty induces major changes in the female breasts owing to the effects of estrogen and progesterone; later, the production of prolactin leads to further breast changes, allowing for lactation. The first clinical sign of puberty in the female child is the breast bud stage, or *thelarche,* normally occurring between 8 and 14 years of age. Breast development that occurs before age 8 years may represent *isolated premature thelarche* or *precocious puberty* and, if starting at ages 13 to 14 years of age, represents *delayed puberty* (see Chapter 13). Breast development in puberty progresses in five stages called the *Tanner stages* or *sexual maturity ratings* (SMRs) (see Chapter 13). This rating system is the product of the research of Stratz (1909), modified by Reynolds and Wines (1948), and finalized by Tanner (1962).

The onset of female breast development, as the first clinical sign of puberty, alerts the adolescent, parents, and others to the emergence of

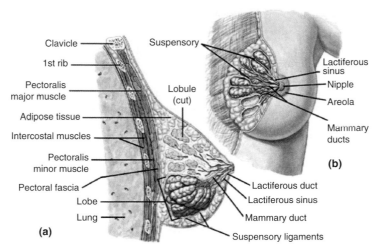

FIGURE 21–2 *Normal Breast Anatomy.*

adolescence, typically occurring 2 (1–3) years prior to menarche. Since society places major emphasis on female breast development and adolescent girls present with growing concerns about the normality or abnormality of this particular body part, clinicians have come to realize the importance of the physical diagnostic process of the adolescent breast.

The development of the breast bud stage heralds the onset of later pubertal changes that occur in a sequential pattern over the next 2 to 4 years. These changes include *pubarche* (development of pubic hair, sometimes occurring before thelarche), height velocity peak (occurring in SMR 2 in contrast to SMR 4 in males), axillary hair development, *menarche* (often 1 to 3 years after thelarche), and then the final pubertal changes. Breasts are modified sweat glands placed within superficial thoracic fascial layers that suspend from the chest by fibrous septa (called *Cooper ligaments*). Normal breast tissue extends from the pectoralis fascia to the dermis (FIGURE 21–2).

History

Breast examination may be part of a normal general examination process or may be necessary because of a specific adolescent or parental concern that an abnormality may exist. Male clinicians may feel more comfortable with a chaperone in the room. A careful, sensitive, and yet thorough examination is important, taking into account the embarrassment that this kind of examination may produce. Ask the adolescent if she has any concerns about her breasts, such as their being too small, too large, asymmetric, or other. Explain to her that there is a wide normal variation regarding the timing of breast development, breast size and shape, and consistency; nipple size can vary as well. Ask if she has felt or noticed any breast tenderness or "lumps" and if the area of concern has changed recently. If there is any specific concern, it is important to ask how long it has been present, if there is any relationship to menstrual cycling, and if there is a family history of breast pathology. The clinician also may ask if there is any discharge from the nipples and if there is any history of breast trauma from sports activity, sexual behavior, or other. If the patient reports a nonbreast lesion, is it along the milk lines? Figure 21-3 visualizes the breast examination in adults; appropriate modification can be applied to the adolescent examination.

Breast Examination

To ensure accurate description of the location of a lesion, the clinician can think of the breast as a circle or "pie" with four sections superimposed on a clock. The lateral breast tissue that extends into the axilla can feel swollen; this *axillary tail of Spence* is normal breast tissue. Areolar hair is normal, and plucking such hairs can lead to ingrown hairs and infection. The areola contains Montgomery tubercles that may produce a small amount of whitish secretion not to be confused with *galactorrhea* (see Chapter 13). Edema fluid in breasts tends to be minimal in the first part of menstruation (follicular phase) and then may increase (50 percent or more) in the luteal, or third, phase of the cycle. The mature breast may increase two to three times its normal size during pregnancy and lactation.

KEY PROBLEM
Breast Mass   The finding of a lump or mass on or near breast tissue may represent a congenital lesion, such as *polythelia* (*extra nipples*) (FIGURE 21–4), *polymastia* (*supernumerary breasts*), or a *combination* of extra breast and nipple tissue. Sometimes these lesions occur in the milk line distribution away from the breasts. A unilateral or bilateral lump in the adolescent male breast area represents *gynecomastia* (see Chapter 13). The most common breast mass found in adolescent girls is the *fibroadenoma* (FIGURE 21–5), found in 70 to 95 percent of breast biopsies done to evaluate a breast lesion. There may be one or more painless, slowly growing lumps. A breast lesion that is growing rapidly may be a *giant fibroadenoma*. The adolescent may present with one or more painful *cystic breast lesions,* as reviewed below in the key problem of breast pain.

A malignant breast lump or mass is unusual in the adolescent female, and if one is found, it is usually *cystosarcoma phyllodes.* In rare cases, *adenocarcoma,* the most common cause of breast cancer in adult females, can be present in the adolescent female. Although breast cancer is rare, it is often the main concern of parents and patients. A unilateral mass under the nipple that presents with a bloody discharge may be an *intraductal papilloma.* Milky nipple discharge apart from lactation is *galactorrhea* (see Chapter 13).

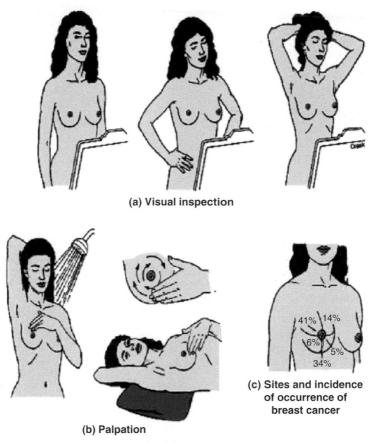

(a) Visual inspection

(b) Palpation

(c) Sites and incidence
of occurrence of
breast cancer

FIGURE 21-3 *The Adult Breast Examination.*

A fine-needle aspiration (FNA), a core needle biopsy (CNB), or an excisional biopsy will elucidate breast lesions. Mammography is often not helpful in breast evaluation of females under age 25 years because of increased breast density owing to fibroglandular tissue. A breast ultrasound is often useful in determining a cystic versus a solid breast mass, whereas a CT scan/MRI may be helpful in differentiating a breast mass from a rib lesion or other chest wall lesion.

KEY PROBLEM
Breast Asymmetry It is common for one breast to start development before the other, although catch-up symmetry usually develops by the end of the adolescent years. However, 25 percent of adult females have visible *breast asymmetry* (FIGURE 21–6). A *breast mass* also can be the cause of breast asymmetry. *Injury* to breast tissue may

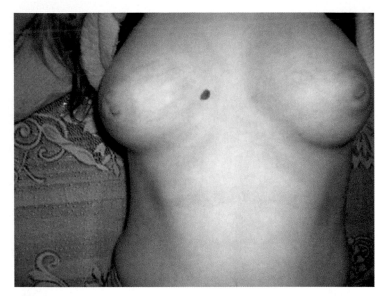

FIGURE 21-4 Polythelia.

cause decreased breast development because of *prepubertal infection* or *trauma* [burns, surgery (biopsy of a "breast lump" that is a normal breast bud), chest tube insertion, or radiation]. *Pseudoasymmetry* may result from a rib cage abnormality or scoliosis. An abnormal breast appearance is associated with the *tuberous breast anomaly* (FIGURE 21–7).

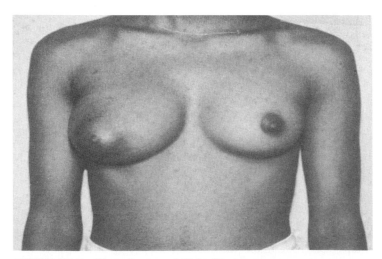

FIGURE 21-5 *Fibroadenoma of Right Breast.*

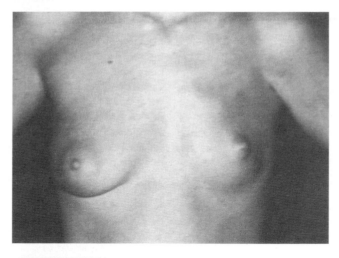

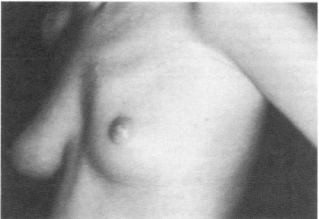

FIGURE 21-6 *Breast Asymmetry in Poland Syndrome.*

KEY PROBLEM
Breast Pain Adolescent females may complain of breast pain when the breasts are growing very rapidly. *Juvenile (virginal* or *idiopathic) hypertrophy* or *mammary hyperplasia* manifests as explosive growth, often occurring after thelarche (FIGURE 21-8). Bilateral hyperplasia may occur in newborn females or males (see Chapter 5). Rapid breast growth in the adolescent female can be massive and is termed *macromastia* or *gigantomastia.* Pain also may arise because of a *breast mass,* solid or cystic. Adult females are more likely to have cystic *breast disease,* but it may occur in adolescent females as well. A common type of adult cystic breast disease is *fibrocystic change,* which also may occur in adolescent females. These painful cystic lesions often change during the menstrual cycle. *Breast pain* or *mastalgia (mastodynia)* also may arise because of physiologic changes in

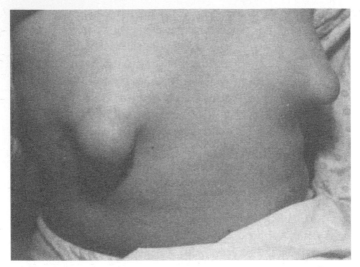

FIGURE 21–7 *Tuberous Breast Anomaly in a 13-year-Old Girl.*

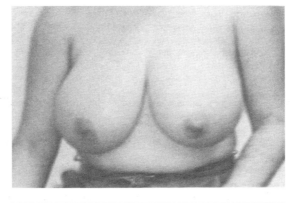

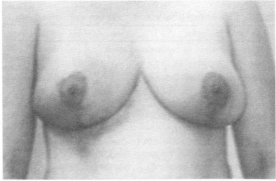

FIGURE 21–8 *Mammary Hyperplasia in a Teenage Girl Showing Appearance Below After a Bilateral Reduction.*

normal breast tissue during menstrual cycles. Painful breasts also may be part of the *premenstrual syndrome. Trauma* to the breast also can result in breast pain, leading to *jogger's nipple, breast contusion, breast abrasion, breast laceration,* or *breast hematoma.* Finally, breast pain may arise from *lactational* or *nonlactational mastitis.*

Synthesizing a Diagnosis

TABLE 21–1 summarizes female breast conditions.

When to Refer

TABLE 21–2 enumerates conditions to refer to surgeons or gynecologists.

THE FEMALE GENITAL SYSTEM AND THE ADOLESCENT

The purposes of this section are

1. To outline the physiology of the adolescent female genital system
2. To outline relevant anatomy
3. To understand the key problems, including pelvic pain, abnormal menstruation, vaginal discharge, and sexually transmitted diseases
4. To learn to perform a complete physical examination referable to the genital system in the adolescent female and develop a list of key findings
5. To synthesize a list of gynecologic diagnoses found in adolescent females
6. To outline confirmatory laboratory and imaging procedures and referrals to specialists with their indications

Physiology of Menstruation

Puberty is the period in which the adolescent attains secondary sex characteristics and the capability for sexual reproduction. This transition occurs between 8–10 and 16+ years of age and involves several hormones that affect the cellular and glandular components of the reproductive system, leading to the anatomic changes of puberty.

For the clinician, parents, and patient, the physical changes in breast development, pubic hair development, and somatic growth indicate the onset of the pubertal process (see Chapter 13). A hormonal process occurs months to years prior to the physical changes of growth. The

TABLE 21-1 Breast Disorders of Adolescent Females

Disorder	Special Comments	Differential Diagnosis	Diagnosis
Polythelia (extra nipple) (FIGURE 21-4)	Seen in 1 to 2 percent of the general population; often asymptomatic and familial; can be associated with cardiovascular and urologic defects; can be located on the milk lines from the axilla to the groin; sometimes seen on the buttocks or back.	Mole, melanoma, hemangioma	Inspection, excisional biopsy
Inverted nipple: nipple that does not project beyond surface of the breast	If present, seen in the newborn at birth; often bilateral and usually reverts to normal in a few weeks; can persist in to the adolescent years; can lead to cosmetic deformity as well as chronic areolar abscesses with swelling, infection, pain.	Bifid nipple; depressed nipple (ducts open in a depressed area within the areolar center); *acute* inversion in adolescence: duct ectasia, malignancy—usually unilateral	Inspection, breast ultrasound
Athelia	Rare congenital anomaly with absence of a nipple; can be unilateral, bilateral, familial, isolated; breast tissue can develop at puberty without a nipple; may be seen after exposure to exogenous androgens taken during pregnancy.		Inspection
Polymastia (super-numerary breast)	Less common than polythelia; seen also along milk line; can be bilateral or unilateral, as well as familial; usual location: below the breast on the chest or upper abdomen; various combinations can occur: nipple, areola, glandular tissue; difficulties often noted during puberty, pregnancy, and/or lactation.	Moles, hidradenitis suppurativa.	Inspection, breast ultrasound

Amastia	Quite rare; often unilateral; association with *Poland syndrome*: amastia, pectoralis muscle aplasia, rib defects, webbed fingers, radial nerve aplasia, brachysyndactyly; *acquired* amastia can be due to breast bud excision, irradiation, injury.		Inspection
Breast asymmetry	Usually normal in which one breast bud develops ahead of the other; catch-up growth usually occurs as puberty continues; however, 25 percent of adult females have visible asymmetry.	*Injury*: prepubertal infection, trauma (burns), surgery (as biopsy of a breast bud), radiation, chest tubes; anterolateral thoracotomies at third to fourth intercostal space; burns; *breast mass*; *pseudoasymmetry*: as scoliosis or rib cage abnormality	Inspection, breast ultrasound
Bilateral breast hypoplasia	Ovarian dysfunction, often with primary amenorrhea, poorly developed nipples	Gonadal dysgenesis (Turner syndrome), congenital adrenal hyperplasia, preadolescent hypothyroidism, androgen-producing tumor, pituitary hypogonadism, radiation effects, bilateral ovariectomy	See Chapter 13 and menstrual disorders section of Chapter 21.

(Continued)

711

TABLE 21-1 *Breast Disorders of Adolescent Females (Continued)*

Disorder	Special Comments	Differential Diagnosis	Diagnosis
Tuberous breasts (FIGURE 21-7)	Anatomic abnormality in which the patient has a small breast volume and the appearance of a protuberant, overdeveloped areola; difficult to provide a Tanner (SMR) stage because nipple-areolar complex appears to be on a thickened stalk; two types noted—type 1 is the classic type.		Inspection, palpation, breast ultrasound
Mammary hyperplasia (FIGURE 21-8)	Explosive growth shortly after thelarche; can be familial; some diagnostic subjectivity involved; cause: tissue sensitivity to estrogen or endogenous hormone (intracellular) production; massive growth can lead to various complications: (a) areolar stretching; tissue necrosis, dermatitis, skin rupture; (b) pain (mastalgia, mastodynia), (c) neck or back strain with poor (kyphotic) posture, headaches, (d) psychological difficulties, including emotional withdrawal, (e) others, such as respiratory distress and spinal curvature in severe cases.	Unilateral: consider breast mass (including giant fibroadenoma; abscess); see Chapter 13 for a consideration of male breast hyperplasia (gynecomastia)	Inspection, palpation, biopsy

Breast atrophy	Significant weight loss leads to decreased breast adipose tissue with decreased size; usually bilateral.	Dieting (crash), including anorexia nervosa (major weight loss), hypoestrogenism (premature ovarian failure) and virilization syndromes, systemic diseases, with weight loss and hypoestrogenic state, *scleroderma* (see localized changes with secondary breast atrophy).	History, inspection, others—depending on the underling cause
Fibroadenoma (FIGURE 21–5)	Most common breast mass of the adolescent female; benign lesion often found in the upper, outer breast quadrant; firm, rubbery, nontender; usually under 5 cm in diameter at discovery; estrogen-sensitive lesion; size may/may not be influenced by cycle of menses; 10 to 20 percent: multiple/bilateral involvement (*fibroadenomatosis*)	Giant (juvenile) fibroadenoma, unilateral virginal hypertrophy, benign breast cyst, cystosarcoma phylloides, adenocarcinoma.	History, inspection, palpation, ultrasound, excisional biopsy
Giant fibroadenoma	Variant of the fibroadenoma that can reach 15 cm in size	See "Fibroadenoma"	See "Fibroadenoma"

(Continued)

TABLE 21-1 *Breast Disorders of Adolescent Females (Continued)*

Disorder	Special Comments	Differential Diagnosis	Diagnosis
Cystosarcoma phyllodes	Rare but most common malignant teen breast tumor (often benign); can see rapid or slow growth, bloody nipple discharge, overlying skin retraction, and necrosis; malignant tumor spreads to the lungs.	Fibroadenoma, giant fibroadenoma, adenocarcinoma, intraductal breast papilloma, mammary duct ectasia, juvenile papillomatosis, papillary duct hyperplasia, infiltrating ductal adenocarcinoma, metastatic cancer, rhabdomysarcoma, neuroblastoma, non-Hodgkin lymphoma.	Ultrasound, fine-needle biopsy, core-needle biopsy, or excisional biopsy
Adenocarcinoma	Very rare cause of breast cancer in adolescent females; main cause of breast cancer in adult females; hard, immobile mass with overlying skin changes (*peau d'orange*), lymphadenopathy (axillary, supraclavicular); may have a positive family history; genetic markers (*BRCA-1*: chromosome 17; *BRCA-2*: chromosome 13)	See "Cystosarcoma phyllodes."	See "Cystosarcoma phyllodes."

Intraductal papilloma	Presents with a unilateral mass under the areola with bloody discharge from the involved nipple; rare and usually benign; galactorrhea as a cause of nipple discharge: see Chapter 13.	Intraductal breast papilloma, mammary duct ectasia, juvenile papillomatosis, papillary duct hyperplasia, papillary carcinoma, infiltrating ductal adenocarcinoma, cystosarcoma phyllodes.	Fine-needle or core-needle biopsy, ultrasound
Benign breast disease	Term applied to a large number of benign breast lesions, especially in adult females; can include normal, physiologic changes in size of teen breasts; pseudolumps; benign cysts can develop; often not fixed to breast tissue; vary over menstrual cycles.	Fibrocystic change, normal breast tissue, postpartum galactocele, traumatic necrosis.	Ultrasound; fine-needle aspiration with cytologic evaluation
Fibrocystic change	Previous term: *fibrocystic/proliferative breast disease;* typically noted in women in the third to fourth decades; nodularity and tenderness that can change during the menstrual cycle.	Benign breast disease, normal breast tissue, postpartum galactocele, traumatic necrosis.	Ultrasound; fine-needle aspiration with cytologic evaluation

(Continued)

TABLE 21-1 *Breast Disorders of Adolescent Females [Continued]*

Disorder	Special Comments	Differential Diagnosis	Diagnosis
Mastalgia (mastodynia)	Breast pain due to hormonally induced process associated with various nodularities and swellings within the breast; can be cyclic; usually develops 18 months after menarche; can be worsened with oral contraceptives; premenstrual mastodynia may develop as part of the premenstrual syndrome.	Sports-trauma nipple or breast pain; erotic stimulation (can lead to nipple irritation and discharge); mastitis; drug side effects (marijuana; phenothiazines; others); costochondritis, cardiac disease, cervical spine disease.	History, inspection, palpation, ultrasound
Mastitis	Most common in lactating females; can be nonlactating as well; precipitants include breast trauma (including sexual) and areolar hair plucking; erythematous, tender, warm breast induration; tender mass (abscess) can occur with or without overt mastitis; microbiologic etiology: *Staphylococcus aureus* (80 to 90 percent); rest: *Streptococcus, E. coli, Pseudomonas, Micrococcus pyogenes,* others.	Consider underlying pregnancy.	History; physical examination, pregnancy test, needle aspiration of abscess with cultures, ultrasound; possible blood culture(s)

Nipple trauma (*jogger nipple; bicyclist's nipple*)	Injured because it is the most prominent breast part; injury to nipple seen in runners or bicycle riders owing to frictional injury of bra or shirts on the nipple; most common in males; can see a bleeding nipple that is raw and painful; can be unilateral or bilateral.	Intraductal papilloma	History, inspection, palpation
Breast trauma	Trauma to the breasts can arise from sports, motor vehicle accidents, others; can lead to breast contusion, abrasion, laceration, or hematoma.	Hematoma: other causes of breast masses (see "Fibroadenoma").	History, inspection, palpation, ultrasound

TABLE 21-2   Breast Conditions to Refer to Gynecologists or Surgeons

Condition	Comment
Polythelia and polymastia	If the patient wishes removal
Bilateral breast hypoplasia	To endocrinologists for workup
Tuberous breasts	For surgical repair
Mammary hyperplasia	If patient wishes breast reduction
Breast mass	For fine-needle aspiration or excisional biopsy
Nipple mass	For fine-needle aspiration or biopsy
Mastitis	For aspiration of underlying abscess
Breast hematoma	For aspiration
Others	Depending on the clinician's expertise

hypothalamic-pituitary-gonadal (HPG) axis has a feedback loop that has both positive (stimulant) and negative (inhibitory) processes. The hypothalamus secretes several hormones, one of which is the gonadotropin-releasing hormone (GnRH). Other hormones released by the hypothalamus include thyrotropin-releasing hormone (TRH), growth hormone-releasing hormone (GHRH), corticotropin-releasing hormone (CRH), and somatostatin. Many of these hormones are short-acting and are released into the hypothalamus portal circulation in a nocturnally increasing pulsatile frequency during late childhood.

The pulsatile GnRH continues until a certain quantity concentrates in the pituitary. The anterior pituitary then is stimulated to release two gonadotropins: luteinizing hormone (LH) and follicle-stimulating hormone (FSH). LH and FSH stimulate the sex (gonadal) steroids; LH stimulates the production of androgens, and FSH stimulates estrogen. The sex steroids further promote the development of secondary sex characteristics such as breast development, pubic hair development, and testicular enlargement (see Chapter 13). Estrogen and progesterone exerts a negative (inhibitory) influence on the hypothalamus.

The menstrual cycle consists of three phases. The first phase is called the *follicular phase,* the second phase is *ovulation,* and the third phase is the *luteal phase.* In between the follicular and luteal phases is the fertile window. GnRH is secreted in a pulsatile nature from the arcuate nuclei in the hypothalamus. The hypothalamus functions as a generator, and GnRH serves as a regulator that governs the cycle of the menstruation. The mature follicular phase generally lasts approximately 14 days, allowing development of the follicle (ovum) and growth of the endometrium.

The ovarian follicles are in a constant state of growth and degeneration. FSH begins to rise just prior to menstruation, triggering the development of ovarian follicles that contain FSH receptors. The follicle that exhibits the highest sensitivity to FSH becomes the dominant follicle for that cycle. This developing follicle releases estrogen and develops increasing numbers of LH receptors. The estrogen then functions to decrease secretions of LH. The follicle also secrets inhibin A and B, which provide feedback on the pituitary. Estrogen levels continue to increase until approximately day 14 of a normal cycle.

The midcycle surge of LH production results in ovulation that lasts a variable amount of time, normally 24 to 48 hours, marking the fertile window as typically 6 days. However, this window of fertility varies with the specific menstrual length, gynecologic age, and several other factors that influence menstrual length. After the midcycle LH surge that triggers release of the dominant mature follicle, this follicle becomes the corpus luteum that produces a sustained progesterone secretion. The corpus luteum has a lifespan of about 12 days unless supported by an implanted pregnancy that produces human chorionic gonadotropin (hCG). At ovulation, progesterone induces an orderly sequence of altered glandular secretion and stromal changes that lead to an endometrium receptive for blastocyte implantation.

If implantation does not occur, the luteal phase continues. Very high levels of progesterone occur during the first 3 days of the luteal phase and remain that way for approximately 12 days. The sustained progesterone level operates as an inhibitory mechanism on the pituitary, signaling a decrease in LH and FSH production and subsequent estrogen and progesterone withdrawal. *Menstruation* (*menstrual period, menses*) is the term that refers to the bleeding event that results when the endometrium desquamates. FIGURE 21–9 provides a timeline for normal menstruation.

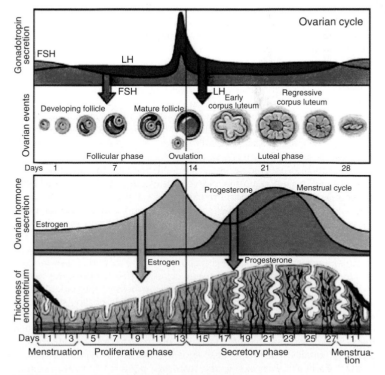

FIGURE 21–9 *The Normal Menstrual Cycle.*

Functional Anatomy

Anatomy of the female genitalia consists of four components: the vulva, vagina, uterus, and pelvic adenexa. The vulva is the external branch of the female pelvis, found below the urogenital diaphragm and below the front of the pubic arch. There is anatomic variability in normal females. The vulva consists of the *mons pubis, labia majora, labia minora, clitoris, vestibule, Skene glands, Bartholin glands, hymen,* and *introitus* (FIGURE 21–10). The *mons pubis* is a hair-covered, rounded eminence in front of the pubic symphysis formed by a collection of fatty tissue beneath the integument. The development of hair is under androgenic hormonal control. Pubic hair grows during puberty in stages referred to as *Tanner staging* (see FIGURE 13–3).

The *labia majora* and *labia minora* are skin folds of adipose tissue that surround the vaginal opening. The labia minora are thinner tissues located medial to the labia majora. The labia majora are two prominent longitudinal cutaneous folds that extend downward and backward from the mons pubis; they form the lateral boundaries of a fissure or cleft, the pudendal cleft or rima, into which the vagina and urethra open. Each labium has two surfaces: an outer, pigmented surface covered with strong, crisp hairs and an inner, smooth surface beset with large sebaceous follicles. Between the two surfaces, there is a considerable quantity of areolar and adipose tissue in addition to vessels, nerves, and glands. Posteriorly, they do not join but appear to become lost in the neighboring integument, ending close to and nearly parallel with each other.

The *labia minora* are two small cutaneous folds situated between the labia majora. They extend from the clitoris in an oblique, downward, lateral, and backward direction for about 4 cm on either side of the vaginal orifice. In the virginal female, the posterior ends of the labia minora are usually joined across the middle line by a fold of skin called the *frenulum* of the labia or the *fourchette.* The upper portion meets and forms a fold over the clitoris; it folds and extends superiorly to form the *prepuce* (i.e., the clitoral hood).

The *clitoris* is an erectile body situated beneath the anterior labial commissure, partially hidden between the anterior ends of the labia minora. It consists of two corpora cavernosa composed of erectile tissue enclosed in a dense layer of fibrous membrane and united together along their medial surfaces by an incomplete fibrous pectiniform septum. It serves as the sensory (sexual) organ in the female. The *vestibule* is the oval-shaped structure between the labia majora. Within the vestibule are the *urethral opening,* the *introitus (vagina),* Skene glands (i.e., *paraurethral glands*), *Bartholin glands,* and the tissue covering the introitus, the *hymen.*

The hymen may or may not be intact regardless of the patient's sexual history. The hymen is a thin fold of mucous membrane situated at the orifice of the vagina; the inner edges of the fold are normally in contact with each other, and the vaginal orifice appears as a cleft between them. There is a considerable variety of normal shapes of the hymen in different females. The *urethra opening* is located in the vestibule inferior to the clitoris and superior to the introitus; posteriorly to it on either side are the paraurethral *Skene glands.* The Bartholin glands' openings lie posteriorly on either side of the vagina and are generally invisible. Their glandular component lie deeper in the vagina, and their function is to maintain moisture within the vagina.

The vagina is a musculomembranous tube between the urethra and rectum. It is situated behind the bladder and in front of the rectum. The vaginal mucosa consists of an internal mucous lining and a muscular coat separated by a layer of erectile tissue. Thick, transverse folds called *rugae* are columns of mucous membrane; furrows of variable depth divide these rugae. The vagina also consists of a muscular coat that is made up of two layers, an external longitudinal and an internal circular layer. The longitudinal fibers are continuous with the superficial muscular fibers of the uterus. The two layers are not distinctly separable from each other. The erectile tissue consists of a layer of loose connective tissue situated between the mucous membrane and the muscular layer. A plexus of large veins and numerous unstriped muscular fibers are imbedded in the tissue. In the adult female, the length of the vagina is approximately 8 cm anteriorly and 9 cm posteriorly. It is capable of expansion and contraction.

The uterus body (*fundus*) divides into two sections: the *corpus* and the *cervix*. The anatomic landmark that joins the body to the cervix is the *isthmus.* The lower part of the uterus, the *cervix*, protrudes into the vagina toward the anterior vaginal wall. During puberty, the uterus descends into the pelvis, the fundus being just below the superior aperture of the pelvic cavity. The opening of the cervix—the *external os*—is a slitlike opening into the endocervical canal. The epithelial surface of the cervix (ectocervix) changes from squamous epithelium to columnar epithelium. The boundary that joins the squamous and columnar epithelium is the squamous columnar junction or transition zone.

The pelvic adenexa consists of the *fallopian tubes* and *ovaries*. The fallopian tubes (oviducts or salpinges) are bilateral and attached to the uterus at the proximal ends, whereas the distal end curves over the ovaries. It is approximately 10 cm long and has three components: the *isthmus*, the *ampulla*, and the *infundibulum.* The infundibulum portion contains ciliated ovarian fimbriae that have a fanlike appearance and wrap around the ovary cilia. They are mobile, open into the peritoneal cavity, and lie within the broad ligament.

The ovaries are almond-shaped organs that consist of three portions: the *outer cortex*, the *central medulla*, and the *rete ovarii*. The *hilum* is the point of attachment of the ovary to the uterus. At birth, the ovary contains approximately 7 million oocytes (gametes or immature ova). This decreases to approximately 500,000 at the start of puberty and continues to decline to near exhaustion by the end of menopause. The ovaries function to secrete hormones that stimulate the vagina and endometrial lining of the uterus as well as development of secondary sex characteristics. The parietal peritoneum consists of the *muscles* and *seven ligaments*. They form the support structure for the uterus, fallopian tubes, ovaries, pelvic organs, and the various blood vessels, nerves, and connective tissues. The seven ligaments are termed the *anterior, posterior, round, broad* (2), and *uterosacral* (2). FIGURES 21–10 and 21–11 illustrate of the external and internal female anatomy.

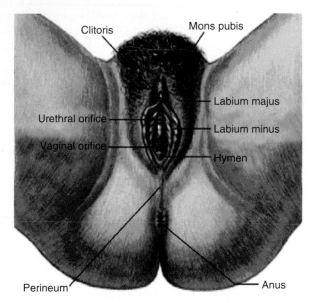

FIGURE 21-10 *The Normal Perineum.*

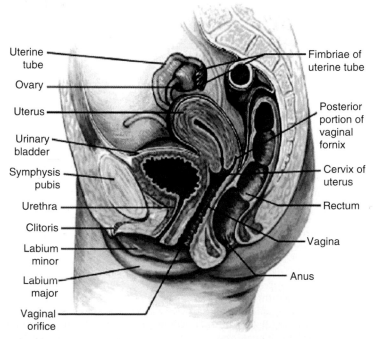

FIGURE 21-11 *Sagittal View of Female Gynecologic Anatomy.*

History

Diagnosis of problems with the gynecology system in adolescents consists mostly of history (see Chapter 1). The clinician must take time using both open- and closed-ended questions, along with an appropriate dose of curiosity and understanding of gynecologic pathophysiology, to acquire the most complete and accurate history and timeline of gynecologic events. There are three factors the provider must be aware of when obtaining the gynecologic sexual history. The *first* is the clinician's personal values, comfort, and ability to speak in terms understandable to the adolescent, the *second* is the ability to understand the developmental age of the adolescent patient, and the *third* is the ability to recognize as well as discuss sensitive and emotional topics. Questions pertaining to the reproductive system often are very uncomfortable for the adolescent. The clinician should modify terminology and questions based on the level of cognitive and psychosocial development of the adolescent.

The gynecologic history should review the adolescent female's sexual development milestones, i.e., age of breast development (*thelarche*), age of axillary and pubic hair growth, and age of menstrual onset (*menarche*). In the menstrual history, determining the age when her menses occurred in a pattern is important. Obtaining the time of her last menses is not always easy because many young adolescents do not make note of their dates. Recommending to the adolescent that she marks a calendar or her electronic date book can improve accuracy. Helping the patient remember will aid the clinician in recognizing an irregular pattern. For very young adolescent (i.e., younger than 14 years old), the clinician may need to get the assistance of a parent, older sibling, or other female adult. Many young females do not recall or understand or are too shy to discuss this information with a health provider.

Additional questions include: What is the interval between cycles? How long does the bleeding last? How heavy is the flow? Adolescents sometimes need assistance to quantify this amount. The number of pads, the type of pads or tampons (light day, regular, or super), the level of saturation (light, regular, or heavy), and the color of bleeding all assist in providing a *quantitative* estimate of blood loss. Determine if the patient has discomfort or pain before, during, or after her period. If she does, identifying the location, quality, radiation, severity, timing, and intensity of the pain is helpful. Other questions include: Does the pain interfere with normal activity? What changes or improves the pain? Are there other symptoms with the pain? (See TABLE 21–3.). *Dysmenorrhea* is the term for pain during menstruation.

Sexual History

Clinicians often avoid or minimize the sexual history (see Chapter 1). It is important not to make assumptions about the patient's gender preference, age of initiating coital behavior (*sexarche*), or level of sexual

TABLE 21–3 *Menstrual History Questions*

Age when monthly/menstrual periods/cycles began (menarche)?

When was your last menstrual period?

How frequent are your periods?

Are the cycles regular (i.e., a defined number of days between the onset of one cycle and the onset of the next)?

What is the length (interval) between cycles?

How many days does the blood flow (or bleeding occur)?

How much is the flow? Heavy? Medium? Light? How many tampons or pads do you use per day?

How saturated are the pads/tampons?

Are there any clots?

Generally, what color is the blood?

Any bleeding between periods? How much?

Any bleeding with intercourse?

Any pain with menstrual periods?

Does the pain interfere with your school or other activities?

---

intimacy. Many adolescents engage in *serial monogamy* or have sexual activity with one partner after another, although staying "faithful" to a specific partner until moving on to another. It is important to identify if sexual abuse or molestation has occurred in the past or is occurring in the present. Some youth are unsure of their sexual orientation and may undergo a gender identity crisis. A detailed and accurate sexual history is essential to discovering the etiology of various problems the patient may present to the clinician, be they medical, behavioral, developmental, psychological, or some combination.

KEY PROBLEM

Abnormal Menstruation A normal menstrual cycle in an adult female involves a mean menstrual interval of 28 days (±7 days), a duration of 4 days (±2 to 3 days), and a median blood loss of 30 ml/month (with an upper limit of normal defined as 60 to 80 ml/month). Since the adolescent may have anovulatory menstrual intervals (menses without ovulation) for 1 to 5 years after menarche, there may be a variety of menstrual patterns until the establishment of a normal pattern based on regular ovulatory menstrual periods. TABLE 21–4 defines basic types of abnormal menstrual patterns.

KEY PROBLEM

Amenorrhea Amenorrhea is *primary* if menstruation has never occurred and *secondary* if menses stop after having occurred for some interval. The term *secondary* applies to adolescents if menses stop for at least 4 to 6 months after regular cycles were established. An alternative definition is absence of menses for a time equivalent to at least three previous menstrual cycles. Primary amenorrhea can occur with or without pubertal delay. Causes of primary amenorrhea with pubertal

TABLE 21–4 *Abnormal Menstrual Patterns*

Condition	Comment
Amenorrhea	Absence of menses; can be *primary* or *secondary.*
Oligomenorrhea	Infrequent, irregular bleeding at >45-day intervals.
Menorrhagia	Prolonged (>7 days) or excessive (>80 ml) uterine bleeding occurring at regular intervals.
Metrorrhagia	Uterine bleeding occurring at irregular but frequent intervals, the amount being variable.
Menometrorrhagia	Prolonged uterine bleeding occurring at irregular intervals.
Hypermenorrhea	Synonymous with menorrhagia.
Polymenorrhea	Uterine bleeding occurring at regular intervals of <21 days.
Break-through bleeding	Small amounts of bleeding between normal menstrual flows.
Dysfunctional uterine bleeding	Abnormal (different from that patient's normal) uterine bleeding that is unrelated to an anatomic lesion.

delay include those due to hypothalamic-pituitary dysfunction. These include *physiologic delay* (the most common), *weight loss, eating disorders, intense exercise, stress, chronic illness, prolactinoma, GnRH deficiency,* and *congenital adrenal hyperplasia* (CAH). Other causes include *Turner syndrome (gonadal dysgenesis)* and *androgen insensitivity syndrome (testicular feminization syndrome).* Causes of primary amenorrhea without pubertal delay include *pseudoamenorrhea* (from *imperforate hymen* or *transverse vaginal septum*), *Mayer-Rokitansky-Kuster-Hauser (MRKH) syndrome* (agenesis of the vagina, cervix, and uterus), *polycystic ovary syndrome (hyperandrogenemia syndrome), obesity,* and *chronic illness* (as thyroid disorders—see secondary amenorrhea). Hypopituitarism from *head trauma, hemochromatosis,* and other causes also can lead to primary amenorrhea. Ovarian failure also may be causative and includes *ovarian tumors, premature failure,* and failure due to *radiation* or *chemotherapy.*

The most common cause of secondary amenorrhea in adolescents is *pregnancy,* and clinicians always should ask about the sexual behavior of adolescents; i.e., ask about the last menstrual period when evaluating *any* adolescent with secondary amenorrhea. Other common causes of secondary amenorrhea include *weight loss, eating disorders (obesity, anorexia nervosa,* or *bulimia nervosa), intense exercise, stress* (including *depression), polycystic ovary syndrome,* and *metabolic* disease such as *thyroid disorders, pituitary adenoma, other pituitary disorders,* and *hypoestrogenemia* (ovarian dysfunction). Also consider *toxic drug effects* [exogenous hormones (oral contraceptive withdrawal, androgens, GnRH analogues), *chronic alcoholism, illicit drugs* (heroin, marijuana), antipsychotics (as phenothiazines), tricyclic antidepressants, antihypertensives (reserpine, methyldopa), and others].

Additional causes of secondary amenorrhea include *systemic illness (cystic fibrosis, inflammatory bowel disease, diabetes mellitus in poor control,* or *cancer), trauma (head trauma* or *spinal cord injury),* and *endocrine-metabolic disorders (hyperprolactinemia, hypo/hyperthyroidism, adrenal insufficiency,* or *Cushing syndrome).* Also consider *tumors (adrenal or ovarian androgen-secreting tumor, granulosa or theca cell tumor of the ovary,* or *adrenocortical carcinoma)* and infiltrative destruction of the hypothalamus *(leukemia, other metastatic malignancy).* Other disorders include *histiocytosis X, sarcoidosis, tuberculosis, radiation, trauma, cerebrovascular accident, pituitary dysfunction [infarction (Sheehan syndrome),* empty sella turcica syndrome, tumors, radiation, trauma (including surgery)], other causes of *ovarian dysfunction [autoimmune, galactosemia, premature menopause, radiation, chemotherapy, surgical oophorectomy, bilateral ovarian torsion or infarction, infection (mumps), sarcoidosis, myotonic dystrophy, ataxia-telangiectasis, 17-α-hydroxylase deficiency],* and *uterine abnormalities [excessive curettage (Asherman syndrome), endometritis (gonococcal infection, tuberculosis,* or *septic abortion), radiation effects,* and *hysterectomy].*

● KEY PROBLEM

■ **Abnormal Vaginal Bleeding** When evaluating abnormal vaginal bleeding, it is important to exclude rectal, urethral, and other perineal bleeding. The most common cause of abnormal vaginal bleeding is uterine bleeding because of abnormal menstruation. Irregular menstrual patterns in young adolescents are often due to failure of ovulation to occur, leading to *dysfunctional uterine bleeding* (DUB) with various menstrual patterns, including *oligomenorrhea, menorrhagia, metrorrhagia, menometrorrhagia, hypermenorrhea,* and *polymenorrhea* (see TABLE 21–4). Ovulatory DUB is much less common than anovulatory DUB and may be due to the *Halban syndrome* (prolonged luteal phase) or *luteal phase abnormalities* (short luteal phase or luteal progesterone insufficiency).

DUB also may be due to chronic anovulation induced by *hypothalamic dysfunction* (from psychological stress or strenuous exercise), *exogenous steroids* (oral contraceptives or progestogens), and various *medications* [anticoagulants, chemotherapy drugs, danocrine, "natural" hormones from plant extracts (DHEA, yam extract), platelet inhibitors, and spironolactone]. Anovulatory DUB also may be due to various *systemic diseases (adrenal insufficiency, chronic liver disease, Cushing syndrome, diabetes mellitus, inflammatory bowel disease, thyroid disease, renal disease, and systemic lupus erythematosus), ovarian failure, androgen excess (ovarian or adrenal tumor), polycystic ovary syndrome, congenital adrenal hyperplasia, or exogenous androgens),* or *estrogen excess* (ovarian granulosa cell–thecal cell tumor).

It is always critical to ask if the adolescent is pregnant and when the last menstrual period was. If the adolescent is sexually active, abnormal vaginal bleeding may be due to *pregnancy complications,* such as *threat-ened or spontaneous abortion, ectopic pregnancy, molar pregnancy,* or *induced abortion.* Abnormal bleeding also may be due to *coagulation disorders* (hemophilia, von Willebrand disease), platelet dysfunction *(Glanzmann thrombasthenia),* and thrombocytopenia *(idiopathic thrombocytopenic pur-pura), aplastic anemia, leukemia, lymphoma,* or *hypersplenism).* In addition, the evaluation should look for such factors as *trauma* (rape or rough vol-untary coital activity), foreign body (IUD or tampon), and *infection:* cervicitis *(Neisseria gonorrhoeae, Chlamydia trachomatis, Trichomonas vagi-nails), endometritis (tuberculosis), pelvic inflammatory disease (PID),* and various other sexually transmitted diseases. Finally, the evaluation should consider *endometriosis* and *genital tumors [botryoid sarcoma, uterine or cervical polyps, ovarian cyst, or tumor (mature teratoma, endometri-oma)], leiomyoma, other ovarian malignancy, and* other malignancies with metastases.

KEY PROBLEM

◢ Excessive Hair Growth or Hirsutism The ado-lescent female who presents with excessive hair growth usually has genetic or familial hirsutism owing to increased androgen sensitivity. However, if the hirsutism is associated with overt virilization, then a number of disorders may be the cause. For example, excess androgen production may occur and be adrenal in origin, *metabolic* such as *CAH (21-hydroxylase deficiency, rarely 3β-hydroxysteroid dehydrogenase deficiency, and 11β-hydroxylase deficiency), adrenal tumors (adrenocortical carcinoma, testosterone-secreting adenoma, and adrenal rest adenoma),* or owing to other metabolic disorders as *Cushing disease.* Hirsutism and virilization also may be due to excessive androgens of ovarian origin, such as from *poly-cystic ovary syndrome* (hyperandrogenemia syndrome), *hyperprolactine-mia, thyroid disease* (hyper- or hypothyroidism), *ovarian tumors* (such as *granulosa cell tumor, arrhenoblastoma, gynandroblastoma, luteoma of preg-nancy,* and others), and *congenital lipoatrophic diabetes.*

Toxic exogenous androgens may induce hirsutism and virilization from medically prescribed drugs (e.g., growth stimulation, ACTH therapy, danocrine prescription, and adrenal replacement) or, in a transsexual, from taking androgens to change from a female to a male appearance. Female athletes may use androgens in the hope of improving their mus-cular strength, but this also may induce unwanted hirsutism and viril-ization. Finally, patients with genetic disorders such as XY females may have testicular androgens, as noted in *5α-reductase deficiency, true her-maphroditism,* or *mixed gonadal dysgenesis.*

KEY PROBLEM

◢ Pelvic Pain *Pelvic pain* is one of the most frequent complaints of the adolescent female. It is important to obtain a good menstrual his-tory (see TABLE 21–3) and determine if it occurs during the menstrual period. What is the duration of the pain? What is its quality, severity (1 to 10 scale, with 10 the most severe)? What is the location of the pain—abdominal, pelvic, not sure? Is it cyclic or noncyclic? What improves the pain, and what makes it worse? Is there a sudden or gradual onset of pain? Is the youth sexually active? How many partners? Any recent partner change? Is there a history of sexually transmitted diseases (STDs) and any previous STD testing? Does she use any type of contraceptive? Does the patient use condoms—*never, occasionally, always*? Have there been any previous pregnancies, miscarriages, or abortions? Is there a history of physical or sexual abuse? Are there any urinary or gastrointestinal symptoms?

The most common pelvic pain associated with ovulatory menstruation is primary dysmenorrhea, usually occurring 1 to 3 years after menarche, when regular ovulation develops. *Secondary dysmenorrhea* refers to pelvic pain owing to overt pelvic pathology, such as *pelvic inflammatory disease, endometriosis, congenital genital tract malformations,* or *obstructions (imperforate hymen, transverse vaginal septum,* or *Mayer-Rokitansky-Kuster-Hauser syndrome—MRKH),* or *endometrial polyps.* The MRKH syndrome involves various degrees of uterine and vaginal agenesis, typically uterine agenesis or a rudimentary uterus with absence of the upper two-thirds of the vagina. The karotype, breasts, ovaries, pubic hair, and hormonal patterns are normal.

The differential diagnosis for dysmenorrhea also includes systems outside the reproductive tract, such as the *urinary system* (obstruction or infection; see Chapter 14), *gastrointestinal tract (irritable bowel syndrome, inflammatory bowel disease, constipation,* or *infections;* see Chapter 10), and the *musculoskeletal system (bone/joint infection of the ileum or sacrum or stress fracture of the pubis or vertebral body.* Pelvic pain starting several days before menses and resolving as menses begins represents the *premenstrual syndrome;* a number of symptoms also may occur, classified as *emotional* (e.g., *depression, crying anger,* and others) and *physical* (e.g., pelvic pain, breast congestion, weight gain, and others). Pain with intercourse, termed *dyspareunia* or *vaginismus,* may involve painful muscle spasms of the lower third of the vagina. There may be a history of rape or other sexual abuse.

Primary and secondary dysmenorrhea are causes of *cyclic* pelvic pain. *Noncyclic* pelvic pain may be due to *endometriosis, pelvic inflammatory disease (PID), pelvic adhesions (owing to PID),* and *ovarian neoplasms.* The location of the pain is also important. A *midline* location may indicate *primary dysmenorrhea, endometriosis, endometritis, normal uterine pregnancy, threatened or septic abortion,* or *cystitis. Lateral* pelvic pain may be related to *endometriosis, PID, ectopic pregnancy, Mittelschmerz syndrome (pain owing to ovulation), ovarian torsion,* and nongynecologic conditions (e.g., *appendicitis, ureteral colic, constipation, psychogenic,* and others).

Endometriosis refers to the presence of endometrial glands and stroma that are outside the uterine cavity. *Pelvic congestion syndrome* is a rare condition of pelvic pain in the adolescent female that can be cyclic or noncyclic and is due to *vascular malformations.* Severe menstrual cramping with minimal menstrual flow suggests the diagnosis of *cervical stenosis. Acute* pain may be due to *ectopic pregnancy, PID,* or *ovarian torsion.*

Pelvic pain also may be due to ovarian masses, benign or malignant. *Ovarian cysts* present with lower abdominal pain, unilateral, rarely bilateral. *Functional ovarian cysts* include *follicular cysts, corpus luteum cyst* and *theca lutein cysts*. Other benign ovarian tumors include *dermoids* (mature *cystic teratomas*) and *sex cord tumors* (*thecomas, fibromas,* and *gonadoblastomas*). Fibromas are associated with the *Meigs syndrome* (ascites, pleural effusion, and fibrous ovarian tumor), usually seen in adult females. *Gonadoblastomas* occur in those with *gonadal dysgenesis* and a Y chromosome. They are at increased risk for a malignant germ cell tumor, and the gonadoblastomas may be associated with primary amenorrhea, virilization, and developmental abnormalities. The most common malignant ovarian neoplasm in adolescent females is the *germ cell carcinoma* [*dysgerminoma* (most common), *embryonal carcinoma, endodermal sinus tumor, polyembryoma, choriocarcinoma,* and *immature teratoma*]. Other malignant ovarian neoplasms include the *Sertoli-Leydig cell tumor* associated with virilization and the *granulosa cell tumor* associated with isosexual precocity. (See Essential Adolescent Medicine, Greydanus DE, Patel DR, Pratt HD, eds. New York: McGraw-Hill, 2006, p. 608–612.)

KEY PROBLEM

Vaginal Discharge TABLE 21–5 reviews various causes of vaginal discharge in adolescent females. Vaginal discharge in an adolescent may be an indication of normal estrogen stimulation or genital infection owing to sexual activity. *Physiologic leukorrhea* develops in young adolescents because of estrogen stimulation, typically appearing some months before menarche and continuing for a number of years after menarche. The discharge can be clear to white, watery to mucoid, and scant to copious in nature; there is no odor or irritation. Nonsexually active adolescents also may develop a vaginal discharge owing to vaginal *foreign-body* retention, *group A streptococcal* infection, genital *contact dermatitis, candidiasis (Candida albicans, C. glabrata),* or *bacterial vaginosis*. Sexual behavior also can be involved with the development of candidiasis, group A streptococcal infection, and bacterial vaginosis.

Sexually active adolescent females may develop a vaginal discharge because of acquisition of an STD or infection (STI). STD agents include *C. trachomatis, N. gonorrhoeae,* herpes simplex virus, and *T. vaginalis*. Adolescents are at increased risk for STDs because of high sexual activity rates, multiple sex partners, use of sex and drugs concomitantly, immature cervix, magical thinking of adolescence (i.e., no harm will come to them despite high-risk behavior), and difficulty dealing with the medical system for treatment. TABLE 21–6 considers STDs not reviewed in TABLE 21–5.

The Pelvic Examination

Most adolescents have unspoken fears and anxiety regarding the pelvic examination. Clinicians also vary in their degree of comfort, skill, and knowledge of performing this examination. Many clinicians use an adult model to perform the pelvic examination. While the technique may not be significantly different, the levels of sensitivity, communication, and patience required for an adolescent are significantly different. The pelvic

TABLE 21-5 *Vaginal Discharge in Adolescent Females*

Cause of Condition or Disorder	Special Comment	Differential Diagnosis	Laboratory Testing
Physiologic leukorrhea (due to estrogen stimulation)	Physiologic process that starts weeks to months before menarche and continues for some years thereafter; can be increased by oral contraception; adolescent may complain of yellow staining of underpants.	STDs if sexually active; bacterial vaginosis if there are symptoms (as vaginal odor)	Saline preparation of vaginal fluid (normal results
Foreign body (tampons, toilet paper, others)	Retained foreign bodies in the vagina can lead to a brown or bloody foul-smelling vaginal discharge.	Group A streptococcal vaginitis	Foreign-body visualization
Group A *Streptococcus*	Vaginal discharge that is sometimes bloody; it may or may not be associated with a streptococcal pharyngitis and sexually activity	Foreign body vaginitis	Vaginal culture
Contact dermatitis	Chemical irritation of the genitalia can lead to a sensitization reaction; can see vaginitis, urethritis, proctitis, or dermatitis of the external genitalia; precipitants can include bubble baths or soaps, vaginal deodorant sprays, douches, perfumes, latex condoms or diaphragms, vaginal spermicides, sexual lubricants, and others.	Scabies, pediculosis, eczema, tinea cruris, psoriasis, eczema, other types of dermatitis (see Chapter 16)	Examine for fungi, scabies, (*Sarcoptes scabiei*) and pediculosis (*Phthirus pubis*).

Candida albicans (other *Candida* spp. such as *C. glabrata*)	Vulvitis with pruritic, red, excoriations; vaginitis with white, thick, curdlike patches on the vaginal wall and cervix; can be precipitated by diabetes mellitus, use of oral corticosteroids, antibiotics, and pregnancy.	Tinea cruris, chemical vaginitis, other STDs if sexually active	Wet mount (saline or 10% KOH to demonstrate yeast or pseudohyphae); Gram stain; fungal culture (Nickerson medium)
Bacterial vaginosis	Clinical syndrome owing to the normal flora of *Lactobacillus* spp. being replaced by anaerobic bacteria such as *Gardnerella vaginalis*, *Mycoplasma hominis*, *Mobiluncus* spp., *Prevotella*; sexually associated disorder; also seen in non-sexually active female adolescent; thin, white, malodorous, nonirritating, and nonpruritic vaginal discharge that clings to vaginal walls.	Chemical vaginitis, candidiasis; if sexually active: trichomoniasis	Wet mount with clue cells [epithelial cells covered ("studded") with many gram-negative bacilli]; "whiff test": fishy odor before and after 10% KOH is added; gram stain; vaginal fluid pH <4.5.

(Continued)

TABLE 21-5 *Vaginal Discharge in Adolescent Females [Continued]*

Cause of Condition or Disorder	Special Comment	Differential Diagnosis	Laboratory Testing
Trichomonas vaginalis (unicellular, flagellated protozoan)	STD that can be asymptomatic; dysuria; vaginitis, cervicitis, secondary vulvitis; copious, intensely pruritic greenish (or gray or yellow-green), frothy ("bubbly") discharge; may be malodorous; pH of 5.0 to 5.5 or higher; vaginocervical ecchymosis ("strawberry marks"); swollen vaginal papillae.	Bacterial vaginitis, chemical vaginitis, candidiasis, urethritis, cystitis.	Saline prep. (moving trichomonads), Pap smear, rare:culture
Chlamydia trachomatis	STD that can be asymptomatic; cervicitis with vaginal red mucosa, hypertrophic cervical erosion, and purulent (mucopurulent) cervical discharge). PID, perihepatitis (Fitz-Hugh-Curtis syndrome), proctitis, pharyngitis, and others; infections in males also include urethritis, nongonococcal urethritis (NGU), prostatitis, and epididymitis.	Gonorrhea, trichomoniasis, bacterial vaginosis *Mycoplasma genitalium*, *U. urealyticum*	Cell culture, nucleic acid amplification tests or NAATs (i.e., polymerase chain reaction, ligase chain reaction, others), enzyme-linked immunoassay (EIA, ELISA), direct fluorescent antibody (DFA), and DNA probe (Gen-Probe PACE 2 assay)

Neisseria gonorrhoeae	Cervicitis [PMNs (polymorphonuclear leukocytes)/1000× magnification]; purulent or mucopurulent cervicitis (MPC); bartholinitis, pharyngitis, PID, perihepatitis (Fitz-Hugh-Curtis syndrome), disseminated gonococcal infection (including dermatitis, arthritis), and others; menorrhagia can be seen; infections in males also include urethritis, nongonococcal urethritis (NGU), prostatitis, orchitis, and epididymitis.	*Chlamydia*, trichomoniasis, bacterial vaginosis, *Mycoplasma genitalium*, *U. urealyticum*	Gram stain of the discharge (pairs of gram-negative, kidney-bean-shaped diplococci); culture with Thayer-Martin medium in a 10% carbon dioxide environment; DNA hybridization techniques (Gen-Probe), and NAATs.
Mucopurulent cervicitis (MPC)	Cervicitis with a purulent or mucopurulent (yellowish) discharge in the cervix and vagina sometimes caused by *N. gonorrhoeae* or *C. trachomatis*; sometimes no microbe identified.		Gram stain of the cervical discharge; laboratory testing for *N. gonorrhoeae* or *C. trachomatis*.

(Continued)

TABLE 21-5 *Vaginal Discharge in Adolescent Females (Continued)*

Cause of Condition or Disorder	Special Comment	Differential Diagnosis	Laboratory Testing
Herpes simplex virus	Herpes genital infection is due to HSV type 2 and type 1; cervicitis (often with a mucopurulent discharge) along with vulvar ulcerations (see Chapter 16); an area of pruritus or hyperesthesia may first develop, followed by small-group vesicles on erythematous bases; these lesions become small, shallow, painful ulcers on the genitals along with inguinal lymphadenopathy.	Primary syphilis (*Treponema pallidum*); chancroid (*Haemophilus ducreyi*); contact dermatitis; molluscum contagiosum	Viral serology, immunofluorescent techniques, and culture with typing are available as diagnostic tests; glycoprotein G-based HSV-2 enzyme-linked immunoassay also available; Giemsa stain or Wright stain (Tzanck test) of material collected from a vesicle or ulcer will reveal balloon cells with intranuclear bodies or multinuclear giant cells; Pap smear also may show the multinuclear giant cells; electron microscopy reveals viral herpetic particles.

Abbreviations: KOH = potassium hydroxide; NAAT = nucleic acid amplification test; U = *Ureaplasma;* Pap = Papanicolaou.

TABLE 21-6 *Sexually Transmitted Diseases*

Cause of Condition or Disorder	Special Comments	Differential Diagnosis	Laboratory
Chancroid	Due to *H. ducreyi* and characterized by genital ulcers, especially in males (penile ulcers); starts as small erosion that is red and becomes a painful ulcer(s); unilateral, suppurative inguinal lymphadenopathy.	Syphilis, granuloma inguinale, lymphogranuloma venereum, genital herpes	Rule out other STD genital ulcers; PCR test for chancroid available; chancroid culture if available.
Syphilis	Due to *T. pallidum;* red ulcer called a *chancre* develops that is not painful unless complicated by secondary infection (see Chapter 16); inguinal lymphadenopathy develops that is nontender and unilateral or bilateral; chancre is the primary stage; untreated, other stages develop: secondary, asymptomatic, early latent, late latent, late (tertiary), neurosyphilis, and relapsing (owing to HIV/AIDS).	Chancroid, granuloma inguinale, lymphogranuloma venereum, genital herpes	Nontreponemal tests (RPR, VDRL), treponemal tests (FTA-ABS, MHA-TP); dark-field examination for *T. pallidum.*
Granuloma inguinale	Due due to *Calymmatobacterium granulomatis;* starts as an erythematous papule (nodule) that becomes a painless ulcer with granulation tissue; inguinal granulomas may look like inguinal lymphadenopathy and are called *pseudobubos;* rare in the United States.	Chancroid, lymphogranuloma venereum, syphilis, genital herpes	Rule out other STD ulcers; Donovan bodies on tissue smear; biopsy.

(Continued)

TABLE 21-6 Sexually Transmitted Diseases *(Continued)*

Cause of Condition or Disorder	Special Comments	Differential Diagnosis	Laboratory
Lympho-granuloma venereum	*C. trachomatis* (serovars L_1, L_2, or L_3; erythematous papule that may be missed and is sometimes painful; inguinal lymphadenopathy with the groove sign (nodes above/below the inguinal ligament); may see fever, malaise, myalgias, arthralgias; rectal sex leads to protocolitis with fistulas and strictures; rare in the United States.	Scabies, pediculosis, eczema, tinea cruris, psoriasis, eczema, other types of dermatitis (see Chapter 16)	Rule out other STD ulcers; complement fixation.
Genital warts	Human papillomavirus (HPV) >100 types; often asymptomatic; warts or condylomas (see Chapter 16) can be seen on the genitals; see link of 15 oncogenic types (such as 16, 18, 31, 45, and others) to cervical neoplasia.	Molluscum contagiosum, condyloma lata (syphilis), urethral prolapse, skin tags (perianal), and benign pearly penile papules (males)	Biopsy; colposcopy; cytology (Pap smear); molecular diagnostic modalities (in situ hybridization, dot-blot [ViraPap/Vira Type]), Southern blot and PCR.

HIV/AIDS (human immuno-acquired virus/deficiency immuno-deficiency syndrome)	HIV-1 in the United States; HIV-2 in other places such as West Africa; transmitted via sexual behavior but also intravenous drug use and breast-feeding; half of new cases in U.S. occur to those under age 25; over 50 million humans are infected globally, with 30 million deaths due to HIV/AIDS.	Broad differential; acute retroviral syndrome of HIV/AIDS develops within first few weeks after infection and presents with fever, malaise, skin rash, and lymphadenopathy	HIV antibody testing (HIV-1, HIV-2): enzyme immunoassay (EIA) as screening test; confirm with Western blot (WB) or IFA (immuno fluorescence assay); plasma HIV RNA
Sexually acquired enteric infections	Mainly seen in homosexuals with oral to anal or oral to oral sex; organisms noted include *Shigella* spp., *Giardia lamblia*, *Entamoeba histolytica*, and *Campylobacter jejuni*; can lead to enterocolitis or proctitis; some have no symptoms.	Differential diagnosis of proctitis and enterocolitis	Stool culture and stool examination for bacteria and parasites
Pinworms	Pinworms travel to the vagina and cause intense pruritus, especially at night; can be sexually acquired; see Chapter 20.	Tinea cruris, chemical vaginitis, candidiasis	Stool examination; cellophane tape test
Pediculosis pubis	Infestation of lice (*Plthirus pubis*) on pubic hair as well as perineal and axillary hair; also seen in eyelashes; intense pruritus can develop, leading to mild to severe skin excoriations; often sexually acquired but also spread via fomites (bedding or clothes).	Scabies, tinea cruris, chemical vulvitis	Pubic hair examination using a hand lens to see the adult form and/or the eggs ("nits").

(Continued)

TABLE 21-6 *Sexually Transmitted Diseases (Continued)*

Cause of Condition or Disorder	Special Comments	Differential Diagnosis	Laboratory
Scabies	Due to the mite *Sarcoptes scabiei*; the female deposits eggs in the skin (stratum corneum), which leads to intense itching, especially at night; various lesions develop: papules, vesicles, pustules, burrows; especially seen over the hands (finger webs; see Chapter 16) but also wrists, axillae, belt line, buttocks, breasts, areolae (females); penis and scrotum in males; sexually acquired.	Pediculosis, tinea curis, chemical vulvitis	Microscopic examination of scraped lesions with immersion oil to find the eggs, adult mites, or feces.
Molluscum contagiosum	Poxvirus infection that leads to a variable number of asymptomatic papules that are white to pearl-colored; larger ones can be umbilicated; can be sexually acquired; found in various places, including genital areas; dermatitis may develop around the lesions; lesions may develop in areas of atopic dermatitis.	Human papillomavirus infections, atopic dermatitis, tinea cruris	

| Tinea cruris | Fungal infection owing to *Trichophyton mentagrophytes* or *Epidermophyton floccosum* that involves crural folds and inner thighs ("jock itch"), usually without infecting the penis or scrotum in males; appears as pruritic, red lesions that are slightly raised and have scaling borders; can be infected by tinea pedis or with infected underwear. | Contact dermatitis (allergic or irritant), erythrasma, (due to *Corynebacterium minutissimum*) candidiasis, intertrigo | Wet mount with 10% KOH; Wood lamp examination; fungal culture. |

Abbreviations: STD = sexually transmitted disease; PCR = polymerase chain reaction; RPR = rapid plasma reagin; VDRL = Venereal Disease Research Laboratory; FTA-ABS = fluorescent treponemal antibody absorption; MHA-TP = microhemagglutination assay; KOH = potassium hydroxide.

examination procedure should be the last component of the complete physical examination.

Performing an age-appropriate pelvic examination must begin with placing the adolescent patient at ease. Begin with establishing a rapport while the patient is fully dressed. Addressing the patient's anxiety, providing knowledge about the female anatomy, and educating the patient on the procedure in a manner that allows her to ask questions is essential. In order to ease patient anxiety, allow the patient to request a female clinician or to have her parent or friend in the room for support.

Reassure the adolescent female that the speculum and other equipment are not large. This may reduce her fears and allow relaxation of her pelvic muscles. Try to discuss some common interesting subject (i.e., school, significant other, or hobbies); this may help to defocus the patient from the procedure and decrease her tension. Having the patient breath deeply is another method for relaxation.

Reviewing her physical findings is important at this point. Many adolescents are not familiar with their bodies and feel uncomfortable with allowing others to view their genitals and breasts. Demystify the female genitalia by allowing the adolescent to take part in the examination. One can do this by having a mirror that the patient can hold and view her genitalia while the clinician is performing the examination. Obtaining knowledge of the internal and external genitals and their function allows the adolescent female to gain a better understanding of the signs and symptoms of disease as well as the importance of preventive health visits.

The equipment required includes a light source, specula, water-based lubricant, Papanicolaou smear testing kit, and other diagnostic test material as indicated by the history. The specula are made of metal or plastic and often come in two types, Pedersen and Graves. They differ in the width of the blades; the Pedersen is generally narrow and best for virgins, younger adolescents, and those with a narrow introitus. The examiner should have knowledge of the mechanism and function of the speculum prior to performing the examination, knowing how to open and close the blades as well as how to lock and release them. This will contribute to diminishing the patient's anxiety.

Prepare and position the patient on the examining table once she undresses and is properly gowned in private. Always keep the patient appropriately covered. The clinician should remind the patient of the steps of the procedure and the reason for the examination. The table's stirrups should be in proper position. Ask the patient to place her heel into the stirrups, and then ask her to slide down to the edge of the table such that her buttocks are slightly over the edge, providing reassurance that she will not fall. The table may be slightly elevated and the examiner may insert a pillow at the back of her head for comfort. Ask her to rotate her thigh externally with abduction and flexion (lithotomy position).

The two main components of the pelvic exam are the internal and external parts.

External
||
Internal
Speculum ⊥ Bimanual

External

Examination of the external genitalia begins with the gloved clinician sitting in a manner that allows him or her to be comfortable and have adequate visualization of the pelvis and the vulva.

Inspection

Do a visualization and assessment of the pubic hair distribution and character over the mons pubis, lower abdomen, and inner thigh. Record this using the Tanner stages (see Chapter 13). Inspect the labia majora, labia minora, clitoris, urethral meatus, and introitus. During inspection, make note of anatomic abnormalities or variation, including evidence of masculinization, inflammation, excoriations, papules, discharge, imperforate hymen, or cystic nodules.

Palpation

Separate the labia majora with the index and thumb of the nondominant hand. Make note of any discharge or signs of disease.

Internal

Release and insert the middle finger inside the introitus, applying pressure to the pelvic floor muscles. This effectively opens the introitus wider, thus allowing a smoother insertion of the speculum.

Speculum

Angle the speculum at about 15 degrees, sliding it over the middle finger; remove the finger. Once past the sensitive urethra, turn the speculum horizontal, and tilt toward the rectum. Slowly open the speculum blades, allowing the cervix to come into view. Secure the speculum in an open position that allows the clinician to obtain any needed specimens.

Obtaining the Papanicolaou smear consist of acquiring endocervical cells by placing the longer end of the wood scraper in the cervical os. Press and turn 360 degrees (a full circle). This should include the transformation zone at the squamous-columnar junction. Remove and place the specimen onto a glass slide. Next, obtain ectocervical cells by placing the endocervical brush inside of the cervical os. Roll it between your fingers (thumb and index) 360 degrees. Remove the brush, and roll the brush against the glass slide. You may use the previous slide that contains the endocervix specimen or another glass slide. Place the slide into an alcohol solution or apply the special fixative. Alternatively, the provider may obtain a liquid-based cytology by placing the specimens directly into preservative.

Inspect the vagina on withdrawal of the speculum slowly making note of color, inflammation, discharge, or ulcers. As the speculum clears the cervix, release the lock on the speculum, close and withdraw, reversing the insertion process.

Bimanual

Next, perform a bimanual examination by lubricating the index and middle fingers of one of your gloved hands. Allow the lubricant to drop to your fingers to avoid contamination. From a standing position, introduce one finger and then, if able, the second finger into the vagina. Abduct the thumb, and with the other hand press downward on the lower abdomen. Palpate the cervix, uterus, and either side of the fallopian tube and ovary. Make note of size, shape, consistency, tenderness, or enlargement of these structures.

Rectovaginal Examination

Withdraw your fingers. Lubricate your glove again. Some clinicians recommend changing gloves or have double gloved initially and remove the contaminated glove prior to performing the rectal component. Inform the patient that the procedure may feel uncomfortable. Reintroduce your index finger in the vagina and the middle finger into the rectum. Repeat the maneuver from the bimanual examination. This component should not be neglected, especially in the evaluation of abdominal pain or in assessing a retrodisplaced uterus. This maneuver also allows palpation of the uterosacral ligaments, cul-de-sac, and the adnexa.

Synthesizing a Diagnosis

TABLE 21–7 lists the clinical high points of adolescent gynecologic diagnosis.

Laboratory and Imaging

TABLE 21–7 also includes laboratory and imaging aids in the right-hand column.

When to Refer

TABLE 21–8 lists indications for specialist referral.

TABLE 21-7 *Gynecologic Disorders of Adolescent Females*

Gynecologic Disorder	Special Comments	Differential Diagnosis	Laboratory Testing
Amenorrhea (primary)	Physiologic is the main cause; MRKH syndrome assoc. with renal abnormalities and spinal malformations; short stature with delayed sexual maturation: Turner syndrome; delayed sexual maturation + hypertension seen in 17α-hydroxylase deficiency; Swyer syndrome; absence of smell sense suggests Kallmann syndrome; visual field deficits suggests brain tumor.	Physiologic, imperforate hymen, Mayer-Rokitansky-Kuster-Hauser (MRKH) syndrome, Turner syndrome (45,XO and mosaicism), chronic illness, hypothalamic: stress, eating disorders, exercise, depression; androgen insensitivity syndrome (46, XY); Swyer syndrome; others (see text).	Serum gonadotropins (FSH, LH), prolactin, TSH; Pelvic ultrasound MRI Head CT/MRI Renal ultrasound/other imaging studies Karyotype Laparoscopy

(Continued)

743

TABLE 21-7 *Gynecologic Disorders of Adolescent Females (Continued)*

Gynecologic Disorder	Special Comments	Differential Diagnosis	Laboratory Testing
Amenorrhea (secondary)	Pregnancy is the main cause: history of sexual activity; may present with a midline "pelvic mass"; causes of oligomenorrhea and secondary amenorrhea are essentially the same; also important is history of dietary habits, exercise, and stress; acne and hirsutism suggest elevated androgen levels; athlete triad syndrome: amenorrhea, dysfunctional eating patterns, osteopenia/porosis.	Pregnancy, lactation, stress, eating disorders, chronic illness, exercise-induced, prolactinoma (headaches, visual field deficits, galactorrhea), PCOS (polycystic ovary syndrome) (see text).	Pregnancy test (β-hCG), progesterone challenge, serum estrogen, FSH, LH; bone mineral densitometry; serum prolactin; thyroid screen; head CT
Dysmenorrhea (primary)	Pelvic pain during normal ovulatory menstruation; no underlying pelvic pathology; may also see gastrointestinal symptoms, headache, myalgia, sweating.	Physiologic	
Dysmenorrhea (secondary)	May be seen at menarche or 3+ years postmenarche.	Endometriosis, PID, reproductive tract anomalies, pelvic adhesions, cervical stenosis, ovarian masses, pelvic congestion syndrome; rule out urinary tract or gastrointestinal causes.	Laparoscopy, STD screen, pelvic ultrasound, MRI

Condition	History/Presentation	Differential	Workup
Dysfunctional uterine bleeding (DUB)	Menstrual calendar useful to get accurate history of menstrual pattern; get sexual activity history; establish presence/absence of *ovulation*: basal body temperature charts, serum progesterone, urinary LH and possibly endometrial biopsy; rule out an STD; virilization evaluation necessary if hirsutism present (See PCOS).	Anovulatory bleeding, pregnancy, ectopic pregnancy, coagulation disorders (such as von Willebrand disease, others), anatomic lesions, endometrial pathology; cervicitis or cervical dysplasia; PID, ovarian cysts, polycystic ovary syndrome, severe stress, rapid or severe weight gain or loss, drug abuse	CBC, platelets, β-hCG, Pap smear, PT, aPTT, PFA, fibrinogen other coagulation disorders screening; thyroid screen; STD screen; ultrasound (transvaginal; pelvic), MRI; hysteroscopy
Ectopic pregnancy	Pain with history of secondary amenorrhea, often with vaginal bleeding.	See DUB differential.	β-hCG; pelvic ultrasound
Endometriosis	Presentation in adolescence not the same as in adults; may have acyclic pain, abnormal uterine bleeding, GI symptomatology.	See secondary dysmenorrhea.	Laparoscopy, laparotomy
Mittelschmerz	Pain associated with ovulation in the middle of a menstrual cycle; may last 1 to 3 days and be mild to severe.	See secondary dysmenorrhea.	Menstrual calendar

(Continued)

TABLE 21-7 *Gynecologic Disorders of Adolescent Females (Continued)*

Gynecologic Disorder	Special Comments	Differential Diagnosis	Laboratory Testing
Ovarian mass	Presents with a lateral location; abnormal menses	Ovarian cysts, ovarian tumors (benign, malignant), polycystic ovary syndrome, ectopic pregnancy, tuboovarian mass	Pregnancy test, pelvic ultrasound; screen for tumor markers: alpha-fetoprotein, estrogen, progesterone, testosterone, LDH.
PID	STD that can lead to uterine tenderness, adnexal tenderness, tenderness on cervical motion, mucopurulent vaginal or cervical discharge; can see fever (T > 101°F, 38.3°C); polymicrobial disorder of the upper genital tract often precipitated by *N. gonorrhoeae, C. trachomatis,* others (*Gardnerella vaginalis, Mycoplasma hominis, Ureaplasma urealyticum, H. influenzae,* coliforms, cytomegalovirus, *Peptostreptococcus,* and other anaerobes); can involve various combinations of endometritis, salpingitis, tuboovarian abscess, and pelvic peritonitis; complications include infertility, chronic pelvic pain, ectopic pregnancy.	Ectopic pregnancy, appendicitis, pyelonephritis, ovarian cyst, septic abortion, others	Nonspecific: WBCs on saline prep; elevated ESR; elevated CRP; lab evidence of *N. gonorrhoeae* or *C. trachomatis*; specific criteria: positive biopsy, endometrium, showing endometritis; evidence of PID on laparoscopy; ultrasound or MRI showing that fallopian tubes are thick and filled with fluid; may be free fluid in the pelvis or a tuboovarian complex.

| Polycystic ovary syndrome (PCOS; hyperandrogenemia syndrome) | Insulin resistance with hyperinsulinemia, hyperandrogenemia, and chronic anovulation; can see irregular menses (secondary amenorrhea, oligomenorrhea, DUB), hirsutism, possible virilization, variable obesity, acanthosis nigricans, possible bilateral enlarged ovaries. | Other causes of hyperandrogenism: HAIR-AN syndrome; congenital adrenal hyperplasia (11β-hydroxylase, 21-hydroxylase, 3β-hydroxysteroid dehydrogenase deficiency); Cushing disease, ovarian hyperthecosis, hyperprolactinemia; ovarian or adrenal tumor; mixed gonadal dysgenesis (45,X/46,XY; gonadal dysgensis with virilization; true hermaphroditism | LH, FSH, T4, prolactin, testosterone (total and free), insulin level, lipid profile, dehydroepiandrosterone sulfate (DHEAS), 17-hydroxyprogesterone, 24-hour urine for free cortisol, dexamethasone suppression test, pelvic ultrasound |

(Continued)

TABLE 21-7 *Gynecologic Disorders of Adolescent Females (Continued)*

Gynecologic Disorder	Special Comments	Differential Diagnosis	Laboratory Testing
Premenstrual syndrome (PMS)	Variety of symptoms start before and end with menses.	Premenstrual dysphoric disorder (PMDD), depression, anxiety, others depending on the presenting symptoms (see text)	DSM-IV (2000) criteria for PMDD

Abbreviations: CBC = complete blood count; Pap = Papanicolaou smear; STD = sexually transmitted disease; MRI = magnetic resonance imaging; GI = gastrointestinal; ESR = erythrocyte sedimentation rate; F = Fahrenheit; C = Centigrade; HAIR-AN = hyperandrogenism, hirsutism, insulin resistance, acanthosis nigricans; DSM-IV = *Diagnostic Statistical Manual*, 4th Edition (American Psychiatric Association); PT = prothrombin time; aPTT = activated partial thromboplastin time; PFA = platelet function analysis; LDH = lactate dehydrogenase.

TABLE 21-8 *Conditions to Refer*

STDs that are unusual or difficult to manage:	Non-STD causes of vaginal discharge difficult to manage:	Complex gynecologic disorders:
HIV/AIDS	Foreign-body vaginitis with foreign bodies not easily removed	Anatomic causes of amenorrhea (e.g., MRKH syndrome)
Syphilis	Contact vaginitis that is severe or resistant to management	Androgen insensitivity syndrome
Chancroid	Chronic vulvovaginal candidiasis	Polycystic ovary syndrome
Granuloma inguinale		Turner syndrome
Lympho-granuloma venereum		Complex endocrine disorders (e.g., congenital adrenal hyperplasia, Cushing)
Human papillo-mavirus (owing to cervical neoplasia potential)		CNS masses (e.g., prolactinoma craniopharyngioma)
PID		Pregnancy and pregnancy complications (e.g., ectopic pregnancy)
		Adrenal and ovarian masses
		Endometriosis and other causes of secondary dysmenorrhea
		Galactorrhea
		Others—depending on the clinician's expertise—as for example, pelvic inflammatory disease (PID)

22 Laboratory Testing Overview

Vinay N. Reddy

Laboratory and other diagnostic studies in pediatrics pose several problems not common in adult medicine. One major problem is that children do not enjoy needle pokes or restraints for imaging procedures and often express their disapproval emphatically. Children also have smaller reserves to call on for laboratory samples; the extreme example of this is in premature infants in intensive care, in whom the most common cause of anemia is phlebotomy for laboratory studies. For these reasons, pediatricians tend to be more parsimonious when ordering diagnostic tests than their adult-practice counterparts—as well we should be.

Choosing a Test

Before ordering a particular test

1. Determine what action you will take if the test is positive.
2. Then determine what action you will take if the test is negative.
3. If $a = b$, do not order the test: it will be a waste of time, money, and patient goodwill.

There are occasions when $a = b$ for the direct care of the patient but not for other purposes, such as public health; in such cases, the test still may be worth obtaining.

Sensitivity and Specificity

A clinician also must know how well a test meets its intended purpose. This can be quantified by the test's *sensitivity* (the probability that the test is positive in a patient known to have the condition being tested for) and *specificity* (the probability that the test is negative in a patient known *not* to have the condition). *Probability*, or the chance of a particular outcome, is expressed as a number between 0 and 1 (or 0 percent and 100 percent), where zero probability represents impossibility and a probability of one represents certainty. Probabilities also can be expressed as odds, or the ratio of two probabilities: The odds of throwing a fair die and having it show a one are the ratio of the probability that a one will appear (1/6) to the probability that a 2, 3, 4, 5, or 6 will appear (5/6), or 1:5. More generally,

$$\text{Odds} = \text{probability} \div (1 - \text{probability}) \quad \text{and}$$
$$\text{Probability} = \text{odds} \div (1 + \text{odds})$$

To determine sensitivity and specificity experimentally, one must have a *gold standard* (a test that is assumed to be perfect); many gold standard tests are more expensive and time-consuming than their not-so-perfect counterparts and are obtained only to confirm the results of initial tests or for research purposes (such as determining the sensitivity and specificity of new tests).

An example is the rapid test for group A streptococcal antigen in throat swabs: In a comparison between a hypothetical rapid test and multiple cultures from the same patient (the gold standard) for 1000 different patients, the following results were obtained:

	One of Multiple Cultures Positive	All Cultures Negative	Total
Rapid test positive	720 (a)	5 (b)	725 ($a + b$)
Rapid test negative	180 (c)	95 (d)	275 ($c + d$)
Total	900 ($a + c$)	100 ($b + d$)	1000 ($a + b + c + d$)

This is an example of a *2 × 2 table*, on which all our definitions will be based. The rows represent the results of the test we are analyzing, whereas the columns represent "truth" (as determined by the gold standard). Using the letters for each of the values in the table,

Sensitivity = $a/(a + c)$ (in our example, 720/900, or 80 percent)
Specificity = $d/(b + d)$ (in our example, 95/100, or 95 percent)

Another way to express sensitivity and specificity is in terms of the error rates:

False-positive rate (or *false-alarm* rate) = $b/(b + d) = 1 - $ specificity, or 5 percent

False-negative rate (or *miss* rate) = $c/(a + c) = 1 - $ sensitivity, or 20 percent[*]

---

[*] The terms *false alarm* and *miss* were coined by the British Royal Air Force, which developed "receiver-operator characteristic curves" to measure the accuracy of radar receivers and their operators during the Battle of Britain in World War II. Specificity was expressed as the probability of a *false alarm*—a British fighter sent aloft to pursue a German bomber that wasn't really there—whereas sensitivity was expressed as the probability of a German bomber being *missed* long enough to drop a bomb on London. The terms *false alarm* and *miss* are still used in the literature of statistical detection theory and are occasionally seen in descriptions of diagnostic tests.

A negative result from a test with high sensitivity is good evidence that the patient does not have the condition being tested for, whereas a negative result from a low-sensitivity test should be confirmed by other means. Similarly, a positive result from a high-specificity test may be taken at face value, whereas confirmation is needed for a negative low-specificity test.

The rapid group A streptococcal antigen test described earlier has fairly high sensitivity and a very high specificity. Therefore, a positive test is sufficient evidence to treat for streptococcal pharyngitis, but a negative test is insufficient proof that the patient is streptococcus free. Many available rapid group A streptococcal antigen tests have similar sensitivity and specificity, so pediatricians routinely obtain a throat culture if the rapid test is negative, depending on how strongly they suspect streptococcal infection.

A perfect test has 100 percent sensitivity and 100 percent specificity and thus has positive and negative predictive values of 100 percent as well. Unfortunately, there are few, if any, perfect tests. Most physiologic measurements are continuous in nature, and their values follow a normal distribution (the bell curve); in many cases, the values are bimodal—two bell curves overlapping, one corresponding to the presence of the condition being tested for and one corresponding to its absence as illustrated in FIGURE 22–1. This overlap region, where the true result and the result of the chosen test may not correspond, is what makes a test imperfect. To decide whether a test is positive or negative, the clinician or the laboratory must choose a *threshold value* to separate positive results from negative results. With some tests, the threshold value between a positive result and a negative result can be selected by the ordering clinician; this allows the clinician some measure of control over the sensitivity and specificity, but not over both individually. The relationship among threshold value, sensitivity, and specificity can be described by a *receiver-operator characteristic* (ROC) *curve* (see preceding footnote), which plots sensitivity against specificity for varying threshold values.

When selecting a threshold value, the ideal goal is to maximize both sensitivity and specificity. Practically, increasing the sensitivity usually lowers the specificity (and vice versa), and the goal is to maximize sensitivity for a given specificity (or vice versa). Any test can have 100 percent sensitivity: just say that the test is positive regardless of the actual results—which, for all but gold standard tests, implies zero specificity and makes the test worthless. In the ROC curve, shown in FIGURE 22–2, sensitivity is plotted against specificity for differing threshold values. (The *x* axis is actually 1 minus the specificity, or the probability of a false alarm.) The upper-right corner represents 100 percent sensitivity and zero specificity, whereas the lower-left corner is the point of zero sensitivity and 100 percent specificity. A perfect test has an ROC curve that passes through a point in the upper-left corner of the graph that corresponds to 100 percent sensitivity and 100 percent specificity. A real test's ROC curve is more likely to rise fairly steeply initially and then curve near the "point of perfection" and continue with little further rise until it reaches the upper-right corner. The diagonal straight line is the ROC curve of a wild guess, which is the worst possible performance for any test. Several different tests for a particular condition can be compared by plotting their ROC curves on the same graph; the test whose ROC curve passes closest to the "point of perfection" will have the best discrimination.

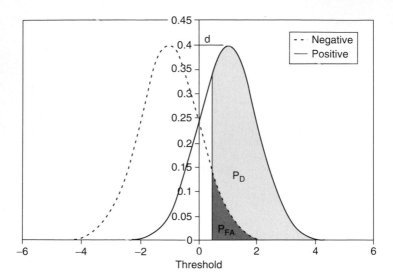

FIGURE 22-1 *These two bell curves represent the possible results of a diagnostic test that yields a single number as a result. The curve on the right shows possible test values for a known (by a gold-standard test) positive result, while the curve on the left shows possible test values for a known negative result. d is the difference between the mean values for positives and negatives; the variance is the same for the two results. For a particular threshold value P_D (the % area under the positive-result curve to the right of the threshold) is the probability of detection of a positive result, while P_{FA} (the % area under the negative-result curve to the right of the threshold) is the probability of a false-negative result. The % area under the positive-result curve to the left of the threshold is the probability of missing a positive result. Increasing the threshold will decrease P_{FA} and will also decrease P_D, while decreasing the threshold increases P_D and also increases P_{FA}.*

Predictive Values and Likelihood Ratios

Strength of suspicion is also important in choosing a test. The *predictive value* of a test (the probability of the test being positive/negative given that the patient does/does not have the condition) depends not only on the sensitivity and specificity but also on the *prevalence* (the probability of the patient having the condition). The *positive predictive value* (PPV) of a given test, which equals $a/(a + b)$ using our preceding notation, rises with increasing prevalence, whereas the *negative predictive value* (NPV), or $d/(c + d)$, falls with increasing prevalence. [The prevalence in the population in which the initial tests were performed is the proportion of test subjects who were positive according to the gold standard test, or $(a + c)/(a + b + c + d)$.] Note that the sensitivity and specificity of a test depend only on the quality of the test, *not* on the prevalence of the condition.

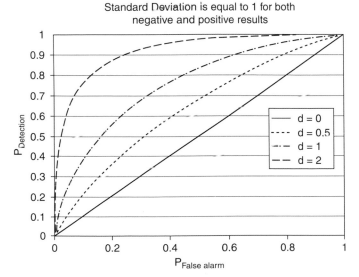

FIGURE 22–2 *Receiver-Operator Characteristics as a Function of the Difference d Between the Means for Negative and Positive Results.*

For the purpose of determining predictive values, the prevalence depends on the clinical level of suspicion, which, in turn, depends on historical information and physical findings, as well as on population prevalence. Returning to our hypothetical group A streptococcal antigen test,

$$PPV = a/(a + b) = 720/725 = 99.3 \text{ percent}$$
$$NPV = d/(c + d) = 95/275 = 34.5 \text{ percent}$$

However, the prevalence of group A streptococcal infection in this "population" is 900/1000 = 90 percent. This is (hopefully!) not the population prevalence of group A streptococcal infection but may very well be the prevalence of such infection *in those patients on whom the rapid strep test is obtained*, more properly termed the *pretest probability* (the probability before the test is performed that the patient has streptococcal infection). If the prevalence of group A streptococcal infection is actually 10 percent, the preceding table will look like this:

	One of Multiple Cultures Positive	All Cultures Negative	Total
Rapid test positive	80 (*a*)	45 (*b*)	125 (*a* + *b*)
Rapid test negative	20 (*c*)	855 (*d*)	875 (*c* + *d*)
Total	100 (*a* + *c*)	900 (*b* + *d*)	1000 (*a* + *b* + *c* + *d*)

For this "population," PPV is $80/(80 + 45) = 80/125 = 64$ percent, and NPV is $855/(20 + 855) = 855/875 = 97.7$ percent. Similar calculations for different prevalence rates, with 95 percent sensitivity and 80 percent specificity, are shown below in table form and graphically in FIGURE 22–3.

Prevalence (percent)	PPV (percent)	NPV (percent)
100	100	0
90	99.3	34.6
75	97.6	61.2
50	94.1	82.6
25	84.2	93.4
10	64	97.7
0	0	100

Screening tests used for large populations, such as occult blood detection in stool as a test for intestinal cancer, need to have high positive predictive values despite low prevalence. This requires sacrificing high specificity in favor of high sensitivity and using confirmatory tests with high specificity to weed out false positives from the initial screening test.

Another way to express predictive value is the *likelihood ratio* (LR). The *positive likelihood ratio* (LR+) of a test is the likelihood (probability) of a positive test in a patient who is known to have the condition (sensitivity) divided by the likelihood of a positive test in a patient who is known *not* to have the condition (1 – specificity, or the false-alarm rate). In the terms of our 2×2 table above,

$$LR+ = [a/(a + c)] \div [b/(b + d)]$$

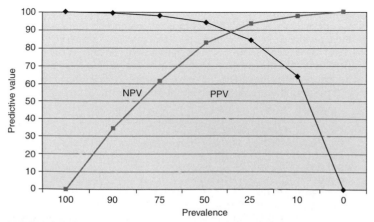

FIGURE 22–3 *Predictive Value as a Function of Prevalence.*

The *negative likelihood ratio* (LR–) is the likelihood of a negative test in a patient with the condition (specificity) divided by the likelihood of a negative test in a patient without the condition (1 – sensitivity, or the miss rate):

$$LR– = [c/(a + c)] \div [d/(b + d)]$$

Likelihood ratios are odds because they are the ratio of two probabilities.

Since the likelihood ratios depend only on the test's sensitivity and specificity, they are independent of prevalence. Also, they can be calculated for a range of test values in those tests which yield a level or count (such as a glucose level), thus giving the ordering physician more information than would result from using a single cutoff value. A larger LR+ indicates that the condition is much more likely, whereas a smaller LR– indicates that the condition is less likely. LRs near 1 (typically between 0.5 and 2.0) are not generally useful, LRs between 0.2 and 0.5 or between 2.0 and 5.0 are suggestive but not conclusive, and LR+ > 5.0 or LR– < 0.2 are strong evidence for or against the condition, respectively.

Using the likelihood ratios, we can calculate a *posttest probability*: the probability that the patient has the condition given the result (positive, negative, or a particular value) of the test. The posttest probability P_{post} is calculated by converting the pretest probability P_{pre} to pretest odds, multiplying by the likelihood ratio (LR+ for a positive result, LR– for a negative result), and converting the resulting posttest odds back to a probability:

$$P_{post} = O_{post}/(1 + O_{post}) \text{ where } O_{post} = (LR \times P_{pre}) \div (1 - P_{pre})$$

Computing the likelihood ratios and posttest probabilities of disease for the tests used in diagnosis allows the physician to quantify the clinical value of those tests and to select tests that will yield the most information at the least cost. Subconsciously, most of us do exactly this when selecting tests to be performed, but it is useful—at times even for experienced physicians and certainly for those in training— to determine explicitly which tests are the best choice for particular clinical situations.

Screening and Case-Finding Tests

Computing likelihood ratios is most important in diagnostic testing. Once a patient is diagnosed, most tests thereafter will be ordered to monitor the progress of the disease and the patient's response to therapy. Another important reason for testing is to detect diseases before clinical signs develop, whether in the general population or in segments of the population at higher-than-average risk for particular diseases. Such tests may reveal patients with higher risk than the general population for a particular disease: One example of a screening test is the measurement of serum bilirubin at 24 hours of age to detect hyperbilirubinemia early enough that treatment will prevent kernicterus. Testing also may be desirable for *case finding*—to detect diseases in their early stages in specific populations at risk. An example is the tuberculin skin test for patients who have been exposed to tuberculosis. (The tuberculin skin test was performed as a screening test for the school-age population as recently as the 1970s. Its use is now limited to case finding in patients at risk.) Some tests may be used for multiple purposes. Urine glucose and ketone tests may be used to screen the general pediatric population for diabetes mellitus, to detect cases of diabetes in high-risk populations' such as obese children, to confirm a diagnosis of diabetes, or to monitor the efficacy of therapy in known diabetics.

Screening tests, because they are used in large populations, should be inexpensive, safe, and easy to perform. A high-cost/high-risk screening test for a particularly common and deadly disease may be acceptable in some populations and circumstances. For example, both the tuberculin skin test and the chest radiograph will detect active pulmonary tuberculosis and can be used for screening. However, the chest radiograph will not detect early infection or extrapulmonary tuberculosis, requires expensive and cumbersome equipment, and requires exposing each screened patient to ionizing radiation. The tuberculin skin test is inexpensive, easy to perform, and cannot be used only in patients allergic to the purified protein derivative preparation (very rare) or who have had tuberculosis in the past (not as rare, but a small segment of the general population). It is therefore better to use the skin test as the primary screening tool for tuberculosis, reserving chest radiographs for those with positive skin tests, a history of tuberculosis, or allergy to the purified protein derivative.

Centers for Disease Control Growth Charts, 2000

CDC Growth Charts: United States

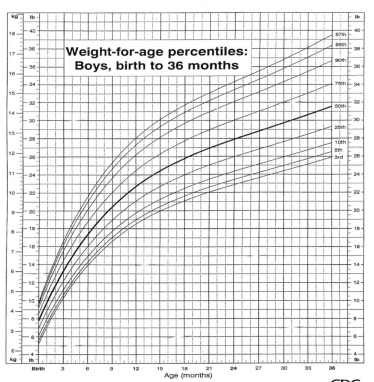

SOURCE: Developed by the National Center for Health Statistics in collaboration with the National Center for Chronic Disease Prevention and Health Promotion (2000).

CDC Growth Charts: United States

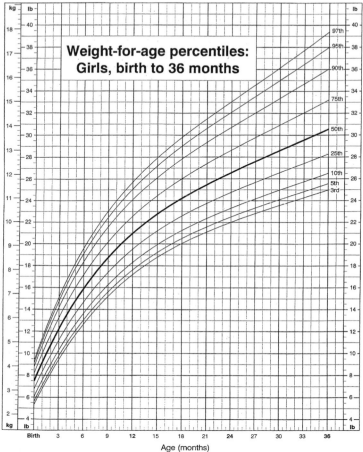

Weight-for-age percentiles:
Girls, birth to 36 months

Age (months)

SOURCE: Developed by the National Center for Health Statistics in collaboration with
the National Center for Chronic Disease Prevention and Health Promotion (2000).

CDC Growth Charts: United States

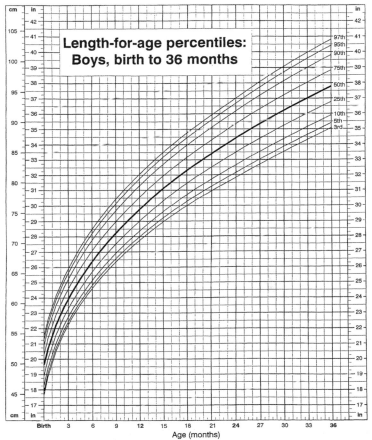

Length-for-age percentiles:
Boys, birth to 36 months

SOURCE: Developed by the National Center for Health Statistics in collaboration with
the National Center for Chronic Disease Prevention and Health Promotion (2000).

CDC Growth Charts: United States

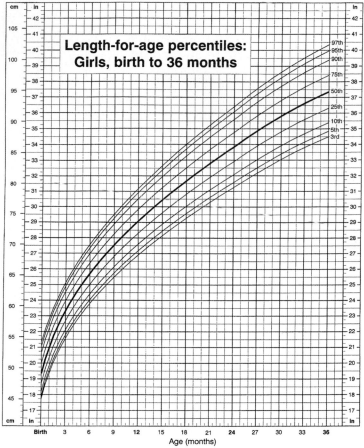

Length-for-age percentiles:
Girls, birth to 36 months

SOURCE: Developed by the National Center for Health Statistics in collaboration with
the National Center for Chronic Disease Prevention and Health Promotion (2000).

CDC Growth Charts: United States

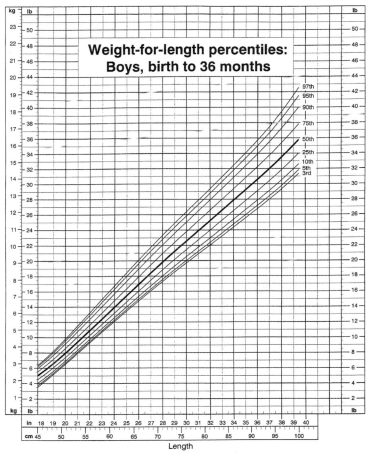

Weight-for-length percentiles: Boys, birth to 36 months

SOURCE: Developed by the National Center for Health Statistics in collaboration with the National Center for Chronic Disease Prevention and Health Promotion (2000).

CDC Growth Charts: United States

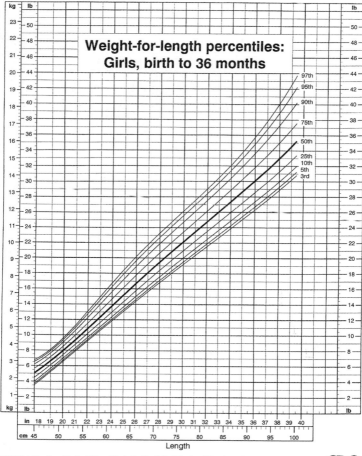

Weight-for-length percentiles: Girls, birth to 36 months

SOURCE: Developed by the National Center for Health Statistics in collaboration with the National Center for Chronic Disease Prevention and Health Promotion (2000).

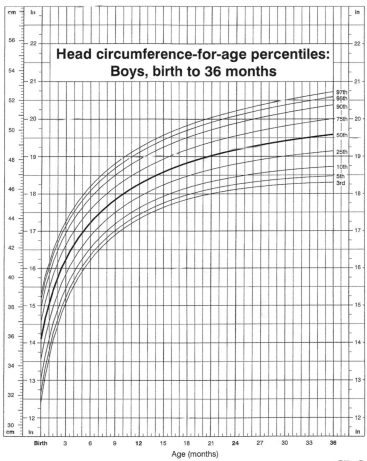

Head circumference-for-age percentiles: Boys, birth to 36 months

SOURCE: Developed by the National Center for Health Statistics in collaboration with the National Center for Chronic Disease Prevention and Health Promotion (2000).

CDC Growth Charts: United States

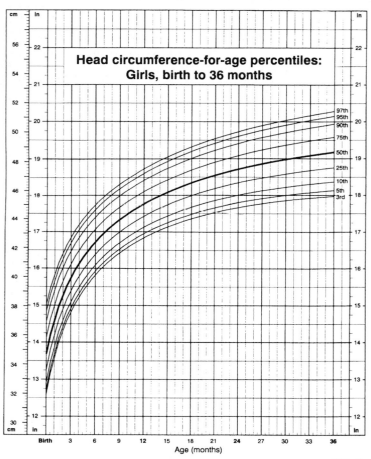

**Head circumference-for-age percentiles:
Girls, birth to 36 months**

Age (months)

SOURCE: Developed by the National Center for Health Statistics in collaboration with
the National Center for Chronic Disease Prevention and Health Promotion (2000).

CDC Growth Charts: United States

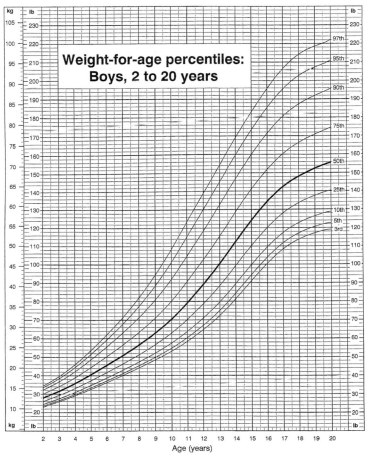

Weight-for-age percentiles:
Boys, 2 to 20 years

SOURCE: Developed by the National Center for Health Statistics in collaboration with
the National Center for Chronic Disease Prevention and Health Promotion (2000).

CDC Growth Charts: United States

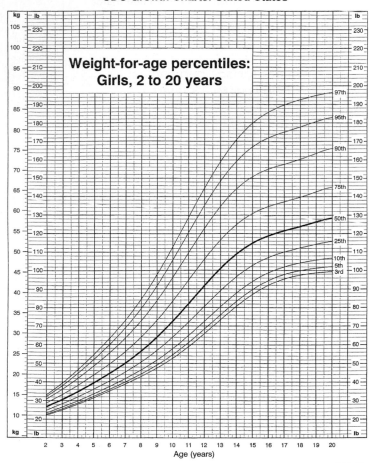

Weight-for-age percentiles: Girls, 2 to 20 years

Age (years)

SOURCE: Developed by the National Center for Health Statistics in collaboration with
the National Center for Chronic Disease Prevention and Health Promotion (2000).

CDC Growth Charts: United States

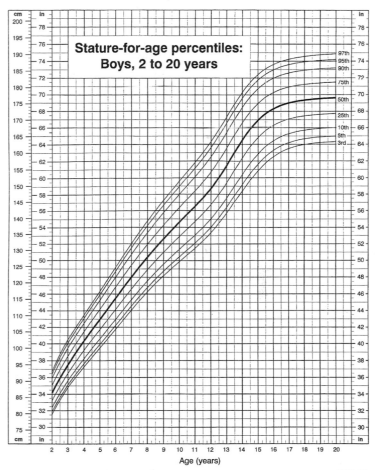

Stature-for-age percentiles:
Boys, 2 to 20 years

SOURCE: Developed by the National Center for Health Statistics in collaboration with
the National Center for Chronic Disease Prevention and Health Promotion (2000).

CDC Growth Charts: United States

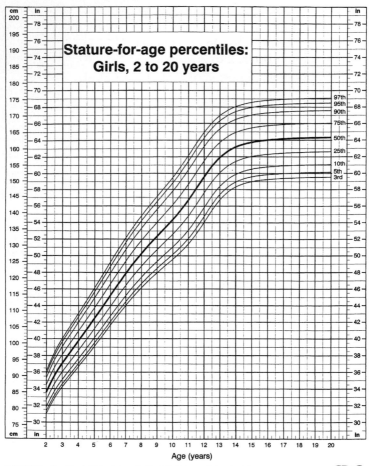

Stature-for-age percentiles: Girls, 2 to 20 years

SOURCE: Developed by the National Center for Health Statistics in collaboration with the National Center for Chronic Disease Prevention and Health Promotion (2000).

CDC Growth Charts: United States

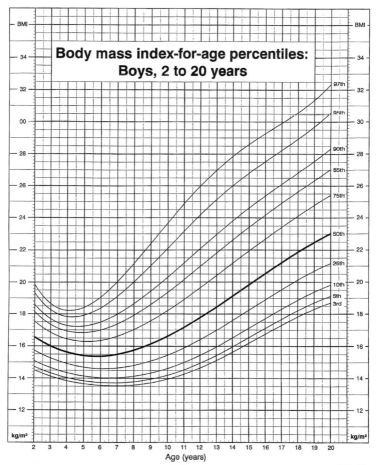

Body mass index-for-age percentiles: Boys, 2 to 20 years

SOURCE: Developed by the National Center for Health Statistics in collaboration with the National Center for Chronic Disease Prevention and Health Promotion (2000).

CDC Growth Charts: United States

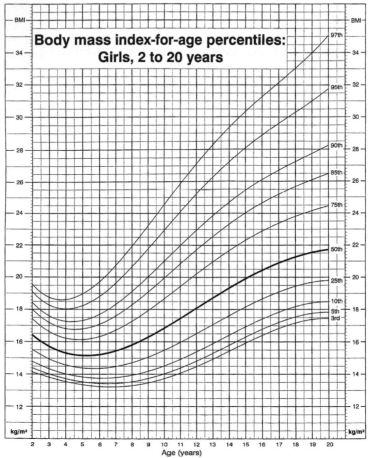

**Body mass index-for-age percentiles:
Girls, 2 to 20 years**

SOURCE: Developed by the National Center for Health Statistics in collaboration with
the National Center for Chronic Disease Prevention and Health Promotion (2000).

Index

Page numbers followed by *f* or *t* indicate figures or tables, respectively.

A

Aarskog syndrome, 125
Abdominal mass
  differential diagnosis, 679*t*
  malignancies associated with,
    522*t*
  in neuroblastoma, 534
Abdominal pain. *See also*
    Gastrointestinal tract
  in adolescents, 278–279, 727–729
  in anemia, 493
  bimanual palpation, 286*f*
  in children, 275–276
  differential diagnosis, 291–295*t*
  in endocrine disorders, 430*t*
  in functional gastrointestinal
    disorders, 280
  iliopsoas test, 287*f*
  in infants, 273
  locations, 287*f*
  nongastrointestinal causes, 64*t*,
    294–295*t*
  obturator test, 287*f*
  referrals/consultation, 290
  in rheumatic diseases, 321*t*
  urinary causes, 663
Abducens nerve (cranial nerve VI),
    355, 376
Abetalipoproteinemia, 400*t*
Acanthosis nigricans, 422, 427*t*,
    558
Accessory nerve (cranial nerve XI),
    355, 378
Accuracy, 45
Acetazolamide, teratogenic effects,
    73*t*
Achilles reflex, 381*t*
Achondroplasia, 120*t*, 123, 135*t*
Acne, 546*f*, 549*f*, 570*t*
Acne rosacea, 556
Acoustic nerve (cranial nerve
    VIII), 355, 377–378
Acquired aphasia, 614
Acrocallosal syndrome, 118

Acrocephaly, 123
Acrocyanosis, 232
Acrodermatitis, 556, 556*f*, 572*t*
Activated partial thromboplastin
    time (aPTT), 512
Acute lymphocytic leukemia
    (ALL), 528
Acute myelogenous leukemia
    (AML), 528
Acute renal failure. *See* Renal
    failure, acute
Acute rheumatic fever
  diagnostic criteria, 261
  diagnostic testing, 254*t*
  epidemiology, 261
  signs and symptoms, 254*t*, 261,
    321*t*, 562*t*, 577*t*
Addison disease
  cutaneous symptoms, 410, 413,
    428*t*, 564*t*, 597
  diagnostic testing, 436*t*
Adductor reflex, 380*t*
Adenocarcinoma, breast, 714*t*
Adjustment disorders, 624
Adolescents
  abdominal pain in, 278–279,
    727–729
  breasts
    endocrine disorders and
      changes in, 414
    key problems, 704–709,
      706–708*f*, 710–717*t*
    physical examination,
      703–704, 705*f*
  cancer. *See* Cancer
  cardiovascular system
    endocrine disorder-related
      symptoms, 413
    functional anatomy,
      physiology, and
      mechanics, 229–230
    history, 230, 231*t*
    physical examination, 41–42,
      241, 251*t*

Adolescents (*Cont.*):
  chest pain in, 208–209
  developmental disorders,
      638–639
  dysmorphology diagnostic
      examination
    history, 116–117
    physical examination, 132
  ears. *See* Ear(s)
  endocrine system
    key problems, 412–415
    physical examination, 422–425
  eyes
    history, 142
    key problems, 146–147
    physical examination, 40, 152
  female genital system. *See*
      Female genital system
  gastrointestinal tract
    key problems, 277–280
    physical examination, 42, 289
  hematopoietic system. *See*
      Hematopoietic system
  hemostatic system. *See*
      Hemostatic system
  history taking
    chief complaint, 17
    consent issues, 17, 21–23
    establishing rapport, 15–16
    health questionnaire, 17, 18–20t
    nonverbal communication, 20
    parental involvement, 16–17
    present illness, 20–23
    sports preparticipation, 22t
  male genital system. *See* Male
      genital system
  musculoskeletal system
    key problems, 315–321
    physical examination, 42,
        329–341, 335–337, 336f, 337f
  neurologic system. *See*
      Neurologic system
  physical examination overview,
      39–43
  psychiatric disorders. *See*
      Psychiatric disorders
  renal system. *See* Renal system
  respiratory system
    key problems, 207–209
    physical examination, 41,
        220–221
  skin
    key problems. *See*
        Dermatologic conditions
    physical examination, 39

Adrenal disorders, 436t, 439–440
Adrenoleukodystrophy, 399t
Affect, 610
Agitation, 65t, 422, 426t
Agranulocytosis, severe infantile,
    503
Alagille syndrome, 274
Albinism, 566t
Alexander disease, 399t
Allergy
  in children, 204–205
  in infants, 200, 201
Alopecia
  differential diagnosis, 321t
    congenital/genetic, 591, 592t
    infectious/inflammatory, 593
    metabolic/toxic, 591, 593
    traumatic, 593
  history, 590–591
  physical examination, 591
Alopecia areata, 593t
Alpers disease, 398t
Alpha$_1$-antitrypsin deficiency, 292t
Alpha-fetoprotein levels, 74, 523t
Alport syndrome, 464
Altered consciousness
  in adolescents, 373
  in children, 367–368
  drug/toxin-induced, 392t
  Glasgow coma scale, 368t
  in infants, 359–360
  non-CNS causes, 65t
Amastia, 711t
Ambiguous genitalia
  categories, 687
  diagnostic testing, 698t
  etiology, 687
  laboratory tests and imaging,
      109t, 681t
  in newborns, 687
  physical examination, 672
  referrals/consultation, 695
Amblyopia, 144, 150
Amenorrhea
  definition, 725t
  primary, 433t, 724–725, 743t
  secondary, 433t, 725–726, 744t
Aminoacidopathies, 397, 398t
Aminoglycosides, teratogenic
      effects, 72t
Amnestic disorder, 617
Amphetamines, teratogenic effects,
      73t
Anabolic steroids, teratogenic
      effects, 72t

Anal reflex, 381*t*, 693
Anaphylaxis, 207
Anemia
  diagnostic synthesis, 493–494
  diagnostic testing, 494, 495*t*, 496*t*
  history, 491–493
  malignancies associated with,
      525*t*
  pathophysiology, 491
  physical examination, 493
  types
    high MCV and low
        reticulocytes, 496
    low MCV and low
        reticulocytes, 494, 496
    normal MCV and high
        reticulocytes, 497–498
    normal MCV and low
        reticulocytes, 496–497
Angelman syndrome, 136*t*
Angiofibroma, 577*t*
Anhedonia, 610
Anisocoria, 144, 146, 154, 157*t*
Ankle. *See* Foot and ankle
Ankyloglossia, 178
Anorexia nervosa, 622
Anosmia, 194–195*t*
Anterior drawer test, 340, 341*f*
Anthropometrics
  body mass index, 771–772*f*
  head circumference, 57,
      765–766*f*
  height/length, 57, 761–762*f*,
      769–770*f*
  weight, 55, 759–760*f*, 763–764*f*,
      767–768*f*
Anti-inflammatory drugs,
      teratogenic effects, 72*t*
Anticancer drugs, teratogenic
      effects, 72*t*
Anticholinergics, poisoning with,
      391*t*
Anticoagulants, teratogenic effects,
      73*t*
Antihypertensive drugs,
      teratogenic effects, 72*t*
Anus, 292*t*, 697*t*. *See also*
      Gastrointestinal tract
Anxiety, 65*t*, 610
Anxiety disorders, 619–621, 620*t*
Aortic stenosis, 257–258
Apert syndrome, 120*t*, 121*t*, 123
Aphasia, acquired, 614
Aphthous ulcers, 171, 183*t*,
      589*t*

Apnea
  causes, 51–52
  in children, 217
  definition, 51
  in infants, 212
  in newborns, 99, 110*t*
Appendicitis, 275, 276, 292*t*
Arachnoid cysts, 385*t*
Arterial blood gas, 222*t*
Arterial thrombosis, 511, 517*t*
Articular cartilage, 302
Ascites, 288, 288*f*
Asperger disorder, 615
Association, in dysmorphology,
      112–113
Asthma
  in adolescents, 208
  in children, 204–205
  in infants, 201
Astigmatism, 152
Ataxia. *See* Clumsiness
Atenolol, teratogenic effects, 72*t*
Athelia, 710*t*
Athetosis, 371
Atrial septal defect (ASD), 252*t*,
      255–256
Atrioventricular (A-V) canals, 252*t*,
      256–257
Attention-deficit/hyperactivity
      disorder, 615
Auditory nerve. *See* Acoustic
      nerve
Auscultation, 27–28, 28*f*. *See also*
      specific systems
Autistic spectrum disorders
  in children, 634–635
  in infants, 634
  screening and diagnosis, 642*f*
  symptoms, 615
Autonomic nervous system. *See*
      Neurologic system

B
Babinski reflex, 95
Back and spine
  key problems
    back pain, 313, 316–317
    scoliosis, 317
  physical examination
    in adolescents, 42, 335–337,
        336*f*, 337*f*
    in dysmorphology diagnostic
        examination, 124, 129
    in infants, 323
    in newborns, 87

Bacterial endocarditis, 262
Bacterial vaginosis, 731*t*
Baker cyst, 338
Balanitis, 589*t*, 668–669
Ballismus, 371
Ballottement, 282, 283*f*
Barium enema, 297*t*
Barlow maneuver, 87, 89*f*
Barotrauma, 182*t*
Beare-Stevenson syndrome, 128
Beau's lines, 262, 597
Becker muscular dystrophy, 399*t*
Beckwith-Wiedemann syndrome
    abdominal defects in, 125
    diagnostic testing, 135*t*
    facial features in, 121*t*
    growth problems in, 96, 122,
        418, 427*t*
    physical examination, 667–668
    plethora in, 101
Behçet syndrome, 171, 183*t*, 321*t*
Bernard-Soulier syndrome, 516*t*
Beta-human chorionic
        gonadotropin, 523
Biceps reflex, 380*t*
Biliary disease, 293*t*. *See also*
        Gastrointestinal tract
Biotin deficiency, 399*t*
Bipolar disorders, 619, 619*t*, 620*t*
Black eye, 522*t*
Bladder
    anatomy, 646–647
    exstrophy, 652, 668, 683*t*
    innervation, 447
    key problems, 680*t*
Blaschko's lines, 556, 557*f*
Bleeding
    disorders. *See* Hemostatic
        system
    dysfunctional uterine, 725*t*,
        726–727, 745*t*
    malignancies associated with,
        525*t*
Blood pressure. *See also*
        Hypertension;
        Hypotension
    measurement, 52–54, 236,
        236*f*
    norms by age and height
        percentile
        boys, 242–244*t*
        girls, 245–248*t*
    orthostatic changes, 55–56
    in shock, 55
Blount disease, 311, 316

Blue baby syndrome
    in methemoglobinemia, 202
    in tetralogy of Fallot, 258
Blue-dot sign, 661, 669
Blue nevus, 563*t*
Body piercing, 666
Bohn nodules, 104
Bone. *See also* Musculoskeletal
        system
    formation, 301–302
    masses, 522*t*
    metabolic diseases, 346*t*
    neoplasms, 347*t*
    pain, 525*t*
Boutonniere deformity, 335
Bowlegs (genu varum)
    in adolescents, 316
    in children, 311, 312*f*
    in endocrine disorders, 426*t*
    physical examination, 329
Brachial plexus neuropathy, 303
Brachioradialis reflex, 380*t*
Bradycardia
    causes, 51, 64*t*
    definition, 51
    in endocrine disorders, 429*t*
    in newborn, laboratory testing,
        107*t*
Bradypnea, 52, 217
Brain. *See also* Neurologic system
    anatomy, 351*f*, 352*f*
    embryologic development,
        349–350
Brain stem aplasias, 385*t*
Brain stem reflexes, 379
Brain tumors
    differential diagnosis, 388–389*t*
    history, 531–532
    imaging, 533
    key findings, 532–533
    physical examination, 532–533
    types, 531
Branched-chain ketoaciduria, 398*t*
Branchio-otorenal syndrome, 122*t*
Breakthrough bleeding, 725*t*
Breast(s)
    anatomy, 703*f*
    development
        normal, 702–703
        premature, 690, 691
    diagnostic synthesis, 710–717*t*
    diagnostic testing, 705
    embryology, 701, 702*f*
    endocrine disorders and
        changes in

in adolescents, 414
in children, 411–412
differential diagnosis,
424–425, 431–432*t*
in infants, 409, 420
history, 703–704
key problems
asymmetry, 705–706, 707*f*,
711*t*
atrophy, 713*t*
hyperplasia, 707, 708*f*
mass, 704–705, 706*f*, 713–715*t*
pain, 707–709, 708*f*, 716*t*
trauma, 717*t*
tuberous anomaly, 706, 708*f*,
712*t*
physical examination
in adolescents, 703–704, 705*f*
in infants and children, 692,
694
referrals/consultation, 718*t*
sexual maturity rating scale,
417*f*
Bronchiectasis, 202–203
Bronchogenic cyst, 208
Bronchomalacia, 201
Bronchopulmonary dysplasia, 200
Bronchoscopy, 224*t*
Bruises, 522*t*. *See also* Hemostatic
system
Budd-Chiari syndrome, 292*t*
Bulimia nervosa, 623
Bullae, 547, 547*f*, 580–582*t*
Bullous dermatosis, 581*t*
Bullous pemphigoid, 581*t*
BUN:creatinine ratio, 486
Bunion, 317
Burkitt lymphoma, 529
Busulfan, teratogenic effects, 72*t*

C
C-reactive protein, 222*t*, 296*t*
Café-au-lait spots, 428*t*, 565*t*
Calcaneovalgus foot, 324
Canavan disease, 399*t*
Cancer
bone tumors, 347*t*. *See also*
Ewing sarcoma;
Osteogenic sarcoma
brain tumors. *See* Brain tumors
breast, 714*t*
diagnostic synthesis, 525*t*
diagnostic testing, 523
history, 521, 522*t*
Hodgkin disease, 530–531

imaging, 523–524
key problems, 521–523, 522*t*,
523*t*
leukemia, 524–528, 526*t*
lymphoma, 528–529
maternal, fetal effects, 70*t*, 72*t*
melanoma, 552*f*, 563*t*, 573*t*, 597
neuroblastoma. *See*
Neuroblastoma
non-Hodgkin lymphoma,
529–530
referrals/consultation, 540
retinoblastoma, 143, 154, 540
rhabdomyosarcoma. *See*
Rhabdomyosarcoma
risk factors, 521
Wilms' tumor (nephroblastoma).
See Wilms' tumor
Candidiasis, vaginal, 731*t*
Capillary blood gas, 222*t*
Captopril, teratogenic effects, 72*t*
Carbamazepine, teratogenic
effects, 72*t*
Carbuncle, 578*t*
Cardinal positions of gaze, 376,
377*f*
Cardiovascular system. *See also*
Congenital heart disease;
Heart disease
cardiac correlates of dysmorphic
syndromes, 232*t*
diagnostic approach, 249–251
diagnostic testing, 252*t*, 254*t*,
262–263, 263*t*
endocrine disorder-related
symptoms
in adolescents, 413
in children, 410
differential diagnosis, 424,
429–430*t*
in infants, 408
functional anatomy, physiology,
and mechanics
children and adolescents,
229–230
newborns and infants,
228–229, 228*f*
history, 230–231*t*
imaging, 252*t*, 254*t*, 262–263,
263*t*
physical examination
in adolescents, 41–42, 241,
251*t*
auscultation
cardiac cycle, 235*f*

Cardiovascular system (*Cont.*):
  general considerations,
    233–236, 234*f*
  innocent murmurs, 238–239
  normal heart sounds,
    235–236
  pathologic heart sounds,
    236–238, 237*t*
  blood pressure
    measurement, 52–54, 236,
      236*f*
    norms by age and height
      percentile, 242–248*t*
  in children, 37, 240–241, 251*t*
  in infants, 33, 240, 250*t*
  inspection, 232
  key findings, 239*t*, 250*t*, 251*t*
  in newborns, 240
  palpation, 233
  percussion, 233
  pulse rates, normal by age,
    233*t*
  referrals/consultation, 264–265,
    265*t*
Carey-Coombs murmur, 261
Caries, 178
Carotenemia, 274
Carpal tunnel syndrome, 347*t*
Cartilage-hair hypoplasia
    syndrome, 592*t*
Case-finding tests, 757–758
Cat scratch fever, 588*t*
Cataracts, in renal disease, 463
Cavus foot, 324
Celiac disease, 291*t*, 297*t*, 426*t*
Cellulitis, 561*t*
Central apnea, 51
Central core disease, 400*t*
Central nervous system. *See*
    Neurologic system
Cephalosporins, teratogenic
    effects, 72*t*
Cerebellar aplasias, 385*t*
Cerebral palsy, 342*t*, 633–634
Ceroid lipofuscinosis, 398*t*
Ceruminosis, 181*t*
Cervical lymphadenopathy, 174
Cervicitis, 733*t*
Chancroid, 677, 735*t*
Charcot-Marie-Tooth disease, 399*t*
CHARGE syndrome, 136*t*, 154,
    157*t*
Chédiak-Higashi syndrome, 504,
    566*t*
Cheilitis, 171, 183*t*

Cherubism, 121*t*, 122*t*
Chest pain
  in adolescents, 208–209
  in children, 205–206
  in infants, 201
  noncardiac causes, 64*t*
  in rheumatic diseases, 321*t*
Chest wall
  developmental and functional
    anatomy, 196
  physical examination, 322–323
  physiology and mechanics, 198
Cheyne-Stokes breathing, 217
Chiari I malformation, 385*t*
Chiari II malformation, 385*t*
Child abuse
  bruising patterns in, 506
  musculoskeletal findings in, 343*t*
  retinal hemorrhages in, 55
  sexually transmitted infections
    in, 699
  skin injuries in, 562*t*
CHILD syndrome, 584*t*, 592*t*
Childhood disintegrative disorder,
    636–637
Children
  cancer. *See* Cancer
  cardiovascular system
    functional anatomy,
      physiology, and
      mechanics, 229–230
    history, 230, 231*t*
    physical examination, 37, 240
  developmental disorders,
      634–638
  developmental timelines, ages 3
    to 6 years, 5*t*
  dysmorphology diagnostic
      examination
    history, 116–117
    physical examination, 132
  ears
    key problems, 168–170
    physical examination, 36, 174
  endocrine system
    key problems, 409–412
    physical examination, 422–425
  eyes
    history, 142
    key problems, 144–146
    physical examination, 36,
      150–152, 151*f*
  female genital system. *See*
      Female genital system
  gastrointestinal tract

key problems, 274–277
physical examination, 37–38, 284–288
hematopoietic system. *See* Hematopoietic system
hemostatic system. *See* Hemostatic system
history taking, 14–15
male genital system. *See* Male genital system
musculoskeletal system
key problems, 309–315
physical examination, 38, 324–329
neurologic system. *See* Neurologic system
nose, throat, and mouth. *See* Mouth and oropharynx; Nose
physical examination overview, 35–38
psychiatric disorders. *See* Psychiatric disorders
renal system. *See* Renal system
respiratory system
key problems, 204–207
physical examination, 37, 215*t*, 217–219
review of systems, 7*t*
skin
disorders. *See* Dermatologic conditions
physical examination, 38
vital signs, 35
Chlamydia trachomatis infections
in females, 732*t*
in males, 677
maternal, fetal effects, 71*t*
Chloroquine, teratogenic effects, 72*t*
Choanal atresia, 193*t*
Cholangitis, 293*t*
Cholecystitis, 293*t*
Cholelithiasis, 293*t*
Cholestasis, 293*t*
Cholesteatoma, 169, 182*t*
Cholinergics, poisoning with, 391*t*
Chordee, 683*t*
Chorea, 371, 392*t*
Chronic inflammatory demyelinating neuropathy, 388*t*
Chvostek sign, 373, 430*t*
Ciliospinal reflex, 379
Cleft palate, 179

Clitoris, 696*t*, 720, 722*f*
Cloacal exstrophy, 668, 683*t*
Clotting disorders. *See* Hemostatic system
Clubbing
digital, 217, 218*f*
nails, 596*t*
Clubfoot (talipes equinovarus), 324, 325*f*
Clumsiness (ataxia)
in children, 370–371
drug/toxin-induced, 392*t*
in infants, 363–364
Cluster headache, 147, 372
Coarctation of the aorta (C/A), 252*t*, 257, 430*t*
Cocaine, teratogenic effects, 73*t*
Coffin-Lowry syndrome, 121*t*
Cognition, assessment, 606–607. *See also* Development; Developmental disorders; Psychiatric disorders
Cold intolerance, 410, 412, 426*t*
Coloboma, 154, 157*t*, 429*t*
Communication disorders, 614
Comparative genomic hybridization (CGH), 133
Compartment syndrome, 316
Complete blood count
in cancer, 523
in leukemia, 527
in respiratory disorders, 222*t*
Complex regional pain syndrome, 345*t*
Compulsions, 611
Computed tomography (CT)
abdominal, 297*t*, 682*t*
in brain tumor diagnosis, 533
in cancer diagnosis, 523
in neuroblastoma diagnosis, 535
in neurologic disorders, 396–397
in respiratory disorders, 223*t*, 224*t*
Conduct disorder, 615
Condylomata. *See* Genital warts
Congenital adrenal hyperplasia, 409, 436*t*, 687
Congenital glaucoma, 143
Congenital heart disease. *See also* Cardiovascular system
cyanotic
Ebstein's anomaly, tricuspid valve, 252*t*, 260
Fontan circulation, 254*t*, 261
hypoplastic left heart syndrome, 252*t*, 260

Congenital heart disease (*Cont.*):
   hypoplastic right heart
      syndrome, 252*t*, 260–261
   patent ductus arteriosus, 252*t*,
      255
   tetralogy of Fallot, 252*t*,
      258–259
   total anomalous pulmonary
      venous return, 252*t*, 259
   transposition of the great
      vessels, 252*t*, 259
   tricuspid atresia, 252*t*, 259–260
   truncus arteriosus, 252*t*, 260
   diagnostic testing, 252*t*, 262–263,
      263*t*
   imaging, 252*t*, 262–263, 263*t*
   maternal, fetal effects, 70*t*
   noncyanotic
      aortic stenosis, 257–258
      atrial septal defect, 252*t*,
         255–256
      atrioventricular canals, 252*t*,
         256–257
      coarctation of the aorta, 252*t*,
         257, 430*t*
      patent ductus arteriosus, 252*t*,
         255
      ventricular septal defect, 252*t*,
         256
   by presentation, 253*t*
   referrals/consultation, 264–265,
      265*t*
Congenital myopathy, 400*t*
Congenital nasolacrimal duct
      obstruction, 142
Congenital vertical talus
      (rockerbottom foot),
      324, 325*f*
Conjunctivitis
   in adolescents, 147
   in children, 145
   differential diagnosis, 156–157
   in infants, 143
   in rheumatic diseases, 321*t*
Conradi syndrome, 121*t*, 130*f*, 584*t*
Constipation
   in adolescents, 278
   in children, 275
   differential diagnosis, 291–295*t*
   in infants, 272
   nongastrointestinal causes, 64*t*,
      294–295*t*
   referrals/consultation, 300
Contact dermatitis, 569*t*, 730*t*
Conversion disorder, 621

Coprolalia, 616
Cornea, clouding, 143, 155
Cornelia de Lange syndrome, 120*t*,
      121*t*, 135*t*
Corrigan pulse, 255
Costochondritis
   in adolescents, 220
   chest pain in, 205, 209
   palpation, 217
Cough
   in adolescents, 207–208
   in children, 202–204
   in infants, 199–200
   nonpulmonary causes, 64*t*
Cover test, 151, 151*f*
Cowden disease, 577*t*
Crackles, 214*t*
Cranial nerves, 354–355. *See also*
      Neurologic system
Craniometaphyseal syndrome,
      121*t*
Craniosynostosis, 123
Cremasteric reflex, 380*t*
Crigler-Najjar syndrome, 273
Crohn disease, 171, 183*t*, 275
Cross-adduction test, 332, 333*f*
Crossed extension reflex, 94
Crouzon syndrome, 120*t*
Cryptorchidism, 125, 432*t*
Cullen sign, 284
Cushing syndrome
   cutaneous symptoms, 410, 427*t*,
      428*t*, 564*t*
   growth problems in, 426*t*
   weight problems in, 418, 427*t*
Cutis marmorata, 104
Cyanosis
   in adolescents, 210
   in children, 206–207
   in infants, 201–202, 250*t*
   in newborns, 101, 108*t*, 232
   noncardiac causes, 64*t*
Cystic fibrosis
   in adolescents, 207
   in children, 202, 204, 205
   gastrointestinal symptoms, 293*t*
   in infants, 199
   laboratory tests, 222*t*
Cystinosis, 469
Cystosarcoma phyllodes, 704, 714*t*
Cysts, 546, 546*f*, 576*t*
Cytomegalovirus (CMV) infection
   cutaneous symptoms, 560*t*
   developmental delay and, 360
   maternal, fetal effects, 71*t*

D

Dandy-Walker syndrome, 385*t*
Darier sign, 543
Deafness. *See* Hearing loss
Deformation, 111
Delirium, 617
Delphian node, 429*t*
Delusions, 609
Dementia, 617
Dentition, 165, 166*t*, 167*f*. *See also*
    Mouth and oropharynx
Denys-Drash syndrome, 472
Depression, 610, 618, 619*t*
Dermatitis, 569*t*, 572*t*
Dermatofibroma, 577*t*
Dermatologic conditions. *See also*
    Skin
  diagnostic synthesis, 559
  diagnostic testing, 597–598
  endocrine disorder-related
    in adolescents, 413, 422–423
    in children, 410, 422–423
    differential diagnosis, 406,
        427–428*t*, 564*t*
    in infants, 407–408
  key findings
    atrophy, 585–586*t*
    bullae, 547, 547*f*, 580–582*t*
    color, 552*f*, 553*f*, 554
    configuration, 543–554,
        544–552*f*
    crusts, 549*f*, 550
    cysts, 546, 546*f*
      dermal, 576*t*
      epidermal, 576*t*
      subdermal, 576*t*
    distribution, 554–559, 555*f*,
        556*f*, 557*f*
    erosions, 549*f*, 550
    excoriations, 549*f*, 550
    fissures, 552*f*, 554
    indurations, 551*f*, 554, 585*t*
    lichenification, 550*f*, 552
    macules, 543, 544*f*
      blue, 563*t*
      blue-black, 574–575*t*
      brown diffuse, 564*t*
      brown localized, 564–566*t*
      purple, 563*t*, 575*t*
      red, 560–563*t*
      white diffuse, 566*t*
      white localized, 566–567*t*
      yellow, 575*t*
    nodules, 545, 545*f*
      flesh and red color, 577*t*

      inflamed red, 578*t*
      juxtaarticular, 577*t*
    papules, 543–544, 544*f*
      brown, 573–574*t*
      flesh colored, 573*t*
      red, 568–572*t*
    pattern, 554
    plaques, 544, 545*f*
    pustules, 548*f*, 549
    scales, 547–548, 547*f*
      ichthyoses, 583–584*t*
    scars, 551*f*, 554
    sclerosis, 585*t*
    ulcers, 550*f*, 552
      painful, 587–589*t*
      painless, 587*t*
    vesicles, 546–547, 546*f*, 579*t*
  in newborns
    benign transient, 104
    developmental abnormalities,
        104
    hamartomas, 106
    hemangiomas, 105–106
    hyperpigmentation, 105
    pigment disorders, 105
    skin peeling, 105
  rheumatic disease-related, 321*t*
Dermatomyositis, 321*t*, 557, 562*t*
Dermatophyte infection, 580*t*
Dermoid cyst, 576*t*
Detrusor muscle, 646
Development
  definitions
    developmental evaluation, 632
    developmental quotient, 631
    developmental screening, 632
    developmental surveillance,
        631–632
    domains, 629–630
    intelligence quotient, 631
    speech and language, 630, 630*t*
  disorders. *See* Developmental
      disorders
  key principles, 629
  timelines
    ages 2 to 9 months, 3*t*
    ages 12 to 24 months, 4*t*
    ages 3 to 6 years, 5*t*
Developmental coordination
    disorder, 614, 638
Developmental disorders
  definitions
    developmental delay, 631
    developmental deviation, 631
    developmental dissociation, 631

Developmental disorders (*Cont.*):
  developmental regression, 631
  global developmental delay,
      631
  mental retardation, 631
  diagnostic synthesis, 639, 640*t*,
      641*f*, 642*f*
  diagnostic testing, 640–641, 642*t*,
      643*t*
  history, 632–633
  key findings
    in adolescents, 638–639
    in children
      atypical language
          development, 634–636,
          637*t*
      early learning difficulties
          and behavioral
          symptoms, 638
      regression of previously
          acquired skills, 636–637
    in infants
      atypical development
          affecting social, cognitive,
          and language milestones,
          360–361, 634
      predominant delay in motor
          milestones, 360–361,
          633–634
  physical examination, 639
  referrals/consultation, 641, 643
Developmental quotient (DQ), 631
Dexamethasone, in labor, fetal
      effects, 73*t*
Diabetes insipidus, 437*t*, 461
Diabetes mellitus
  cutaneous symptoms, 586*t*
  diagnostic testing, 437*t*, 440–441
  eye abnormalities in, 429*t*
  maternal, fetal effects, 70*t*
Diabetic embryopathy, 134*t*
Diadochokinesia, 375
Diagnostic tests. *See also specific
      systems*
  case-finding, 757–758
  likelihood ratios, 756–757
  predictive value, 754–756, 756*f*
  screening, 757–758
  selection, 751
  sensitivity and specificity,
      751–753, 754*f*
Diaper rash, 557, 566*t*, 669
Diarrhea
  in adolescents, 278
  in children, 274–275

differential diagnosis, 291–295*t*
  in infants, 271–272
  malignancies associated with,
      522*t*
  nongastrointestinal causes, 64*t*,
      294–295*t*
  referrals/consultation, 300
Differential diagnosis
  computers in, 67–68
  medical reasoning and, 61–63,
      66–67
  steps, 60–61
Diffusing capacity, lung, 225*t*
DiGeorge syndrome, 232*t*, 260,
      420, 429*t*
DIGFAST, mnemonic for manic
      episode, 619*t*
Digital clubbing, 217, 218*f*
Diphtheria, 172
Disaccharidase deficiency, 271
Disruption, 111–112
Disseminated intravascular
      coagulation (DIC), 518*t*
Dissociative disorders, 621–622
Diuretics, teratogenic effects, 73*t*
Down syndrome
  cardiac anomalies in, 232*t*, 256,
      258
  diagnostic testing, 134*t*
  facial features in, 120*t*, 121*t*
Drug eruption, 561*t*, 569*t*
Dubin-Johnson syndrome, 273
Duchenne muscular dystrophy,
      399*t*
Duodenum, 291*t*. *See also*
      Gastrointestinal tract
Dysarthria, speech disorders and,
      637*t*
Dysfunctional uterine bleeding,
      725*t*, 726–727, 745*t*
Dyshidrosis, 547*f*, 552*f*, 559, 572*t*
Dysmenorrhea, 728, 744*t*
Dysmetria, 375
Dysmorphology diagnostic
      examination
  history
    adolescent, 118
    childhood, 117–118
    family, 113–114
    gestational, 114–115
    infant, 116–117
    neonatal, 116
  laboratory evaluation, 133,
      134–136*t*
  physical examination

adolescents, 132
children, 132
facial features, 119–121*t*, 119*f*
general considerations,
118–119
infants
chest/back/abdomen,
128–130
face, 127–128
genitalia, 130
growth, 127
limbs, 130–131
neurologic, 127
skin, 131–132
newborns
chest/back/abdomen,
124–125
cranium, 123
face, 124
genitalia, 125
growth, 122
limbs, 125–126
neurologic, 123
skin, 127
referrals/consultation, 133
terminology, 111–113
Dysphagia
in brain tumors, 533
causes, 172–173
in children, 206–207
in rheumatic diseases, 321*t*
Dysplasia, 112
Dyspnea
in anemia, 493
in rheumatic diseases, 321*t*
Dyssynergia, 375
Dystonia, drug/toxin-induced,
392*t*

E
Eagle-Barrett syndrome, 295*t*
Ear(s)
developmental and functional
anatomy, 159–161, 160*f*,
161*f*
diagnostic testing
audiometry, 186
tympanocentesis, 186
tympanometry, 180, 185–186,
185*f*
differential diagnoses
auricle, 181*t*
canal, 181*t*
inner ear, 182–183*t*
middle ear, 182*t*

drainage/ache, malignancies
associated with, 522*t*
endocrine disorder-related
abnormalities
in children, 410
differential diagnosis, 429*t*
in infants, 408, 420
key problems
hearing loss, 169–170
otalgia, 168–169
otorrhea, 169
tinnitus, 170
vertigo, 170
low-set, in newborns, 108*t*
physical examination
in adolescents, 40–41
auricle, 175
canal, 175
in children, 36, 174
in dysmorphology diagnostic
examination, 121*t*
in infants, 32–33, 174
inner ear, 176
middle ear, 175–176
in newborns, 81–82
physiology and mechanics,
158–159
referrals/consultation, 187
renal disease-associated
abnormalities, 464
Eating disorders, 295*t*, 622–623
Ebstein's anomaly, tricuspid valve,
252*t*, 260
Ecchymoses, 563*t*
Ecthyma gangrenosum, 574*t*
Ectopic pregnancy, 745*t*
Eczema
ear, 181*t*
flexural distribution in, 554,
555*f*
lichenification in, 550*f*
scales/crusts in, 548*f*, 565*t*, 569*t*
Eczema herpeticum, 572*t*, 579*t*
Egophony, 219
Ehlers-Danlos syndrome
cardiac anomalies in, 232*t*
cutaneous symptoms, 508, 586*t*
diagnostic testing, 135*t*
neurologic characteristics, 123
Ehrlichiosis, 560*t*
Eisenmenger complex, 255
Elbow. *See* Upper extremity
Elimination disorders, 616
Encopresis, 616, 676
Endocarditis, bacterial, 262

Endocrine system
  anatomy, 403, 404*f*
  developmental physiology,
    403–405
  diagnostic testing
    adrenal disorders, 439–440
    calcium metabolism disorders,
      440
    diabetes insipidus, 440
    hypoglycemia, 441
    puberty disorders, 439
    thyroid, 434, 439
    type 1 diabetes mellitus,
      440–441
    type 2 diabetes mellitus, 441
  history, 405–407
  key problems
    abdominal symptoms
      in adolescents, 414
      in children, 410
      differential diagnosis, 430*t*
      in infants, 408
    breast changes
      in adolescents, 414
      in children, 411–412
      differential diagnosis,
        431–432*t*
      in infants, 409
    cardiovascular symptoms
      in adolescents, 413
      in children, 410
      differential diagnosis,
        429–430*t*
      in infants, 408
    constitutional symptoms
      in adolescents, 412
      in children, 409–410
      differential diagnosis,
        425–426*t*
      in infants, 407
    ear abnormalities
      in children, 410
      differential diagnosis, 429*t*
      in infants, 408
    eye abnormalities
      in adolescents, 413
      in children, 410
      differential diagnosis,
        428–429*t*
      in infants, 408
    female external genitalia
      abnormalities
      in adolescents, 414
    growth issues
      in adolescents, 413

      in children, 410
      differential diagnosis,
        426–427*t*
      in infants, 407
    head abnormalities
      in adolescents, 413
      in children, 410
      differential diagnosis, 428*t*
      in infants, 408
    heat or cold intolerance
      in adolescents, 412
      in children, 410
    male genitalia abnormalities
      in adolescents, 414
      in children, 412
      differential diagnosis,
        432–433*t*
      in infants, 409
    menstrual disturbances
      in adolescents, 414, 415
      differential diagnosis, 433*t*
      vaginal bleeding in infants,
        409
    neck abnormalities
      in adolescents, 413
      in children, 410
      differential diagnosis, 429*t*
      in infants, 408
    neurologic symptoms
      in adolescents, 414
      in children, 410
      differential diagnosis, 430*t*
      in infants, 408–409
    polyuria and polydipsia
      in adolescents, 414
      in children, 412
      differential diagnosis, 433*t*
      in infants, 409
    premature pubarche, 433*t*
    pubic hair, premature
      development, 409
    respiratory symptoms, 408
    skin and cutaneous
      appendage abnormalities
      in adolescents, 413
      in children, 410
      differential diagnosis,
        427–428*t*, 564*t*
      in infants, 407–408
    weight issues, 410, 427*t*
  physical examination
    in children and adolescents
      abdominal, 424
      agitation, tremors, 422
      breasts, 424–425

cardiovascular, 424
constitutional, 422
ears, 423
eyes, 423
general observation, 422
male genitalia, 425
measurements, 422
neck, 423–424
neurologic, 424
skin and cutaneous
    appendages, 422–423
genital measurement, 416
growth measurement, 415,
    416t
in infants
    breasts, 420–421
    cardiovascular, 420
    constitutional, 416–417
    ears, 420
    eyes, 420
    female genitalia, 421
    general observation, 417
    head, 419–420
    male genitalia, 421
    measurements, 417–418
    neck, 420
    neurologic, 420
    premature pubarche, 421
    skin and cutaneous
        appendages, 419
    thyroid, 415–416
Endometriosis, 295t, 728, 745t
Enterobius vermicularis. See
    Pinworms
Enterovirus infection, maternal,
    fetal effects, 71t
Enuresis, 616, 663, 684t
Epidermoid cyst, 576t
Epidermolysis bullosa acquisita,
    581t
Epidermolysis bullosa letalis, 581t
Epidermolysis bullosa simplex,
    581t
Epidermolytic hyperkeratosis, 584t
Epididymitis, 660
Epiglottitis, 172, 200
Epilepsy, 358, 364–365. *See also*
    Seizures
Epispadias, 125, 683t
Epistaxis, 194t
Epstein's pearls, 104
Erb palsy, 87, 88f
Erosions, skin, 549f, 550
Erysipelas, 561t
Erythema infectiosum, 557, 560t

Erythema multiforme, 171, 183t,
    582t
Erythema nodosum, 557, 578t
Erythrocyte sedimentation rate,
    222t, 296t
Erythrocytosis (polycythemia)
    diagnostic testing, 498–499
    differential diagnosis, 498
    history and physical
        examination, 498
Escherichia coli infection, maternal,
    fetal effects, 71t
Esophagus. *See also*
        Gastrointestinal tract
    differential diagnosis, 291t
    key problems and findings,
        291t
    obstruction, 172, 184t
Esophoria, 150
Esotropia, 143, 150
Euphoria, 610
Eustachian tube dysfunction,
    168, 182t
Euthymia, 610
Ewing sarcoma
    clinical presentation, 347t, 538
    diagnostic testing, 347t, 538
    history, 538
    imaging, 538
    physical examination, 538
Excoriations, skin, 549f, 550
Exophoria, 150
Exotropia, 143, 150
Expressive language disorder,
    614, 635
External rotation test, 341
Eye(s)
    brain tumor-associated
        abnormalities, 532
    differential diagnoses
        anisocoria, 154
        corneal clouding, 155
        diagnostic tests and imaging,
            157t
        funduscopic abnormalities,
            155
        irregular pupil, 154
        lens abnormalities, 155
        leukocoria, 154
        lid ptosis, 153
        lid swelling, 153–154
        nystagmus, 156
        opsoclonus, 156
        red eye, 156–157
        strabismus, 156

Eye(s) (*Cont.*):
  endocrine disorder-related
      abnormalities
    in adolescents, 413
    in children, 410
    differential diagnosis, 423,
        428–429*t*
    in infants, 408, 420
  functional anatomy, 138–141,
      139–140*f*, 140*t*, 141*f*
  history, 141–142
  key problems
    in adolescents, 146–147
      eye pain, 147
      headache, 147
      ocular misalignment, 147
      "pink eye," 147
      poor vision, 146
    in children, 144–146
      difference in pupil size, 146
      eyelid lesions, 146
      headache, 145–146
      ocular misalignment, 145
      pain, 145
      "pink eye," 145
      poor vision, 144–145
      trauma, 146
    in infants, 142–144
      abnormal eye movements,
          144
      anomalous head posture,
          144
      corneal clouding, 143
      difference in pupil size, 144
      ocular misalignment, 143
      "pink eye," 143
      poor tracking, 142
      tearing, 142–143
      trauma, 144
      tumor/mass, 144
      white pupil, 143
  physical examination
    in adolescents, 40, 152
    in children, 36, 150–152, 151*f*
    in dysmorphology diagnostic
        examination, 119*t*
    in infants, 32, 148–150
    in newborns, 80–81, 81*f*
    overview, 147–148, 148*f*, 149*f*,
        150*f*
  physiology and mechanics,
      137–138
  referrals/consultation, 157–158
  renal disease-associated
      abnormalities, 463–464

F
Facial nerve (cranial nerve VII),
      355, 376–377
Factitious disorders, 621
Factor V Leiden mutation, 210, 362
Failure to thrive
  definition, 57–58
  in endocrine disorders, 427*t*
  referrals/consultation, 299
  in renal disease, 455, 457*t*, 458*t*
Familial Mediterranean fever, 171,
      183*t*
Family history
  in dysmorphology diagnostic
      examination, 113–114
  in psychodiagnostic
      examination, 604–605
Fanconi syndrome, 469
FAPA syndrome, 171, 183*t*
Facioscapulohumeral dystrophy,
      399*t*
Fatigue
  in anemia, 492
  in endocrine disorders, 409, 412,
      425*t*
  in rheumatic diseases, 321*t*
Febrile seizure, 358
Feeding problems
  in anemia, 492
  in infants, 273
  pica, 615
  rumination disorder, 615–616
Female genital system. *See also*
      Breast(s)
  anatomy, 686, 720–721, 722*f*
  diagnostic synthesis
    in adolescents, 743–748*t*
    in infants and children,
        696–697*t*
  diagnostic testing, 698*t*
  endocrine-related abnormalities,
      414, 421
  history
    in adolescents, 723–724, 724*t*
    in infants and children,
        686–687
  key problems
    in adolescents
      abnormal vaginal bleeding,
          726–727
      menstrual cycle
          disturbances. *See*
          Menstrual cycle,
          disturbances
      pelvic pain, 727–729

sexually transmitted
infections, 735–739*t*
vaginal discharge, 729,
730–734*t*
in infants and children
ambiguous genitalia. *See*
Ambiguous genitalia
breast development, 690
precocious puberty, 691
pubic/axillary hair
development, 690–691
vaginal bleeding, 687–689
vulvar/vulvovaginal mass,
689–690
vulvitis, 689
measurements, 416
physical examination
in adolescents, 729, 740–742
in children, 693–695
in newborns and infants, 86,
691–693
physiology, 685–686
referrals/consultation, 695,
698–699, 749*t*
Female pseudohermaphroditism,
687. *See also* Ambiguous
genitalia
Fetal alcohol syndrome, 120*t*, 134*t*
Fetal hydantoin syndrome, 134*t*
Fetor hepaticus, 281
Fever
causes, 48
definition, 48
diagnostic work-up, 48
in Hodgkin disease, 530
malignancies associated with,
522*t*, 525*t*
in rheumatic diseases, 321*t*
Fibrinogen, 512
Fibroadenoma, 704, 706*f*, 713*t*
Fibrocystic breast disease, 715*t*
Fibromas, 179
Fibromyalgia, 321*t*, 345*t*
Field defect, in dysmorphology, 113
Fifth disease. *See* Erythema
infectiosum
Fissures, skin, 552*f*, 554
Fitz-Hugh-Curtis syndrome,
289, 295*t*
Flank mass, 536
Flat feet, 312
Flight of ideas, 608
Fluid wave, 288, 288*f*
Fluorescent in situ hybridization
(FISH), 133

Fluoroscopy, 223*t*
Fluoxetine, teratogenic effects, 73*t*
Folliculitis, 568*t*
Fontan circulation, 254*t*, 261
Foot and ankle. *See also* Lower
extremity
anatomy, 310*f*, 311*f*
ankle clonus, 95
key problems
club foot, 324, 325*f*
flat feet, 312
heel pain, 315
in-toeing, 309–310
metatarsus adductus, 324, 324*f*
out-toeing, 310–311
pain, 317–318
rockerbottom foot, 324, 325*f*
movements, 306–307*f*
physical examination
in adolescents, 340–341, 341*f*
in infants, 324–325
Foreign body
aspiration, 205
nasal, 193*t*
vaginal, 688, 730*t*
Fractional excretion of sodium
(FENa), 485
Fractional excretion of urea
nitrogen (FEUN), 486
Fragile-X syndrome
diagnostic testing, 134*t*
facial features in, 121*t*
genital malformations in, 125
mental retardation in, 635
Friedreich ataxia, 400*t*
Frontonasal dysplasia, 120*t*
Functional dyspepsia, Rome II
criteria, 280*t*
Funduscopic examination, 40,
155
Fungal infections, cutaneous, 566*t*,
568*t*
Furunculosis, 181*t*

G
Gag reflex, 378
Gait
in adolescents, 329
assessment, 374–375
in children, 325–326
Galactorrhea, 414, 424
Galant response, 92, 93*f*
Galeazzi sign, 87, 89*f*
Gambling, pathological, 624
Gamekeeper's thumb, 335

Gastroesophageal reflux disease
(GERD)
in children, 206–207
in infants, 201
signs and symptoms, 291*t*
Gastrointestinal tract
anatomy, 269, 270*f*
diagnostic testing, 296–297*t*
differential diagnosis, 290,
291–293*t*
endocrine disorders and, 408,
410, 414
imaging, 296*t*
key problems
in adolescents
constipation, 278
diarrhea, 278
jaundice, 279–280
pain, 278–279
vomiting, 277–278
in children
constipation, 275
diarrhea, 274–275
jaundice, 276–277
pain, 275–276
vomiting, 274
functional disorders, Rome II
criteria, 280*t*
in infants
constipation, 272
diarrhea, 271–272
jaundice, 273–274
pain, 273
poor feeding, 273
vomiting, 269–271
physical examination
in adolescents, 42, 289
anatomic regions, 282*f*
ascites, 288, 288*f*
ballottement of abdominal
masses, 283*f*
in children
auscultation, 288
observation, 284–285
overview, 37–38
palpation, 285–288, 286*f*
percussion, 288
in dysmorphology diagnostic
examination, 124–125,
129–130
iliopsoas test, 287*f*
in infants
auscultation, 284
inspection, 280–281
overview, 34

palpation, 281–283
percussion, 284
key findings, 289
locations of acute abdominal
pain, 287*f*
in newborns, 84–85
obturator test, 287*f*
palpation, 286*f*
physiology and mechanics,
267–269
Gaucher type II disease, 399*t*
Gender identity disorders, 622
Generalized anxiety disorder, 621
Genital warts, 589*t*, 669, 677, 690,
696*t*, 736*t*
Genitals
ambiguous. *See* Ambiguous
genitalia
female. *See* Female genital
system
male. *See* Male genitourinary
system
Genu valgum (knock-knees), 311,
313*f*, 329
Genu varum. *See* Bowlegs
Geographic tongue, 178–179
German measles, 560*t*
Gianotti-Crosti syndrome, 556*f*,
568*t*
Gilbert syndrome, 273
Glanzmann thrombasthenia, 516*t*
Glasgow coma scale, 368*t*
Glaucoma, congenital, 143
Global developmental delay,
631, 641*f*. *See also*
Developmental
disorders
Glossopharyngeal nerve (cranial
nerve IX), 355, 378
Goldenhar syndrome
diagnostic testing, 134*t*
symptoms, 117
vertebral malformations, 124
Gonorrhea
cutaneous symptoms, 589*t*
in females, 733*t*
in males, 677
maternal, fetal effects, 71*t*
Gower sign, 384
Gram stain, 597
Grammar, 630
Granuloma annulare, 558, 571*t*
Granuloma inguinale, 735*t*
Granulomas, 587*t*
Grasp reflex, 91

Graves disease
  eye abnormalities in, 411, 428, 428*t*
  nail abnormalities in, 428*t*
  neck abnormalities in, 408
  neurologic signs and symptoms, 424
  tachycardia in, 429*t*
Gray matter degeneration, 386*t*, 398*t*
Grey-Turner's sign, 284
Groin pain, 319
Group A streptococcal infections
  pharyngitis, 172
  vaginal, 730*t*
Group B streptococcal infection, maternal, fetal effects, 71*t*
"Growing pains," 314
Growth
  assessment. *See also* Anthropometrics
    in dysmorphology diagnostic examination, 122, 127
    in physical examination for endocrine disorders, 415, 416*t*
  failure
    in endocrine disorders
      in adolescents, 413
      in children, 410
      diagnostic testing, 435*t*
      differential diagnosis, 426–427*t*
      in infants, 407
      nonendocrine causes, 65
    in renal disease, 455, 457*t*, 458*t*
Guillain-Barré syndrome, 388*t*
Gynecomastia, 424–425

H
Hair
  developmental anatomy, 559
  endocrine-related abnormalities, 422–423, 427–428*t*
  history, 590
  key findings
    hair loss. *See* Alopecia
    hirsutism. *See* Hirsutism
    hypertrichosis. *See* Hypertrichosis
  physiology, 590
Hallermann-Streiff syndrome, 592*t*
Hallucinations, 609
Hallucinogens, toxidrome, 391*t*

Hallux valgus, 317
Halo nevus, 567*t*
Haloperidol, teratogenic effects, 73*t*
Hamartomas, in newborns, 106
Hamstring reflex, 380*t*
Hand-foot-mouth disease, 171, 183*t*, 579*t*
Hand and wrist. *See also* Upper extremity
  anatomy, 308*f*
  movements, 304–305*f*
Harlequin color change/effect, 104, 232
Hawkins-Kennedy test, 331, 331*f*
Head
  endocrine-related abnormalities
    in adolescents, 413
    in children, 410
    differential diagnosis, 428*t*
    in infants, 408
  physical examination
    in adolescents, 39
    in children, 36
    in infants, 32, 322
    in newborns, 78–79
Headache
  in adolescents, 147, 372
  in anemia, 493
  in brain tumors, 531–532
  in children, 145–146, 366–367
  in endocrine disorders, 428*t*
  malignancies associated with, 522*t*, 525*t*
  non-CNS causes, 65*t*
  in rheumatic diseases, 321*t*
Hearing loss
  causes, 169–170, 182*t*
  developmental disabilities and, 638
  diagnostic testing, 640
  drug/toxin-induced, 392*t*
Heart disease. *See also* Cardiovascular system
  acquired
    bacterial endocarditis, 262
    diagnostic testing, 254*t*, 262–263, 263*t*
    Fontan circulation, 254*t*, 261
    imaging, 254*t*, 262–263, 263*t*
    Kawasaki disease/syndrome, 254*t*, 261–262
    myocarditis/myocardiomyopathy, 254*t*, 262
    referrals/consultation, 264–265, 265*t*

Heart disease (*Cont.*):
  rheumatic heart disease, 254*t*,
    261
  signs and symptoms, 254*t*
  congenital. *See* Congenital heart
    disease
Heart murmurs. *See also*
    Congenital heart disease
  Carey-Coombs, 261
  innocent, 238–239
  in newborns, 102, 108*t*
  pathologic, 236–238, 237*f*
Heart rate
  endocrine disorders and, 408,
    411, 413
  lability, 51
  measurement, 50
  orthostatic changes, 55
Heart rhythm, 50–51
Heat cramps, 49
Heat exhaustion, 49
Heat intolerance, 410, 412, 426*t*
Heat stroke, 49
HEEADSSS, 21
Helicobacter pylori, 296*t*
Hemangiomas
  erosion and crust secondary to,
    549*f*
  laryngeal, 201
  nasal, 194*t*
  in newborns, 105–106
  strawberry, 572*t*
Hematemesis, 64*t*, 291*t*
Hematochezia, 291–292*t*
Hematopoietic system
  malignancies. *See* Leukemia;
    Lymphoma
  platelet disorders
    history and physical
      examination, 499
    key findings, 499
    key problems, 499
    thrombocytopenia, 499–500
    thrombocytosis, 500–501
  red blood cell disorders
    anemia
      diagnostic synthesis,
        493–494
      diagnostic testing, 494, 495*t*,
        496*t*
      high MCV and low
        reticulocytes, 496
      history, 491–493
      low MCV and low
        reticulocytes, 494, 496

  normal MCV and high
    reticulocytes, 497–498
  normal MCV and low
    reticulocytes, 496–497
  pathophysiology, 491
  physical examination, 493
components, 490–491
erythrocytosis (polycythemia)
  diagnostic testing, 498–499
  differential diagnosis, 498
  history and physical
    examination, 498
  physiology and mechanics,
    489–490
  sickle cell disease, 501, 502*t*
white blood cell disorders
  leukocytosis, 505
  leukopenia, 501, 503
  lymphocytopenia, 504
  lymphocytosis, 505–506
  neutropenia
    acquired causes, 504
    definition, 503, 503*t*
    intrinsic causes, 503–504
  neutrophilia, 505
Hematuria
  causes, 462*t*, 465, 466*t*
  differential diagnosis, 466*t*,
    653–654, 662, 666,
    679–680*t*, 684*t*
  evaluation, 462
  malignancies associated with,
    522*t*
  nonurinary causes, 65*t*
Hemifacial microsomia, 121*t*
Hemochromatosis, 564*t*
Hemoglobin/hematocrit
  indications, 296*t*, 681*t*
  normal values by age group and
    gender, 495*t*
Hemoglobinuria, 462, 463*t*
Hemolytic anemia, 497–498
Hemolytic-uremic syndrome,
    294*t*, 518*t*
Hemophilia
  findings, 511, 514–515*t*
  history, 506, 509, 514*t*
Hemoptysis, 321*t*
Hemostatic system
  bleeding disorders
    birth history, 508–509
    developmental history, 509
    diagnostic algorithm, 519*f*
    differential diagnosis,
      514–517*t*

family history, 509
imaging, 520
past history, 508
presenting complaint, 506–507
referrals/consultation, 520
social history, 509
clotting disorders
birth history, 509
diagnostic algorithm, 519*f*
differential diagnosis,
517–518*t*
family history, 509
imaging, 520
past history, 508
presenting complaint, 507–508
referrals/consultation, 520
components, 491
diagnostic testing, 512
key problems
in adolescents, 511
in children, 511
in infants
excess bruising or
ecchymoses, 510
excessive bleeding, 510
pain, 511
rash or discoloration, 511
swelling, 511
physical examination, 513*t*
physiology and mechanics, 490
terminology, 507
Henoch-Schönlein purpura
bruising in, 510
cutaneous symptoms, 321*t*, 345*t*,
557, 676
gastrointestinal symptoms, 294*t*,
321*t*
musculoskeletal symptoms, 345*t*
Hepatitis B, maternal, fetal effects,
71*t*
Hepatitis C, maternal, fetal effects,
71*t*
Hereditary hemorrhagic
telangiectasia, 506
Hermansky-Pudlak syndrome,
566*t*
Hernias, 659
Herpangina, 183*t*
Herpes hominis infection,
maternal, fetal effects, 71*t*
Herpes simplex virus infections
cutaneous, 579*t*, 589*t*
encephalitis, 359
genital, 677, 693, 734*t*
oral cavity, 177, 183*t*

Herpes zoster infection
chest pain in, 205
dermatomal distribution in, 554,
555*f*
scars from, 551*f*
vesicles in, 579*t*
Hip. *See also* Lower extremity
developmental dysplasia, 87, 89*f*
pain, 319
physical examination
in adolescents, 337
in infants, 323–324
rotation, 326, 327*f*, 327*t*
Hirschsprung disease, 271, 272,
292*t*, 300
Hirsutism, 422–423, 427*t*, 594, 727
History. *See also specific systems*
in developmental diagnosis,
632–633
in diagnostic framework, 60–63
initial interview
data gathering, 1–2
developmental landmarks, 3*t*,
4*t*, 5*t*
family history, 2, 6–7
intake form, 8–9*t*
past medical history, 2
review of systems, 2, 6*t*, 7*t*
present illness
adolescents, 15–23
children, 14–15
focused interview, 10–13, 11*t*
general comments, 10
infants, 13–14
in psychodiagnostic
examination, 600
in psychodiagnostic
examination, 599–605
HIV/AIDS, 737*t*
Hoarseness, 173
Hodgkin disease, 530–531
Holoprosencephaly, 120*t*
Homicidal acts, 611
Homicidal ideation, 609
Hoover sign, 384
Horner syndrome
in brain tumors, 533
causes, 154
diagnostic testing, 157*t*
in neuroblastoma, 535
Hydradenitis suppurativa,
578*t*
Hydrocele, 659, 659*f*, 673–674
Hydrocephalus, 294*t*, 385*t*
Hydronephrosis, 652, 672, 683*t*

Hymen
  anatomy, 720
  bleeding, 697*t*
  cysts, 689, 697*t*
  imperforate, 295*t*, 689–690, 697*t*
  mass, 697*t*
Hypercalcemia, 436*t*, 440
Hyperextension test, 335, 336*f*
Hypermenorrhea, 725*t*
Hypermobility syndrome, 345*t*
Hyperopia, 152
Hyperparathyroidism, maternal,
      fetal effects, 70*t*
Hyperpigmentation, 105
Hyperpnea, in infants, 212
Hypersomnia, 623
Hypersplenism, 504
Hypertelorism, 108*t*
Hypertension
  in endocrine disorders, 430*t*
  maternal, fetal effects, 70*t*
  neonatal, 453, 454*t*, 481
  noncardiac causes, 64*t*
  in Wilms' tumor, 536
Hyperthermia, 48–49
  maternal, teratogenic effects, 73*t*
  in newborns, 96–97, 110*t*
Hyperthyroidism
  cutaneous symptoms, 564*t*
  gastrointestinal symptoms, 294*t*
  maternal, fetal effects, 70*t*
  menstrual disturbances in, 433*t*
Hypertrichosis, 427*t*
Hypertrophic cardiomyopathy,
      254*t*, 262
Hyphema, 157
Hypocalcemia
  diagnostic testing, 436*t*, 440
  neurologic signs and symptoms,
      408, 420, 424, 430*t*
  respiratory symptoms, 408
Hypoglossal nerve (cranial nerve
      XII), 355, 378
Hypoglycemia, 438*t*, 441
Hypomelanosis of Ito, 400*t*, 557*f*
Hypopigmentation,
      postinflammatory, 567*t*
Hypoplastic left heart syndrome,
      252*t*, 260
Hypoplastic right heart syndrome,
      252*t*, 260–261
Hypopnea, in infants, 212
Hypospadias, 125, 670*f*, 672, 683*t*
Hypotelorism, 108*t*
Hypotension, 55

  in anemia, 493
  in endocrine disorders, 430*t*
  noncardiac causes, 64*t*
Hypothermia, 49–50, 97, 110*t*
Hypothyroidism
  bradycardia in, 429*t*
  cutaneous symptoms, 407, 428
  hair abnormalities in, 428*t*
  maternal, fetal effects, 70*t*
  menstrual disturbances in, 433*t*
Hypotonia
  in children, 368–370
  in infants, 362–363

I
Ibuprofen, teratogenic effects, 72*t*
Ichthyosis, 105, 583–584*t*
Iliopsoas test, 287*f*
Illusions, 608
Immune thrombocytopenic purpura
  history and findings, 516*t*
  maternal, fetal effects, 70*t*
Immunoglobulin E, 222*t*
Impetigo, 181*t*, 183*t*, 580*t*
In-toeing, 309–310
Inborn errors of metabolism
  altered consciousness in, 359
  clinical characteristics, 398*t*
  developmental delay and, 360
  history and CNS locations, 386*t*
  odors in, 373, 398*t*
  referrals/consultation, 397
Incontinentia pigmenti, 400*t*, 567*t*
Indomethacin, teratogenic effects,
      72*t*
Indurations, skin, 551*f*, 554, 585*t*
Infant(s). *See also* Newborn(s);
      Newborn assessment
  cardiovascular system
    functional anatomy,
      physiology, and
      mechanics, 228–229, 228*f*
    history, 230, 230*t*
    physical examination, 33, 240
  developmental disorders,
      633–634
  developmental timelines
    2 to 9 months, 3*t*
    12 to 24 months, 4*t*
  dysmorphology diagnostic
      examination
    history, 116–117
    physical examination
      chest/back/abdomen,
      128–130

face, 127–128
genitalia, 130
growth, 127
limbs, 130–131
neurologic, 127
skin, 131–132
ears, 32–33
endocrine system, 416–421
key problems, 405–409
physical examination, 416–421
eyes
history, 142
key problems, 142–144
physical examination, 32,
148–150
gastrointestinal tract
key problems, 269–274
physical examination, 34
genitalia, 34
head, 32
history taking, 13–14
musculoskeletal system
key problems, 303–309
physical examination, 34,
322–324
neurologic system
key problems, 358–364
physical examination, 34–35
nose, mouth, and throat, 33
physical examination overview,
31–35
respiratory system
key problems, 199–202
physical examination, 33,
211–216, 215*t*
review of systems, 6*t*
skin, 34. *See also* Dermatologic
conditions
vital signs, 32
Infantile spasms, 358, 396*t*
Infections, maternal, fetal effects,
69–70, 71*t*
Inflammatory bowel disease, 321*t*
Insect bites, 569*t*
Insomnia, 623
Insulin resistance, 427*t*
Intelligence quotient (IQ), 631
Intermittent explosive disorder,
623–624
Intersex. *See* Ambiguous genitalia
Intertrigo, 563*t*
Intravenous pyelogram (IVP),
682*t*
Intussusception, 275, 283, 291*t*
Iritis, in rheumatic diseases, 321*t*

Iron-deficiency anemia, 494, 496,
595
Irritability/jitteriness, 100–101,
110*t*, 493
Irritable bowel syndrome, 280*t*
Isotretinoin, teratogenic effects,
73*t*
Isovaleric acidemia, 398*t*

J
Janeway lesions, 575*t*
Jaundice
in adolescents, 279–280
in anemia, 493
in children, 276–277
differential diagnosis, 291–295*t*
in infants, 273–274
in newborns, 102–103, 109*t*
nongastrointestinal causes, 64*t*
physiology, 268–269
Jaw reflex, 378
Jeune thoracic dystrophy, 124
Jobe relocation test, 331, 331*f*
Johanson-Blizzard syndrome, 591
Joint pain, 525*t*. *See also*
Musculoskeletal
system
Jones criteria, rheumatic fever, 261
Juvenile myalgia, 314
Juvenile rheumatoid arthritis, 562*t*,
570*t*, 577*t*

K
Kabuki syndrome, 136*t*
Kallmann syndrome, 420, 430*t*
Kawasaki disease/syndrome
complications, 262
cutaneous symptoms, 558, 570*t*
diagnostic testing and imaging,
254*t*
musculoskeletal findings, 345*t*
signs and symptoms, 254*t*,
261–262, 295*t*, 321*t*
strawberry tongue, 178
Kayser-Fleischer ring, 276
Kearns-Sayre syndrome, 398*t*
Keloids, 573*t*
Keratosis pilaris, 571*t*
KID syndrome, 584*t*
Kidney(s). *See also* Renal system
agenesis, 450–451
anatomy, 443, 445–446, 445*f*, 446*f*
blood supply and lymphatic
drainage, 446–447
changes at birth, 448–449

Kidney(s) (*Cont.*):
  congenital anomalies, 451–452,
      451*t*
  development, 449–450
  ectopia, 450
  failure. *See* Renal failure
  innervation, 447
  malformation, 679*t*
  mass/swelling, 664, 679*t*
  microcirculation, 447–448
  palpation, 464
  prenatal ultrasonography, 450*t*
  weight by age, 445*t*
Klebsiella infection, maternal, fetal
      effects, 71*t*
Kleptomania, 624
Klinefelter syndrome
  breast changes in, 431*t*
  diagnostic testing, 134*t*
  growth problems in, 413, 427*t*
Klippel-Feil syndrome
  anomalies, 118
  facial features, 122*t*
  musculoskeletal features, 124,
      306
Klippel-Trenaunay syndrome,
      126
Klumpke's palsy, 87, 88*f*, 304
Knee. *See* Lower extremity
Knock-knees (genu valgum), 311,
      313*f*, 329
Koilonychia, 596*t*
Korotkoff sounds, 53, 53*f*
Kugelberg-Welander syndrome,
      399*t*
Kussmaul breathing, 217

L
Labia, 686, 689, 720, 722*f*
Laboratory tests. *See* Diagnostic
      tests
Labyrinthine tests, 375
Labyrinthitis, 182*t*
Lachman test, 338, 338*f*
Landau-Kleffner syndrome, 396*t*,
      637
Langerhans histiocytosis, 574*t*
Language
  definitions, 629–630, 630*t*
  developmental disorders
    in children, 634–636
    in infants, 634
Large for gestational age
      newborns. *See also*
        Newborn assessment

  causes, 78, 96
  definition, 77
  laboratory tests and imaging,
      108*t*
Large intestine, 292*t*. *See also*
        Gastrointestinal tract
Laryngomalacia, 201
Laryngotracheal bronchitis, 199
Larynx
  developmental and functional
        anatomy, 190, 192, 192*f*
  physiology and mechanics, 197
Laurence-Moon-Biedl syndrome,
      463
Lawrence-Seip syndrome, 586*t*
Learning disorders, 613, 638–639
Leigh disease, 398*t*
Lennox-Gastaut syndrome, 396*t*
Lentigo syndromes, 565*t*
LEOPARD syndrome, 232*t*, 565*t*
Lesch-Nyhan syndrome, 361, 398*t*,
      595
Lethargy
  in anemia, 492
  in endocrine disorders, 425*t*
  non-CNS causes, 65*t*
Leukemia, 526–528, 526*t*
Leukemoid reaction, 505
Leukocoria, 143, 154, 157*t*, 540
Leukocytosis, 505, 525*t*
Leukopenia, 501, 503, 525*t*
Leukorrhea, physiologic, 729,
      730*t*
Lexical deficit disorder, 636
Lichen nitidus, 573*t*
Lichen planus, 558, 575*t*
Lichen sclerosus, 689, 698
Lichen sclerosus et atrophicus,
      558, 573*t*
Lichen striatus, 572*t*
Lichenification, skin, 550*f*, 552
Likelihood ratio, 756–757
Limp
  in adolescents, 315–316
  in children, 313–314
Lindsay nails, 597
Linear nevus sebaceous, 400*t*
Lithium, teratogenic effects, 73*t*
Liver disease, 293*t*. *See also*
        Gastrointestinal tract
  dermatologic signs, 284
  fetor hepaticus in, 281
  key problems and findings,
      292*t*
  referrals/consultation, 300

Liver function studies, 297*t*
Load and shift test, 332, 332*f*
Lower extremity. *See also* Foot and
ankle
anatomy, knee, 309*f*
key problems
bowlegs, 311, 312*f*, 316
hip, groin pain, 319
joint pain, 315, 318
joint swelling, 320
knee pain, 319–320
knock-knees, 311, 313*f*
leg-length inequality, 314
leg pain, 314, 316
limp, 313–314, 315–316
stiffness, 320
toe walking, 314
weakness, 320–321
physical examination
in adolescents
knees, 337–340, 338*f*, 339*f*
legs, 340
in children, 329
gait, 325–326
torsional profile, 326–327,
327–328*f*
in dysmorphology diagnostic
examination, 125–126,
130–131
in infants, 323–324
in newborns, 87–88, 89*f*
Ludwig angina, 172, 184*t*
Lung(s). *See also* Respiratory
system
developmental and functional
anatomy, 192, 196
physiology and mechanics,
197–198
Lung sounds, 214*t*
Lupus erythematosus. *See*
Systemic lupus
erythematosus
Lupus nephritis, 474
Lupus panniculitis, 578*t*
Lyme disease, 568*t*
Lymphadenopathy
causes, 174
in lymphoma, 528
malignancies associated with,
522*t*, 525*t*
Lymphatic system, 34, 38
Lymphocytopenia, 504
Lymphocytosis, 505–506
Lymphogranuloma venereum,
736*t*

Lymphoma
clinical presentation, 528–529
diagnosis, 528
Hodgkin disease, 530–531
neck mass in, 174
non-Hodgkin, 529–530

M
Macrocephaly, 108*t*
Macromastia, 707
Macules, 543, 544*f*
blue, 563*t*
blue-black, 574–575*t*
brown diffuse, 564*t*
brown localized, 564–566*t*
purple, 563*t*, 575*t*
red, 560–563*t*
white diffuse, 566*t*
white localized, 566–567*t*
yellow, 575*t*
Madelung deformity, 426*t*
Magnesium sulfate, in labor, fetal
effects, 73*t*
Magnet response, 92, 94*f*
Magnetic resonance imaging (MRI)
in brain tumors, 533
in cancer diagnosis, 523
in Ewing sarcoma, 538
in neuroblastoma, 535
in neurologic disorders, 396–397
in osteogenic sarcoma, 538
in respiratory disorders, 224*t*
in soft-tissue sarcoma, 540
spine, 682*t*
urogram, 683*t*
Major anomaly, 112
Male genitourinary system
anatomy, 645–650, 646*f*
diagnostic synthesis, 679–680*t*
diagnostic testing, 681*t*
endocrine disorder-related
abnormalities
in adolescents, 414
in children, 412
differential diagnosis, 425,
432–433*t*
in infants, 412, 421
imaging, 682–683*t*
key problems
in adolescents, 665–667
in children
abdominal/pelvic/genital
pain, 663
hematuria or urine
discoloration, 662

Male genitourinary system (*Cont.*):
    kidney mass or swelling, 664
    lower urinary tract
      symptoms, 662
    penis, pain/mass/swelling,
      664
    scrotum,
      pain/mass/swelling,
      664–665
    testicle maldevelopment,
      664
    umbilical discharge, 662
    urine retention, 662
    voiding habit changes, 663
   in newborns and infants
    antenatal hydronephrosis,
      652
    antenatally detected
      malformation, 652
    hematuria or urine
      discoloration, 653–654
    oligohydramnios, 652
    penis, mass/swelling/pain
      in, 657, 657*f*, 660
    scrotum,
      mass/swelling/pain in,
      657–660, 661
    umbilical discharge,
      654–655
    undescended testicle, 658
    urine retention, 652–653
    voiding habit changes,
      655–656
  pathophysiology, 649–650
  measurements, 416
  physical examination
   in adolescents, 42, 677–678
   in children
    inspection, 676
    palpation, 676–677
   in newborns and infants
    auscultation, 675
    in dysmorphology
     diagnostic examination,
     125
    inspection, 667–672, 670*f*, 671*f*
    overview, 34, 86
    palpation, 672–675, 673*f*,
     674*f*
    percussion, 675
    transillumination, 675
  referrals/consultation, 683–684*t*
  sexual maturity rating scale, 419*f*
Malformation, 111
Malignant hyperthermia, 49

Mallet finger, 335
Mallory-Weiss tear, 291*t*
Mammary ridges, 702*f*
Marcus Gunn jaw winking, 153
Marfan syndrome
  cardiac anomalies in, 232*t*
  diagnostic testing, 134*t*
  facial features in, 120*t*, 122*t*
Mastalgia, 707, 716*t*
Mastitis, 716*t*
Mathematics disorder, 613, 639
Mayer-Rokitansky-Kuster-Hauser
    syndrome, 728
McCune-Albright syndrome
  cutaneous symptoms in, 407,
    410, 428*t*, 565*t*
  precocious puberty in, 691
McMurray test, 339, 339*f*
MCAD, 398*t*
Measles, 560*t*
Meckel's diverticulum, 275, 291*t*
Mees nails, 595
Meier-Gorlin syndrome, 121*t*
Melanoma, 552*f*, 563*t*, 573*t*, 597
MELAS syndrome, 398*t*
Meniere disease, 183*t*
Meningoencephalitis, 294*t*
Menkes syndrome, 398*t*, 592*t*
Menometrorrhagia, 725*t*
Menorrhagia, 725*t*
Menstrual cycle
  disturbances
   abnormal patterns, 724, 725*t*
   amenorrhea. *See* Amenorrhea
   dysmenorrhea, 728, 744*t*
   in endocrine disorders
    in adolescents, 414, 415
    differential diagnosis, 433*t*
  history, 723, 724*t*
  physiology, 709, 718–719, 719*f*
Mental retardation
  causes, 635
  characteristics, 635
  definition/classification, 624,
    624*t*, 631
Mental status examination,
    605–607
Mercury, teratogenic effects, 73*t*
MERFF syndrome, 398*t*
Meta-iodobenzylguanidine (MIBG)
    scintigraphy, 535
Metabolic panel, 296*t*
Metachromatic leukodystrophy,
    399*t*
Metatarsus adductus, 324, 324*f*

Methimazole, teratogenic effects, 73*t*
Methylmalonic acidemia, 398*t*
Metrorrhagia, 725*t*
Microcephaly, 108*t*, 123
Migraine, 366. *See also* Headache
Miliaria crystallina, 104, 570*t*
Miliaria rubra, 104, 570*t*
Mini Mental Status Examination, 374*t*
Minimal residual disease, 528
Minor anomaly, 112
Minor variant, 112
Mitochondrial disorders, 386*t*, 398*t*
Mittelschmerz, 295*t*, 728, 745*t*
Moebius syndrome
   facial features in, 120*t*, 122*t*
   neurologic characteristics, 123, 361
   strabismus in, 156
Molluscum contagiosum, 544*f*, 573*t*, 738*t*
Mongolian spots, 544*f*
Monilethrix, 592*t*
Monilial rash, 558
Mononucleosis, 560*t*
Mood disorders
   assessment, 606, 610
   bipolar, 619, 619*t*, 620*t*
   depressive, 618, 619*t*
Moro reflex, 91, 91*f*
Morphea, 586*t*
Morphology, language, 630*t*
Motor development. *See*
         Development;
         Developmental disorders
Mouth and oropharynx
   developmental and functional
         anatomy, 162–165, 163*t*, 164*f*
   diagnostic testing, 186–187
   differential diagnoses
      lips, 183*t*
      oral cavity, 183*t*
      pharynx, 184*t*
   key problems
      dysphagia, 172–173
      pain
         lips and tongue, 170–171
         mouth, 171
         pharynx, 171–172
   physical examination
      in adolescents, 41, 176
      in children, 36, 176
      in dysmorphology diagnostic
            examination, 120*t*
      in infants, 33, 176

   in newborns, 82–83
   oral cavity, 176–179
   oropharynx, 179–180
   physiology and mechanics, 159
   referrals/consultation, 188
Movement disorders
   in children, 371
   drug/toxin-induced, 392*t*
   in infants, 364
Mowat-Wilson syndrome, 125
Mucoceles, 179
Mucopolysaccharidoses, 399*t*
Multiple endocrine neoplasia
         (MEN) 2b, 429*t*
Murmurs. *See* Heart murmurs
Murphy's sign, 289
Muscular dystrophy, 386*t*, 399*t*
Musculoskeletal system
   diagnostic synthesis, 341–342
   diagnostic testing, 344–348*t*
   functional anatomy, 302, 303–311*f*
   imaging, 344–348*t*
   key problems and findings
      acute trauma, 348*t*
      in adolescents
         back pain, 316–317
         bowlegs, 316
         constitutional symptoms, 321, 321*t*
         deterioration of function, 321
         elbow pain, 319
         foot and ankle pain, 317–318
         hip, groin pain, 319
         joint pain, 318
         joint swelling, 320
         knee pain, 319–320
         leg pain, 316
         limp, 315–316
         neck pain, 316
         rheumatic diseases, 321*t*
         shoulder pain, 318–319
         stiffness, 320
         weakness, 320–321
         wrist pain, 319
      bone neoplasms, 347*t*
      cerebral palsy, 342*t*
      in children
         back pain, 313
         bowlegs, 311, 312*f*
         flat feet, 312
         heel pain, 315
         in-toeing, 309–310

Musculoskeletal system (*Cont.*):
joint pain, 315
knock-knees, 311, 313*f*
lack of arm movement, 314
leg-length inequality, 314
leg pain, 314
limp, 313–314
out-toeing, 310–311
toe walking, 314
chronic pain syndromes, 345*t*
club foot, 324, 325*f*
congenital conditions, 344*t*
developmental variations,
344*t*
in infants
delayed walking, 305
lack of arm movement,
303–304
torticollis, 305–306, 309
infections, 345*t*
metabolic bone disease, 346*t*
metatarsus adductus, 324, 324*f*
muscle disease, 348*t*
nonaccidental trauma, 343*t*
orthopedic conditions, 346*t*
overuse syndromes, 346*t*
peripheral neuropathy, 347*t*
psychosomatic disorders, 347*t*
rheumatic diseases, 344*t*
rockerbottom foot, 324, 325*f*
systemic disease, 346*t*
vasculitis, 345*t*
physical examination
in adolescents
ankle, 340–341, 341*f*
elbow, 332, 334
foot, 341
gait and posture, 329
hand and wrist, 335
hips and pelvis, 337
knees, 337–340, 338*f*, 339*f*
legs, 340
shoulders, 329–332,
330–334*f*
spine and back, 335–337,
336*f*, 337*f*
in children, 38
gait, 325–326
lower limb, 329
neck, 328
posture, 326
torsional profile, 327*f*, 327*t*,
328*f*, 328*t*
in infants, 34
chest wall, 322–323

foot and ankle, 324, 324*f*, 325*f*
head, 322
hips and groin, 323–324
knee, 324
lower limbs, 323
neck, 322
shoulders, clavicles, 322
spine and back, 323
upper limbs, 323
in newborns, 87–88, 88*f*, 89*f*
physiology and mechanics,
301–302
referrals/consultation, 343
renal disease-related symptoms,
465
Mutism, selective, 616
Myasthenia gravis
history and CNS locations,
388*t*
in infants, 363
maternal, fetal effects, 70*t*
Mycoplasma pneumoniae infections
laboratory testing, 222*t*
maternal, fetal effects, 71*t*
Myocarditis/myocardiomyopathy,
254*t*, 262
Myoclonic seizures, 358
Myopia, 152
Myotonic dystrophy, 123

N
Nails
acquired disorders, 595, 597
congenital/genetic disorders,
595, 596*t*
developmental anatomy, 594
endocrine-related disorders,
428*t*
history, 594
key findings, 595
NAME syndrome, 565*t*
Narcolepsy, 623
Near-drowning, 206
Neck
developmental and functional
anatomy, 162*f*, 165,
167*f*
diagnostic testing, 187
endocrine disorder-related
abnormalities
in adolescents, 413
in children, 410
differential diagnosis,
423–424, 429*t*
in infants, 410, 420

key problems
  hoarseness and stridor, 173
  masses, 173–174
  pain, 316
  torticollis, 173
physical examination
  in adolescents, 41
  in children, 36 37, 328
  in dysmorphology diagnostic
    examination, 122*t*
  in infants, 33, 322
  lymph nodes, 180
  in newborns, 83
  palpation, 180
  range of motion, 180
physiology and mechanics, 159
referrals/consultation, 188
Necrobiosis lipoidica
  diabeticorum, 586*t*
Neer test, 330, 330*f*
Negative predictive value, 754
Neisseria gonorrhoeae. See
  Gonorrhea
Nemaline myopathy, 400*t*
Nephroblastoma. *See* Wilms' tumor
Nephron, 446, 446*f*, 447–448
Nephrophthisis–medullary cystic
  disease complex, 461
Nephrotic syndrome
  in children and adolescents,
    474–475, 474*t*
  congenital, 471–472, 472*t*
Netherton syndrome, 584*t*
Neural tube defects, 349
Neuroblastoma, 294*t*
  clinical presentation by primary
    site, 533–534, 533*t*
  diagnostic testing, 535
  distant spread, 535
  history, 534
  imaging, 535
  key points, 535–536
  physical examination
    abdomen, 534
    spine, 535
    thorax, 535
Neurocutaneous syndromes,
  400*t*, 401
Neurofibroma, 577*t*
Neurofibromatosis I
  cutaneous symptoms, 428*t*, 565*t*
  diagnostic testing, 134*t*
  facial features, 120*t*
  history and CNS locations, 387*t*
Neurofibromatosis II, 387*t*

Neurologic system
congenital malformations
  diagnostic testing, 393*t*
  history and CNS locations, 385*t*
  referrals/consultation, 397,
    398–400*t*
cranial nerves, 354–355
diagnostic synthesis, 384
diagnostic testing, 394–395*t*
EEG findings, 392, 396*t*
embryologic development,
  349–350
endocrine-related symptoms
  in adolescents, 414
  in children, 410
  differential diagnosis, 424, 430
  in infants, 408–409, 420
functional anatomy, 350–356,
  351–353*f*
genetic/metabolic disorders
  diagnostic testing, 393*t*
  history and CNS locations,
    386–387*t*
  patterns of onset and course,
    357*f*
  referrals/consultation, 397,
    398–400*t*, 401
history, 356–357*f*, 356–358
imaging, 396–397
infectious/inflammatory
  conditions
  diagnostic testing, 394*t*
  history and CNS locations,
    387–388*t*
  patterns of onset and course,
    357*f*
  referrals/consultation, 401
key problems
  in adolescents
    altered consciousness, 372
    headache, 372
    seizures, 371–372
  in children, 364–366
    altered consciousness, 367–368
    clumsiness (ataxia), 370–371
    developmental
      delay/regression, 368
    focal weakness, 370
    headache, 366–367
    hypotonia, 368–370
    movement disorders, 371
  in infants
    altered consciousness,
      359–360
    clumsiness (ataxia), 363–364

Neurologic system (*Cont.*):
    developmental
        delay/regression, 360–361
        focal weakness, 361–362
        hypotonia, 362–363
        movement disorders, 364
        seizures, 358–359
    motor pathways, 353*f*
    neoplastic disease. *See also* Brain
            tumors
        diagnostic testing, 395*t*
        history and CNS locations,
            388–389*t*
        patterns of onset and course,
            357*f*
        referrals/consultation, 401
    physical examination
        in adolescents, 43
        brain/cranial nerves, 375–378
        cerebellar, 374–375
        cerebral, 373–374, 374*t*
        in children, 38
        in dysmorphology diagnostic
            examination, 123, 127
        in infants, 34–35
        motor, 382–384
        in newborns, 89–95, 90–95*f*
        overview, 373
        sensory, 381–382, 382*f*, 383*f*
        spinal reflexes, 379, 379*f*, 379*t*,
            380–381*t*
    physiology and mechanics,
        349–350
    referrals/consultation, 397,
        398–400*t*, 401
    renal disease-related symptoms,
        464
    sensory pathways, 353*f*
    toxidromes
        causative agents, 391*t*, 392*t*
        diagnostic testing, 394*t*
        patterns of onset and course,
            357*f*
        presentation and vital signs, 391*t*
        symptoms, 392*t*
    traumatic/hypoxic disorders
        history and CNS locations, 388*t*
        referrals/consultation, 401
    vascular disorders
        diagnostic testing, 395*t*
        history and CNS locations,
            389–390*t*
        patterns of onset and course,
            356*f*
        referrals/consultation, 401

Neuroma, 577*t*
Neuropathy
    congenital causes, 399*t*
    drug/toxin-induced, 392*t*
Neutropenia
    acquired causes, 504
    definition, 503, 503*t*
    intrinsic causes, 503–504
    in leukemia, 527
Neutrophilia, 505
Nevi, 563*t*, 565*t*, 574*t*
Nevus depigmentosus, 567*t*
Newborn(s). *See also* Infant(s)
    assessment. *See* Newborn
            assessment
    cardiovascular system
        functional anatomy,
            physiology, and
            mechanics, 228–229, 228*f*
        physical examination, 240
    common problems
        apnea, 99
        cyanosis, 101, 232
        heart murmurs, 102
        irritability/jitteriness, 100–101
        jaundice, 102–103
        large for gestational age, 96
        pallor or plethora, 101
        poor feeding/lethargy, 99
        seizures, 101
        small for gestational age, 96
        tachypnea
            cardiac causes, 98
            infectious causes, 99
            metabolic causes, 99
            neurologic causes, 98
            respiratory causes, 97–98
        temperature instability
            hyperthermia, 96–97
            hypothermia, 97
        vomiting, 99–100
    dermatologic conditions
        benign transient, 104
        developmental abnormalities,
            104
        hamartomas, 106
        hemangiomas, 105–106
        hyperpigmentation, 105
        pigment disorders, 105
        skin peeling, 105
    dysmorphology diagnostic
            examination
        chest/back/abdomen, 124–125
        cranium, 123
        face, 124

genitalia, 125
growth, 122
limbs, 125–126
neurologic, 123
skin, 127
renal disorders
acute renal failure, 453, 455, 456t
clinical manifestations, 452t
extrarenal abnormalities associated with, 452t
hypertension, 453, 454t
prenatal detection, 451–452, 451t
Newborn assessment
general considerations
Apgar score, 76, 77t
gestational age assessment, 78
initial impression, 76, 77f
measurements, 75f, 77–78
transition, 76–77
laboratory tests and imaging, 106–107, 107t
based on initial physical assessment, 108–109t
based on key signs, 110t
based on prenatal history, 107t
screening, 106–107
physical examination
abdomen
auscultation, 85
inspection, 84–85
palpation, 85
percussion, 85
back, 87
ears, 81–82
eyes, 80–81, 81f
form, 78f
head, 78–79
mouth, tongue, and throat, 82–83
neck, 83
neurologic
cerebral, 89–90
cranial nerves, 354–355
motor, 91
reflexes, 91–95, 91–95f
sensory, 90
nose, 82
thorax
auscultation, 84
inspection, 83
palpation, 84
prenatal examination

intrauterine growth patterns, 75f
monitoring pregnancy, labor, and delivery, 74–75
testing, 74, 76t
prenatal history
infectious maternal conditions, 69–70, 71t
noninfectious maternal conditions, 70–71, 70t
teratogenic exposures, 72–73t
Niemann-Pick disease, 399t
Nightmare disorder, 623
Nipple
inverted, 710t
trauma, 717t
Nitrofurantoin, teratogenic effects, 72t
Nodules
characteristics, 545, 545f
flesh and red color, 577t
inflamed red, 578t
juxtaarticular, 577t
Non-Hodgkin lymphoma
clinical presentation, 529
diagnostic testing, 530
key points, 530
physical examination, 529–530
Noonan syndrome
cardiac anomalies in, 118, 232t, 257
diagnostic testing, 134t
facial features in, 120t, 122t
genital malformations in, 125
Nose
developmental and functional anatomy, 189–190, 190f
key problems
anosmia, 194–195t
epistaxis, 194t
masses, 194t
obstruction, 193t
septal defects, 193–194t
physical examination
in adolescents, 41
in children, 36
in dysmorphology diagnostic examination, 120t
in infants, 33
in newborns, 82–83
physiology and mechanics, 196–197
Nuclear imaging
in cancer diagnosis, 523
male genitourinary system, 683t

Nystagmus
  differential diagnosis, 156, 157*t*
  in endocrine disorders, 429*t*
  in infants, 144
  testing, 375

O

Obesity
  endocrine causes, 410, 427*t*
  maternal, fetal effects, 70*t*
Obsessions, 608
Obsessive-compulsive disorder, 620
Obstructive apnea, 51
Obstructive sleep apnea, 217
Obturator test, 287*f*
Oculomotor nerve (cranial nerve III), 355, 376, 377*f*
Olfactory nerve (cranial nerve I), 354, 375
Oligohydramnios, 76*t*, 107*t*, 652
Oligomenorrhea, 725*t*
Oliguria, 65*t*, 460, 460*t*
Onychomycoses, 597
Opiates
  teratogenic effects, 73*t*
  toxidrome, 391*t*
Oppositional defiant disorder, 615
Opsoclonus, 156, 157*t*
Optic nerve (cranial nerve II), 354, 376–377
Orbital cellulitis, 153
Orbital tumor/mass, 144, 153–154
Orchitis, 660
Organic acidemias, 398*t*
Orthostatic hypotension, 55–56
Ortolani maneuver, 87, 90*f*
Oscillotonometry, 53–54
Osler's nodes, 575*t*
Osteogenesis imperfecta, 123, 135*t*
Osteogenic sarcoma
  clinical presentation, 347*t*, 537
  diagnostic testing, 537
  history, 537
  imaging, 347*t*, 537–538
  physical examination, 537
Ostium primum, 255
Ostium secundum, 255
Otahara syndrome, 396*t*
Otalgia, 168–169
Otitis externa, 168, 169, 181*t*
Otitis media, 168, 169, 182*t*
Otorrhea, 169
Out-toeing, 310–311

Ovaries
  anatomy, 721, 722*f*
  cyst/torsion, 295*t*, 728
  mass, 728–729, 746*t*
Oxytocin in labor, fetal effects, 73*t*

P

Pachyonychia congenita, 596*t*
Paget-Schrotter syndrome, 319
Pain assessment scale, 12*f*
Pain disorder, 621
Pallor, 101, 110*t*, 493
Palpation, 26. *See also specific systems*
Palpitations, in endocrine disorders, 426*t*
Pancreas, 293*t*. *See also* Gastrointestinal tract
Pancreatitis, 293*t*
Panic disorder, 620, 620*t*
Panniculitis, 578*t*
Papanicolaou smear, 741
Papilledema, 155
Papilloma, intraductal, 704, 715*t*
Papules
  brown, 573–574*t*
  characteristics, 543–544, 544*f*
  flesh colored, 573*t*
  red, 568–572*t*
  vulvar, 696*t*
Paraneoplastic syndromes, 534
Paraphilias, 622, 622*t*
Paraphimosis, 657*f*, 670, 683*t*
Parathyroid gland disorders, 436*t*
Paronychia, 597
Parulis, 178
Parvovirus B-19, maternal, fetal effects, 71*t*
Patellar apprehension test, 338
Patellofemoral syndrome, 319–320
Patent ductus arteriosus (PDA), 252*t*, 255
Pathological gambling, 624
Patrick test, 337, 337*f*
Pectoralis reflex, 380*t*
Pectus carinatum, 207, 211*f*, 216
Pectus excavatum, 207, 211*f*, 216
Pediculosis pubis, 737*t*
Pelizaeus-Merzbacher disease, 399*t*
Pelvic examination
  in adolescents, 729, 740–742
  in children, 693–695
Pelvic inflammatory disease, 295*t*, 746*t*
Pelvic pain, in adolescent female, 727–729

Pemphigus foliaceus, 581*t*
Pemphigus vulgaris, 580*t*
Pendred syndrome, 408, 429*t*
Penis
    anatomy, 648–649, 648*f*, 649*f*
    anomalies, 669–672, 670*f*, 6701*f*
    buried, 670
    mass/discharge, 666–667, 680*t*
    pain and swelling, 657, 657*f*,
        666–667, 680*t*
Peptic ulcer disease, 291*t*
Percussion, 27. *See also specific*
        systems
Perez response, 92
Perichondritis, 181*t*
Perineum, 697*t*
Periodic breathing, 212
Peripheral nervous system. *See*
        Neurologic system
Peripheral pulse, 50
Peritonsillar abscess, 172, 179, 184*t*
Personality disorders, 625, 625*t*
Pertussis, 199, 203
Pervasive developmental
        disorders, 614–615
Petechiae, 562*t*, 563*t*, 570*t*
Peutz-Jeghers syndrome, 565*t*
Pharyngitis, 171–172, 184*t*
Phenobarbital, teratogenic effects,
        72*t*
Phenylketonuria (PKU), 373, 398*t*,
        566*t*
Phenytoin, teratogenic effects, 72*t*
Phimosis, 657*f*, 683*t*
Phobias, 608, 620
Phonological disorder, 614,
        635–636
Phonology, 630*t*
Phrenic nerve trauma, 213
Physical examination. *See also*
        specific systems
    in adolescents, 39–43
    auscultation, 27–28, 28*f*
    in children, 35–38
    in diagnostic framework, 60–63
    general considerations, 29–30,
        30*f*
    in infants, 31–35
    inspection, 25–26
    olfaction, 26
    palpation, 26
    percussion, 27
Pica, 615
Piebaldism, 566*t*
Pierre Robin syndrome, 121*t*, 178

Ping pong ball skull, 408, 419, 428*t*
Pinworms, 689, 698*t*, 737*t*
Pituitary tumors, 428*t*
Pityriasis alba, 567*t*
Pityriasis rosea, 558, 558*f*, 571*t*
Placing response, 92–93, 94*f*
Plagiocephaly, 123
Plantar fasciitis, 317
Plantar reflex, 381*t*
Plaques, skin, 544, 545*f*
Platelet count, 296*t*, 527
Platelet disorders
    acquired, 516*t*
    congenital, 516*t*
    history and physical
        examination, 499, 516*t*
    key findings, 499, 516*t*
    key problems, 499
    thrombocytopenia, 499–500
    thrombocytosis, 500–501
Platelet functional analysis (PFA),
        512
Plethora, 101
Pleural rub, 214*t*
Pneumothorax, 205
Poikiloderma, 586*t*
Poisoning
    causative agents, 391*t*, 392*t*
    diagnostic testing, 394*t*
    patterns of onset and course,
        357*f*
    presentation and vital signs,
        391*t*
    symptoms, 392*t*
Poland anomaly, 124
Poland syndrome, 211, 707*f*
Polycystic ovary syndrome, 427*t*,
        564*t*, 747*t*
Polycythemia. *See* Erythrocytosis
Polyhydramnios, 76*t*, 107*t*
Polymastia, 704, 710*t*
Polymenorrhea, 725*t*
Polyps, nasal, 193*t*
Polythelia, 704, 706*f*, 710*t*
Polyuria and polydipsia
    in adolescents, 414
    causes, 460–461, 461*t*
    in children, 412
    differential diagnosis, 433*t*, 461
    in infants, 409
    nonrenal causes, 65*t*
Portal hypertension, 292*t*
Porter's tip syndrome, 87
Positive predictive value, 754
Posttraumatic stress disorder, 621

Posture
in adolescents, 329
in children, 326
Potassium hydroxide (KOH)
preparation, 598
PQRST system, 11, 11*t*
Prader-Willi syndrome
diagnostic testing, 135*t*
growth problems in, 426*t*
neurologic characteristics, 123
weight problems in, 427*t*
Pragmatics, language, 630*t*
Preauricular sinus, 181*t*
Precision, 45
Precocious puberty, 690–691, 698
Precordial catch syndrome, 209
Predictive value, 754–756, 756*f*
Prednisone, teratogenic effects use,
72*t*
Premenstrual syndrome, 728, 748*t*
Preseptal cellulitis, 153
Pressure sores, 580*t*, 587*t*
Pretest probability, 755
Prevalence, 755–756
Priapism, 657, 681*t*
Primary ciliary dyskinesia,
202–203, 207
Probability, 751
Progeria, 586*t*
Progesterone, teratogenic effects,
72*t*
Progressive ataxias, 400*t*
Pronator reflex, 380*t*
Propionic acidemia, 398*t*
Propranolol, teratogenic effects,
72*t*
Propylthiouracil, teratogenic
effects, 73*t*
Prostate, 650
Protein C deficiency, 510
Proteinuria
causes, 467
definition, 484*t*
diagnostic testing, 482, 484, 484*t*
orthostatic, 467
pathophysiology, 465
transient, 467
Proteus infection, maternal, fetal
effects, 71*t*
Proteus syndrome, 126
Prothrombin time, 512
Prune-belly syndrome, 668, 683*t*
Pseudomonas infection, maternal,
fetal effects, 71*t*
Pseudotumor cerebri, 294*t*, 372

Pseudoxanthoma elasticum, 575*t*
Psoriasis, 547*f*, 571*t*
Psychiatric disorders
axis I disorders, 613*t*
adjustment disorders, 624
anxiety disorders, 619–621,
620*t*
attention-deficit and
disruptive behavior
disorders, 615
cognitive disorders, 617
communication disorders, 614
dissociative disorders, 621–622
eating disorders, 622–623
elimination disorders, 616
factitious disorders, 621
feeding and eating disorders,
615–616
impulse-control disorders,
623–624
learning disorders, 613
mood disorders, 618–619,
619*t*, 620*t*
motor skills disorders,
613–614
pervasive developmental
disorders, 614–615
psychotic disorders, 618
reactive attachment disorder,
616
selective mutism, 616
separation anxiety disorder,
616
sexual and gender identity
disorders, 622, 622*t*
sleep disorders, 623
somatoform disorders, 621
substance-related disorders,
617–618
tic disorders, 616
axis II disorders
mental retardation, 624, 624*t*
personality disorders, 625,
625*t*
diagnostic process, 612
diagnostic testing, 626–627
domains of impairment
behavior disturbances,
611–612
feeling disturbances
affect, 610
mood, 610
thought disturbances
content, 608–609
process, 607–608

history, 599–605, 602*t*
imaging, 626
mental status examination,
605–607
Psychosis, 65*t*, 618
Psychotropic drugs, teratogenic
effects, 73*t*
Ptosis, 153, 157*t*
Puberty. *See also* Menstrual cycle
delayed
diagnostic testing, 435*t*, 439
nonendocrine causes, 65
precocious
characteristics, 690–691
referrals/consultation, 698
premature
diagnostic testing, 435*t*, 439
differential diagnosis, 433*t*
sexual maturity rating scales
breasts, 417*f*
male genitalia, 419*f*
pubic hair, 418*f*
Pubic hair
premature development, 433*t*,
690–691
sexual maturity rating scale,
418*f*
Pulmonary function tests, 221, 225*t*
Pulse rates, normal by age, 233*t*
Pupillary reflex, 378
Pure white cell aplasia, 504
Purpura, 563*t*
Pustules, 548*f*, 549
Pyloric stenosis, 283, 291*t*
Pyogenic granuloma, 471*t*
Pyromania, 624

Q
Quadriceps reflex, 380*t*
Quinine, teratogenic effects, 72*t*

R
Radial head subluxation, 314
Radiography
in cancer diagnosis, 523
in Ewing sarcoma, 538
in gastrointestinal disorders, 298*t*
male genitourinary system, 682*t*
in osteogenic sarcoma, 538
in respiratory disorders,
223–224*t*
Ramsay-Hunt syndrome, 181*t*
Raynaud phenomenon, 321*t*
Reactive attachment disorder,
616–617

Reading disorder, 613, 639
Receiver-operator characteristic
(ROC) curve, 753, 755*f*
Red blood cells, 495*t*. *See also*
Anemia
Referential thinking, 609
Reflexes
brain stem, 379
newborn, 91–95, 91–95*f*
spinal, 379, 379*f*, 379*t*, 380–381*t*
Refsum disease, 400*t*, 584*t*
Reiger syndrome, 121*t*
Reiter syndrome, 321*t*, 677
Renal agenesis, 450
Renal colic, 459–460, 459*t*
Renal ectopia, 450
Renal failure
acute
in children and adolescents
causes, 478*t*
diagnostic approach, 479
diagnostic testing, 484–486,
485*t*
pathophysiology, 476, 478
in infants and newborns
causes, 456*t*
classification, 455
clinical manifestations, 453,
455
diagnostic testing, 481
differential diagnosis, 653
chronic
causes, 479–480, 480*t*
definition and classification,
479, 479*t*
diagnostic testing, 486–487,
487*t*, 488*t*
maternal, fetal effects, 70*t*
Renal system
anatomy, 443–445, 444*f*
blood supply and lymphatic
drainage, 446–447
changes at birth, 448–449
development, 449–450
diagnostic testing
acute renal failure, 481,
484–486, 485*t*
chronic renal failure, 486–487,
487*t*, 488*t*
neonatal hypertension, 481
proteinuria, 482, 484, 484*t*
renal tubular acidosis, 482,
483*t*
urinary tract infection, 482
urolithiasis, 485*t*

Renal system (*Cont.*):
  history, 457–458
  innervation, 447
  key problems
    in children
      clinical manifestations, 473*t*
      discolored urine. *See*
        Hematuria
      dysuria. *See* Urinary tract
        infection
      enuresis. *See* Enuresis
      flank pain, 459
      frequency. *See* Urinary
        frequency
      oliguria, 460, 461*t*
      polyuria, 460–461, 461*t*
      renal colic, 459–460, 459*t*
    in infants and newborns
      clinical manifestations, 452*t*
      extrarenal abnormalities
        associated with, 452*t*
      growth retardation, poor
        feeding, and failure to
        thrive, 455, 457*t*, 458*t*
    in prenatal period, 450–451, 450*t*
  key syndromes
    in children and adolescents
      acquired disease, 473
      congenital disease, 472–473
      nephrotic syndrome,
        474–475, 474*t*
      renal failure. *See* Renal
        failure
      urolithiasis, 475–476, 475*t*,
        477*t*, 485*t*
    in infants and newborns
      congenital disorders,
        451–452, 451*t*
      glomerulonephritis, 471
      hypertension, 453, 454*t*, 481
      nephrotic syndrome,
        471–472, 472*t*
      renal failure. *See* Renal
        failure
      renal tubular acidosis,
        468–472, 469*t*, 470*t*, 471*t*
      urinary tract infection, 467
  physical examination
    general assessment, 462–463
    hematuria, 462, 462*t*
    hypertension, 462
    palpation, 464
    proteinuria, 465, 467
  physiology, 447–448
  referrals/consultation, 488*t*

Renal tubular acidosis (RTA)
  diagnostic testing, 482, 483*t*
  distal (type 1), 470–471, 470*t*
  distal (type 4), 471
  proximal (type 2), 468–470, 469*t*
  syndrome associated with,
    469*t*
Repeatability, 46
Reserpine, teratogenic effects, 72*t*
Resonance disorders, 637*t*
Respiratory rate
  key findings and syndromes,
    51–52
  measurement, 51
  normal, by age, 212*f*
Respiratory syncytial virus (RSV)
    infection, 200
Respiratory system
  developmental and functional
    anatomy
    lung, intrathoracic airways,
      and thorax, 192, 196
    nose, sinuses, and larynx,
      189–192, 190*f*, 191*f*
  diagnostic testing
    imaging, 221, 223–224*t*
    laboratory, 221, 222*t*
    pulmonary function testing,
      221, 225*t*
  history, 198–199
  key problems
    in adolescents
      chest pain, 208–209
      cough, 207–208
      cyanosis, 209
      wheezing and stridor, 208
    in children
      chest pain, 205–206
      cough, 202–204
      cyanosis, 206–207
      wheezing and stridor,
        204–205
    in infants
      chest pain, 201
      cough, 199–200
      cyanosis, 201–202
      wheezing and stridor,
        200–201
  physical examination
    in adolescents
      auscultation, 220–221
      inspection, 220
      overview, 41
      palpation, 220
      percussion, 221

in children
  auscultation, 218–219
  inspection, 216–217
  overview, 37
  palpation, 217
  percussion, 219, 219*f*
  tips for performing, 215*t*
in infants
  auscultation, 213–216
  inspection, 211–213, 211*f*
  overview, 33
  palpation, 213
  percussion, 216
  tips for performing, 215*t*
lung sounds, 214*t*
respiratory rates by age, 212*f*
by pulmonary function
  abnormality, 225*t*
referrals/consultation, 221,
  225–226
Retinoblastoma, 143, 154, 540
Retractions, 212–213
Retropharyngeal abscess, 172,
  184*t*, 205
Rett syndrome
  developmental delays in, 636
  diagnostic testing, 136*t*
  neurologic symptoms, 361, 364,
    398*t*
Review of systems
  in children, 7*t*
  in infants, 6*t*
Reye syndrome, 292*t*
Rhabdomyosarcoma
  clinical presentation, 153–154,
    539
  diagnostic testing, 539
  differential diagnosis, 194*t*
  embryonal, 689
  history, 539
  imaging, 539
  paratesticular, 661
  physical examination, 539
Rheumatic diseases, 321*t*. *See also*
    Juvenile rheumatoid
    arthritis
Rheumatic fever. *See* Acute
    rheumatic fever
Rheumatic heart disease, 254*t*, 261
Rhonchus, 214*t*
Rickets
  diagnostic testing, 436*t*
  head abnormalities in, 408, 428
  physical characteristics, 426*t*
Ringworm, 566*t*

Riva-Rocci method, 52–53, 53*f*
Roberts syndrome, 121*t*
Rockerbottom foot (congenital
    vertical talus), 324, 325*f*
Rocky Mountain spotted fever,
    557, 560*t*
Rolandic epilepsy, 365, 396*t*
Romberg sign, 374
Roseola, 560*t*
Rotor syndrome, 273
Rubella syndrome, 71*t*, 232*t*
Rumination, 608
Rumination disorder, 615–616
Russell-Silver syndrome, 122, 122*t*,
    131*f*, 426*t*

S
Saethre-Chotzen syndrome, 136*t*
Salicylates, teratogenic effects, 72*t*
Sandhoff gangliosidosis, 399*t*
Sarcoma botryoides, 689, 697*t*
Scabies, 558, 568*t*, 738*t*
Scales, 547–548, 547*f*, 583–584*t*
Scaphoid abdomen, 109*t*
Scarlatiniform rashes, 557
Scarlet fever, 172, 567*t*
Scars, 551*f*, 554, 586*t*
Schamroth's sign, 217, 218*f*
Schizophrenia, 618
Schwachman-Diamond-Oski
    syndrome, 504
Schwartz equation, for renal
    disease progression, 486,
    487*t*
Sclerae, blue, in newborns, 108*t*
Sclerederma, 585*t*
Scleroderma, 551*f*, 585*t*
Sclerosis, 585*t*
Scoliosis, 317
Screening tests, 757–758
Scrotum
  anatomy, 649
  key problems, 680*t*, 684*t*
  mass, 660–661, 674*f*
  swelling/pain, 658–661, 664–665,
    674*f*
  transillumination, 659*f*, 675
Sebaceous nevus, 545*f*
Sebaceous nevus of Jadassohn,
    106
Seborrhea, 559, 571*t*
Seckel syndrome, 120*t*
Sedative/hypnotics, toxidrome,
    391*t*
Seesaw respirations, 213

Seizures
  in adolescents, 371–372
  in brain tumors, 532
  in children, 364–366
  drug/toxin-induced, 392*t*
  EEG patterns, 396*t*
  in endocrine disorders, 426*t*
  in infants, 358–359
  in newborns, 101, 110*t*
  non-CNS causes, 65*t*
Selective mutism, 616, 636
Self-injurious behavior, 611
Semantic-pragmatic deficit
       disorder, 636
Semantics, 630*t*
Sensitivity, 751–753, 754*f*
Sensory testing, 381–382, 382*f*, 383*f*
Separation anxiety disorder, 616
Sepsis, neonatal, 96–97
Septo-optic dysplasia, 408, 411
Sequence, in dysmorphology, 112
Sever disease, 315
Sexual differentiation, 404, 647. *See
       also* Ambiguous genitalia
Sexual disorders, 622, 622*t*
Sexually transmitted diseases
  in adolescents, 677, 729
  in children, 699
  differential diagnosis, 735–739*t*
  referrals/consultation, 749*t*
  signs and symptoms, 735–739*t*
Shock, 55
Short stature. *See* Growth
       disorders
Shoulder. *See* Upper extremity
Sickle cell disease
  clinical features, 502*t*
  maternal, fetal effects, 70*t*
  pathophysiology, 501
  prevalence, 501
SIGECAPS, mnemonic for
       depression, 619*t*
Sinovenous thrombosis, 517*t*
Sinus(es)
  key problems, 195*t*
  paranasal, 190, 191*f*
Sinus arrhythmia, 50
Sinusitis
  in children, 203
  differential diagnosis, 195*t*
  history and examination, 195*t*
  in infants, 200
Sirenomelia, 450
Sjögren-Larsson syndrome, 584*t*
Skier's thumb, 335

Skin
  disorders. *See* Dermatologic
       conditions
  functional anatomy, 542–543,
       542*f*
  history, 543
  physical examination
    in adolescents, 39
    in children, 38
    in dysmorphology diagnostic
       examination, 127, 131–132
    in infants, 34
  physiology, 541–542
Skin reflexes, 380*t*
Sleep disorders, 623
Sleep terror disorder, 623
Sleepwalking disorder, 623
Slipped capital femoral epiphysis,
       315
Slipping rib syndrome, 209, 220
Small for gestational age
       newborns. *See also*
       Newborn assessment
  causes, 77, 96
  definition, 78
  laboratory tests and imaging,
       108*t*
Small intestine, 291*t*. *See also*
       Gastrointestinal tract
Smith-Lemli-Opitz syndrome, 125,
       136*t*
Smith-Magenis syndrome, 122*t*,
       136*t*
Social history
  in developmental diagnosis, 633
  in psychodiagnostic
       examination, 603–604
Social phobia, 620
Soft-tissue mass, 522*t*
Somatoform disorders, 621
Sotos syndrome, 96, 122*t*, 131*f*,
       135*t*
Specificity, 751–753, 754*f*
Speech
  definitions, 630
  developmental disorders,
       635–636, 637*t*
Speech sound disorder, 637*t*
Speed test, 332, 334*f*
Spermatoceles, 665
Sphygmomanometry, 52–53, 53*f*
Spina bifida, 385*t*
Spinal accessory nerve (cranial
       nerve XI), 355, 378
Spinal dysraphism, 294*t*

Spinal muscle atrophy, 386*t*, 399*t*
Spinal reflexes, 379, 379*f*, 379*t*,
    380–381*t*
Spine. *See* Back and spine
Spirometry, 225*t*
Spondylolysis, 317
Sporotrichosis, 589*t*
Sports, preparticipation history, 22*t*
Sprague stethoscope, 28, 28*f*
Squeeze test, 340
Staphylococcal infection
    nails, 597
    pustules from, 548*f*
    scalded skin syndrome, 580*t*
Startle response, 91
Static lung volumes, 225*t*
Stationary testing, 374
Steatocystoma, 576*t*
Stepping reflex, 93, 95*f*
Steroid medications, teratogenic
        effects, 72*t*
Stevens-Johnson syndrome, 582*t*
Stickler syndrome, 135*t*
Stiff baby syndrome, 362
Stomach, 291*t*. *See also*
        Gastrointestinal tract
Stool tests, 297*t*
Storage diseases, 386*t*, 399*t*
Strabismus, 145, 147, 150, 156
Strawberry hemangioma, 572*t*
Streptoccocal infections, 557
Stress fracture, 316, 317
Stress injuries, 315
Stretch marks, 427*t*
Striae, 586*t*
Stridor
    in adolescents, 208
    characteristics, 214
    in children, 204–205
    in infants, 200–201
    nonpulmonary causes, 64*t*
Stuttering, 614, 637*t*
Subglottic stenosis, 208
Substance abuse
    criteria, 618
    maternal, fetal effects, 73*t*
Substance dependence, 617–618
Subungual hematoma, 597
Suck reflex, 91
Suicidal acts, 611
Suicidal ideation, 609
Sulfonamides, teratogenic effects,
        72*t*
Superior mesenteric artery
        syndrome, 277

Superior vena cava syndrome, 535
Supporting reaction, 92
Supraspinatus test, 332, 333*f*
Sweat test, 222*t*, 297*t*
Sympathomimetics
    in labor, fetal effects, 73*t*
    toxidrome, 391*t*
Syncope, 366, 426*t*
Syndrome, 112
Synovial cyst, 576*t*
Syntax, 630*t*
Syphilis
    maternal, fetal effects, 71*t*
    primary, 589*t*, 677, 735*t*
    secondary, 568*t*
Syringoma, 576*t*
Systemic lupus erythematosus
    cutaneous symptoms, 557, 562*t*,
        570*t*, 585*t*
    maternal, fetal effects, 70*t*
    oral lesions in, 171, 183*t*
    systemic signs and symptoms,
        321*t*

T
Tachycardia
    in anemia, 493
    causes, 50–51, 64*t*
    definition, 50–51
    in endocrine disorders, 429*t*
    in infants, 250*t*
    in newborn, laboratory testing,
        107*t*
Tachypnea
    causes, 52, 64*t*
    in children, 216–217
    definition, 52
    in infants, 212
    in newborns
        cardiac causes, 98
        infectious causes, 99
        laboratory tests and imaging,
            110*t*
        metabolic causes, 99
        neurologic causes, 98
        respiratory causes, 97–98
Talar tilt, 340
Talipes equinovarus (clubfoot),
        324, 325*f*
Tall stature. *See* Growth disorders
Tardive dyskinesia, 371
Tarsal tunnel syndrome, 347*t*
Tattoo, 563*t*, 666
Tay-Sachs disease, 399*t*
Tearing, 142–143

Teeth. *See* Dentition
Telangiectasias, 561*t*
Temperature
 measurement, 46–48
 signs and syndromes, 48–50
Temporomandibular joint
  dysfunction, 169
Tendon reflexes, 380–381*t*
Tension headache, 147
Testicles
 anatomy, 648
 differences in size, 683*t*
 maldevelopment, 664
 neoplasms, 661, 674, 674*f*
 referrals/consultation, 683*t*
 retractile, 658, 668
 torsion, 658, 661
 undescended, 658, 664, 668,
   673, 673*f*, 683*t*
Tetracyclines, teratogenic effects,
  72*t*
Tetralogy of Fallot, 252*t*, 258–259
Texidor's twinge, 209
Thalidomide, teratogenic effects,
  73*t*
Thiazide diuretics, teratogenic
  effects, 73*t*
Third nerve palsy, 153, 157*t*
Thorax, physical examination
 in adolescents, 41
 in children, 37
 in infants, 33
 in newborns, 83–84
Thought disturbances. *See also*
  Psychiatric disorders
 assessment, 606
 content, 606, 608–609
 process, 606, 607–608
Thrombocytopenia
 diagnostic testing, 500
 key findings/problems, 499
 in leukemia, 527
 malignancies associated with,
   525*t*
 pathophysiology, 499–500
Thrombocytosis, 500, 501
Thrombotic thrombocytopenic
  purpura, 518*t*
Thrush, 171
Thumb, movements, 304–305*f*
Thyroglossal duct cyst, 408
Thyroid gland
 anatomy, 165
 developmental physiology,
   404–405

 diagnostic testing, 434, 435*t*, 439
 enlarged, 173, 429*t*
 palpation, 180
Thyroid medications, teratogenic
  effects, 73*t*
Tic disorders, 371, 616
Tietze syndrome, 209, 217, 220
Tinea barbis, 568*t*
Tinea capitis, 566*t*, 593*t*
Tinea corporis, 566*t*
Tinea cruris, 566*t*, 568*t*, 739*t*
Tinea versicolor, 558, 566*t*, 567*t*,
   568*t*, 598
Tinnitus, 170
Titubation, 375
Tobacco, teratogenic effects, 73*t*
Tocolytics, in labor, fetal effects,
   73*t*
Toe walking, 314
Tongue. *See also* Mouth and
   oropharynx
 anatomy, 164, 164*f*
 physical examination, 178–179
Tonic neck reflex, 92, 92*t*
TORCH infections
 developmental delay and, 360
 diagnostic testing, 297*t*
 gastrointestinal symptoms, 281,
   292*t*
Torsional profile
 foot progression angle, 326
 foot shape, 327
 hip rotation, 326, 327*f*, 327*t*
 thigh-foot angle, 327, 328*f*, 328*t*
Torticollis, 144, 173, 305–306, 309
Total anomalous pulmonary
   venous return, 252*t*, 259
Tourette syndrome, 371, 618
Toxic epidermal necrolysis, 582*t*
Toxic shock syndrome, 561*t*
Toxoplasmosis, maternal, fetal
   effects, 71*t*
Tracheoesophageal fistula, 203,
   205, 291*t*
Tracheomalacia, 201
Traction reflex, 92, 93*f*
Transient tachypnea of the
   newborn, 52, 98
Transillumination, scrotum, 659*f*,
   675
Transposition of the great vessels
   (TGV), 252*t*, 259
Trauma
 breast/nipple, 709, 717*t*
 mouth, 171

musculoskeletal, 348*t*
nonaccidental, 343*t*. *See also*
　Child abuse
ocular, 144, 146, 157*t*
Treacher Collins syndrome, 117,
　120*t*, 121*t*, 128*f*
Trendelenburg test, 335–336
Triceps reflex, 380*t*
Trichoepithelioma, 576*t*
Trichomonas vaginalis, 732*t*
Trichorhinophalangeal syndrome,
　120*t*, 592*t*
Trichothiodystrophy, 592*t*
Trichotillomania, 593, 624
Tricuspid atresia, 252*t*, 259–260
Trigeminal nerve (cranial nerve V),
　355, 376, 377*f*
Trimethadione, teratogenic effects,
　72*t*
Trismus, 169
Trisomy-13, 121*t*, 135*t*
Trisomy-18, 121*t*, 134*t*
Trisomy-21. *See* Down syndrome
Trochlear nerve (cranial nerve IV),
　355, 376
Trousseau sign, 373, 430*t*
Truncus arteriosus, 252*t*, 260
Tuberculosis, 202
Tuberous sclerosis
　cutaneous symptoms, 567*t*,
　　596*t*
　diagnostic testing, 136*t*, 598
　history and CNS locations,
　　387*t*
Tularemia, 588*t*
Turner syndrome
　cardiac anomalies in, 232*t*, 257
　diagnostic testing, 134*t*
　facial features in, 121*t*, 122*t*
　hand deformities in, 126
　horseshoe kidney in, 118
　menstrual disturbances in,
　　414, 415
　nail abnormalities in, 408, 410,
　　428*t*
　physical characteristics, 417, 426*t*
Twenty-nail dystrophy, 597
Tyrosinemia, 292*t*, 373, 399*t*
Tzanck smear, 598

U
Ulcers, skin
　characteristics, 550*f*, 552
　painful, 587–589*t*
　painless, 587*t*

Ultrasonography
　bladder and kidneys, 682*t*
　in cancer diagnosis, 523
　in neuroblastoma, 535
　in neurologic disorders, 396
　prenatal, 74, 450
　in respiratory disorders, 224*t*
　scrotum, 682*t*
　spine, 682*t*
Umbilicus, discharge from,
　654–655, 665
Underweight, endocrine
　causes, 410
Upper extremity
　anatomy, 308*f*
　key problems
　　elbow injuries, 315
　　elbow pain, 319
　　joint pain, 315, 318
　　joint swelling, 320
　　lack of movement, 303–304, 314
　　shoulder pain, 318–319
　　stiffness, 320
　　stress injury, 315
　　wrist pain, 319
　movements, 303*f*
　physical examination
　　in adolescents
　　　elbow, 332, 334
　　　hand and wrist, 335
　　　shoulder, 329–332, 330–334*f*
　　in dysmorphology diagnostic
　　　examination, 125–126,
　　　130–131
　　in infants, 322, 323
　　in newborns, 87, 88*f*
Urachal sinus/tract/cyst, 654–655,
　683*t*
Urea cycle defects, 397, 398*t*
Ureter
　innervation, 447
　mass/swelling, 679*t*
　pain, 680*t*
Urethra, 696*t*
Urinalysis
　hematuria. *See* Hematuria
　indications, 296*t*, 681*t*
　proteinuria. *See* Proteinuria
　routine, 465
Urinary frequency
　nonurinary causes, 65*t*
　normal, by age, 460*t*
Urinary incontinence, 663
Urinary retention, 65*t*, 652–653,
　662, 684*t*

Urinary system. *See also* Renal
system
anatomy, 444–445, 444*f*, 645–647
changes at birth, 448–449
innervation, 447
Urinary tract infection
differential diagnosis, 684*t*
in infants, 467, 482
symptoms, 662, 663
Urine
discoloration, 653–654. *See also*
Hematuria
normal volume by age, 460*t*
Urine culture, 296*t*
Urine determination of neutrophil
gelatinase–associated
lipocalcine (NGAL), 486
Urolithiasis
clinical presentation, 475–476
diagnostic testing, 485*t*
disorders associated with, 477*t*
risk factors, 475*t*
Urticaria, 561*t*, 569*t*
Urticaria pigmentosa, 561*t*
Uterus, 721, 722*f*
Uveitis, 157*t*

V
Vagina
anatomy, 686, 721
bleeding
abnormal, in adolescents,
726–727, 745*t*
in infants and children,
687–689, 698*t*
discharge
in adolescents, 729, 730–734*t*
in infants and children, 697*t*,
698
malignancies associated with,
522*t*
referrals/consultation, 748*t*
Vagus nerve (cranial nerve X), 355,
378
Valproate, teratogenic effects, 72*t*
Van der Woude syndrome, 121*t*
Varicella
cutaneous symptoms, 546*f*, 557,
579*t*
maternal, fetal effects, 71*t*
Varicocele, 664–665, 674*f*, 676, 684*t*
Varus and valgus stress test, 340
Vasculitis, 587*t*
VATER/VACTERL association

characteristics, 113
diagnostic testing, 134*t*
vertebral malformations in, 124
Vellus hair cyst, 576*t*
Velocardiofacial syndrome, 118,
120*t*, 129*f*, 134*t*
Venous thrombosis, 507, 517*t*
Ventricular septal defect (VSD),
252*t*, 256
Verbal dyspraxia, 635, 637*t*
Vertigo, 170
Vesicles, 546–547, 546*f*, 579*t*
Vestibular neuronitis, 182*t*
Viral croup syndrome, 199
Virilization, in newborns, 109*t*
Vision problems
in adolescents, 146
in children, 144–145, 152, 638
developmental disabilities and,
638
Vital signs
children, 35
consistency, 45–46
heart rate and rhythm, 50–51
infants, 32
peripheral blood pressure, 52–53
respiratory rate, 51–52
temperature, 46–50
Vitamin D, teratogenic effects, 73*t*
Vitiligo, 553*f*, 567*t*, 598
Vocal cord dysfunction, 208
Voiding
change in habits, 655–656, 663
difficulty/dysfunction, 522*t*, 684*t*
Voiding cystourethrogram
(VCUG), 682*t*
Volvulus, 294*t*
Vomiting
in adolescents, 277–278, 299
in brain tumors, 532
in children, 274, 299
differential diagnosis, 291–295*t*
in infants, 269–271, 299
malignancies associated with,
522*t*
in newborns, 99–100, 110*t*
nongastrointestinal causes, 64*t*,
294–295*t*
Von Willebrand disease, 515*t*
Vulva
anatomy, 720, 722*f*
erythema/irritation/pruritus,
689, 696*t*, 698*t*
mass, 689–690, 696*t*
papules, 696*t*

W

Waardenburg syndrome, 117, 120*t*, 566*t*
Walking, delayed, 305
Warfarin, teratogenic effects, 73*t*
Warts, 568*t*
Water-hammer pulse, 255
Weakness
  focal
    in children, 370
    in infants, 361–362
  generalized. *See* Hypotonia
Weight
  gain, endocrine causes, 410, 427*t*
  loss
    in endocrine disorders, 427*t*
    in Hodgkin disease, 530
    in rheumatic diseases, 321*t*
  normal
    body mass index-for-age percentiles, 771–772*f*
    weight-for-age percentiles, 759–760*f*, 767–768*f*
    weight-for-length percentiles, 763–764*f*
Werdnig-Hoffman syndrome, 399*t*
Werner syndrome, 586*t*
Wheeze/wheezing
  in adolescents, 208
  characteristics, 214*t*
  in children, 204–205
  in infants, 200–201
  nonpulmonary causes, 64*t*
White blood cell (WBC) count, 296*t*, 503*t*
White blood cell (WBC) differential, 296*t*

White blood cell (WBC) disorders
  leukocytosis, 505
  leukopenia, 501, 503
  lymphocytopenia, 504
  lymphocytosis, 505–506
  neutropenia
    acquired causes, 504
    definition, 503, 503*t*
    intrinsic causes, 503–504
  neutrophilia, 505
White matter degeneration, 386*t*, 399*t*
Wilkie disease, 277, 291*t*
Williams syndrome, 117, 118, 120*t*, 136*t*
Wilms' tumor (nephroblastoma), 672
  diagnostic testing, 536
  history, 536
  imaging, 537
  incidence, 536
  key points, 537
  physical examination, 536, 672
  syndromes associated with, 536
Wilson disease, 276, 294*t*, 297*t*, 564*t*
Wiskott-Aldrich syndrome, 572*t*
Wood's lamp, 598
Wooly hair syndrome, 592*t*
Wrist. *See* Hand and wrist
Written expression disorder, 613, 639

X

Xanthomas, 575*t*
Xyphoid syndrome, 209